GRAY'S

# ATLAS
## OF ANATOMY

**Richard L. Drake, PhD**

Director of Anatomy
Professor of Surgery
Cleveland Clinic Lerner College of Medicine
Cleveland, Ohio, USA

**A. Wayne Vogl, PhD**

Professor of Anatomy and Cell Biology
Director of Gross Anatomy
Department of Cellular and Physiological Sciences
Faculty of Medicine
University of British Columbia
Vancouver, British Columbia, Canada

**Adam W. M. Mitchell, MBBS, FRCS, FRCR**

Joint Head of Graduate Entry Anatomy
Imperial College
University of London
Consultant Radiologist
Department of Imaging
Charing Cross Hospital
London, UK

*Illustrated by*

**Richard M. Tibbitts**

Saffron Walden, UK

**Paul E. Richardson**

Cambridge, UK

*Photographs by*

**Ansell Horn**

# GRAY'S

# ATLAS
## OF ANATOMY

Richard L. Drake

A. Wayne Vogl

Adam W. M. Mitchell

Richard M. Tibbitts

Paul E. Richardson

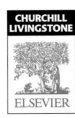

CHURCHILL
LIVINGSTONE

ELSEVIER

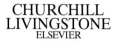

1600 John F. Kennedy Blvd.
Ste 1800
Philadelphia, PA 19103-2899

GRAY'S ATLAS OF ANATOMY                                            ISBN: 978-0-443-06721-1

---

**Notice**

Knowledge and best practice in this field are constantly changing. As new research and experience broaden our knowledge, changes in practice, treatment, and drug therapy may become necessary or appropriate. Readers are advised to check the most current information provided (i) on procedures featured or (ii) by the manufacturer of each product to be administered, to verify the recommended dose or formula, the method and duration of administration, and contraindications. It is the responsibility of the practitioner, relying on experience and knowledge of the patient, to make diagnoses, to determine dosages and the best treatment for each individual patient, and to take all appropriate safety precautions. To the fullest extent of the law, neither the Publisher nor the Authors assume any liability for any injury and/or damage to persons or property arising out of or related to any use of the material contained in this book.

The Publisher

---

**Library of Congress Cataloging-in-Publication Data**

Gray's Atlas of anatomy / Richard L. Drake . . . [et al.]. – 1st ed.
    p. ; cm.
    Companion to: Gray's anatomy for students / Richard L. Drake, Wayne Vogl, Adam W.M. Mitchell. 2005.
    Includes bibliographical references and index.
    ISBN 978-0-443-06721-1
   1. Anatomy–Atlases.   I. Drake, Richard L., Ph.D.   II. Drake, Richard L., Ph.D. Gray's anatomy for students.   III. Gray, Henry, 1825–1861. Gray's anatomy.   IV. Title: Atlas of anatomy.
    [DNLM:   1. Anatomy–Atlases. QS 17 G784 2008]
QM25.G72 2008
611.0022'3–dc22                                                    2007017928

*Acquisitions Editor:* William Schmitt
*Developmental Editor:* Rebecca Gruliow
*Publishing Services Manager:* Linda Van Pelt
*Project Manager:* Francisco Morales
*Design and Art Direction:* Antbits Ltd.
*Marketing Manager:* Theresa Dudas

Printed in Canada
Last digit is the print number:   9  8  7  6  5  4  3  2  1

To my wife who supports me and to my parents who are always with me.
*Richard L. Drake*

To my family, to my professional colleagues and role models, and to my students.
*Wayne Vogl*

Thanks, to Cathy, Max and Elsa
*Adam W. M. Mitchell*

To my family – my inspiration, Evi, Zoë, and Nicholas x
*Richard M. Tibbitts*

To Lesley and Maja and in memory of AMR and JER
*Paul Richardson*

# ACKNOWLEDGMENTS

The following reviewers helped enormously with their detailed critiques and suggestions for every chapter. Their assistance was invaluable.

Mark Hankin, PhD, University of Toledo College of Medicine, Toledo, Ohio

Marios Loukas, MD, PhD, St. George's University School of Medicine, Grenada

James J. Rechtien, DO, PhD, Michigan State University School of Medicine, East Lansing, Michigan

William A. Roy, PT, PhD, Touro University, Henderson, Nevada

Susan Standring, PhD, DSc, Professor of Experimental Neurobiology and Head, Division of Anatomy, Cell and Human Biology, Guy's, King's and St Thomas' School of Biomedical Sciences, King's College London, London

William Swartz, PhD, Louisiana State University Health Sciences Center, Baton Rouge, Louisiana

Mark F. Teaford, PhD, Johns Hopkins University School of Medicine, Baltimore, Maryland

We want to thank Dr. Bruce Crawford for a radiograph of the head and neck and Dr. Murray Morrison for laryngoscopic images of the larynx; Dr. Jerry Healy for three images in the Abdomen section: the celiac artery, the bile duct system, and a three-dimensional view of abdominal vessels; and Siemens Medical Solutions USA and the following individuals with that company: Mollie Beaver, Director, CT Clinical Solutions, and Dr. Louise McKenna, Global Clinical Marketing Manager, CT Oncology, who supplied a *syngo* Multi-modality Workplace, which was used to acquire the majority of the clinical images.

Stuart Morrison, MD, helped with all aspects of coordinating the collection of the radiographic material. Radiological assistance and images were contributed in each of the following areas:

**Back**

Mark Kayanja, MD, PhD
Jeffrey S. Ross, MD

**Thorax**

Mario Garcia, MD
A. Michael Lincoff, MD

**Abdomen**

Namita Gandhi, MD
Michelle Inkster, MD, PhD
Brian R. Lane, MD
Anand Rao, MD
James S. Wu, MD

**Pelvis**

Matthew Barber, MD, MHS
Tommaso Falcone, MD
J. Stephen Jones, MD
Eunice Moon, MD
James S. Newman, MD, PhD

**Extremities**

Hakan Ilaslan, MD
Bradford J. Richmond, MD
Joshua Polster, MD

**Head and Neck**

Todd W. Stultz, DDS, MD
J. Martin Paloma, DDS, MSD
Cindy McConnaughy
Ronald Lemmo, DDS

A working knowledge of anatomy is not an "optional extra" for health care professionals – it is fundamental. Acquiring that knowledge has always challenged even the most motivated students. Over many generations, learning materials that aid the process effectively have been warmly welcomed by students and their teachers (and by patients, who are the ultimate beneficiaries of that knowledge). I remember my own students' response when I first included illustrations from *Gray's Anatomy for Students* in a lecture—afterward, I was asked repeatedly for the source of the marvelous pictures. Looking beyond the "wow" factor that leapt from the pages of the book, it was clear that an enormous amount of thought and skill had gone into producing the artwork.

This atlas contains a series of additional outstanding pieces of anatomical art from the illustrative team of Richard Tibbitts and Paul Richardson that will complement those in *Gray's Anatomy for Students*, combined with relevant clinical pictures, surface anatomy, and images from a range of modern imaging procedures. Of course, anatomy cannot be learned from books and interactive DVDs alone, no matter how excellent they may be. Anatomy is a practical subject, best learned by gaining hands-on experience of the body. Students should spend as much time as they can examining cadaveric dissections (if they do not have the opportunity to dissect themselves) and should always read from screen or page with the appropriate bones in front of them. They need to combine and correlate information from a wide variety of sources in order to gain the working knowledge mentioned earlier.

This atlas will provide a valuable companion to their studies, and I am confident that it will remain in their libraries long after they have completed the early stages of their training.

Susan Standring
Division of Anatomy, Cell and Human Biology
King's College, London

We began working on *Gray's Atlas of Anatomy* in 2005 following the publication of our textbook, *Gray's Anatomy for Students*. We wanted to produce an atlas that would build on themes and concepts established in the textbook and that would couple artistic renderings of "internal" gross anatomy with actual "living" anatomy, as visualized with modern imaging techniques and with surface anatomy. We believe that the final atlas presents a fresh and integrated approach to anatomy that is accessible to entry-level students in anatomy, as well as to students at more advanced levels.

Because an atlas is used in a much different way than a textbook, we could not simply repackage figures used in *Gray's Anatomy for Students* and put them in the atlas. Consequently, most of the figures in the atlas are new and were designed to present structures in a more complete context than in the textbook, even though the color palate and overall look of the figures in both the atlas and textbook are similar. Also, figures in the atlas provide additional detail not included in the textbook and directly correlate artistic representations of anatomy with computed tomography (CT) and magnetic resonance imaging (MRI). Where appropriate, we have included endoscopic, laryngoscopic, and laparoscopic views of the anatomy and have included examples of ultrasound images. In a number of regions, we also have reconstructed the internal anatomy of patients by abstracting specific information from multiple MR or CT images, and we present these reconstructions together with artwork of the same anatomy. Although the artwork was done independently of the reconstructed images, the two types of representations are strikingly similar.

Each page of this atlas was planned prior to beginning work on the figures, and all of the artwork was generated digitally. Most of the figures were created from an extensive digital database created for the textbook. Each figure was reviewed for accuracy and revised accordingly.

We hope that the textbook and atlas used together will provide new and powerful learning tools for students of human gross anatomy.

The Authors

# CONTENTS

# CONTENTS

# CONTENTS

# 6 LOWER LIMB

# CONTENTS

## 7 UPPER LIMB

# CONTENTS

## 8 HEAD AND NECK

# CONTENTS

# 1

# THE BODY

## CONTENTS

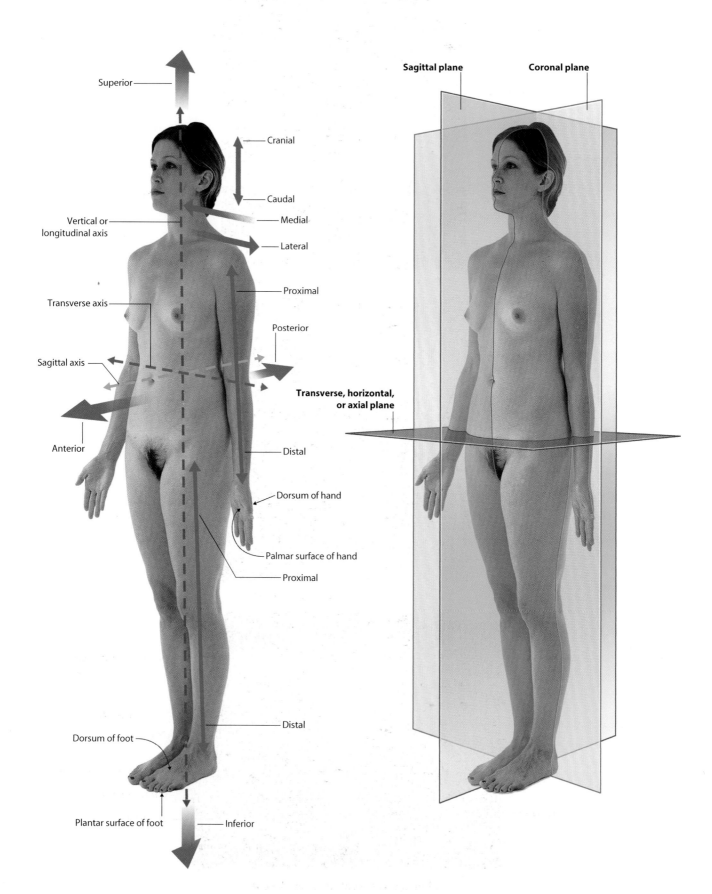

Superior

Cranial

Caudal

Medial

Vertical or longitudinal axis

Lateral

Proximal

Transverse axis

Posterior

Sagittal axis

Transverse, horizontal, or axial plane

Anterior

Distal

Dorsum of hand

Palmar surface of hand

Proximal

Distal

Dorsum of foot

Plantar surface of foot

Inferior

Sagittal plane

Coronal plane

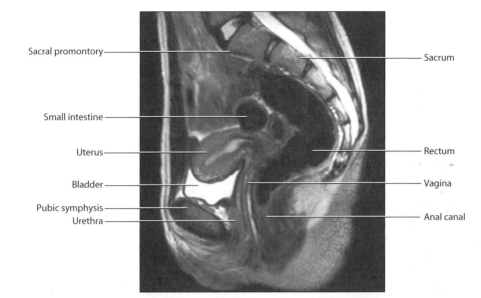

Sacral promontory

Small intestine

Uterus

Bladder

Pubic symphysis

Urethra

Sacrum

Rectum

Vagina

Anal canal

**T2-weighted MR image, in sagittal plane**

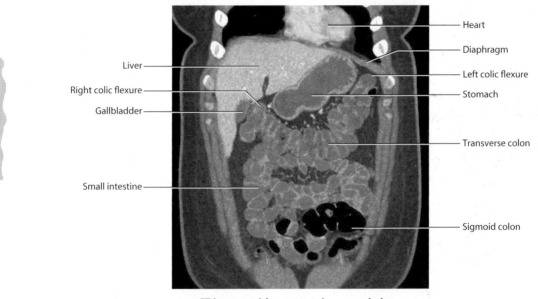

Liver

Right colic flexure

Gallbladder

Small intestine

Heart

Diaphragm

Left colic flexure

Stomach

Transverse colon

Sigmoid colon

**CT image, with contrast, in coronal plane**

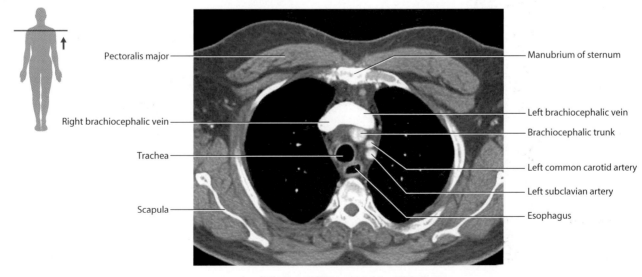

Pectoralis major

Right brachiocephalic vein

Trachea

Scapula

Manubrium of sternum

Left brachiocephalic vein

Brachiocephalic trunk

Left common carotid artery

Left subclavian artery

Esophagus

**CT image, with contrast, in axial plane**

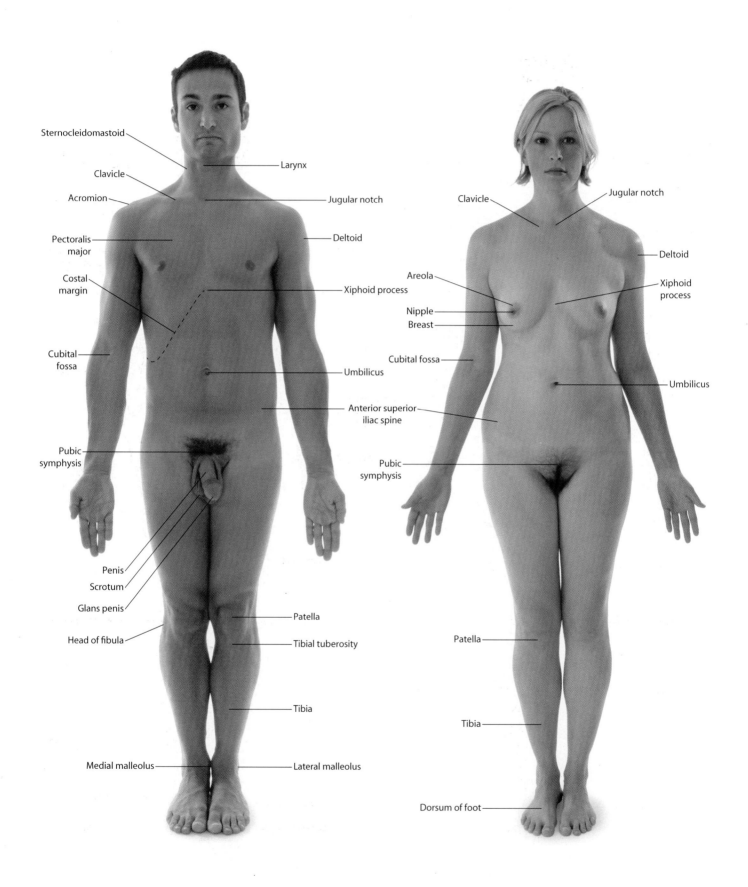

Sternocleidomastoid

Clavicle

Acromion

Pectoralis major

Costal margin

Cubital fossa

Pubic symphysis

Penis

Scrotum

Glans penis

Head of fibula

Medial malleolus

Larynx

Jugular notch

Deltoid

Xiphoid process

Umbilicus

Anterior superior iliac spine

Patella

Tibial tuberosity

Tibia

Lateral malleolus

Clavicle

Areola

Nipple

Breast

Cubital fossa

Pubic symphysis

Patella

Tibia

Jugular notch

Deltoid

Xiphoid process

Umbilicus

Dorsum of foot

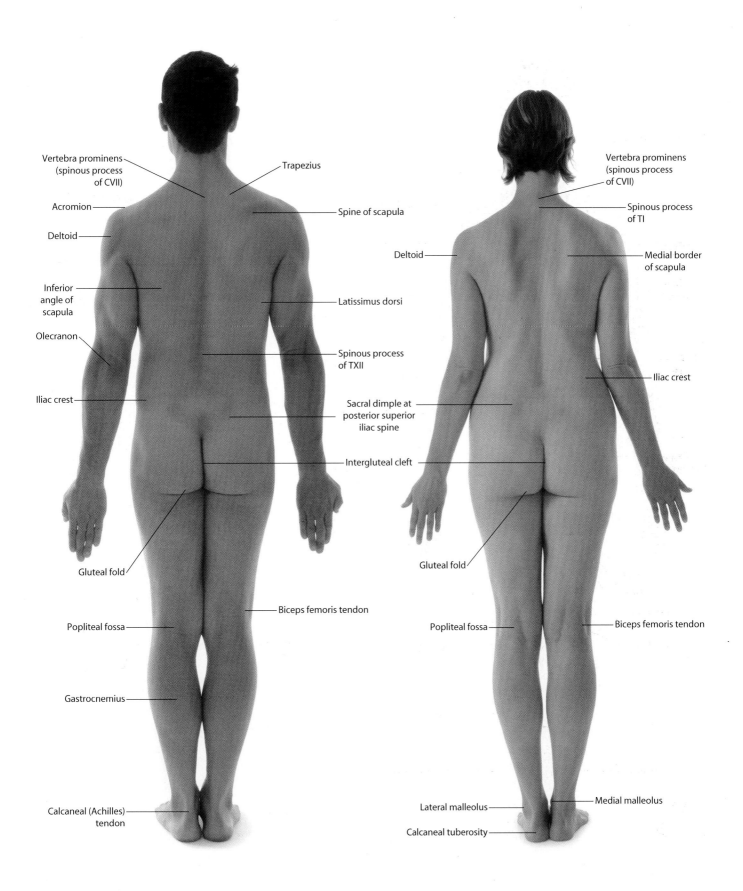

Vertebra prominens (spinous process of CVII)

Trapezius

Acromion

Spine of scapula

Deltoid

Inferior angle of scapula

Latissimus dorsi

Olecranon

Spinous process of TXII

Iliac crest

Sacral dimple at posterior superior iliac spine

Intergluteal cleft

Gluteal fold

Biceps femoris tendon

Popliteal fossa

Gastrocnemius

Calcaneal (Achilles) tendon

Vertebra prominens (spinous process of CVII)

Spinous process of TI

Deltoid

Medial border of scapula

Iliac crest

Gluteal fold

Popliteal fossa

Biceps femoris tendon

Lateral malleolus

Medial malleolus

Calcaneal tuberosity

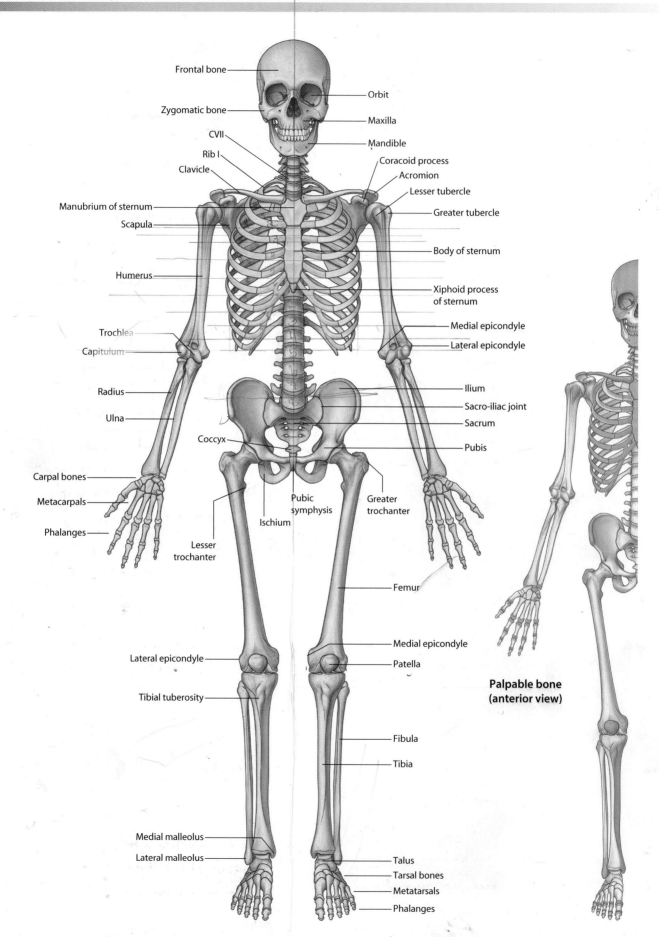

Frontal bone

Orbit

Zygomatic bone

Maxilla

CVII

Mandible

Rib I

Coracoid process

Clavicle

Acromion

Lesser tubercle

Manubrium of sternum

Greater tubercle

Scapula

Body of sternum

Humerus

Xiphoid process
of sternum

Trochlea

Medial epicondyle

Capitulum

Lateral epicondyle

Radius

Ilium

Ulna

Sacro-iliac joint

Sacrum

Coccyx

Pubis

Carpal bones

Metacarpals

Pubic
symphysis

Greater
trochanter

Phalanges

Ischium

Lesser
trochanter

Femur

Medial epicondyle

Lateral epicondyle

Patella

Tibial tuberosity

Fibula

Tibia

Medial malleolus

Lateral malleolus

Talus

Tarsal bones

Metatarsals

Phalanges

**Palpable bone
(anterior view)**

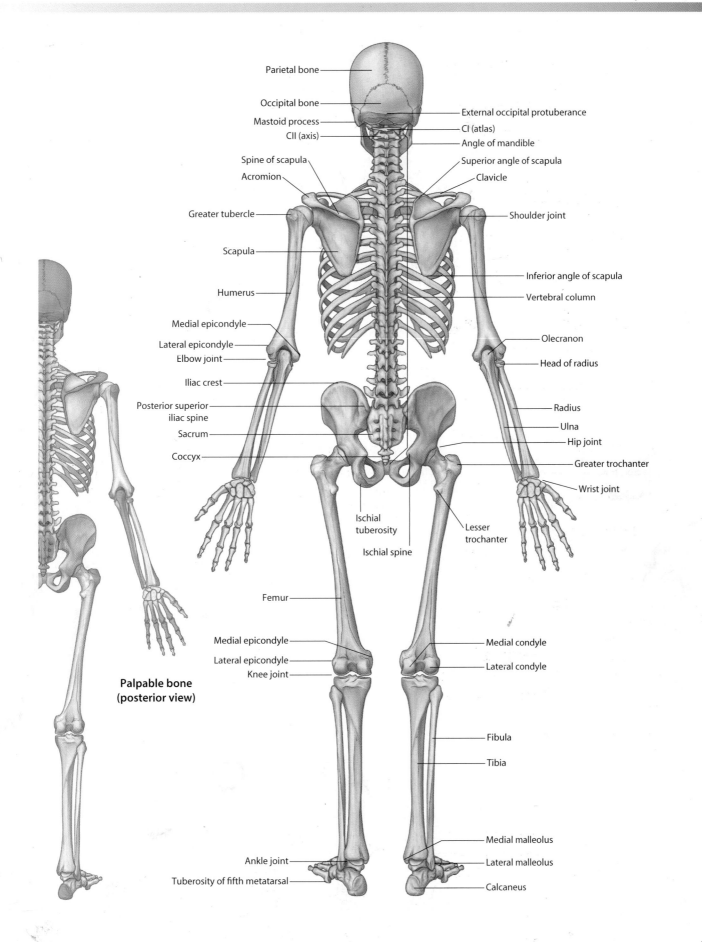

Parietal bone

Occipital bone

External occipital protuberance

Mastoid process

CI (atlas)

CII (axis)

Angle of mandible

Spine of scapula

Superior angle of scapula

Acromion

Clavicle

Greater tubercle

Shoulder joint

Scapula

Inferior angle of scapula

Humerus

Vertebral column

Medial epicondyle

Olecranon

Lateral epicondyle

Head of radius

Elbow joint

Iliac crest

Radius

Posterior superior
iliac spine

Ulna

Sacrum

Hip joint

Coccyx

Greater trochanter

Wrist joint

Ischial
tuberosity

Lesser
trochanter

Ischial spine

Femur

Medial epicondyle

Medial condyle

Lateral epicondyle

Lateral condyle

Knee joint

**Palpable bone
(posterior view)**

Fibula

Tibia

Medial malleolus

Ankle joint

Lateral malleolus

Tuberosity of fifth metatarsal

Calcaneus

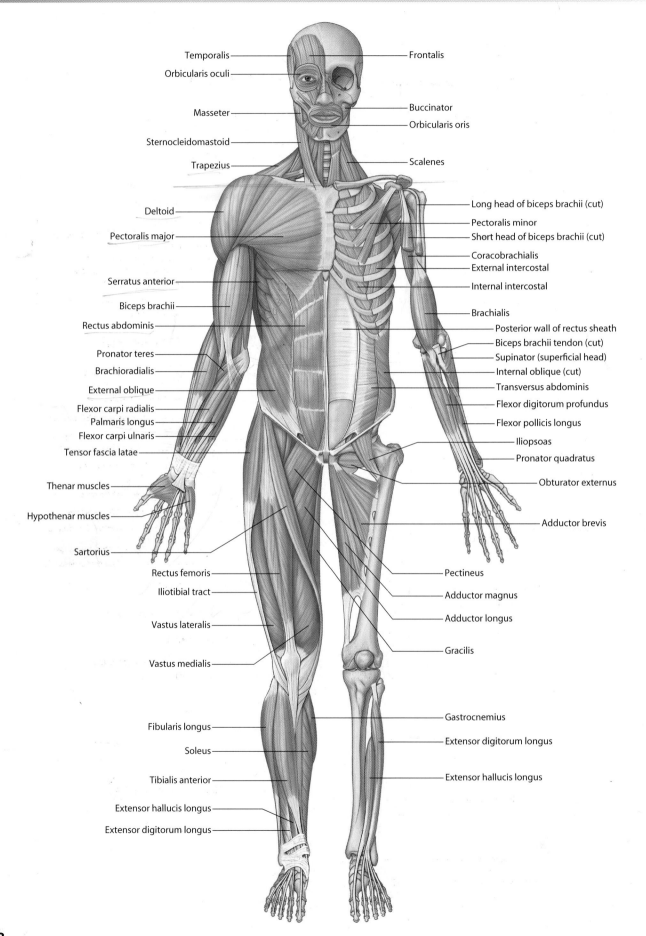

Temporalis

Orbicularis oculi

Masseter

Sternocleidomastoid

Trapezius

Deltoid

Pectoralis major

Serratus anterior

Biceps brachii

Rectus abdominis

Pronator teres

Brachioradialis

External oblique

Flexor carpi radialis

Palmaris longus

Flexor carpi ulnaris

Tensor fascia latae

Thenar muscles

Hypothenar muscles

Sartorius

Rectus femoris

Iliotibial tract

Vastus lateralis

Vastus medialis

Fibularis longus

Soleus

Tibialis anterior

Extensor hallucis longus

Extensor digitorum longus

Frontalis

Buccinator

Orbicularis oris

Scalenes

Long head of biceps brachii (cut)

Pectoralis minor

Short head of biceps brachii (cut)

Coracobrachialis

External intercostal

Internal intercostal

Brachialis

Posterior wall of rectus sheath

Biceps brachii tendon (cut)

Supinator (superficial head)

Internal oblique (cut)

Transversus abdominis

Flexor digitorum profundus

Flexor pollicis longus

Iliopsoas

Pronator quadratus

Obturator externus

Adductor brevis

Pectineus

Adductor magnus

Adductor longus

Gracilis

Gastrocnemius

Extensor digitorum longus

Extensor hallucis longus

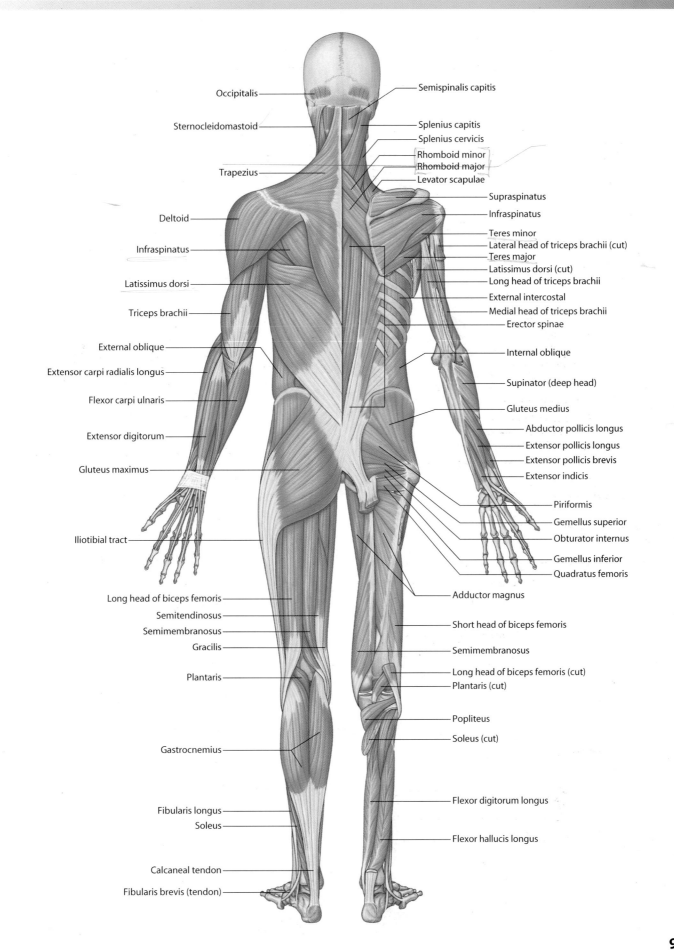

Occipitalis

Semispinalis capitis

Sternocleidomastoid

Splenius capitis

Splenius cervicis

Rhomboid minor

Rhomboid major

Levator scapulae

Trapezius

Supraspinatus

Infraspinatus

Deltoid

Teres minor

Lateral head of triceps brachii (cut)

Infraspinatus

Teres major

Latissimus dorsi (cut)

Latissimus dorsi

Long head of triceps brachii

Triceps brachii

External intercostal

Medial head of triceps brachii

Erector spinae

External oblique

Internal oblique

Extensor carpi radialis longus

Supinator (deep head)

Flexor carpi ulnaris

Gluteus medius

Extensor digitorum

Abductor pollicis longus

Extensor pollicis longus

Extensor pollicis brevis

Gluteus maximus

Extensor indicis

Piriformis

Gemellus superior

Obturator internus

Iliotibial tract

Gemellus inferior

Quadratus femoris

Long head of biceps femoris

Adductor magnus

Semitendinosus

Semimembranosus

Short head of biceps femoris

Gracilis

Semimembranosus

Plantaris

Long head of biceps femoris (cut)

Plantaris (cut)

Popliteus

Soleus (cut)

Gastrocnemius

Flexor digitorum longus

Fibularis longus

Soleus

Flexor hallucis longus

Calcaneal tendon

Fibularis brevis (tendon)

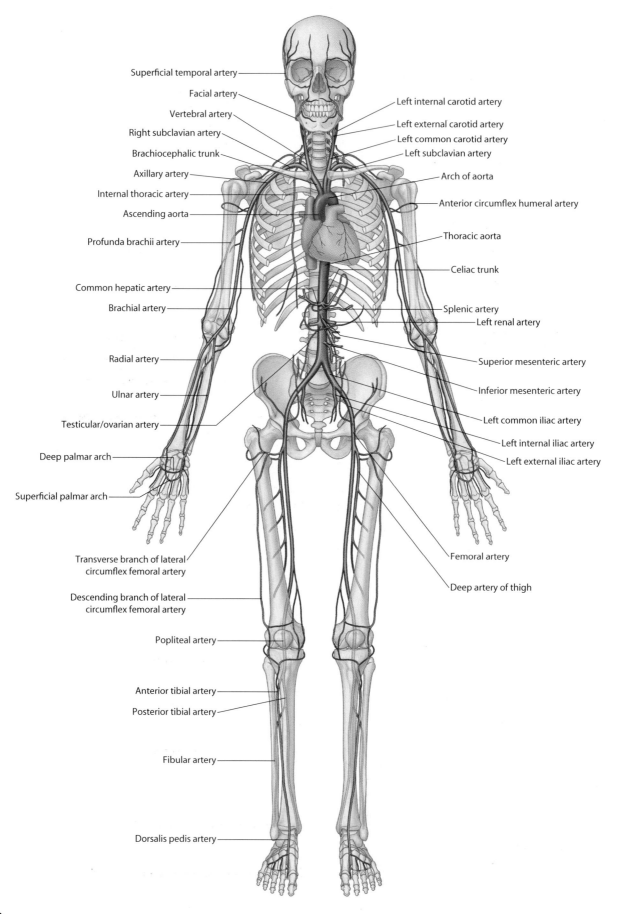

Superficial temporal artery

Facial artery

Vertebral artery

Right subclavian artery

Brachiocephalic trunk

Axillary artery

Internal thoracic artery

Ascending aorta

Profunda brachii artery

Common hepatic artery

Brachial artery

Radial artery

Ulnar artery

Testicular/ovarian artery

Deep palmar arch

Superficial palmar arch

Transverse branch of lateral circumflex femoral artery

Descending branch of lateral circumflex femoral artery

Popliteal artery

Anterior tibial artery

Posterior tibial artery

Fibular artery

Dorsalis pedis artery

Left internal carotid artery

Left external carotid artery

Left common carotid artery

Left subclavian artery

Arch of aorta

Anterior circumflex humeral artery

Thoracic aorta

Celiac trunk

Splenic artery

Left renal artery

Superior mesenteric artery

Inferior mesenteric artery

Left common iliac artery

Left internal iliac artery

Left external iliac artery

Femoral artery

Deep artery of thigh

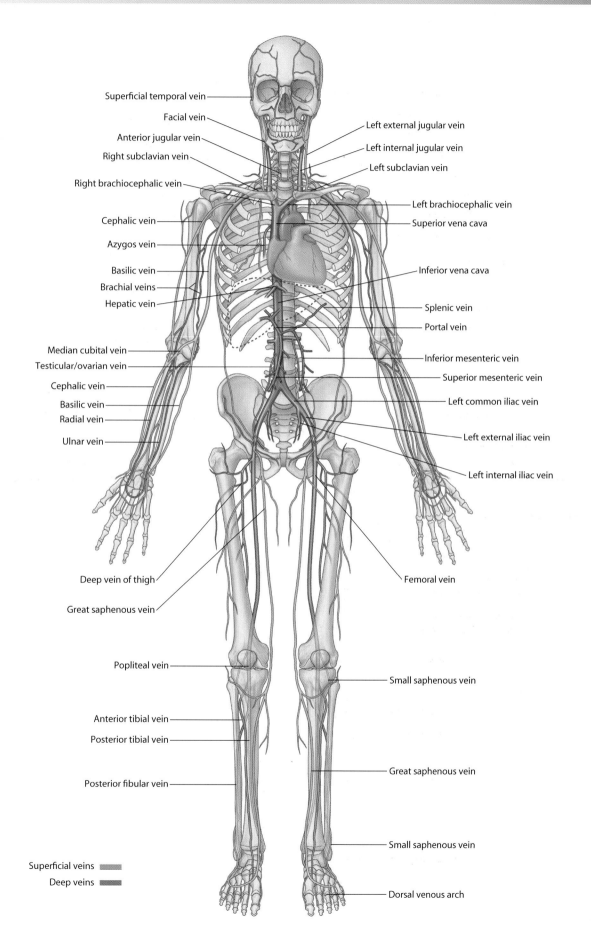

Superficial temporal vein

Facial vein

Anterior jugular vein

Right subclavian vein

Right brachiocephalic vein

Cephalic vein

Azygos vein

Basilic vein

Brachial veins

Hepatic vein

Median cubital vein

Testicular/ovarian vein

Cephalic vein

Basilic vein

Radial vein

Ulnar vein

Deep vein of thigh

Great saphenous vein

Popliteal vein

Anterior tibial vein

Posterior tibial vein

Posterior fibular vein

Left external jugular vein

Left internal jugular vein

Left subclavian vein

Left brachiocephalic vein

Superior vena cava

Inferior vena cava

Splenic vein

Portal vein

Inferior mesenteric vein

Superior mesenteric vein

Left common iliac vein

Left external iliac vein

Left internal iliac vein

Femoral vein

Small saphenous vein

Great saphenous vein

Small saphenous vein

Dorsal venous arch

Superficial veins

Deep veins

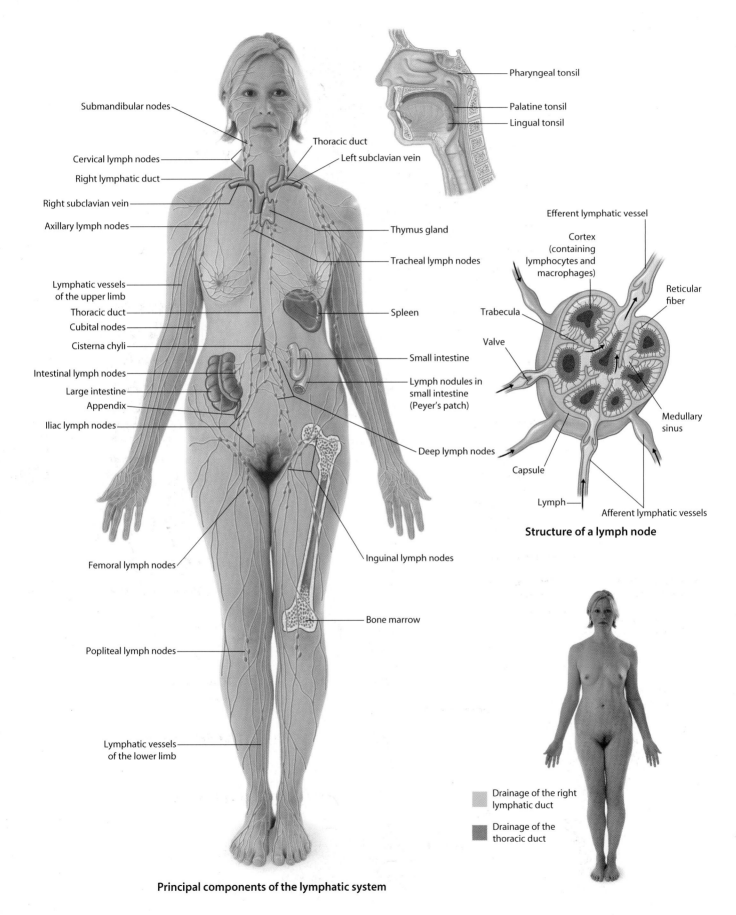

Submandibular nodes

Cervical lymph nodes

Right lymphatic duct

Right subclavian vein

Axillary lymph nodes

Lymphatic vessels
of the upper limb

Thoracic duct

Cubital nodes

Cisterna chyli

Intestinal lymph nodes

Large intestine

Appendix

Iliac lymph nodes

Femoral lymph nodes

Popliteal lymph nodes

Lymphatic vessels
of the lower limb

Pharyngeal tonsil

Palatine tonsil

Lingual tonsil

Thoracic duct

Left subclavian vein

Thymus gland

Tracheal lymph nodes

Spleen

Small intestine

Lymph nodules in
small intestine
(Peyer's patch)

Deep lymph nodes

Inguinal lymph nodes

Bone marrow

Efferent lymphatic vessel

Cortex
(containing
lymphocytes and
macrophages)

Reticular
fiber

Trabecula

Valve

Medullary
sinus

Capsule

Lymph

Afferent lymphatic vessels

**Structure of a lymph node**

Drainage of the right
lymphatic duct

Drainage of the
thoracic duct

**Principal components of the lymphatic system**

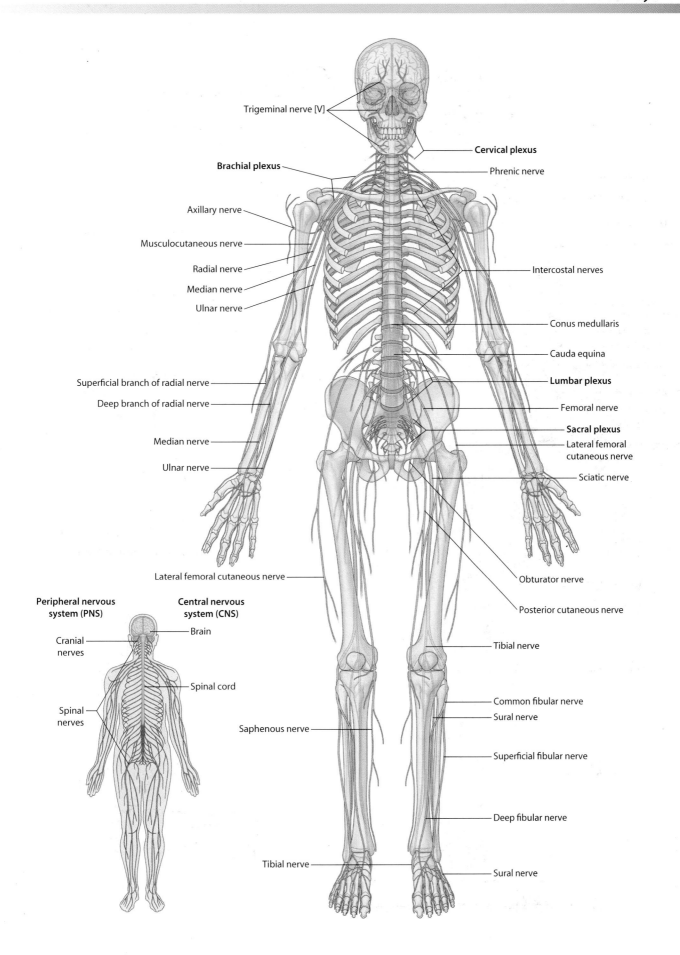

Trigeminal nerve [V]

**Cervical plexus**

**Brachial plexus**

Phrenic nerve

Axillary nerve

Musculocutaneous nerve

Radial nerve

Median nerve

Ulnar nerve

Intercostal nerves

Conus medullaris

Cauda equina

**Lumbar plexus**

Superficial branch of radial nerve

Deep branch of radial nerve

Femoral nerve

**Sacral plexus**

Median nerve

Lateral femoral
cutaneous nerve

Ulnar nerve

Sciatic nerve

Obturator nerve

Lateral femoral cutaneous nerve

Posterior cutaneous nerve

Tibial nerve

Peripheral nervous
system (PNS)

Central nervous
system (CNS)

Brain

Cranial
nerves

Spinal cord

Common fibular nerve

Sural nerve

Spinal
nerves

Superficial fibular nerve

Saphenous nerve

Deep fibular nerve

Tibial nerve

Sural nerve

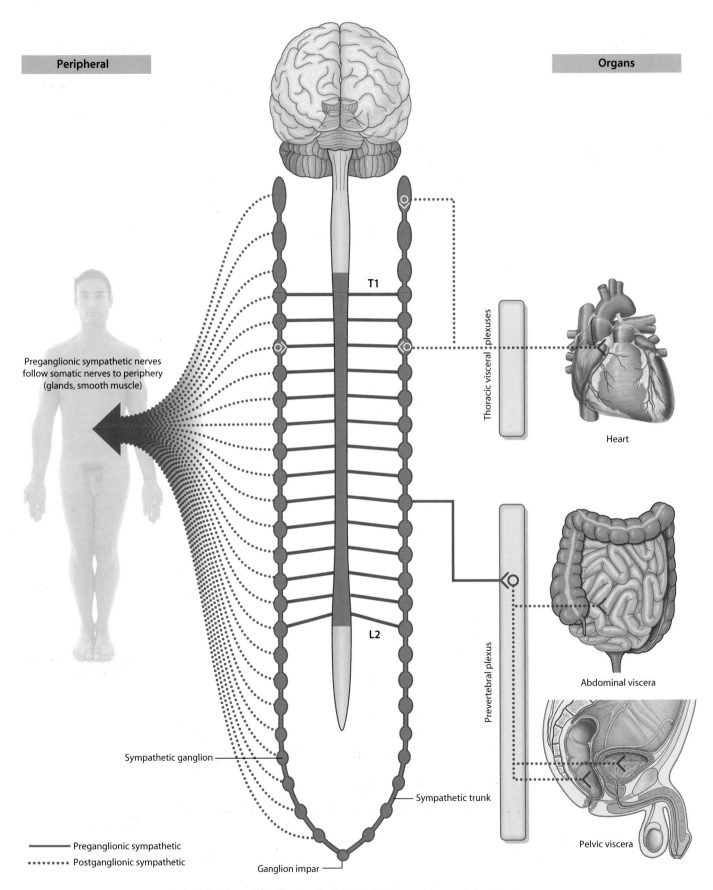

**Peripheral**

**Organs**

T1

Preganglionic sympathetic nerves
follow somatic nerves to periphery
(glands, smooth muscle)

Thoracic visceral plexuses

Heart

L2

Prevertebral plexus

Abdominal viscera

Sympathetic ganglion

Sympathetic trunk

Pelvic viscera

—— Preganglionic sympathetic

········ Postganglionic sympathetic

Ganglion impar

**All sympathetic visceral efferent (motor) nerves originate from
spinal levels T1–L2 and pass into the associated spinal nerves**

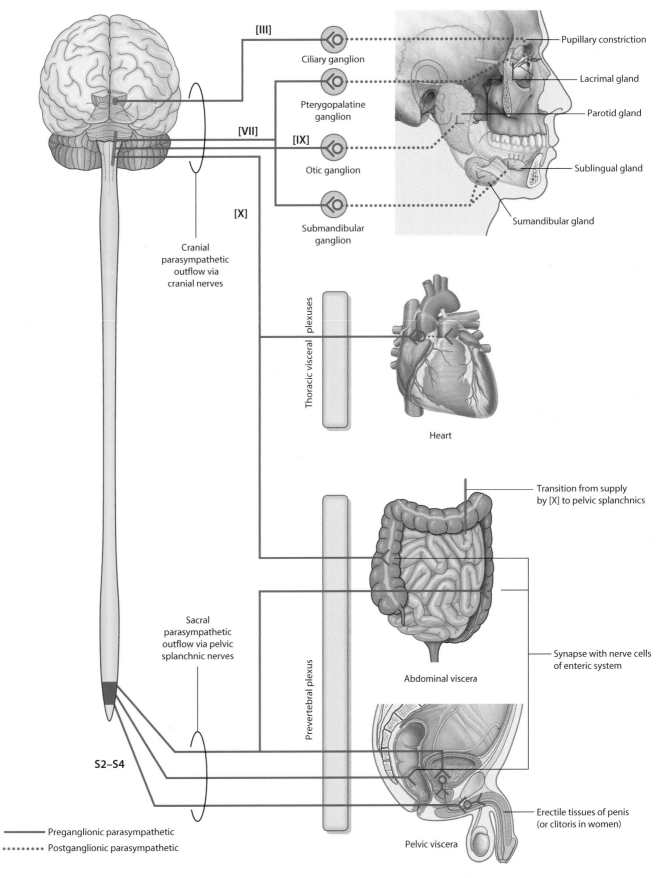

[III]
Ciliary ganglion

Pupillary constriction

Lacrimal gland

Pterygopalatine ganglion

[VII]

[IX]

Parotid gland

Otic ganglion

Sublingual gland

[X]

Sumandibular gland

Submandibular ganglion

Cranial parasympathetic outflow via cranial nerves

Thoracic visceral plexuses

Heart

Transition from supply by [X] to pelvic splanchnics

Sacral parasympathetic outflow via pelvic splanchnic nerves

Prevertebral plexus

Synapse with nerve cells of enteric system

Abdominal viscera

S2–S4

—— Preganglionic parasympathetic
········· Postganglionic parasympathetic

Erectile tissues of penis (or clitoris in women)

Pelvic viscera

**All paraympathetic visceral efferent (motor) nerves emerge from the brain in
cranial nerves III, VII, IX, and X and from spinal levels S2–S4**

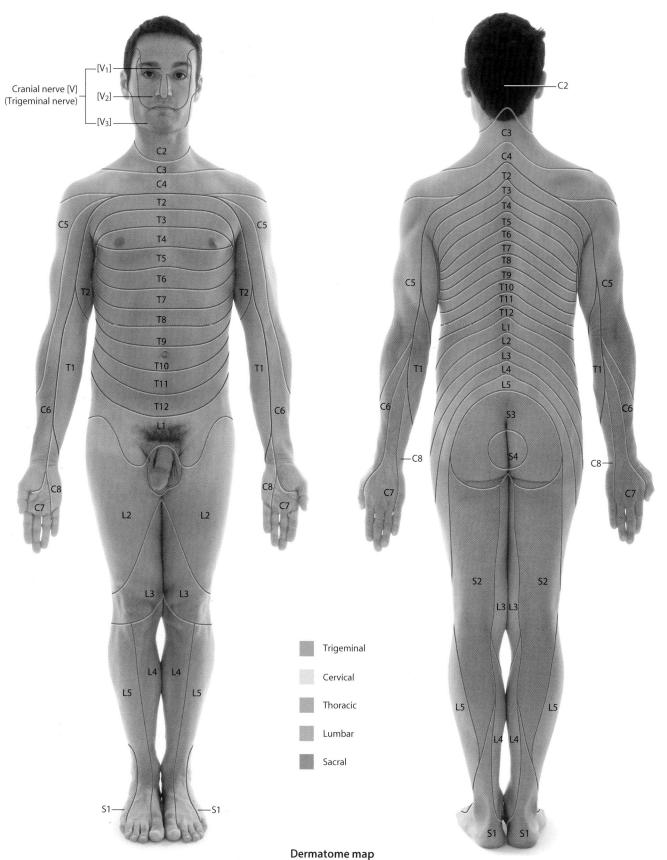

Cranial nerve [V]
(Trigeminal nerve)

[V₁]

[V₂]

[V₃]

Trigeminal

Cervical

Thoracic

Lumbar

Sacral

**Dermatome map
(cutaneous distribution of nerves)**

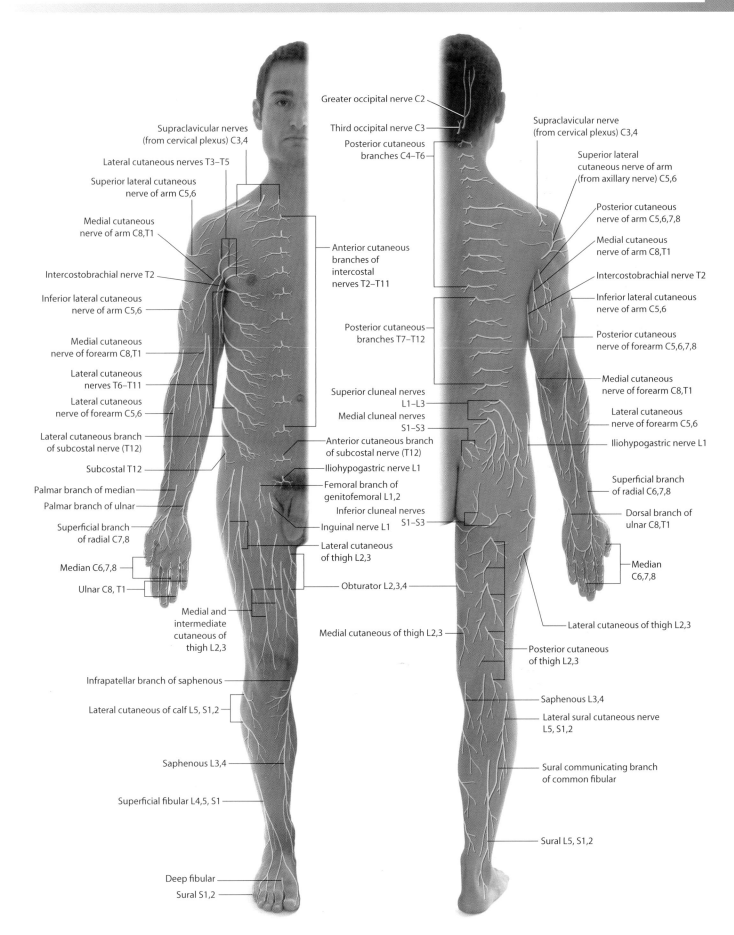

Greater occipital nerve C2

Third occipital nerve C3

Supraclavicular nerves (from cervical plexus) C3,4

Lateral cutaneous nerves T3–T5

Superior lateral cutaneous nerve of arm C5,6

Medial cutaneous nerve of arm C8,T1

Intercostobrachial nerve T2

Inferior lateral cutaneous nerve of arm C5,6

Medial cutaneous nerve of forearm C8,T1

Lateral cutaneous nerves T6–T11

Lateral cutaneous nerve of forearm C5,6

Lateral cutaneous branch of subcostal nerve (T12)

Subcostal T12

Palmar branch of median

Palmar branch of ulnar

Superficial branch of radial C7,8

Median C6,7,8

Ulnar C8, T1

Medial and intermediate cutaneous of thigh L2,3

Infrapatellar branch of saphenous

Lateral cutaneous of calf L5, S1,2

Saphenous L3,4

Superficial fibular L4,5, S1

Deep fibular

Sural S1,2

Posterior cutaneous branches C4–T6

Anterior cutaneous branches of intercostal nerves T2–T11

Posterior cutaneous branches T7–T12

Superior cluneal nerves L1–L3

Medial cluneal nerves S1–S3

Anterior cutaneous branch of subcostal nerve (T12)

Iliohypogastric nerve L1

Femoral branch of genitofemoral L1,2

Inferior cluneal nerves S1–S3

Inguinal nerve L1

Lateral cutaneous of thigh L2,3

Obturator L2,3,4

Medial cutaneous of thigh L2,3

Supraclavicular nerve (from cervical plexus) C3,4

Superior lateral cutaneous nerve of arm (from axillary nerve) C5,6

Posterior cutaneous nerve of arm C5,6,7,8

Medial cutaneous nerve of arm C8,T1

Intercostobrachial nerve T2

Inferior lateral cutaneous nerve of arm C5,6

Posterior cutaneous nerve of forearm C5,6,7,8

Medial cutaneous nerve of forearm C8,T1

Lateral cutaneous nerve of forearm C5,6

Iliohypogastric nerve L1

Superficial branch of radial C6,7,8

Dorsal branch of ulnar C8,T1

Median C6,7,8

Lateral cutaneous of thigh L2,3

Posterior cutaneous of thigh L2,3

Saphenous L3,4

Lateral sural cutaneous nerve L5, S1,2

Sural communicating branch of common fibular

Sural L5, S1,2

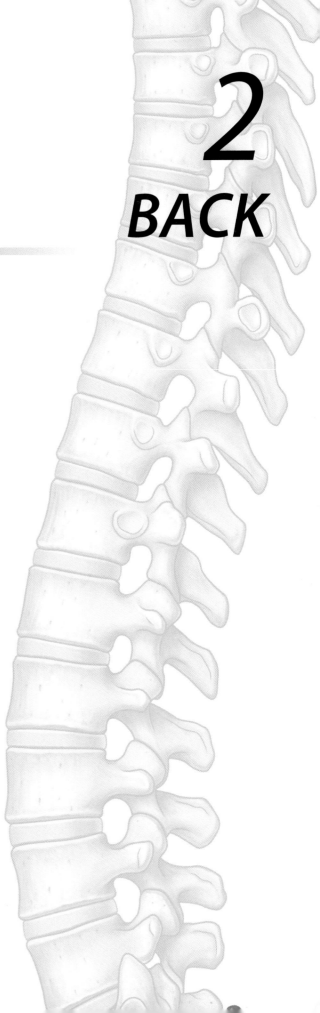

# 2
# *BACK*

## CONTENTS

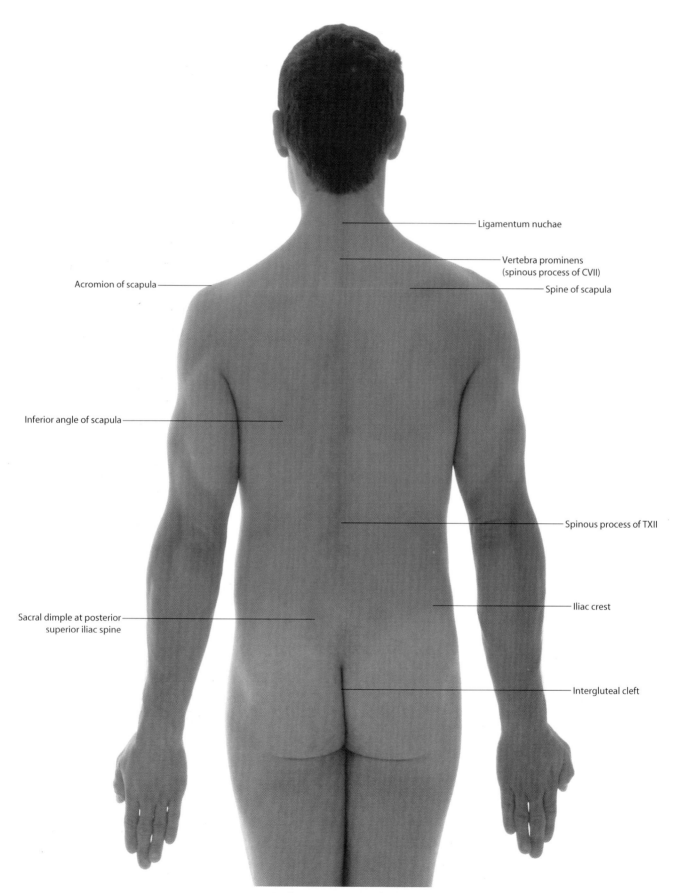

Ligamentum nuchae

Vertebra prominens
(spinous process of CVII)

Spine of scapula

Acromion of scapula

Inferior angle of scapula

Spinous process of TXII

Sacral dimple at posterior
superior iliac spine

Iliac crest

Intergluteal cleft

**Surface anatomy of the back**

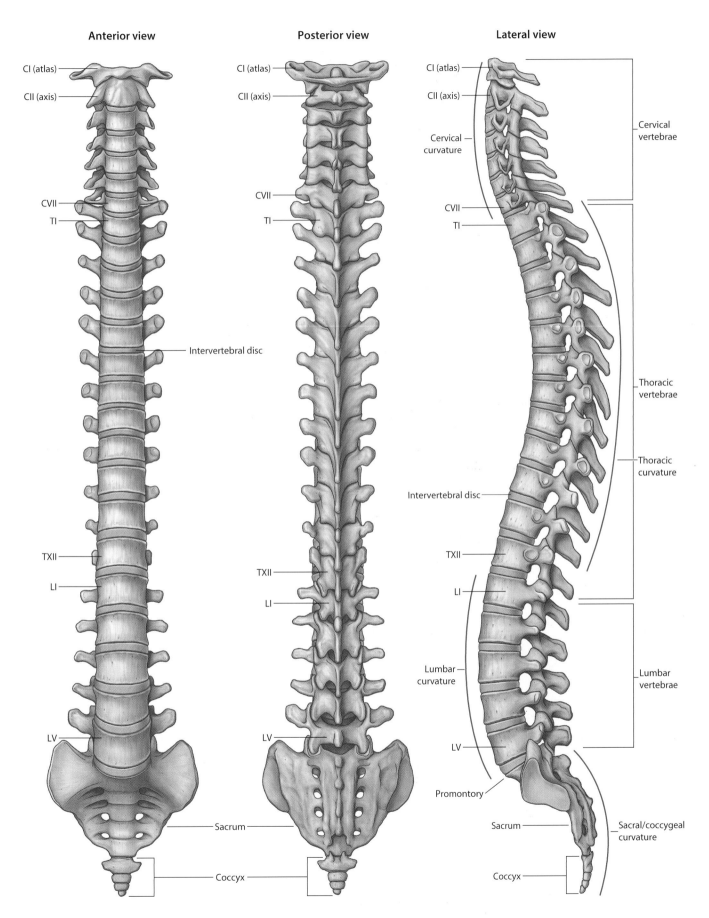

**Anterior view**

CI (atlas)
CII (axis)
CVII
TI
Intervertebral disc
TXII
LI
LV
Sacrum
Coccyx

**Posterior view**

CI (atlas)
CII (axis)
CVII
TI
TXII
LI
LV
Sacrum
Coccyx

**Lateral view**

CI (atlas)
CII (axis)
Cervical curvature
CVII
TI
Cervical vertebrae
Intervertebral disc
Thoracic vertebrae
Thoracic curvature
TXII
LI
Lumbar curvature
Lumbar vertebrae
LV
Promontory
Sacrum
Sacral/coccygeal curvature
Coccyx

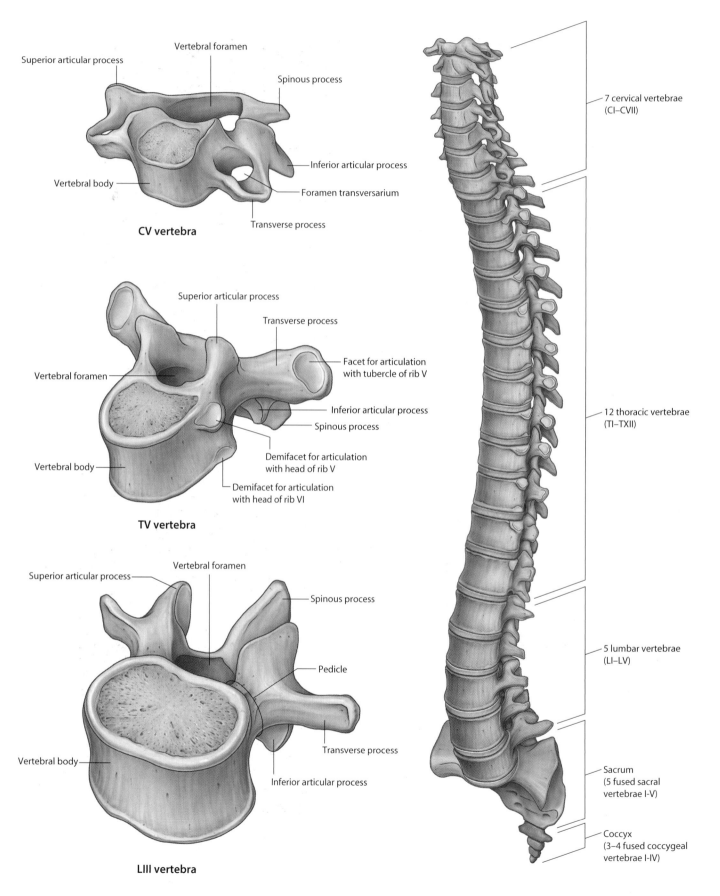

Superior articular process

Vertebral foramen

Spinous process

Inferior articular process

Foramen transversarium

Vertebral body

Transverse process

**CV vertebra**

Superior articular process

Transverse process

Facet for articulation with tubercle of rib V

Vertebral foramen

Inferior articular process

Spinous process

Demifacet for articulation with head of rib V

Vertebral body

Demifacet for articulation with head of rib VI

**TV vertebra**

Superior articular process

Vertebral foramen

Spinous process

Pedicle

Transverse process

Vertebral body

Inferior articular process

**LIII vertebra**

7 cervical vertebrae (CI–CVII)

12 thoracic vertebrae (TI–TXII)

5 lumbar vertebrae (LI–LV)

Sacrum (5 fused sacral vertebrae I-V)

Coccyx (3–4 fused coccygeal vertebrae I-IV)

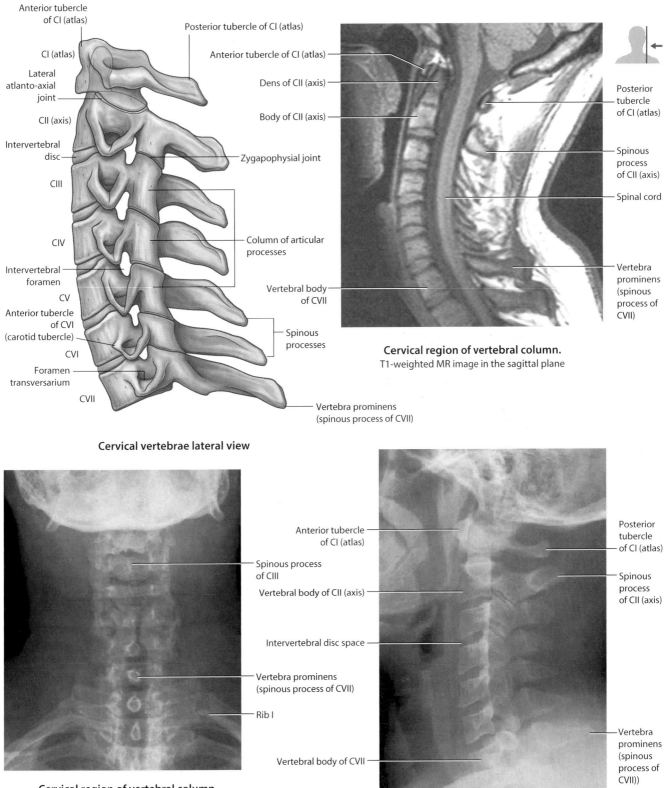

Anterior tubercle of CI (atlas)

CI (atlas)

Lateral atlanto-axial joint

CII (axis)

Intervertebral disc

CIII

CIV

Intervertebral foramen

CV

Anterior tubercle of CVI (carotid tubercle)

CVI

Foramen transversarium

CVII

Posterior tubercle of CI (atlas)

Zygapophysial joint

Column of articular processes

Spinous processes

Vertebra prominens (spinous process of CVII)

**Cervical vertebrae lateral view**

Anterior tubercle of CI (atlas)

Dens of CII (axis)

Body of CII (axis)

Vertebral body of CVII

Posterior tubercle of CI (atlas)

Spinous process of CII (axis)

Spinal cord

Vertebra prominens (spinous process of CVII)

**Cervical region of vertebral column.**
T1-weighted MR image in the sagittal plane

Spinous process of CIII

Vertebra prominens (spinous process of CVII)

Rib I

**Cervical region of vertebral column.**
Radiograph, AP view

Anterior tubercle of CI (atlas)

Vertebral body of CII (axis)

Intervertebral disc space

Vertebra prominens (spinous process of CVII)

Vertebral body of CVII

Posterior tubercle of CI (atlas)

Spinous process of CII (axis)

Vertebra prominens (spinous process of CVII))

**Cervical region of vertebral column.**
Radiograph, lateral view

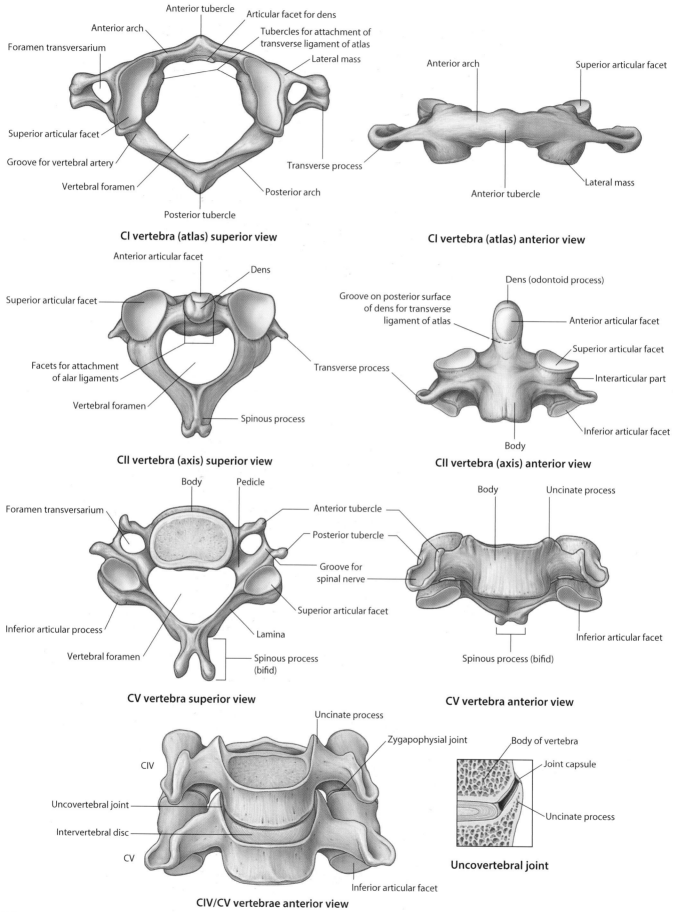

Anterior tubercle
Anterior arch
Articular facet for dens
Foramen transversarium
Tubercles for attachment of transverse ligament of atlas
Lateral mass
Superior articular facet
Groove for vertebral artery
Vertebral foramen
Transverse process
Posterior arch
Posterior tubercle

**CI vertebra (atlas) superior view**

Anterior arch
Superior articular facet
Lateral mass
Anterior tubercle

**CI vertebra (atlas) anterior view**

Anterior articular facet
Dens
Superior articular facet
Facets for attachment of alar ligaments
Vertebral foramen
Transverse process
Spinous process

**CII vertebra (axis) superior view**

Dens (odontoid process)
Groove on posterior surface of dens for transverse ligament of atlas
Anterior articular facet
Superior articular facet
Interarticular part
Inferior articular facet
Body

**CII vertebra (axis) anterior view**

Body
Pedicle
Foramen transversarium
Anterior tubercle
Posterior tubercle
Groove for spinal nerve
Superior articular facet
Inferior articular process
Lamina
Vertebral foramen
Spinous process (bifid)

**CV vertebra superior view**

Body
Uncinate process
Spinous process (bifid)
Inferior articular facet

**CV vertebra anterior view**

Uncinate process
Zygapophysial joint
Body of vertebra
CIV
Joint capsule
Uncovertebral joint
Intervertebral disc
Uncinate process
CV
Inferior articular facet

**Uncovertebral joint**

**CIV/CV vertebrae anterior view**

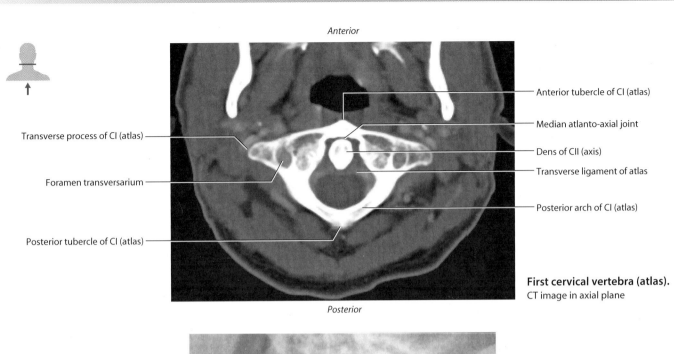

*Anterior*

Transverse process of CI (atlas)

Foramen transversarium

Posterior tubercle of CI (atlas)

Anterior tubercle of CI (atlas)

Median atlanto-axial joint

Dens of CII (axis)

Transverse ligament of atlas

Posterior arch of CI (atlas)

*Posterior*

**First cervical vertebra (atlas).**
CT image in axial plane

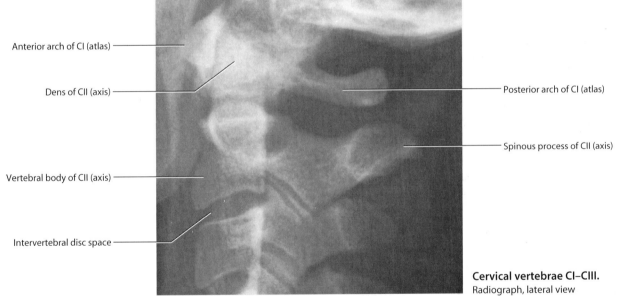

Anterior arch of CI (atlas)

Dens of CII (axis)

Vertebral body of CII (axis)

Intervertebral disc space

Posterior arch of CI (atlas)

Spinous process of CII (axis)

**Cervical vertebrae CI–CIII.**
Radiograph, lateral view

*Anterior*

Foramen transversarium

Vertebral foramen

Lamina

Vertebral body

Anterior tubercle

Posterior tubercle

Spinous process

**Typical cervical vertebra.**
CT image in axial plane

*Posterior*

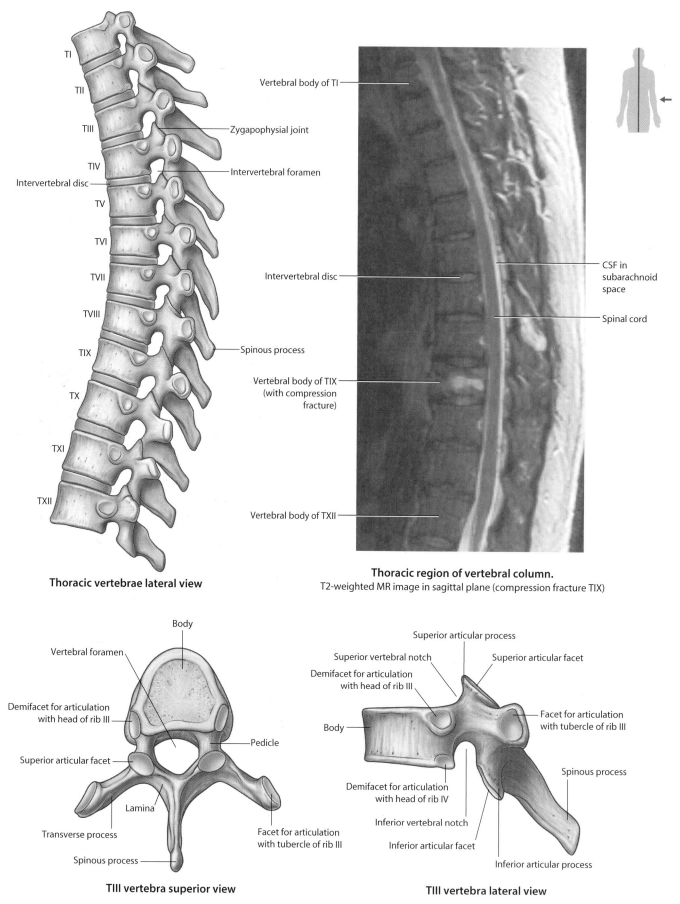

TI

TII

TIII — Zygapophysial joint

TIV — Intervertebral foramen

Intervertebral disc

TV

TVI

TVII

TVIII

TIX — Spinous process

TX

TXI

TXII

**Thoracic vertebrae lateral view**

Vertebral body of TI

Intervertebral disc

Vertebral body of TIX (with compression fracture)

Vertebral body of TXII

CSF in subarachnoid space

Spinal cord

**Thoracic region of vertebral column.**
T2-weighted MR image in sagittal plane (compression fracture TIX)

Body

Vertebral foramen

Demifacet for articulation with head of rib III

Superior articular facet

Transverse process

Lamina

Spinous process

Pedicle

Facet for articulation with tubercle of rib III

**TIII vertebra superior view**

Superior articular process

Superior vertebral notch

Demifacet for articulation with head of rib III

Body

Superior articular facet

Facet for articulation with tubercle of rib III

Demifacet for articulation with head of rib IV

Inferior vertebral notch

Inferior articular facet

Spinous process

Inferior articular process

**TIII vertebra lateral view**

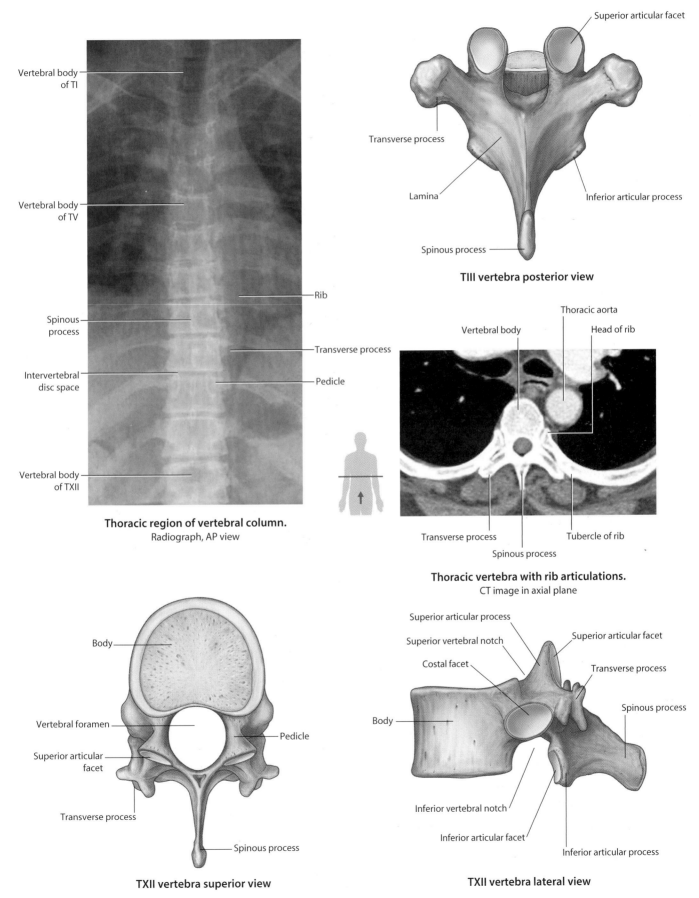

Vertebral body of TI

Vertebral body of TV

Spinous process

Intervertebral disc space

Vertebral body of TXII

Rib

Transverse process

Pedicle

**Thoracic region of vertebral column.**
Radiograph, AP view

Superior articular facet

Transverse process

Lamina

Inferior articular process

Spinous process

**TIII vertebra posterior view**

Vertebral body

Thoracic aorta

Head of rib

Transverse process

Spinous process

Tubercle of rib

**Thoracic vertebra with rib articulations.**
CT image in axial plane

Body

Vertebral foramen

Superior articular facet

Transverse process

Pedicle

Spinous process

**TXII vertebra superior view**

Superior articular process

Superior vertebral notch

Costal facet

Body

Inferior vertebral notch

Inferior articular facet

Superior articular facet

Transverse process

Spinous process

Inferior articular process

**TXII vertebra lateral view**

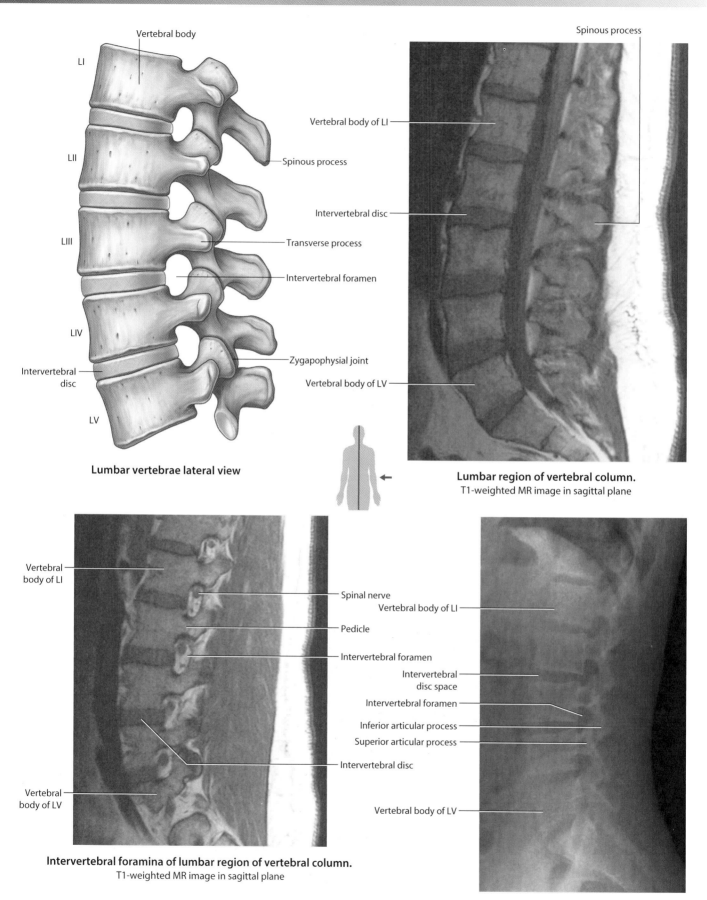

**Lumbar vertebrae lateral view**

Vertebral body

LI

Spinous process

LII

LIII

Transverse process

Intervertebral foramen

LIV

Intervertebral disc

Zygapophysial joint

Vertebral body of LV

LV

**Lumbar region of vertebral column.**
T1-weighted MR image in sagittal plane

Spinous process

Vertebral body of LI

Intervertebral disc

**Intervertebral foramina of lumbar region of vertebral column.**
T1-weighted MR image in sagittal plane

Vertebral body of LI

Spinal nerve

Pedicle

Intervertebral foramen

Intervertebral disc

Vertebral body of LV

**Lumbar region of vertebral column.**
Radiograph, lateral view

Vertebral body of LI

Intervertebral disc space

Intervertebral foramen

Inferior articular process

Superior articular process

Vertebral body of LV

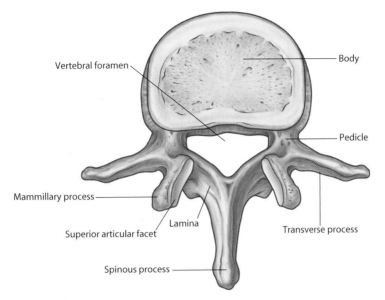

Vertebral foramen

Body

Pedicle

Mammillary process

Lamina

Superior articular facet

Transverse process

Spinous process

**LIV vertebra superior view**

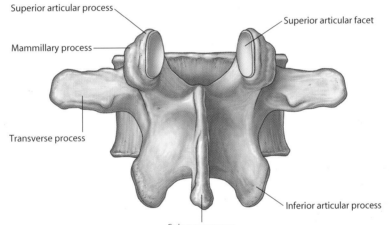

Superior articular process

Superior articular facet

Mammillary process

Transverse process

Inferior articular process

Spinous process

**LIV vertebra posterior view**

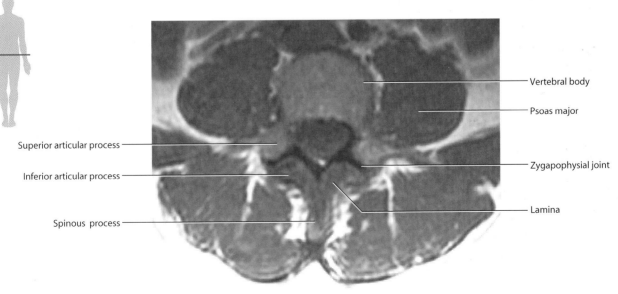

Vertebral body

Psoas major

Superior articular process

Inferior articular process

Zygapophysial joint

Lamina

Spinous process

**Articulation of lumbar vertebrae.**
T1-weighted MR image in axial plane

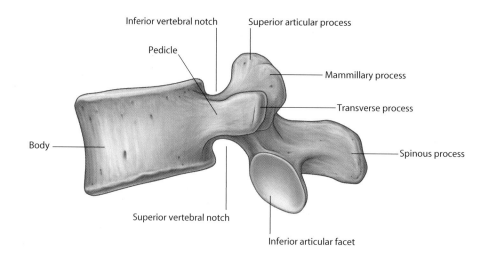

Inferior vertebral notch

Pedicle

Superior articular process

Mammillary process

Transverse process

Body

Spinous process

Superior vertebral notch

Inferior articular facet

**LIV vertebra lateral view**

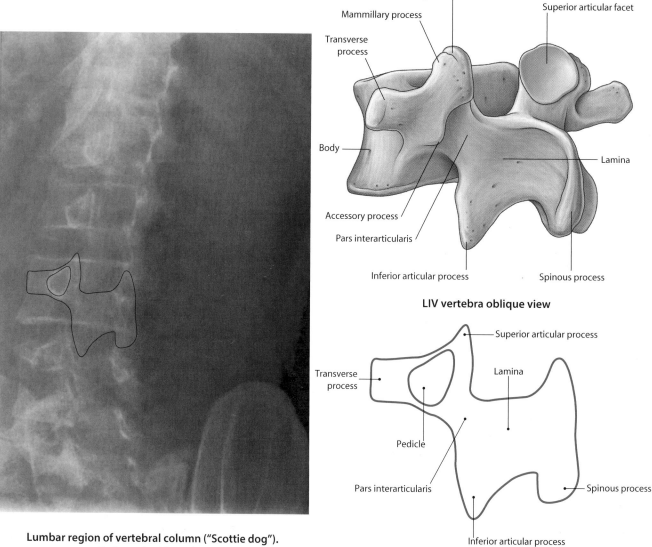

Superior articular process

Mammillary process

Transverse process

Superior articular facet

Body

Lamina

Accessory process

Pars interarticularis

Inferior articular process

Spinous process

**LIV vertebra oblique view**

Transverse process

Superior articular process

Lamina

Pedicle

Pars interarticularis

Inferior articular process

Spinous process

**Lumbar region of vertebral column ("Scottie dog").**
Radiograph, oblique view

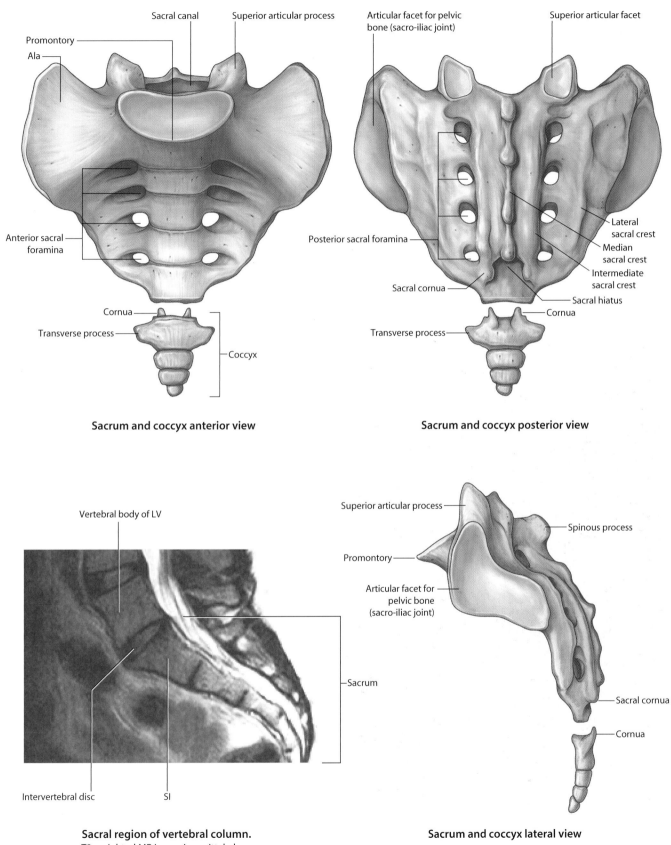

Sacral canal
Promontory
Ala
Superior articular process

Anterior sacral foramina

Cornua
Transverse process

Coccyx

**Sacrum and coccyx anterior view**

Articular facet for pelvic bone (sacro-iliac joint)
Superior articular facet

Posterior sacral foramina

Sacral cornua

Lateral sacral crest
Median sacral crest
Intermediate sacral crest
Sacral hiatus
Cornua

Transverse process

**Sacrum and coccyx posterior view**

Vertebral body of LV

Sacrum

Intervertebral disc
SI

**Sacral region of vertebral column.**
T2-weighted MR image in sagittal plane

Superior articular process
Spinous process
Promontory
Articular facet for pelvic bone (sacro-iliac joint)

Sacral cornua
Cornua

**Sacrum and coccyx lateral view**

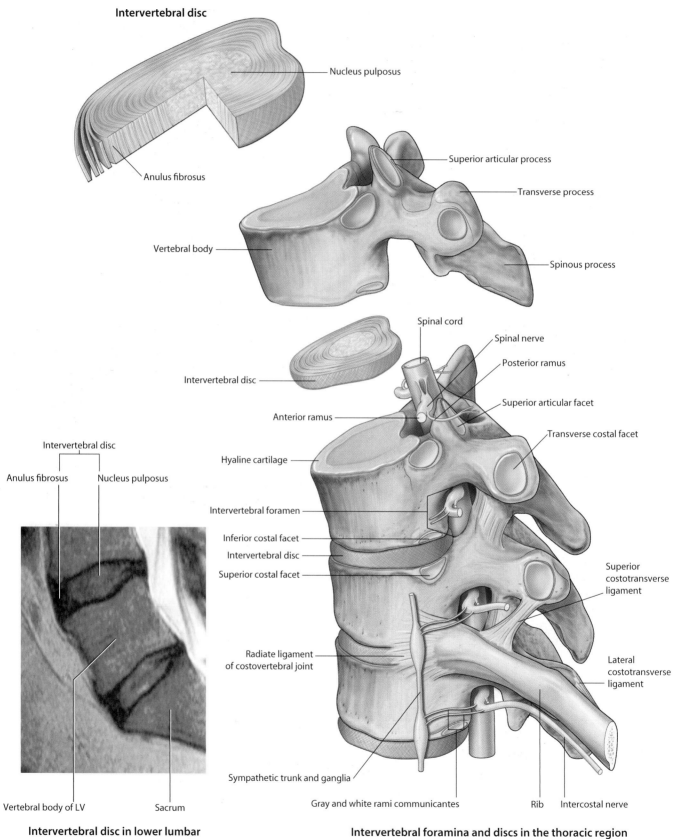

**Intervertebral disc**

Nucleus pulposus

Anulus fibrosus

Superior articular process

Transverse process

Vertebral body

Spinous process

Spinal cord

Spinal nerve

Posterior ramus

Intervertebral disc

Anterior ramus

Superior articular facet

Transverse costal facet

Intervertebral disc

Anulus fibrosus    Nucleus pulposus

Hyaline cartilage

Intervertebral foramen

Inferior costal facet

Intervertebral disc

Superior costal facet

Superior costotransverse ligament

Radiate ligament of costovertebral joint

Lateral costotransverse ligament

Sympathetic trunk and ganglia

Vertebral body of LV          Sacrum

Gray and white rami communicantes          Rib    Intercostal nerve

**Intervertebral disc in lower lumbar region of vertebral column.**
T2-weighted MR image in sagittal plane

**Intervertebral foramina and discs in the thoracic region**

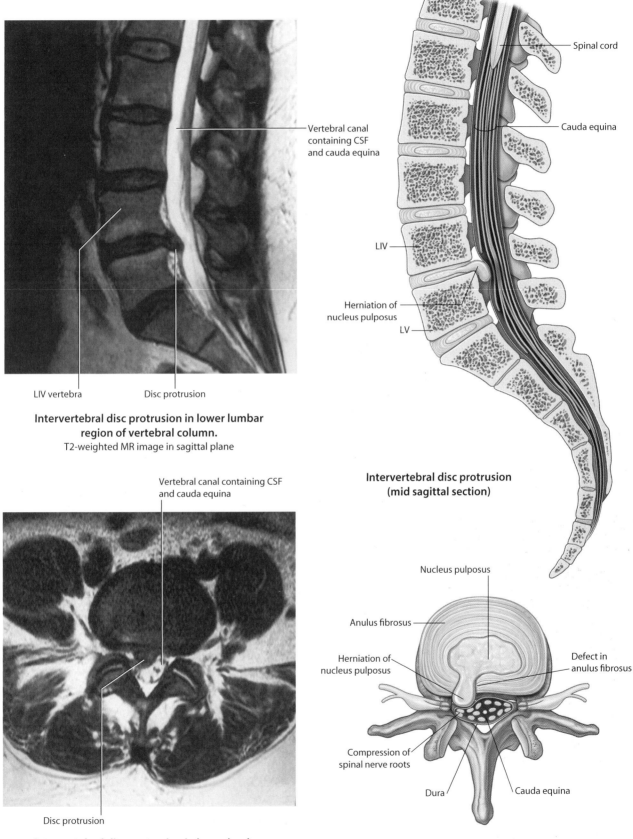

Vertebral canal
containing CSF
and cauda equina

LIV vertebra    Disc protrusion

**Intervertebral disc protrusion in lower lumbar
region of vertebral column.**
T2-weighted MR image in sagittal plane

Spinal cord

Cauda equina

LIV

Herniation of
nucleus pulposus

LV

**Intervertebral disc protrusion
(mid sagittal section)**

Vertebral canal containing CSF
and cauda equina

Disc protrusion

**Intervertebral disc protrusion in lower lumbar
region of vertebral column.**
T2-weighted MR image in axial plane

Nucleus pulposus

Anulus fibrosus

Herniation of
nucleus pulposus

Defect in
anulus fibrosus

Compression of
spinal nerve roots

Dura    Cauda equina

**Intervertebral disc protrusion (superior view)**

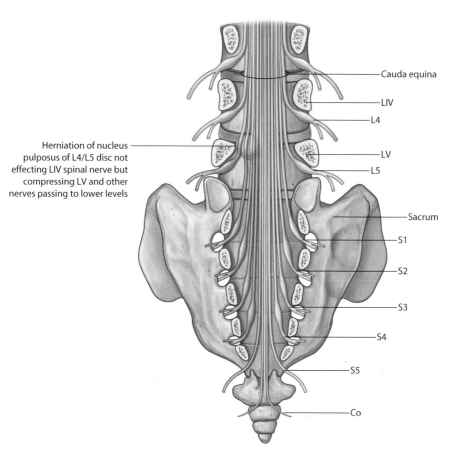

Cauda equina

LIV

L4

Herniation of nucleus
pulposus of L4/L5 disc not
effecting LIV spinal nerve but
compressing LV and other
nerves passing to lower levels

LV

L5

Sacrum

S1

S2

S3

S4

S5

Co

Intervertebral disc protrusion (posterior view)

| Nerve root | Main weakness | Reflex decreased | Area of sensory decrease | Disc involved |
|---|---|---|---|---|
| C5 | Deltoid (biceps) | (biceps, pectoralis) | Shoulder, upper lateral arm | C4–C5 |
| C6 | Wrist extension | (biceps, brachioradialis) | 1st and 2nd digits (lateral forearm) | C5–C6 |
| C7 | Triceps | Triceps | Third finger | C6–C7 |
| C8 | Intrinsic hand muscles | | 4th and 5th digits (medial forearm) | C7–T1 |

Clinically important nerve roots in the upper limb

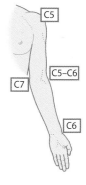

| Nerve root | Main weakness | Reflex decreased | Area of sensory decrease | Disc involved |
|---|---|---|---|---|
| L4 | Iliopsoas and quadriceps | Patellar tendon (knee jerk) | Knee, medial lower leg | L3–L4 |
| L5 | Dorsiflexion of foot at ankle (big toe extension, foot eversion and inversion | | Dorsum of foot, big toe | L4–L5 |
| S1 | Plantar flexion of foot at ankle | Achilles tendon (ankle jerk) | Lateral foot, small toe, sole | L5–S1 |

Clinically important nerve roots in the lower limb

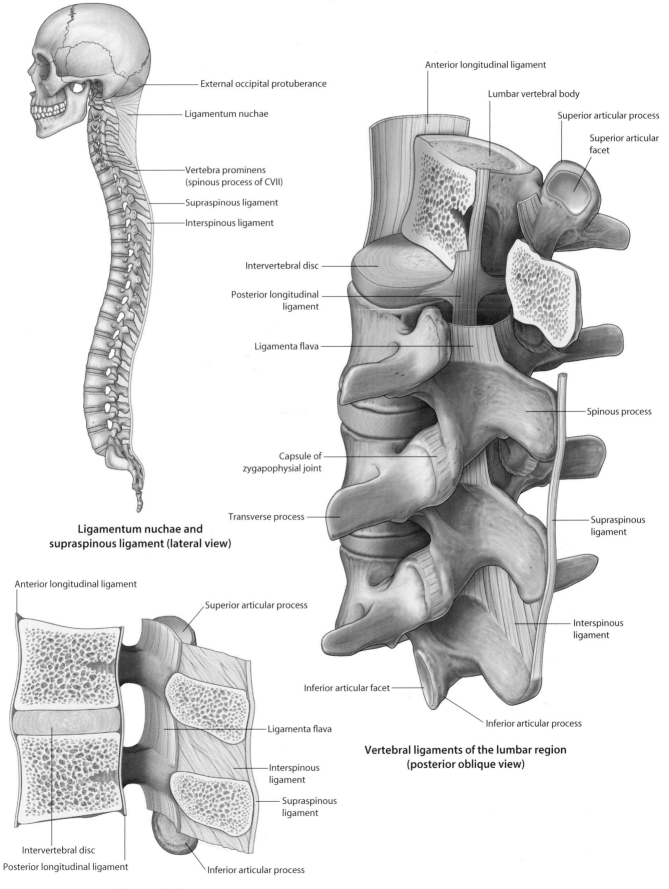

External occipital protuberance

Ligamentum nuchae

Vertebra prominens
(spinous process of CVII)

Supraspinous ligament

Interspinous ligament

**Ligamentum nuchae and
supraspinous ligament (lateral view)**

Anterior longitudinal ligament

Lumbar vertebral body

Superior articular process

Superior articular
facet

Intervertebral disc

Posterior longitudinal
ligament

Ligamenta flava

Spinous process

Capsule of
zygapophysial joint

Transverse process

Supraspinous
ligament

Interspinous
ligament

Inferior articular facet

Inferior articular process

**Vertebral ligaments of the lumbar region
(posterior oblique view)**

Anterior longitudinal ligament

Superior articular process

Ligamenta flava

Interspinous
ligament

Supraspinous
ligament

Intervertebral disc

Posterior longitudinal ligament

Inferior articular process

**Ligamenta flava**

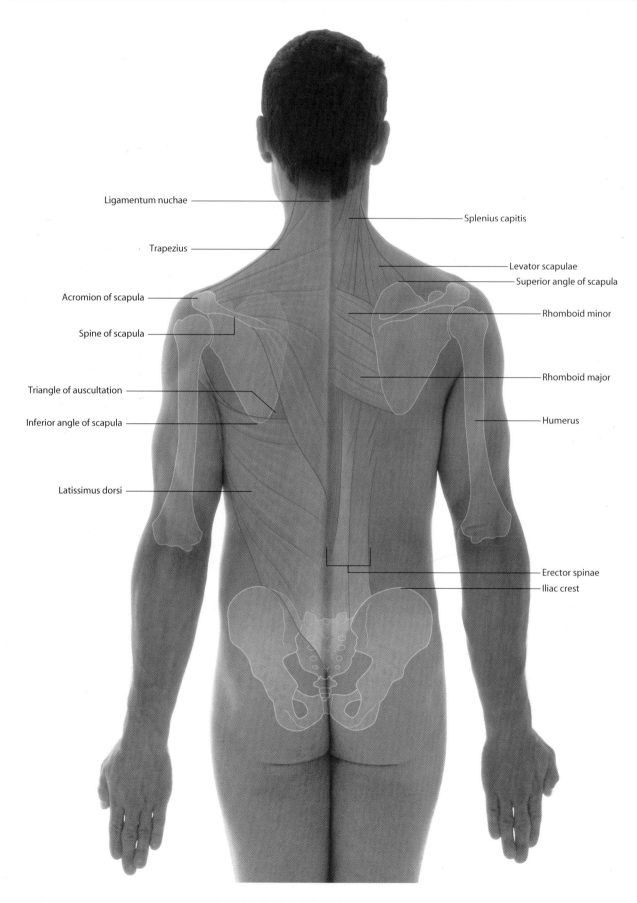

Ligamentum nuchae

Trapezius

Acromion of scapula

Spine of scapula

Triangle of auscultation

Inferior angle of scapula

Latissimus dorsi

Splenius capitis

Levator scapulae

Superior angle of scapula

Rhomboid minor

Rhomboid major

Humerus

Erector spinae

Iliac crest

**Posterior view of male showing surface projections of back muscles**

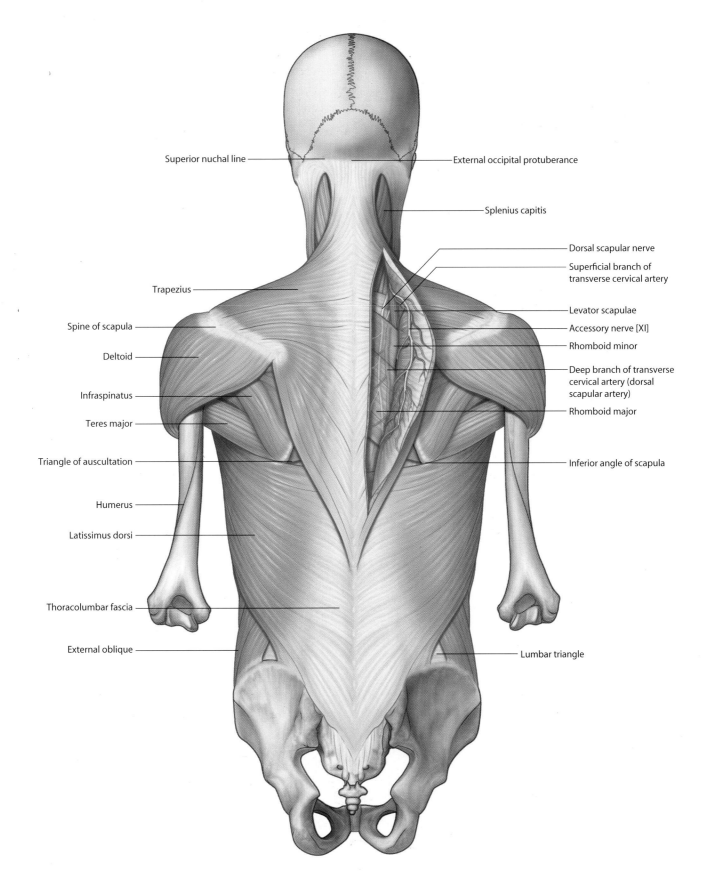

Superior nuchal line

External occipital protuberance

Splenius capitis

Dorsal scapular nerve

Superficial branch of transverse cervical artery

Trapezius

Levator scapulae

Spine of scapula

Accessory nerve [XI]

Deltoid

Rhomboid minor

Infraspinatus

Deep branch of transverse cervical artery (dorsal scapular artery)

Teres major

Rhomboid major

Triangle of auscultation

Inferior angle of scapula

Humerus

Latissimus dorsi

Thoracolumbar fascia

External oblique

Lumbar triangle

**Superficial musculature – trapezius and latissimus dorsi**

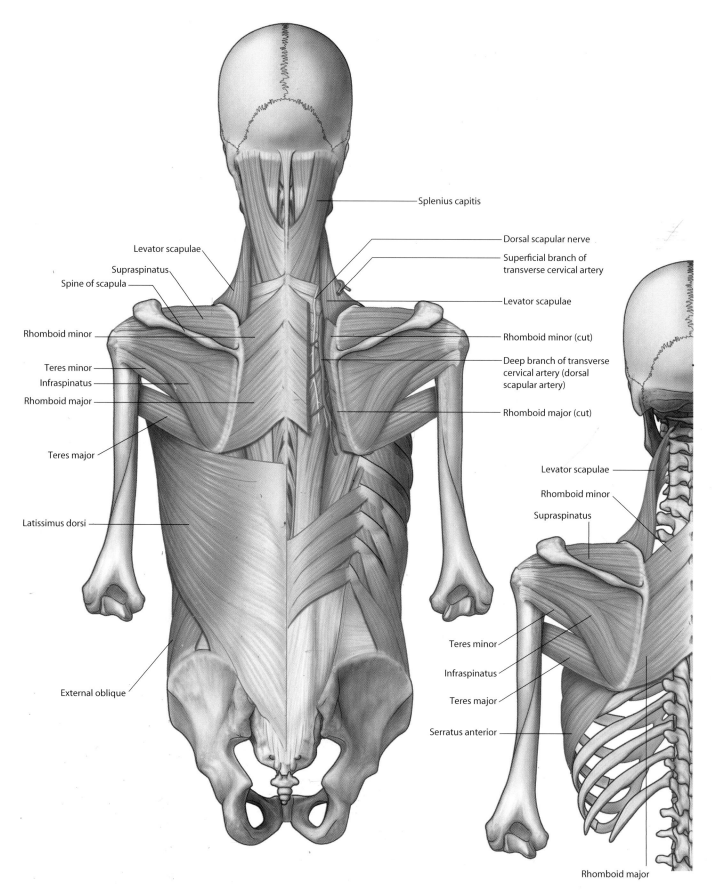

Splenius capitis

Dorsal scapular nerve

Superficial branch of transverse cervical artery

Levator scapulae

Rhomboid minor (cut)

Deep branch of transverse cervical artery (dorsal scapular artery)

Rhomboid major (cut)

Levator scapulae

Supraspinatus

Spine of scapula

Rhomboid minor

Teres minor

Infraspinatus

Rhomboid major

Teres major

Latissimus dorsi

External oblique

Levator scapulae

Rhomboid minor

Supraspinatus

Teres minor

Infraspinatus

Teres major

Serratus anterior

Rhomboid major

**Superficial musculature – levator scapulae and rhomboid major and minor**

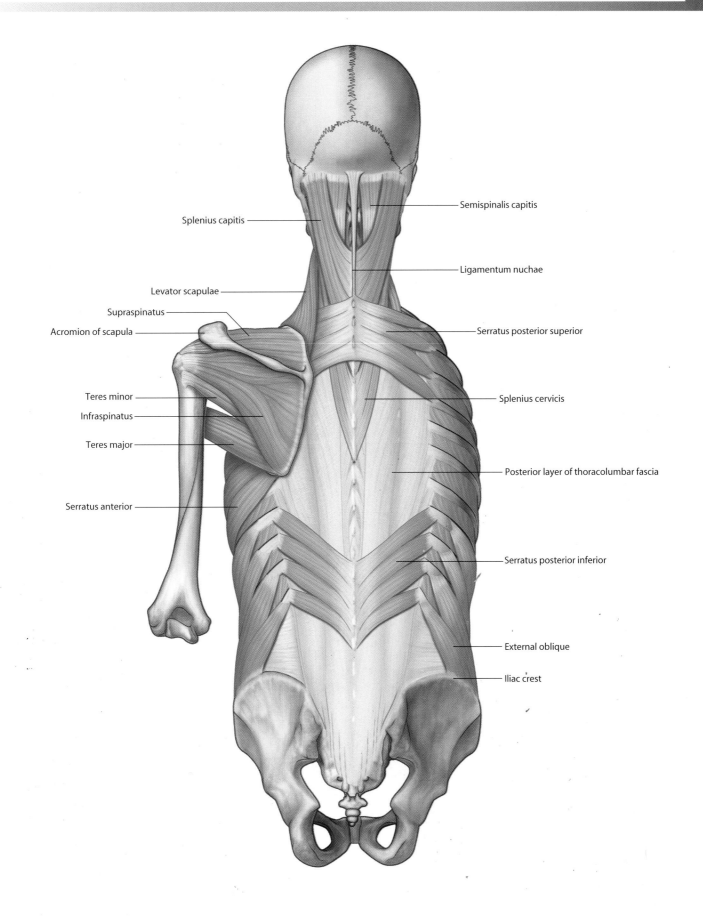

Splenius capitis

Levator scapulae

Supraspinatus

Acromion of scapula

Teres minor

Infraspinatus

Teres major

Serratus anterior

Semispinalis capitis

Ligamentum nuchae

Serratus posterior superior

Splenius cervicis

Posterior layer of thoracolumbar fascia

Serratus posterior inferior

External oblique

Iliac crest

**Intermediate musculature**

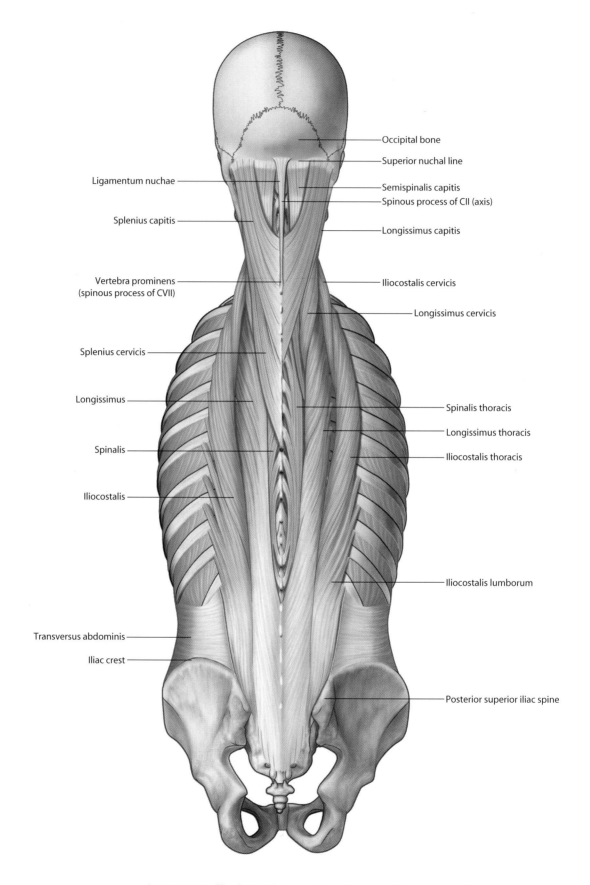

Occipital bone

Superior nuchal line

Ligamentum nuchae

Semispinalis capitis

Spinous process of CII (axis)

Splenius capitis

Longissimus capitis

Vertebra prominens
(spinous process of CVII)

Iliocostalis cervicis

Longissimus cervicis

Splenius cervicis

Longissimus

Spinalis thoracis

Longissimus thoracis

Spinalis

Iliocostalis thoracis

Iliocostalis

Iliocostalis lumborum

Transversus abdominis

Iliac crest

Posterior superior iliac spine

**Deep group of back muscles – erector spinae muscles**

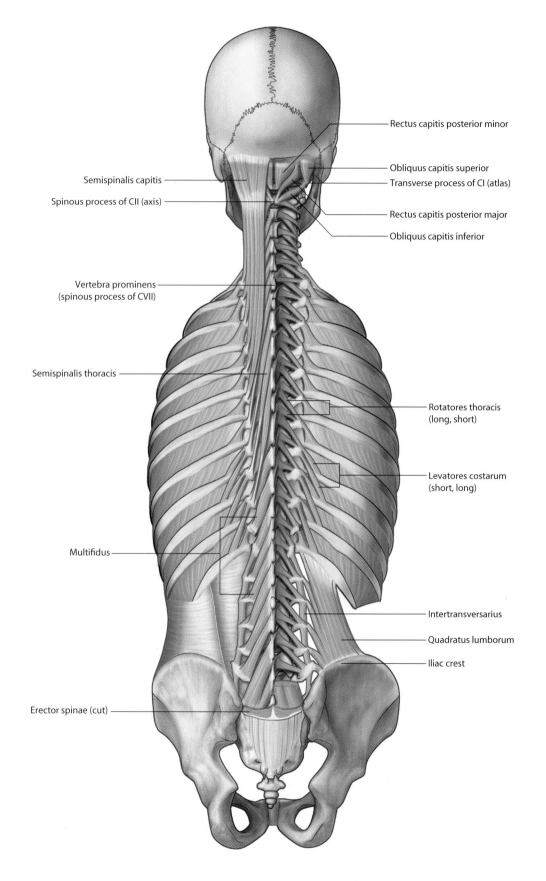

Rectus capitis posterior minor

Semispinalis capitis

Obliquus capitis superior
Transverse process of CI (atlas)

Spinous process of CII (axis)

Rectus capitis posterior major
Obliquus capitis inferior

Vertebra prominens
(spinous process of CVII)

Semispinalis thoracis

Rotatores thoracis
(long, short)

Levatores costarum
(short, long)

Multifidus

Intertransversarius
Quadratus lumborum
Iliac crest

Erector spinae (cut)

**Deep group of back muscles – transversospinales and segmental muscles**

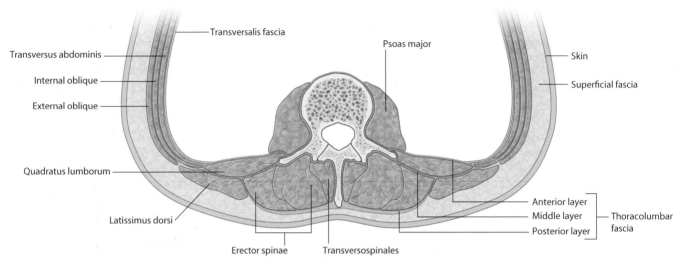

Transversalis fascia

Transversus abdominis

Internal oblique

External oblique

Psoas major

Skin

Superficial fascia

Quadratus lumborum

Latissimus dorsi

Anterior layer

Middle layer

Posterior layer

Thoracolumbar fascia

Erector spinae

Transversospinales

**Thoracolumbar fascia and the deep back muscles
(transverse section – lumbar region)**

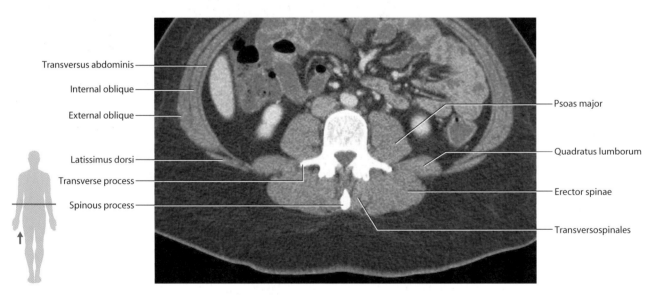

Transversus abdominis

Internal oblique

External oblique

Latissimus dorsi

Transverse process

Spinous process

Psoas major

Quadratus lumborum

Erector spinae

Transversospinales

**Lumbar region (LIII) showing back musculature.**
CT image in axial plane

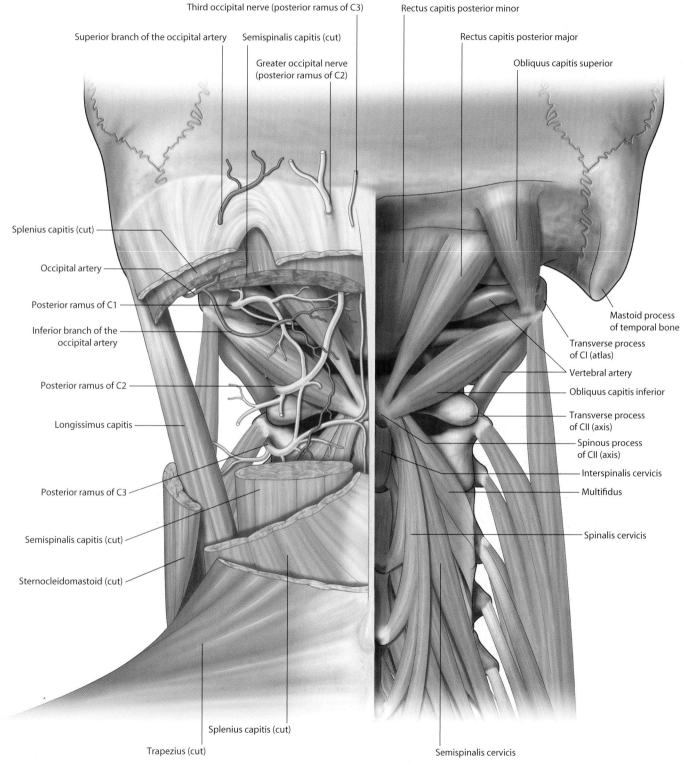

Third occipital nerve (posterior ramus of C3)

Superior branch of the occipital artery

Semispinalis capitis (cut)

Greater occipital nerve (posterior ramus of C2)

Rectus capitis posterior minor

Rectus capitis posterior major

Obliquus capitis superior

Splenius capitis (cut)

Occipital artery

Posterior ramus of C1

Inferior branch of the occipital artery

Posterior ramus of C2

Longissimus capitis

Posterior ramus of C3

Semispinalis capitis (cut)

Sternocleidomastoid (cut)

Mastoid process of temporal bone

Transverse process of CI (atlas)

Vertebral artery

Obliquus capitis inferior

Transverse process of CII (axis)

Spinous process of CII (axis)

Interspinalis cervicis

Multifidus

Spinalis cervicis

Splenius capitis (cut)

Trapezius (cut)

Semispinalis cervicis

**Suboccipital region**

**43**

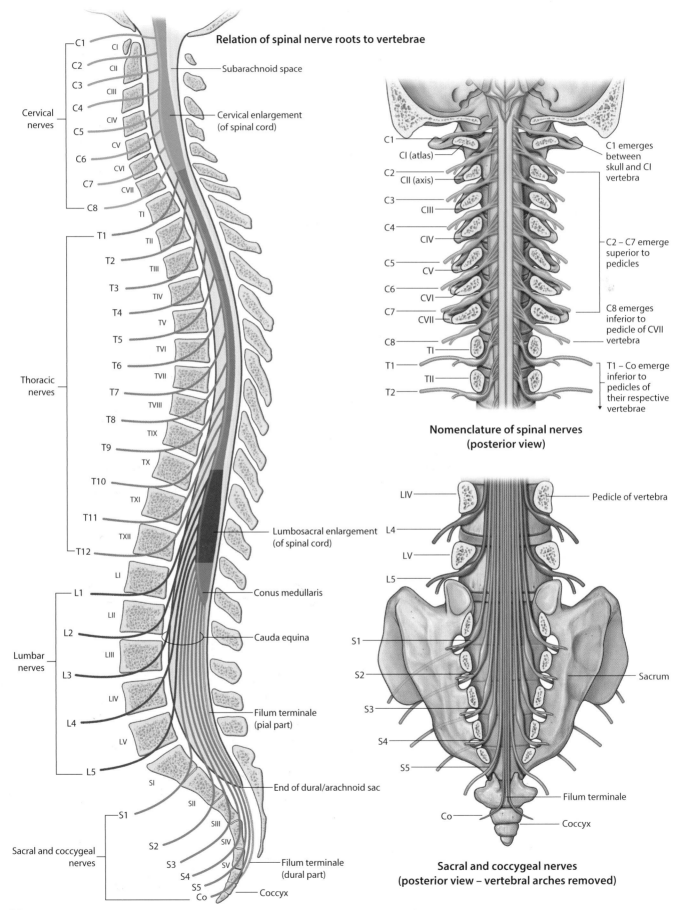

**Relation of spinal nerve roots to vertebrae**

Cervical nerves
- C1 — CI
- C2 — CII
- C3 — CIII
- C4 — CIV
- C5 — CV
- C6 — CVI
- C7 — CVII
- C8

Subarachnoid space

Cervical enlargement (of spinal cord)

Thoracic nerves
- T1 — TI
- T2 — TII
- T3 — TIII
- T4 — TIV
- T5 — TV
- T6 — TVI
- T7 — TVII
- T8 — TVIII
- T9 — TIX
- T10 — TX
- T11 — TXI
- T12 — TXII

Lumbosacral enlargement (of spinal cord)

Lumbar nerves
- L1 — LI
- L2 — LII
- L3 — LIII
- L4 — LIV
- L5 — LV

Conus medullaris

Cauda equina

Filum terminale (pial part)

End of dural/arachnoid sac

Sacral and coccygeal nerves
- S1 — SI
- S2 — SII
- S3 — SIII
- S4 — SIV
- S5 — SV
- Co

Filum terminale (dural part)

Coccyx

**Nomenclature of spinal nerves (posterior view)**

- C1
- CI (atlas)
- C2
- CII (axis)
- C3
- CIII
- C4
- CIV
- C5
- CV
- C6
- CVI
- C7
- CVII
- C8
- TI
- T1
- TII
- T2

C1 emerges between skull and CI vertebra

C2 – C7 emerge superior to pedicles

C8 emerges inferior to pedicle of CVII vertebra

T1 – Co emerge inferior to pedicles of their respective vertebrae

**Sacral and coccygeal nerves (posterior view – vertebral arches removed)**

- LIV
- L4
- LV
- L5
- S1
- S2
- S3
- S4
- S5
- Co

Pedicle of vertebra

Sacrum

Filum terminale

Coccyx

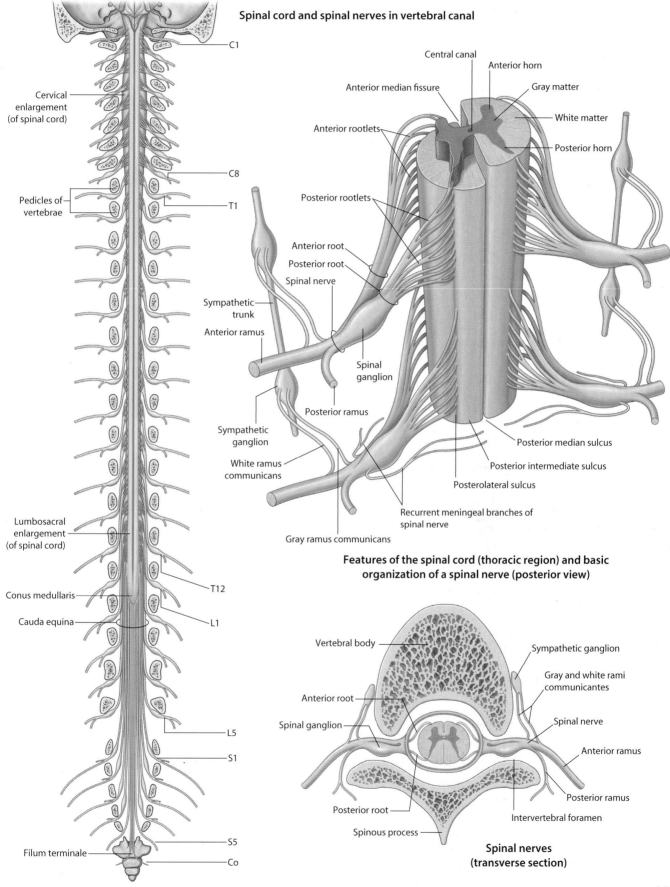

C1

Cervical
enlargement
(of spinal cord)

C8

Pedicles of
vertebrae

T1

Lumbosacral
enlargement
(of spinal cord)

Conus medullaris

Cauda equina

T12

L1

L5

S1

Filum terminale

S5

Co

**Spinal cord and spinal nerves in vertebral canal**

Central canal

Anterior horn

Anterior median fissure

Gray matter

Anterior rootlets

White matter

Posterior horn

Posterior rootlets

Anterior root

Posterior root

Spinal nerve

Sympathetic
trunk

Anterior ramus

Spinal
ganglion

Sympathetic
ganglion

Posterior ramus

Posterior median sulcus

White ramus
communicans

Posterior intermediate sulcus

Posterolateral sulcus

Recurrent meningeal branches of
spinal nerve

Gray ramus communicans

**Features of the spinal cord (thoracic region) and basic
organization of a spinal nerve (posterior view)**

Vertebral body

Sympathetic ganglion

Gray and white rami
communicantes

Anterior root

Spinal ganglion

Spinal nerve

Anterior ramus

Posterior ramus

Posterior root

Intervertebral foramen

Spinous process

**Spinal nerves
(transverse section)**

**45**

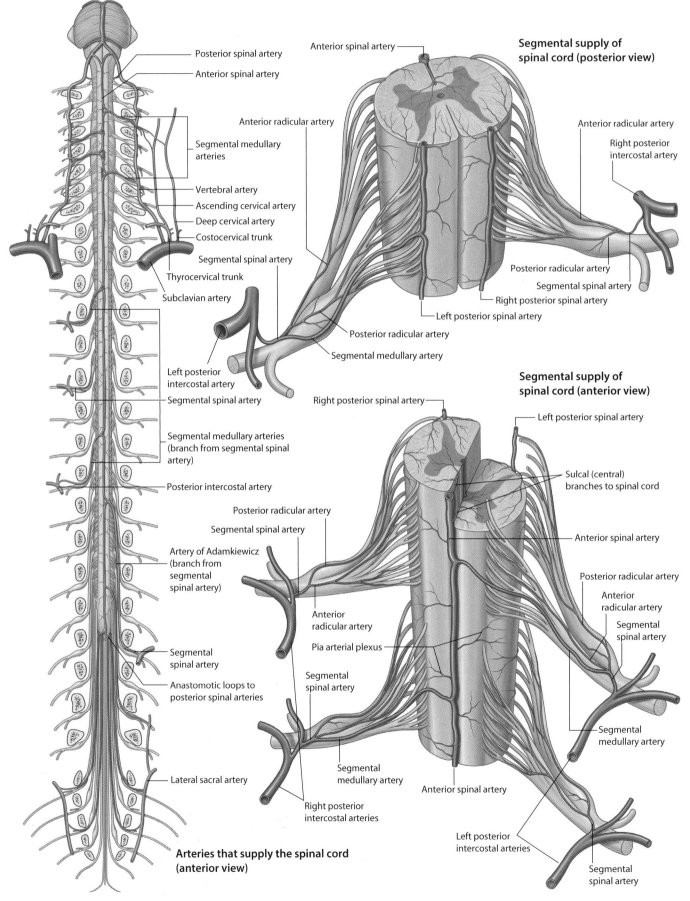

Posterior spinal artery

Anterior spinal artery

Segmental medullary arteries

Vertebral artery

Ascending cervical artery

Deep cervical artery

Costocervical trunk

Segmental spinal artery

Thyrocervical trunk

Subclavian artery

Left posterior intercostal artery

Segmental spinal artery

Segmental medullary arteries (branch from segmental spinal artery)

Posterior intercostal artery

Artery of Adamkiewicz (branch from segmental spinal artery)

Segmental spinal artery

Anastomotic loops to posterior spinal arteries

Lateral sacral artery

**Arteries that supply the spinal cord (anterior view)**

Anterior spinal artery

**Segmental supply of spinal cord (posterior view)**

Anterior radicular artery

Anterior radicular artery

Right posterior intercostal artery

Posterior radicular artery

Segmental spinal artery

Right posterior spinal artery

Left posterior spinal artery

Posterior radicular artery

Segmental medullary artery

**Segmental supply of spinal cord (anterior view)**

Right posterior spinal artery

Left posterior spinal artery

Sulcal (central) branches to spinal cord

Anterior spinal artery

Posterior radicular artery

Posterior radicular artery

Segmental spinal artery

Anterior radicular artery

Segmental spinal artery

Anterior radicular artery

Pia arterial plexus

Segmental spinal artery

Segmental medullary artery

Segmental medullary artery

Anterior spinal artery

Right posterior intercostal arteries

Left posterior intercostal arteries

Segmental spinal artery

46

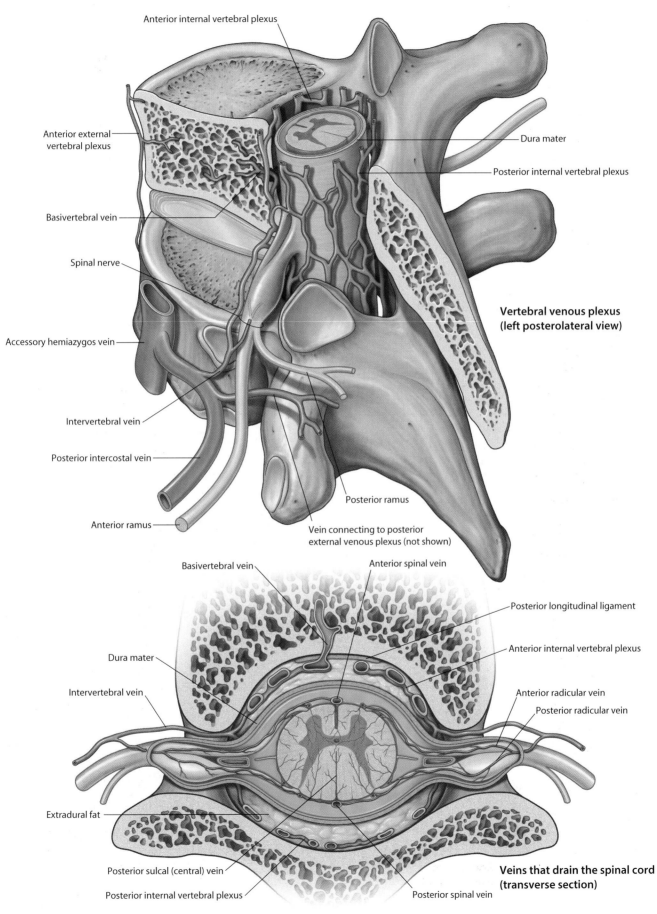

Anterior internal vertebral plexus

Anterior external vertebral plexus

Basivertebral vein

Spinal nerve

Accessory hemiazygos vein

Intervertebral vein

Posterior intercostal vein

Anterior ramus

Dura mater

Posterior internal vertebral plexus

**Vertebral venous plexus (left posterolateral view)**

Posterior ramus

Vein connecting to posterior external venous plexus (not shown)

Basivertebral vein

Anterior spinal vein

Dura mater

Intervertebral vein

Posterior longitudinal ligament

Anterior internal vertebral plexus

Anterior radicular vein

Posterior radicular vein

Extradural fat

Posterior sulcal (central) vein

Posterior internal vertebral plexus

Posterior spinal vein

**Veins that drain the spinal cord (transverse section)**

**47**

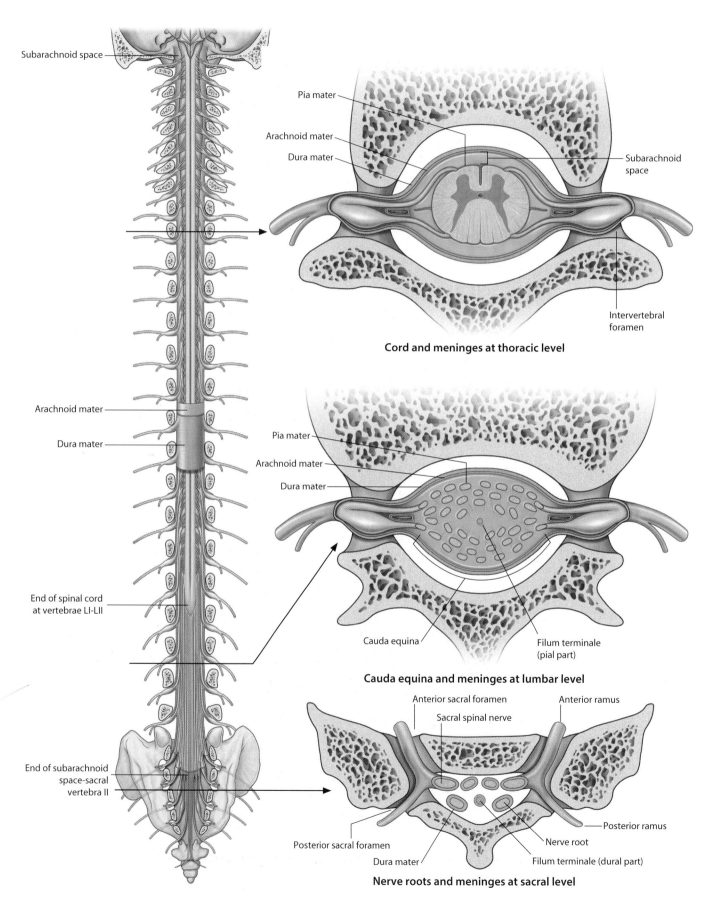

Subarachnoid space

Arachnoid mater

Dura mater

End of spinal cord
at vertebrae LI-LII

End of subarachnoid
space-sacral
vertebra II

Pia mater

Arachnoid mater

Dura mater

Subarachnoid
space

Intervertebral
foramen

**Cord and meninges at thoracic level**

Pia mater

Arachnoid mater

Dura mater

Cauda equina

Filum terminale
(pial part)

**Cauda equina and meninges at lumbar level**

Anterior sacral foramen

Sacral spinal nerve

Anterior ramus

Posterior ramus

Posterior sacral foramen

Nerve root

Dura mater

Filum terminale (dural part)

**Nerve roots and meninges at sacral level**

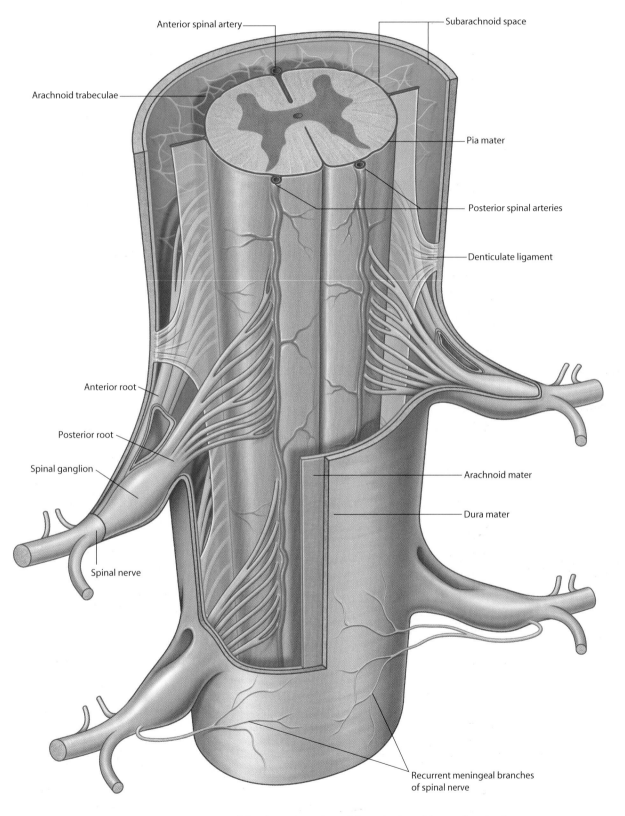

Anterior spinal artery

Subarachnoid space

Arachnoid trabeculae

Pia mater

Posterior spinal arteries

Denticulate ligament

Anterior root

Posterior root

Spinal ganglion

Arachnoid mater

Dura mater

Spinal nerve

Recurrent meningeal branches
of spinal nerve

**Meninges covering parts of the thoracic region of the spinal cord (posterior view)**

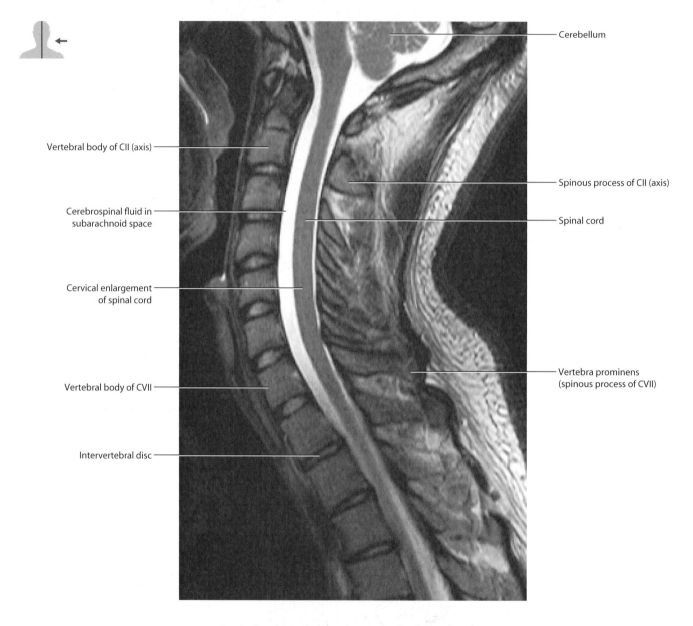

Cerebellum

Vertebral body of CII (axis)

Spinous process of CII (axis)

Cerebrospinal fluid in subarachnoid space

Spinal cord

Cervical enlargement of spinal cord

Vertebral body of CVII

Vertebra prominens (spinous process of CVII)

Intervertebral disc

**Cervical and upper thoracic vertebral column showing upper and middle portions of spinal cord.**
T2-weighted MR image in sagittal plane

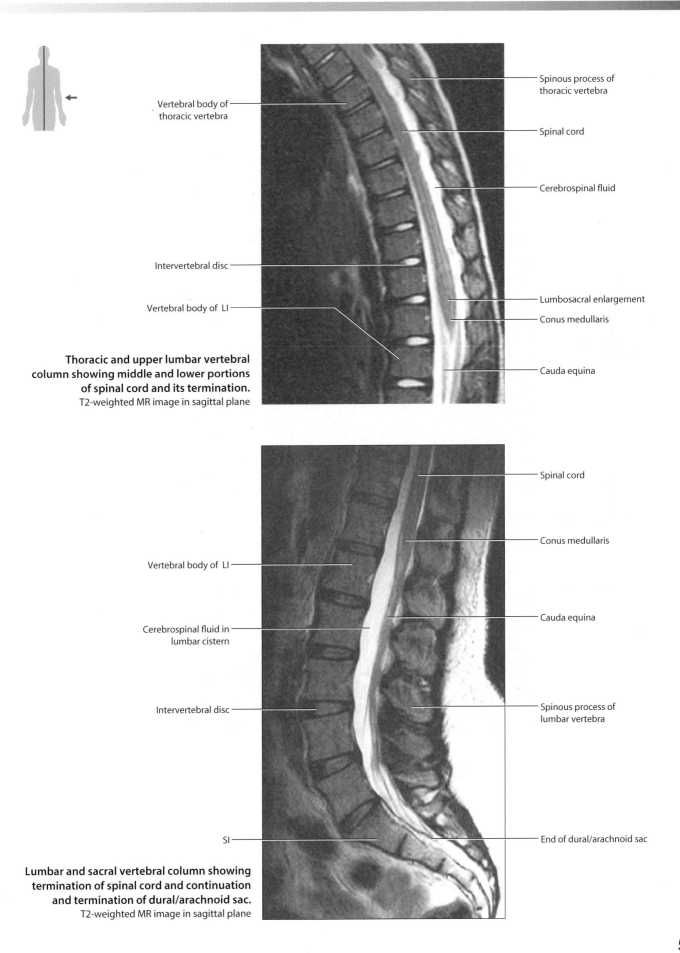

Vertebral body of thoracic vertebra

Spinous process of thoracic vertebra

Spinal cord

Cerebrospinal fluid

Intervertebral disc

Vertebral body of LI

Lumbosacral enlargement

Conus medullaris

Cauda equina

**Thoracic and upper lumbar vertebral column showing middle and lower portions of spinal cord and its termination.**
T2-weighted MR image in sagittal plane

Spinal cord

Conus medullaris

Vertebral body of LI

Cerebrospinal fluid in lumbar cistern

Cauda equina

Intervertebral disc

Spinous process of lumbar vertebra

SI

End of dural/arachnoid sac

**Lumbar and sacral vertebral column showing termination of spinal cord and continuation and termination of dural/arachnoid sac.**
T2-weighted MR image in sagittal plane

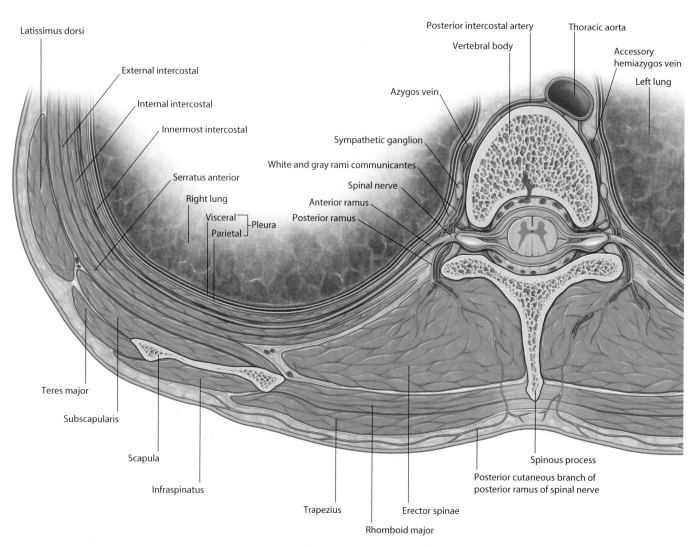

Latissimus dorsi

External intercostal

Internal intercostal

Innermost intercostal

Serratus anterior

Right lung

Visceral ⌉
          ⌐ Pleura
Parietal ⌋

Teres major

Subscapularis

Scapula

Infraspinatus

Trapezius

Rhomboid major

Erector spinae

Posterior intercostal artery

Vertebral body

Thoracic aorta

Accessory hemiazygos vein

Left lung

Azygos vein

Sympathetic ganglion

White and gray rami communicantes

Spinal nerve

Anterior ramus

Posterior ramus

Spinous process

Posterior cutaneous branch of posterior ramus of spinal nerve

**Transverse section through thoracic region of vertebral column**

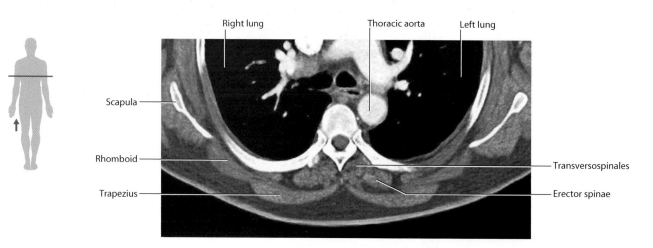

Right lung

Thoracic aorta

Left lung

Scapula

Rhomboid

Trapezius

Transversospinales

Erector spinae

**Thoracic region of back.**
CT image in axial plane

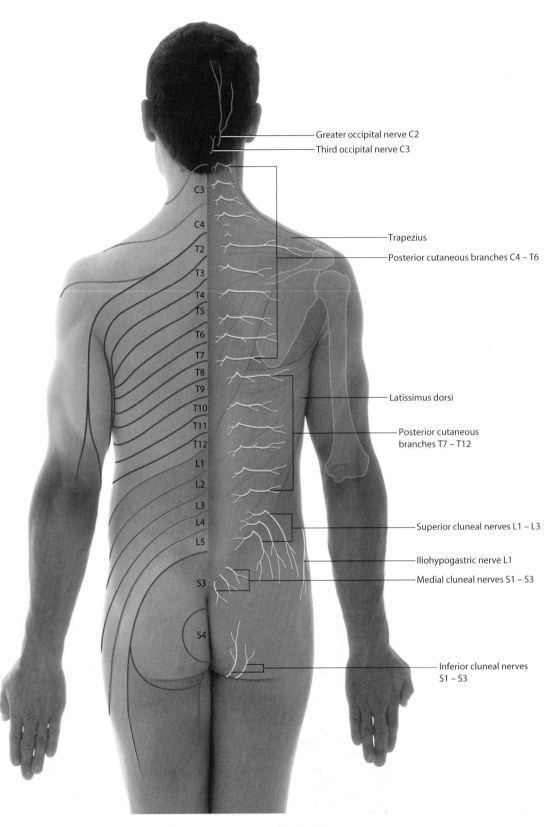

Greater occipital nerve C2

Third occipital nerve C3

C3

C4

T2

T3

T4

T5

T6

T7

T8

T9

T10

T11

T12

L1

L2

L3

L4

L5

S3

S4

Trapezius

Posterior cutaneous branches C4 – T6

Latissimus dorsi

Posterior cutaneous branches T7 – T12

Superior cluneal nerves L1 – L3

Iliohypogastric nerve L1

Medial cluneal nerves S1 – S3

Inferior cluneal nerves S1 – S3

**Dermatomes and cutaneous nerves of the back**

# 3
# THORAX

## CONTENTS

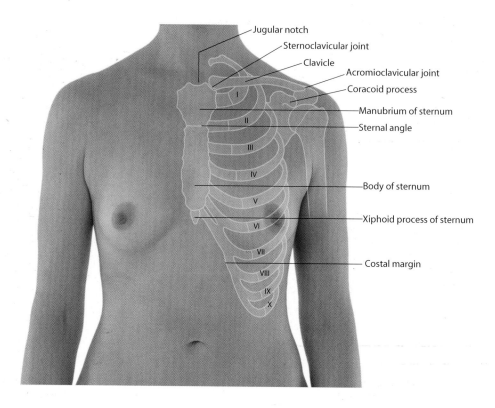

Jugular notch
Sternoclavicular joint
Clavicle
Acromioclavicular joint
Coracoid process
Manubrium of sternum
Sternal angle
Body of sternum
Xiphoid process of sternum
Costal margin

**Anterior chest wall in a woman**

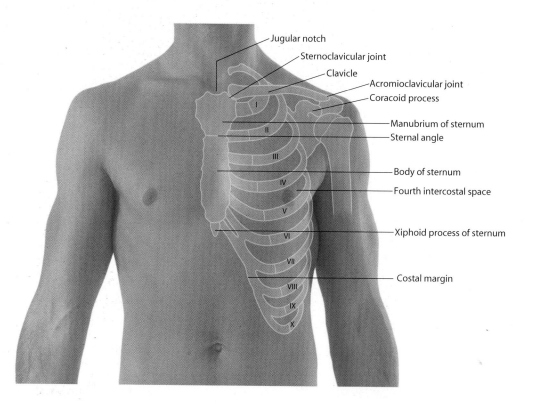

Jugular notch
Sternoclavicular joint
Clavicle
Acromioclavicular joint
Coracoid process
Manubrium of sternum
Sternal angle
Body of sternum
Fourth intercostal space
Xiphoid process of sternum
Costal margin

**Anterior chest wall in a man**

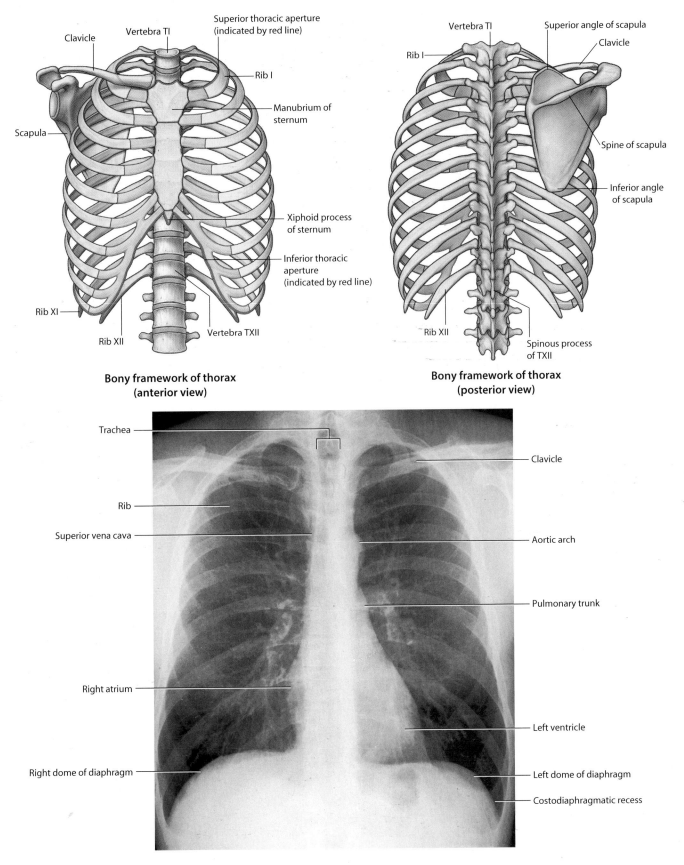

**Bony framework of thorax
(anterior view)**

**Bony framework of thorax
(posterior view)**

**Positioning of structures in chest.**
Radiograph, AP view

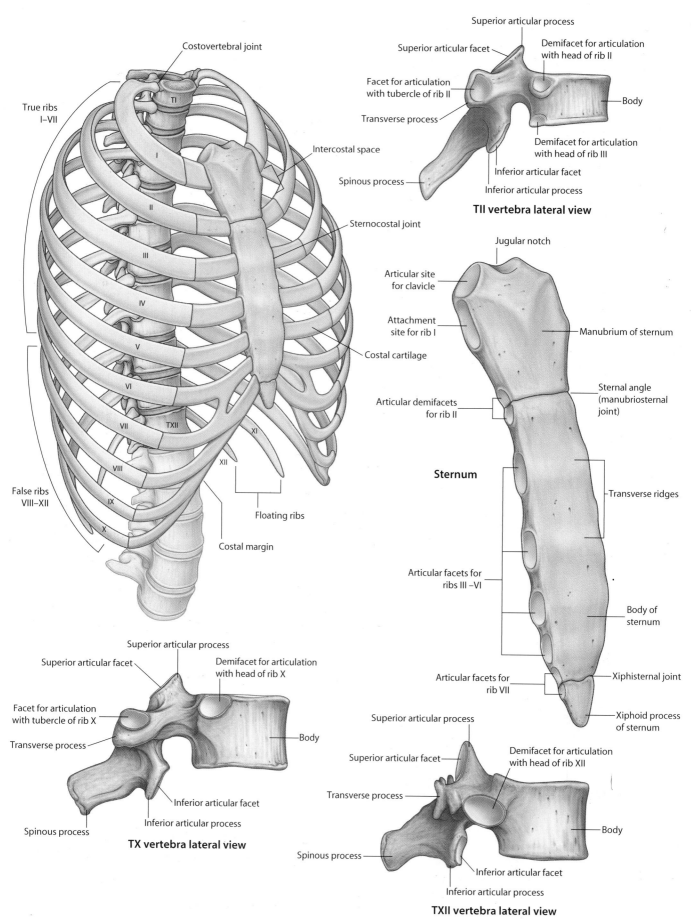

Costovertebral joint

True ribs
I–VII

TI

I

II

III

IV

V

VI

VII          TXII

VIII

IX

X

XI

XII

False ribs
VIII–XII

Intercostal space

Sternocostal joint

Costal cartilage

Floating ribs

Costal margin

**Superior articular process**

Superior articular facet

Facet for articulation
with tubercle of rib II

Transverse process

Spinous process

Demifacet for articulation
with head of rib II

Body

Demifacet for articulation
with head of rib III

Inferior articular facet

Inferior articular process

**TII vertebra lateral view**

Jugular notch

Articular site
for clavicle

Attachment
site for rib I

Articular demifacets
for rib II

**Sternum**

Articular facets for
ribs III –VI

Articular facets for
rib VII

Manubrium of sternum

Sternal angle
(manubriosternal
joint)

Transverse ridges

Body of
sternum

Xiphisternal joint

Xiphoid process
of sternum

Superior articular process

Superior articular facet

Facet for articulation
with tubercle of rib X

Transverse process

Spinous process

Demifacet for articulation
with head of rib X

Body

Inferior articular facet

Inferior articular process

**TX vertebra lateral view**

Superior articular process

Superior articular facet

Transverse process

Spinous process

Demifacet for articulation
with head of rib XII

Body

Inferior articular facet

Inferior articular process

**TXII vertebra lateral view**

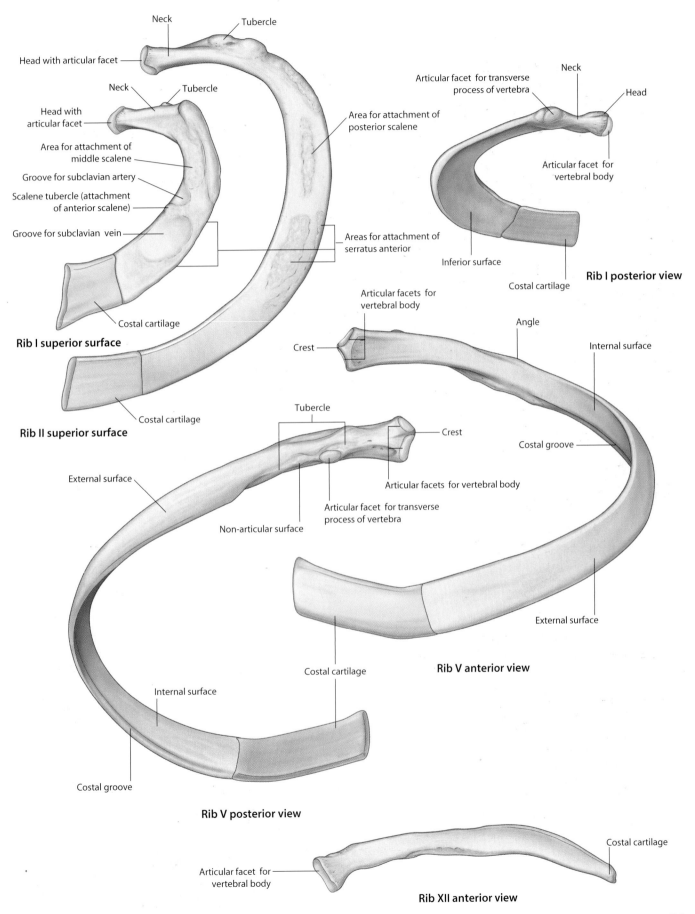

Neck

Tubercle

Head with articular facet

Neck

Tubercle

Head with
articular facet

Area for attachment of
middle scalene

Groove for subclavian artery

Scalene tubercle (attachment
of anterior scalene)

Groove for subclavian vein

Area for attachment of
posterior scalene

Areas for attachment of
serratus anterior

**Rib I superior surface**

Costal cartilage

Costal cartilage

**Rib II superior surface**

Articular facet for transverse
process of vertebra

Neck

Head

Articular facet for
vertebral body

Inferior surface

Costal cartilage

**Rib I posterior view**

Articular facets for
vertebral body

Crest

Angle

Internal surface

Costal groove

Tubercle

Crest

External surface

Articular facets for vertebral body

Non-articular surface

Articular facet for transverse
process of vertebra

External surface

**Rib V anterior view**

Internal surface

Costal cartilage

Costal cartilage

Costal groove

**Rib V posterior view**

Costal cartilage

Articular facet for
vertebral body

**Rib XII anterior view**

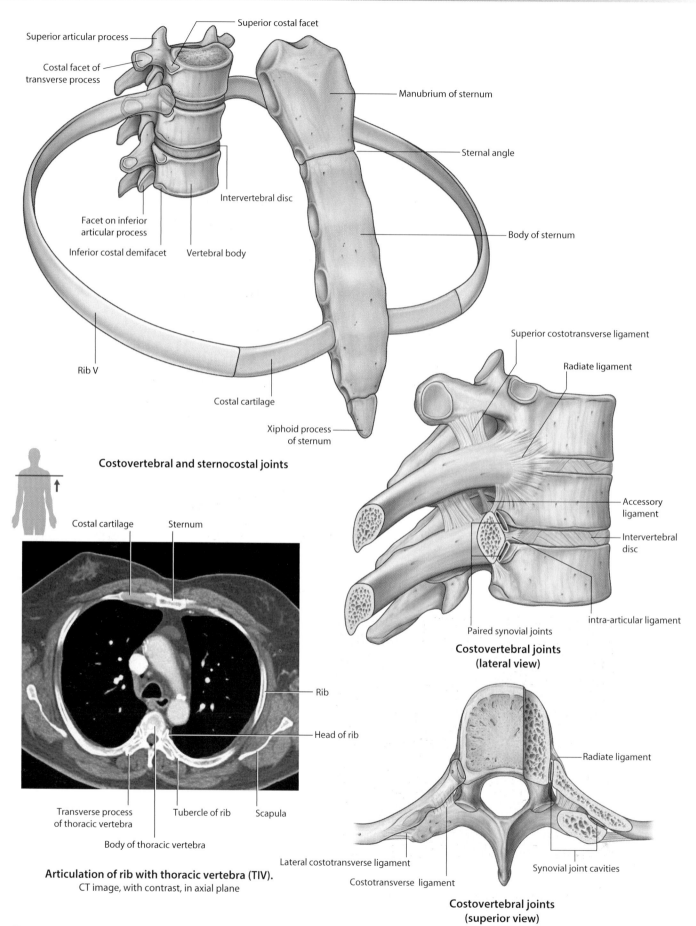

Superior articular process

Costal facet of transverse process

Superior costal facet

Manubrium of sternum

Sternal angle

Intervertebral disc

Facet on inferior articular process

Body of sternum

Inferior costal demifacet

Vertebral body

Rib V

Costal cartilage

Xiphoid process of sternum

**Costovertebral and sternocostal joints**

Superior costotransverse ligament

Radiate ligament

Accessory ligament

Intervertebral disc

Paired synovial joints

intra-articular ligament

**Costovertebral joints
(lateral view)**

Costal cartilage    Sternum

Rib

Head of rib

Transverse process of thoracic vertebra

Tubercle of rib    Scapula

Body of thoracic vertebra

**Articulation of rib with thoracic vertebra (TIV).**
CT image, with contrast, in axial plane

Radiate ligament

Lateral costotransverse ligament

Costotransverse ligament

Synovial joint cavities

**Costovertebral joints
(superior view)**

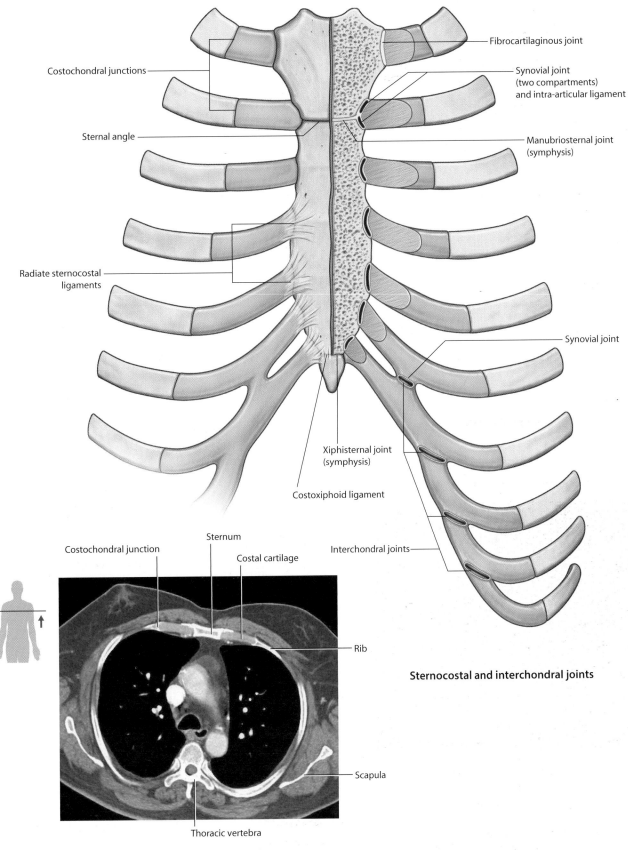

Costochondral junctions

Sternal angle

Radiate sternocostal
ligaments

Fibrocartilaginous joint

Synovial joint
(two compartments)
and intra-articular ligament

Manubriosternal joint
(symphysis)

Synovial joint

Xiphisternal joint
(symphysis)

Costoxiphoid ligament

Interchondral joints

**Sternocostal and interchondral joints**

Costochondral junction

Sternum

Costal cartilage

Rib

Scapula

Thoracic vertebra

**Articulation of costal cartilage with sternum.**
CT image, with contrast, in axial plane

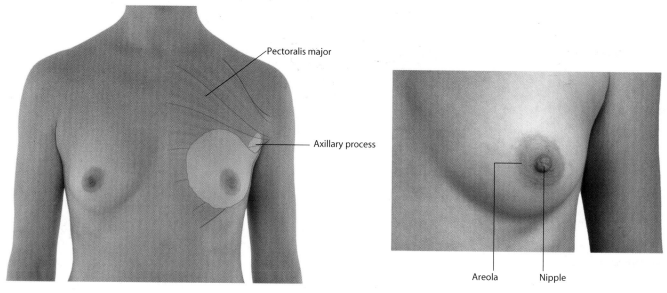

Pectoralis major

Axillary process

Areola    Nipple

**Anterior view**

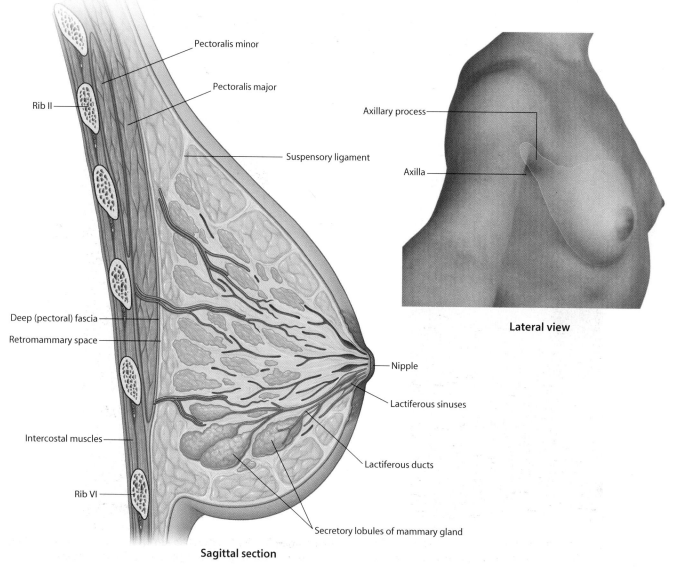

Pectoralis minor

Pectoralis major

Rib II

Suspensory ligament

Axillary process

Axilla

Deep (pectoral) fascia

Retromammary space

Nipple

Lactiferous sinuses

Lactiferous ducts

Intercostal muscles

Rib VI

Secretory lobules of mammary gland

**Sagittal section**

**Lateral view**

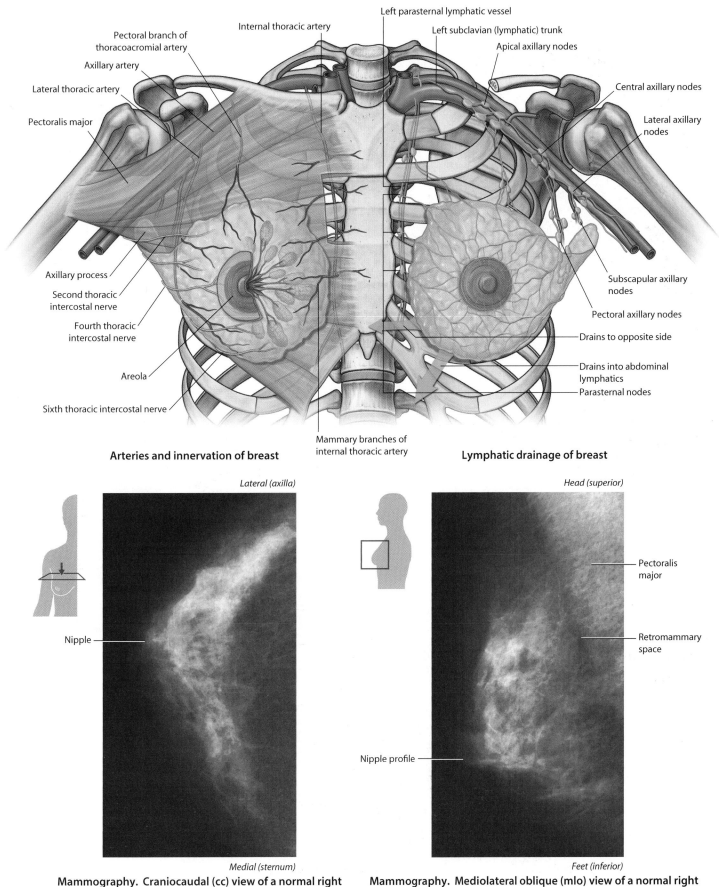

Left parasternal lymphatic vessel

Left subclavian (lymphatic) trunk

Apical axillary nodes

Internal thoracic artery

Pectoral branch of thoracoacromial artery

Axillary artery

Lateral thoracic artery

Pectoralis major

Central axillary nodes

Lateral axillary nodes

Axillary process

Second thoracic intercostal nerve

Fourth thoracic intercostal nerve

Areola

Sixth thoracic intercostal nerve

Subscapular axillary nodes

Pectoral axillary nodes

Drains to opposite side

Drains into abdominal lymphatics

Parasternal nodes

Mammary branches of internal thoracic artery

**Arteries and innervation of breast**

**Lymphatic drainage of breast**

*Lateral (axilla)*

Nipple

*Medial (sternum)*

**Mammography. Craniocaudal (cc) view of a normal right breast showing a heterogeneously dense appearance**

*Head (superior)*

Pectoralis major

Retromammary space

Nipple profile

*Feet (inferior)*

**Mammography. Mediolateral oblique (mlo) view of a normal right breast showing a heterogeneously dense appearance**

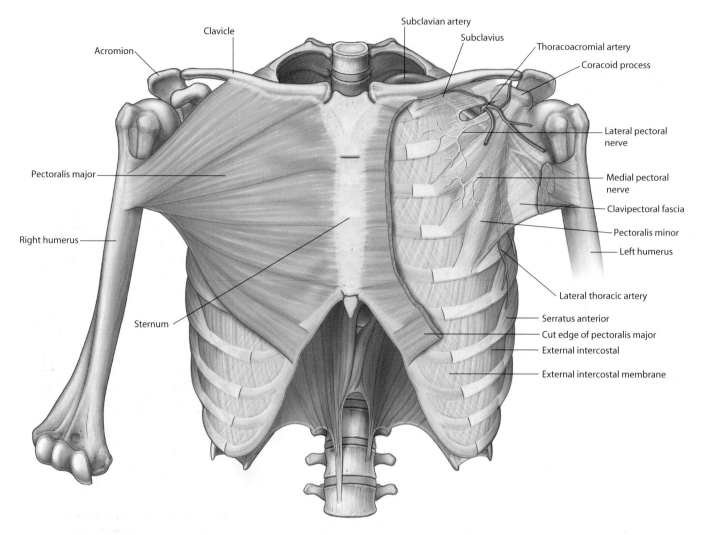

**Pectoralis major muscle and related deep structures**

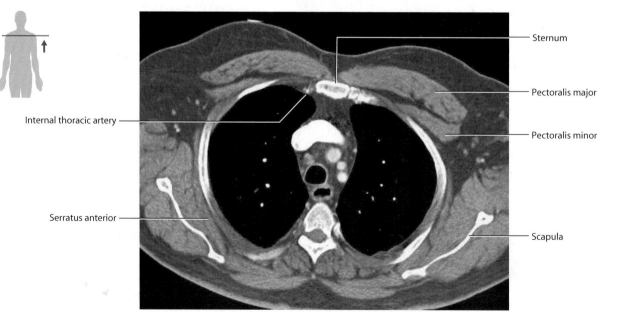

**Pectoralis major and minor muscles on anterior thoracic wall.**
CT image, with contrast, in axial plane

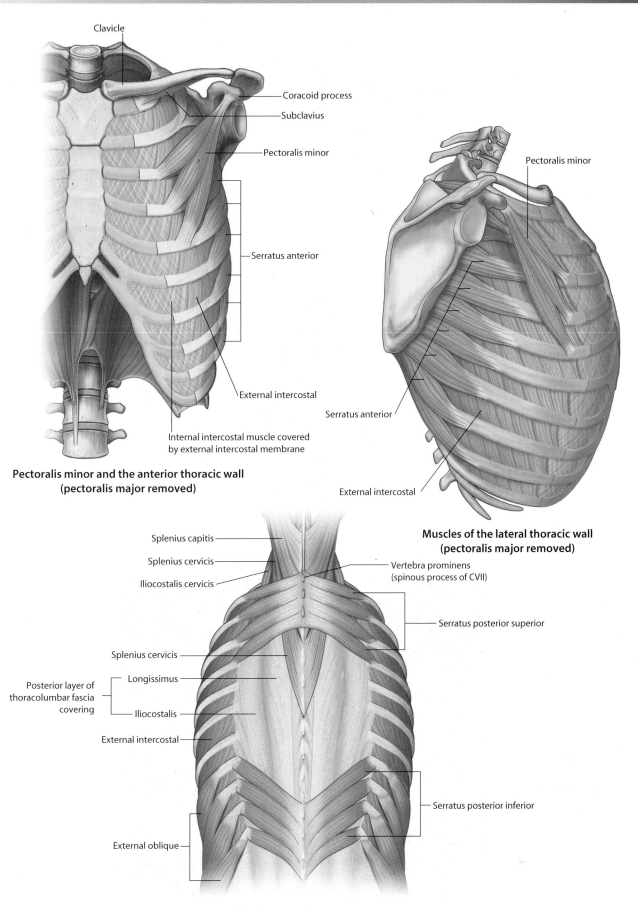

Clavicle

Coracoid process

Subclavius

Pectoralis minor

Serratus anterior

External intercostal

Internal intercostal muscle covered
by external intercostal membrane

**Pectoralis minor and the anterior thoracic wall
(pectoralis major removed)**

Pectoralis minor

Serratus anterior

External intercostal

**Muscles of the lateral thoracic wall
(pectoralis major removed)**

Splenius capitis

Splenius cervicis

Iliocostalis cervicis

Vertebra prominens
(spinous process of CVII)

Serratus posterior superior

Splenius cervicis

Longissimus

Posterior layer of
thoracolumbar fascia
covering

Iliocostalis

External intercostal

Serratus posterior inferior

External oblique

**Muscles of the posterior thoracic wall**

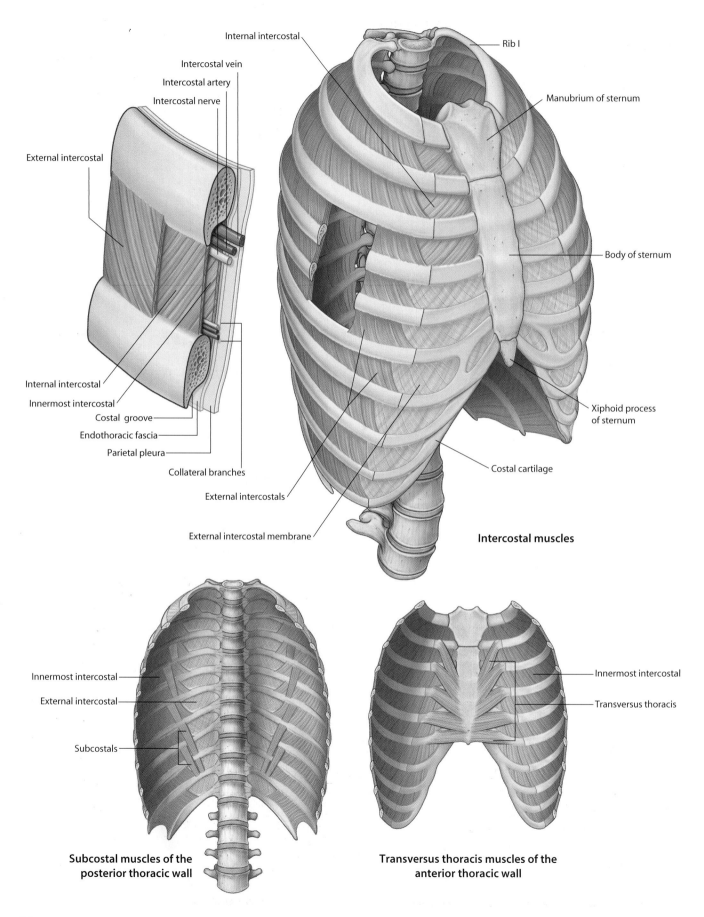

Internal intercostal

Intercostal vein

Intercostal artery

Intercostal nerve

External intercostal

Internal intercostal

Innermost intercostal

Costal groove

Endothoracic fascia

Parietal pleura

Collateral branches

External intercostals

External intercostal membrane

Rib I

Manubrium of sternum

Body of sternum

Xiphoid process of sternum

Costal cartilage

**Intercostal muscles**

Innermost intercostal

External intercostal

Subcostals

**Subcostal muscles of the posterior thoracic wall**

Innermost intercostal

Transversus thoracis

**Transversus thoracis muscles of the anterior thoracic wall**

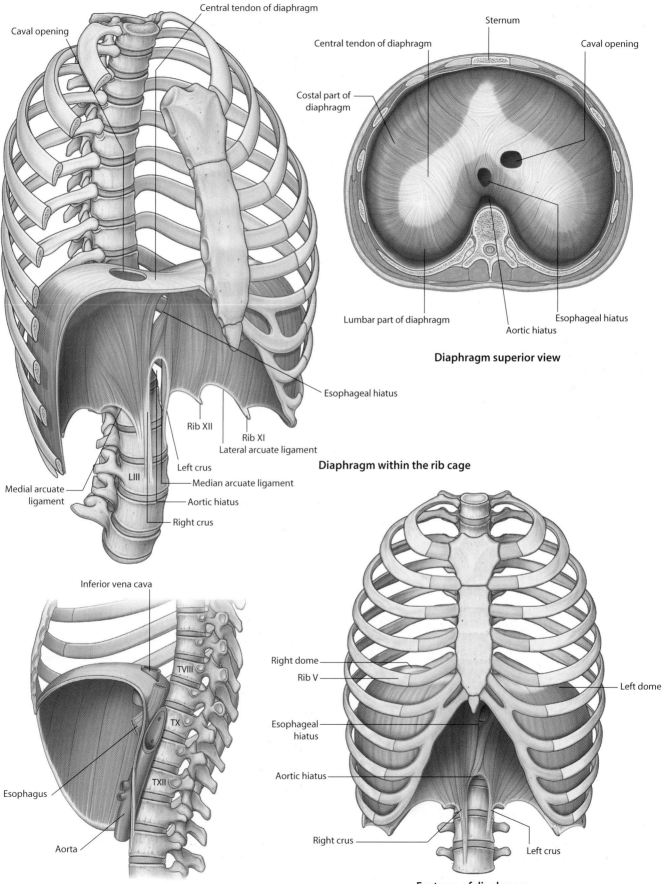

Caval opening

Central tendon of diaphragm

Esophageal hiatus

Rib XII

Rib XI

Lateral arcuate ligament

Medial arcuate ligament

LIII

Left crus

Median arcuate ligament

Aortic hiatus

Right crus

**Diaphragm within the rib cage**

Central tendon of diaphragm

Sternum

Caval opening

Costal part of diaphragm

Lumbar part of diaphragm

Aortic hiatus

Esophageal hiatus

**Diaphragm superior view**

Inferior vena cava

TVIII

TX

TXII

Esophagus

Aorta

**Major structures that pass through the diaphragm**

Right dome

Rib V

Esophageal hiatus

Aortic hiatus

Right crus

Left dome

Left crus

**Features of diaphragm**

**67**

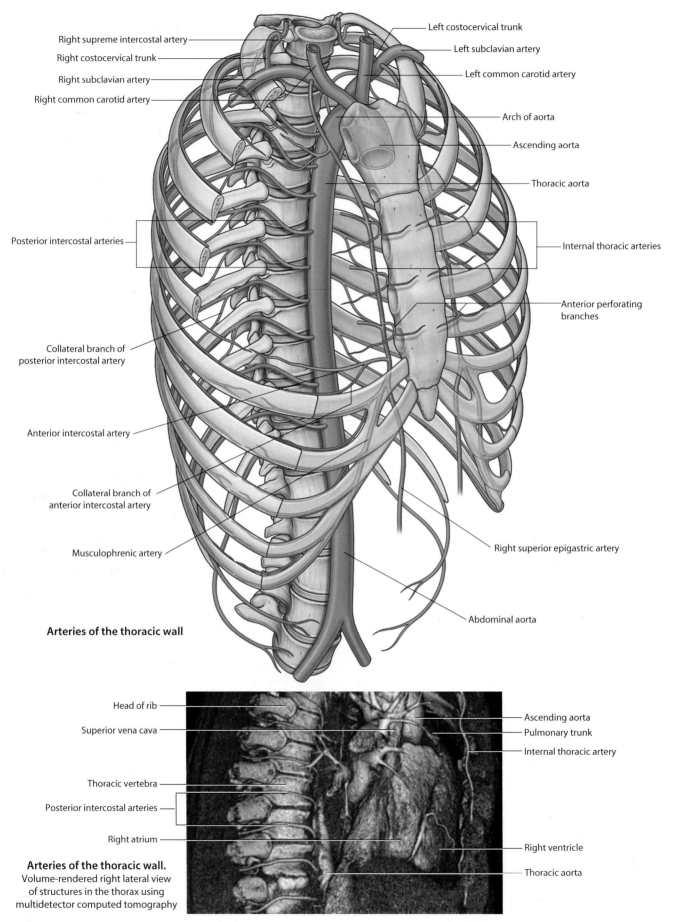

Right supreme intercostal artery

Right costocervical trunk

Right subclavian artery

Right common carotid artery

Left costocervical trunk

Left subclavian artery

Left common carotid artery

Arch of aorta

Ascending aorta

Thoracic aorta

Posterior intercostal arteries

Internal thoracic arteries

Anterior perforating branches

Collateral branch of posterior intercostal artery

Anterior intercostal artery

Collateral branch of anterior intercostal artery

Musculophrenic artery

Right superior epigastric artery

Abdominal aorta

**Arteries of the thoracic wall**

Head of rib

Superior vena cava

Thoracic vertebra

Posterior intercostal arteries

Right atrium

Ascending aorta

Pulmonary trunk

Internal thoracic artery

Right ventricle

Thoracic aorta

**Arteries of the thoracic wall.**
Volume-rendered right lateral view of structures in the thorax using multidetector computed tomography

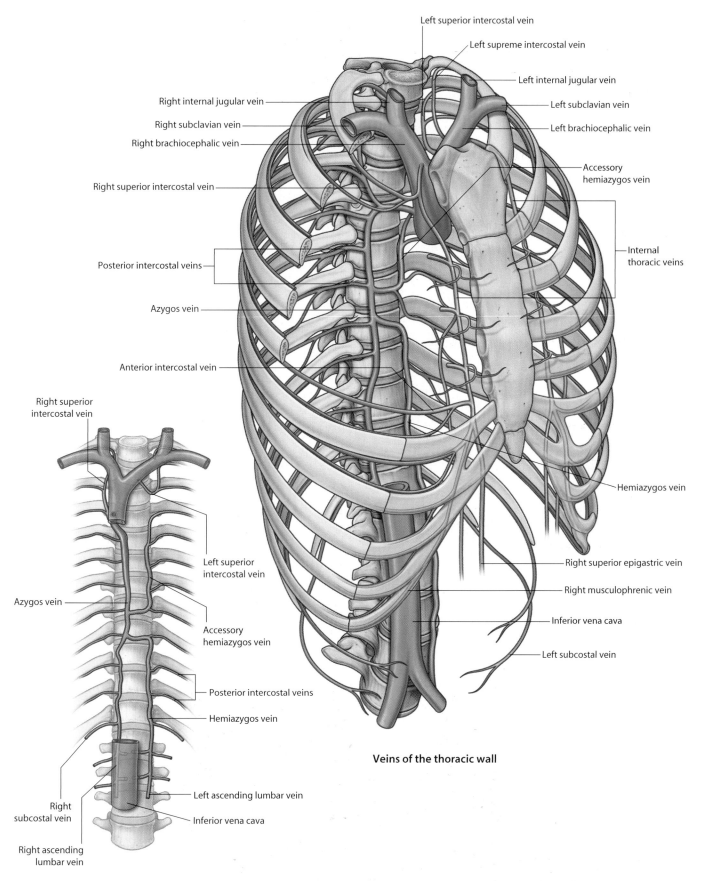

Left superior intercostal vein

Left supreme intercostal vein

Left internal jugular vein

Right internal jugular vein

Left subclavian vein

Right subclavian vein

Left brachiocephalic vein

Right brachiocephalic vein

Accessory hemiazygos vein

Right superior intercostal vein

Posterior intercostal veins

Internal thoracic veins

Azygos vein

Anterior intercostal vein

Hemiazygos vein

Right superior intercostal vein

Right superior epigastric vein

Left superior intercostal vein

Right musculophrenic vein

Azygos vein

Inferior vena cava

Accessory hemiazygos vein

Left subcostal vein

Posterior intercostal veins

Hemiazygos vein

**Veins of the thoracic wall**

Left ascending lumbar vein

Right subcostal vein

Inferior vena cava

Right ascending lumbar vein

**Azygos system of veins**

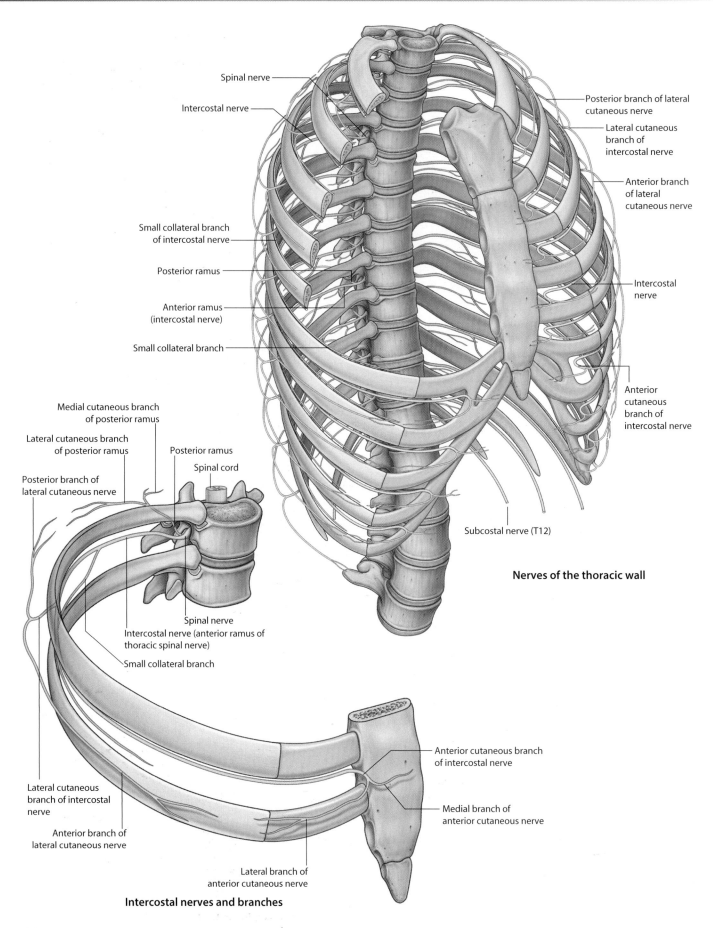

Spinal nerve

Intercostal nerve

Posterior branch of lateral cutaneous nerve

Lateral cutaneous branch of intercostal nerve

Anterior branch of lateral cutaneous nerve

Small collateral branch of intercostal nerve

Posterior ramus

Anterior ramus (intercostal nerve)

Small collateral branch

Intercostal nerve

Anterior cutaneous branch of intercostal nerve

Subcostal nerve (T12)

**Nerves of the thoracic wall**

Medial cutaneous branch of posterior ramus

Lateral cutaneous branch of posterior ramus

Posterior ramus

Spinal cord

Posterior branch of lateral cutaneous nerve

Spinal nerve

Intercostal nerve (anterior ramus of thoracic spinal nerve)

Small collateral branch

Anterior cutaneous branch of intercostal nerve

Medial branch of anterior cutaneous nerve

Lateral cutaneous branch of intercostal nerve

Anterior branch of lateral cutaneous nerve

Lateral branch of anterior cutaneous nerve

**Intercostal nerves and branches**

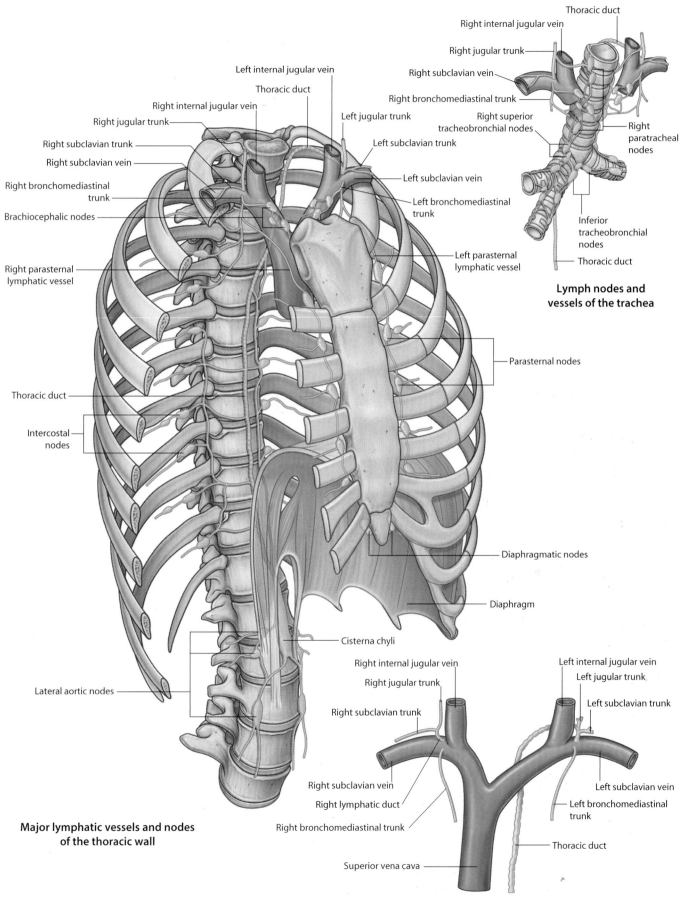

Thoracic duct

Right internal jugular vein

Right jugular trunk

Right subclavian vein

Right bronchomediastinal trunk

Right superior
tracheobronchial nodes

Right
paratracheal
nodes

Inferior
tracheobronchial
nodes

Thoracic duct

**Lymph nodes and
vessels of the trachea**

Left internal jugular vein

Thoracic duct

Right internal jugular vein

Right jugular trunk

Right subclavian trunk

Right subclavian vein

Right bronchomediastinal
trunk

Brachiocephalic nodes

Left jugular trunk

Left subclavian trunk

Left subclavian vein

Left bronchomediastinal
trunk

Right parasternal
lymphatic vessel

Left parasternal
lymphatic vessel

Thoracic duct

Intercostal
nodes

Parasternal nodes

Diaphragmatic nodes

Diaphragm

Cisterna chyli

Lateral aortic nodes

Right internal jugular vein

Right jugular trunk

Right subclavian trunk

Left internal jugular vein

Left jugular trunk

Left subclavian trunk

Right subclavian vein

Right lymphatic duct

Right bronchomediastinal trunk

Left subclavian vein

Left bronchomediastinal
trunk

Thoracic duct

Superior vena cava

**Major lymphatic vessels and nodes
of the thoracic wall**

**Termination of the lymphatic trunks**

71

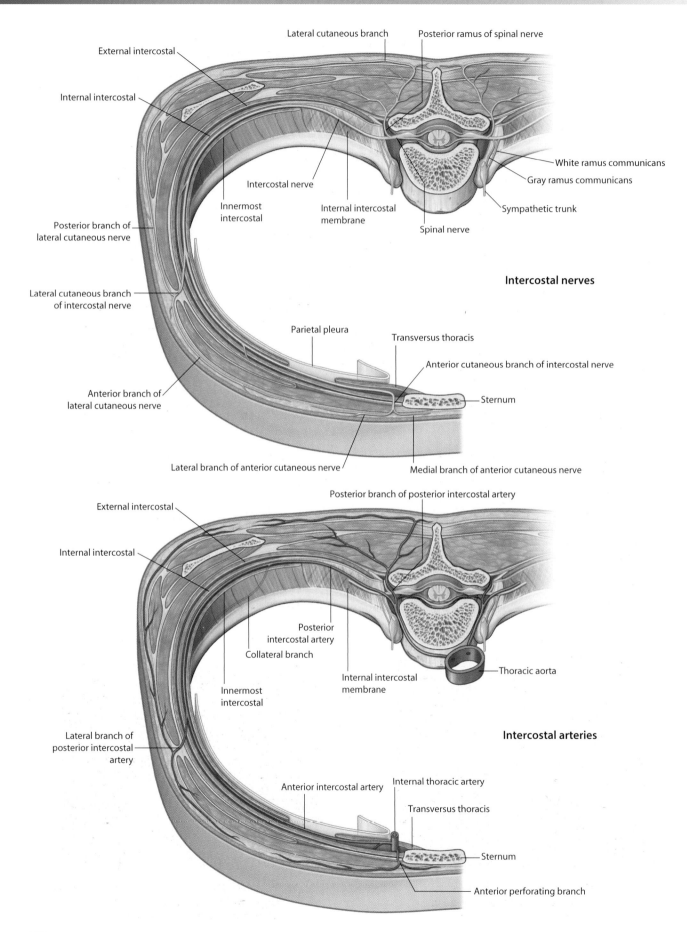

Lateral cutaneous branch

Posterior ramus of spinal nerve

External intercostal

Internal intercostal

Intercostal nerve

Innermost intercostal

Internal intercostal membrane

White ramus communicans

Gray ramus communicans

Sympathetic trunk

Spinal nerve

Posterior branch of lateral cutaneous nerve

**Intercostal nerves**

Lateral cutaneous branch of intercostal nerve

Parietal pleura

Transversus thoracis

Anterior cutaneous branch of intercostal nerve

Sternum

Anterior branch of lateral cutaneous nerve

Lateral branch of anterior cutaneous nerve

Medial branch of anterior cutaneous nerve

Posterior branch of posterior intercostal artery

External intercostal

Internal intercostal

Posterior intercostal artery

Collateral branch

Innermost intercostal

Internal intercostal membrane

Thoracic aorta

**Intercostal arteries**

Lateral branch of posterior intercostal artery

Anterior intercostal artery

Internal thoracic artery

Transversus thoracis

Sternum

Anterior perforating branch

72

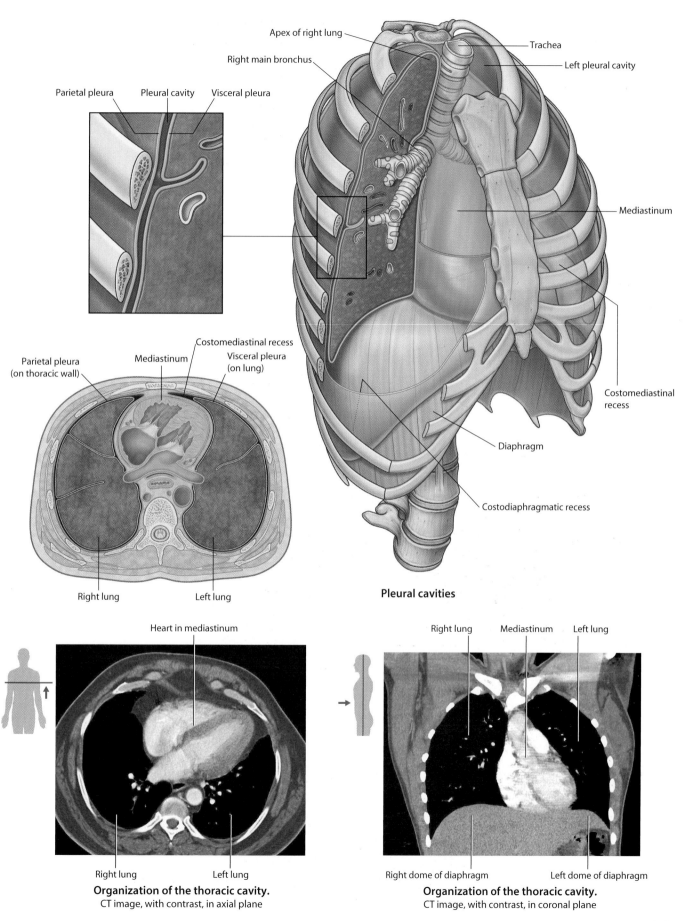

Apex of right lung

Right main bronchus

Trachea

Left pleural cavity

Parietal pleura    Pleural cavity    Visceral pleura

Mediastinum

Costomediastinal recess

Parietal pleura    Mediastinum    Costomediastinal recess
(on thoracic wall)
Visceral pleura
(on lung)

Diaphragm

Right lung    Left lung

Costodiaphragmatic recess

**Pleural cavities**

Heart in mediastinum

Right lung    Mediastinum    Left lung

Right lung    Left lung

Right dome of diaphragm    Left dome of diaphragm

**Organization of the thoracic cavity.**
CT image, with contrast, in axial plane

**Organization of the thoracic cavity.**
CT image, with contrast, in coronal plane

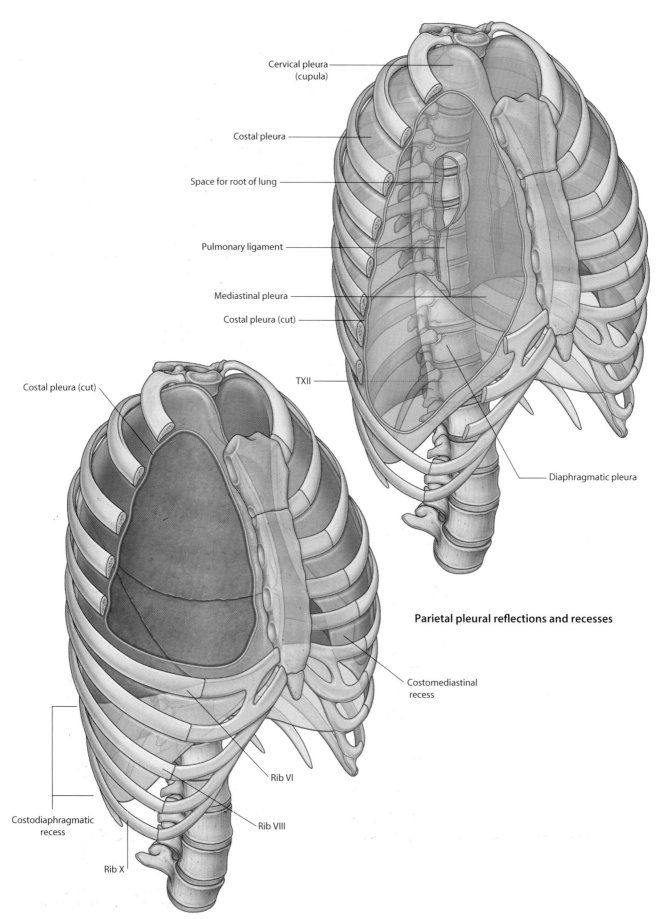

Cervical pleura
(cupula)

Costal pleura

Space for root of lung

Pulmonary ligament

Mediastinal pleura

Costal pleura (cut)

TXII

Diaphragmatic pleura

Costal pleura (cut)

**Parietal pleural reflections and recesses**

Costomediastinal
recess

Rib VI

Rib VIII

Costodiaphragmatic
recess

Rib X

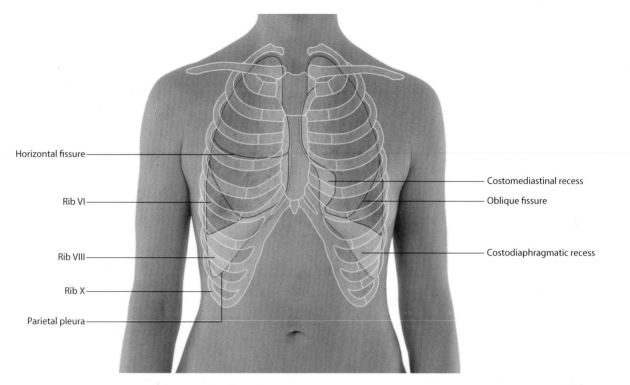

Horizontal fissure

Rib VI

Rib VIII

Rib X

Parietal pleura

Costomediastinal recess

Oblique fissure

Costodiaphragmatic recess

**Surface projections of the pleura and lungs (anterior view)**

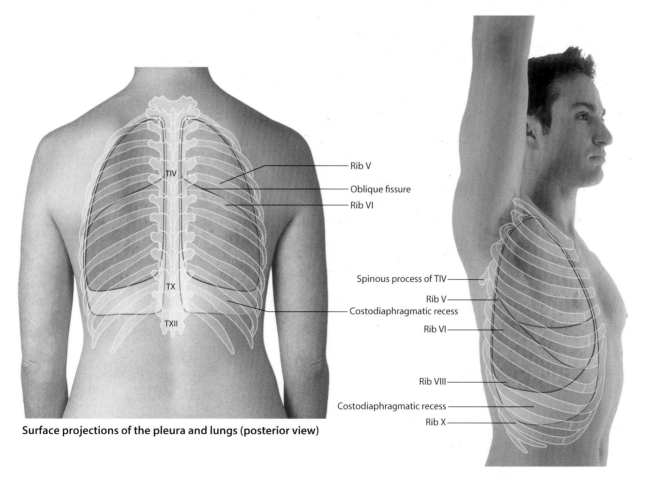

TIV

TX

TXII

Rib V

Oblique fissure

Rib VI

**Surface projections of the pleura and lungs (posterior view)**

Spinous process of TIV

Rib V

Costodiaphragmatic recess

Rib VI

Rib VIII

Costodiaphragmatic recess

Rib X

**Surface projections of the pleura and right lung (lateral view)**

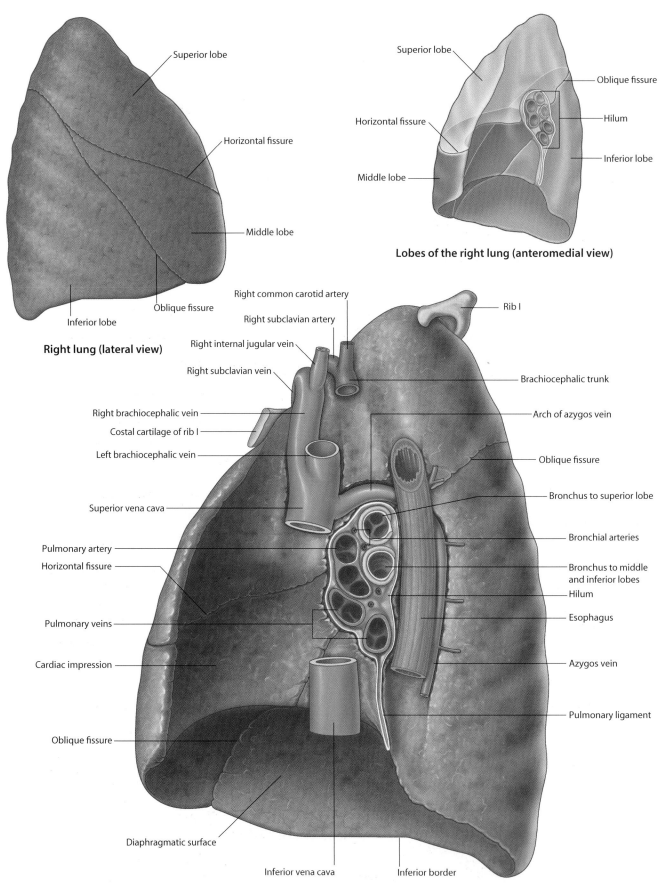

Superior lobe

Horizontal fissure

Middle lobe

Inferior lobe

Oblique fissure

**Right lung (lateral view)**

Superior lobe

Horizontal fissure

Middle lobe

Oblique fissure

Hilum

Inferior lobe

**Lobes of the right lung (anteromedial view)**

Right common carotid artery

Right subclavian artery

Right internal jugular vein

Right subclavian vein

Right brachiocephalic vein

Costal cartilage of rib I

Left brachiocephalic vein

Superior vena cava

Pulmonary artery

Horizontal fissure

Pulmonary veins

Cardiac impression

Oblique fissure

Diaphragmatic surface

Inferior vena cava

Rib I

Brachiocephalic trunk

Arch of azygos vein

Oblique fissure

Bronchus to superior lobe

Bronchial arteries

Bronchus to middle and inferior lobes

Hilum

Esophagus

Azygos vein

Pulmonary ligament

Inferior border

**Right lung and related structures (medial view)**

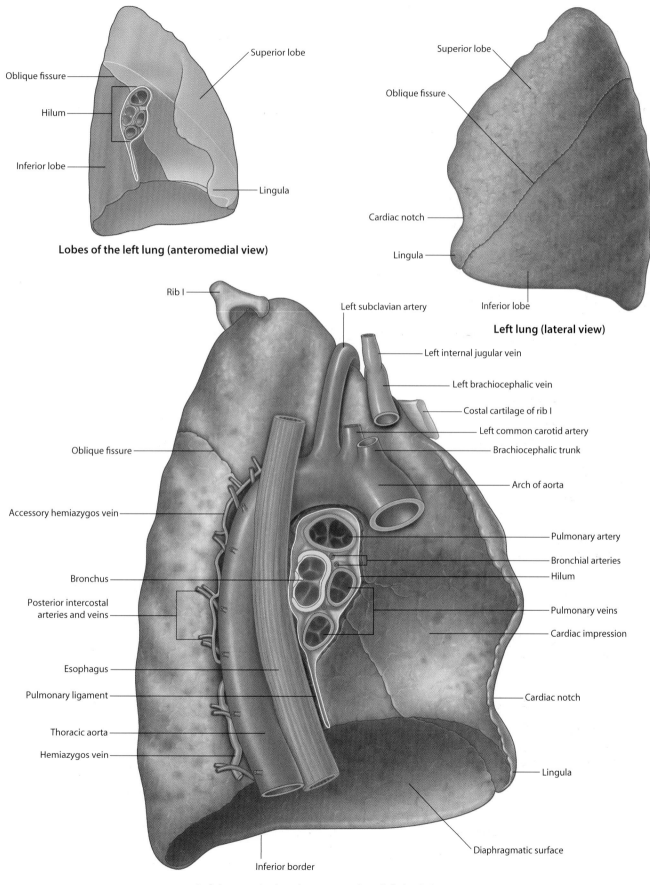

Lobes of the left lung (anteromedial view)

Oblique fissure

Hilum

Inferior lobe

Superior lobe

Lingula

Superior lobe

Oblique fissure

Cardiac notch

Lingula

Inferior lobe

**Left lung (lateral view)**

Rib I

Left subclavian artery

Left internal jugular vein

Left brachiocephalic vein

Costal cartilage of rib I

Left common carotid artery

Brachiocephalic trunk

Arch of aorta

Oblique fissure

Accessory hemiazygos vein

Pulmonary artery

Bronchial arteries

Hilum

Bronchus

Posterior intercostal
arteries and veins

Pulmonary veins

Cardiac impression

Esophagus

Pulmonary ligament

Cardiac notch

Thoracic aorta

Hemiazygos vein

Lingula

Diaphragmatic surface

Inferior border

**Left lung and related structures (medial view)**

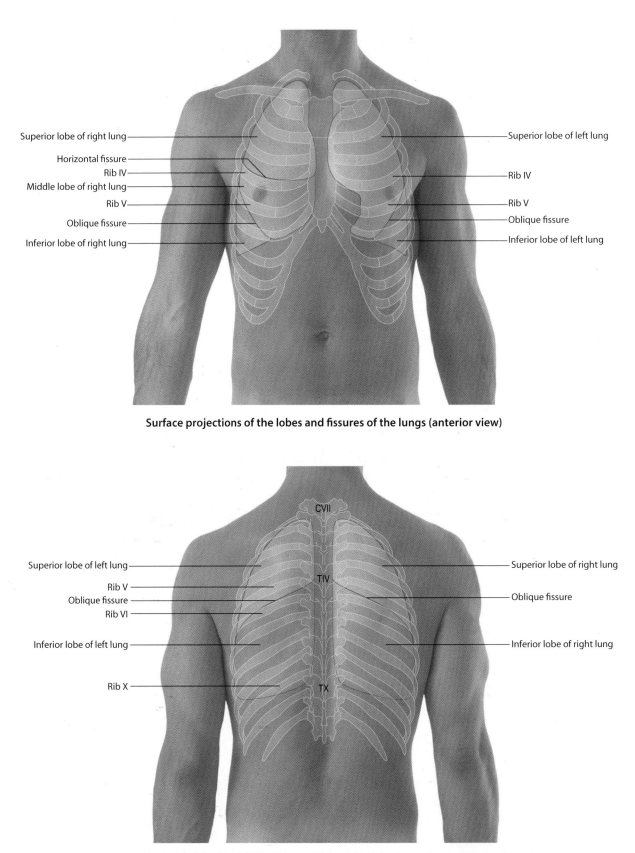

Superior lobe of right lung

Horizontal fissure

Rib IV

Middle lobe of right lung

Rib V

Oblique fissure

Inferior lobe of right lung

Superior lobe of left lung

Rib IV

Rib V

Oblique fissure

Inferior lobe of left lung

**Surface projections of the lobes and fissures of the lungs (anterior view)**

CVII

Superior lobe of left lung

Rib V

Oblique fissure

Rib VI

Inferior lobe of left lung

Rib X

TIV

TX

Superior lobe of right lung

Oblique fissure

Inferior lobe of right lung

**Surface projections of the lobes and fissures of the lungs (posterior view)**

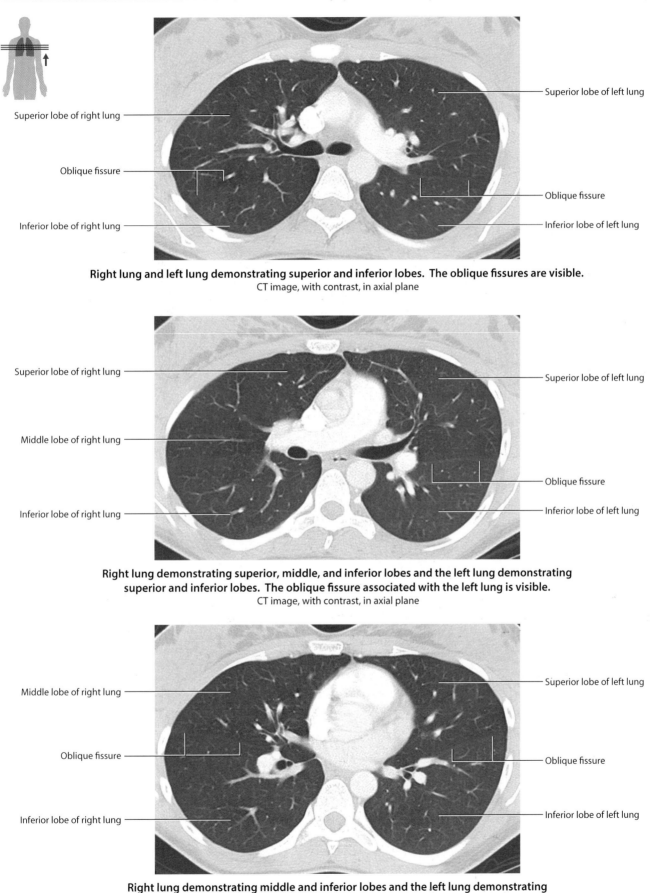

Superior lobe of right lung

Superior lobe of left lung

Oblique fissure

Oblique fissure

Inferior lobe of right lung

Inferior lobe of left lung

**Right lung and left lung demonstrating superior and inferior lobes. The oblique fissures are visible.**
CT image, with contrast, in axial plane

Superior lobe of right lung

Superior lobe of left lung

Middle lobe of right lung

Oblique fissure

Inferior lobe of right lung

Inferior lobe of left lung

**Right lung demonstrating superior, middle, and inferior lobes and the left lung demonstrating superior and inferior lobes. The oblique fissure associated with the left lung is visible.**
CT image, with contrast, in axial plane

Middle lobe of right lung

Superior lobe of left lung

Oblique fissure

Oblique fissure

Inferior lobe of right lung

Inferior lobe of left lung

**Right lung demonstrating middle and inferior lobes and the left lung demonstrating superior and inferior lobes. The oblique fissures are visible.**
CT image, with contrast, in axial plane

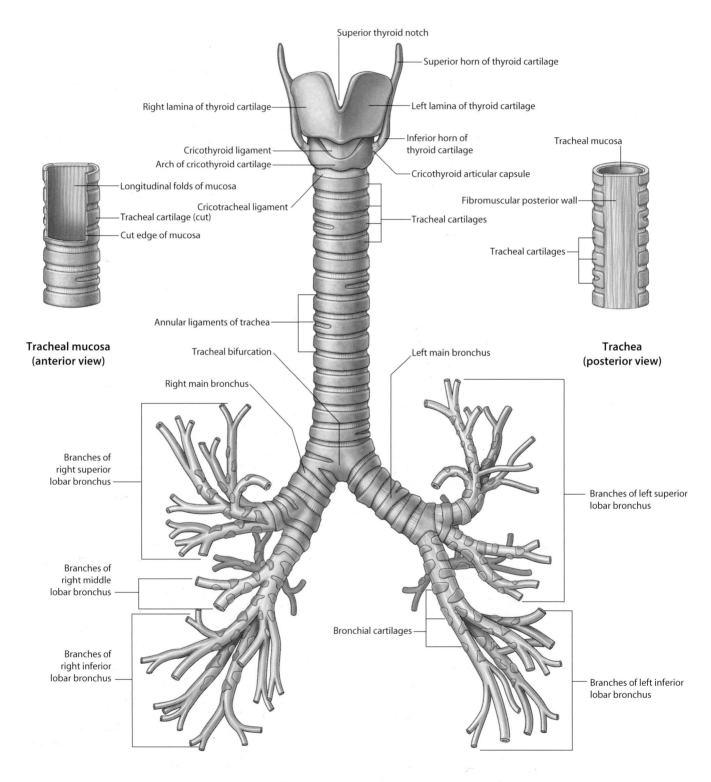

Superior thyroid notch

Superior horn of thyroid cartilage

Right lamina of thyroid cartilage

Left lamina of thyroid cartilage

Cricothyroid ligament

Inferior horn of thyroid cartilage

Arch of cricothyroid cartilage

Cricothyroid articular capsule

Tracheal mucosa

Longitudinal folds of mucosa

Tracheal cartilages

Cricotracheal ligament

Tracheal cartilage (cut)

Fibromuscular posterior wall

Cut edge of mucosa

Tracheal cartilages

**Tracheal mucosa
(anterior view)**

Annular ligaments of trachea

**Trachea
(posterior view)**

Left main bronchus

Tracheal bifurcation

Right main bronchus

Branches of
right superior
lobar bronchus

Branches of left superior
lobar bronchus

Branches of
right middle
lobar bronchus

Bronchial cartilages

Branches of
right inferior
lobar bronchus

Branches of left inferior
lobar bronchus

**Trachea and bronchial tree**

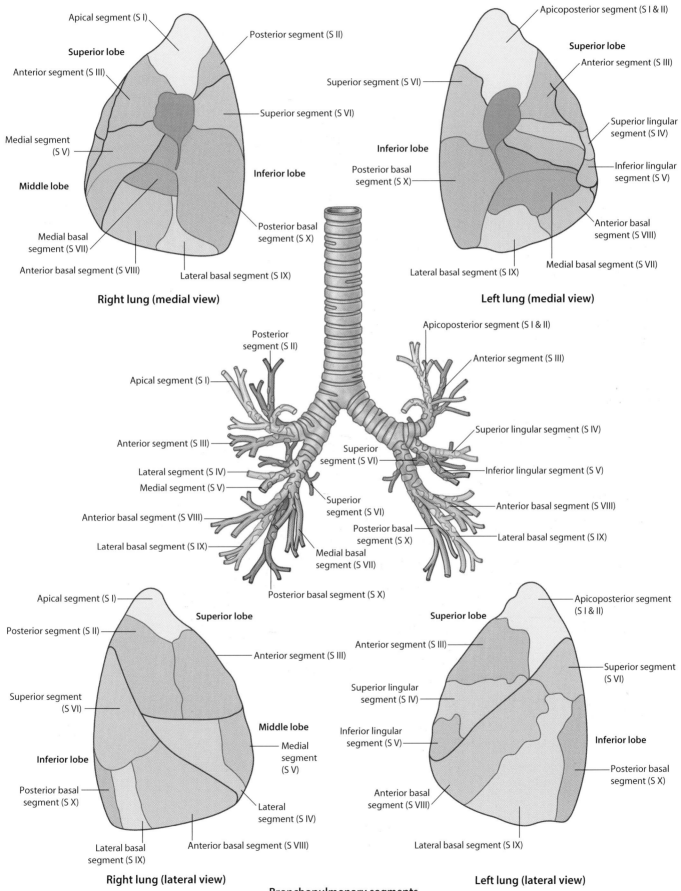

Apical segment (S I)

**Superior lobe**

Posterior segment (S II)

Anterior segment (S III)

Medial segment (S V)

**Middle lobe**

Superior segment (S VI)

Medial basal segment (S VII)

Anterior basal segment (S VIII)

**Inferior lobe**

Posterior basal segment (S X)

Lateral basal segment (S IX)

**Right lung (medial view)**

Apicoposterior segment (S I & II)

**Superior lobe**

Anterior segment (S III)

Superior segment (S VI)

Superior lingular segment (S IV)

**Inferior lobe**

Posterior basal segment (S X)

Inferior lingular segment (S V)

Anterior basal segment (S VIII)

Medial basal segment (S VII)

Lateral basal segment (S IX)

**Left lung (medial view)**

Posterior segment (S II)

Apical segment (S I)

Anterior segment (S III)

Lateral segment (S IV)

Medial segment (S V)

Anterior basal segment (S VIII)

Lateral basal segment (S IX)

Superior segment (S VI)

Superior segment (S VI)

Medial basal segment (S VII)

Posterior basal segment (S X)

Apicoposterior segment (S I & II)

Anterior segment (S III)

Superior lingular segment (S IV)

Inferior lingular segment (S V)

Anterior basal segment (S VIII)

Lateral basal segment (S IX)

Posterior basal segment (S X)

Apical segment (S I)

**Superior lobe**

Posterior segment (S II)

Anterior segment (S III)

Superior segment (S VI)

**Middle lobe**

Medial segment (S V)

**Inferior lobe**

Posterior basal segment (S X)

Lateral segment (S IV)

Lateral basal segment (S IX)

Anterior basal segment (S VIII)

**Right lung (lateral view)**

**Superior lobe**

Apicoposterior segment (S I & II)

Anterior segment (S III)

Superior segment (S VI)

Superior lingular segment (S IV)

Inferior lingular segment (S V)

**Inferior lobe**

Posterior basal segment (S X)

Anterior basal segment (S VIII)

Lateral basal segment (S IX)

**Left lung (lateral view)**

**Bronchopulmonary segments**

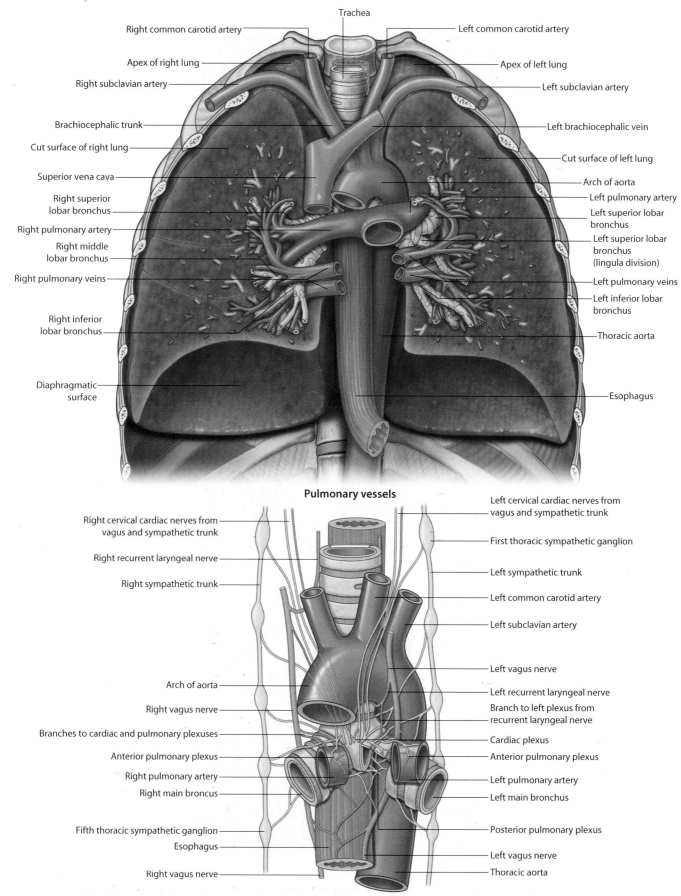

Trachea

Right common carotid artery

Apex of right lung

Right subclavian artery

Brachiocephalic trunk

Cut surface of right lung

Superior vena cava

Right superior lobar bronchus

Right pulmonary artery

Right middle lobar bronchus

Right pulmonary veins

Right inferior lobar bronchus

Diaphragmatic surface

Left common carotid artery

Apex of left lung

Left subclavian artery

Left brachiocephalic vein

Cut surface of left lung

Arch of aorta

Left pulmonary artery

Left superior lobar bronchus

Left superior lobar bronchus (lingula division)

Left pulmonary veins

Left inferior lobar bronchus

Thoracic aorta

Esophagus

**Pulmonary vessels**

Right cervical cardiac nerves from vagus and sympathetic trunk

Right recurrent laryngeal nerve

Right sympathetic trunk

Arch of aorta

Right vagus nerve

Branches to cardiac and pulmonary plexuses

Anterior pulmonary plexus

Right pulmonary artery

Right main broncus

Fifth thoracic sympathetic ganglion

Esophagus

Right vagus nerve

Left cervical cardiac nerves from vagus and sympathetic trunk

First thoracic sympathetic ganglion

Left sympathetic trunk

Left common carotid artery

Left subclavian artery

Left vagus nerve

Left recurrent laryngeal nerve

Branch to left plexus from recurrent laryngeal nerve

Cardiac plexus

Anterior pulmonary plexus

Left pulmonary artery

Left main bronchus

Posterior pulmonary plexus

Left vagus nerve

Thoracic aorta

**Pulmonary plexus**

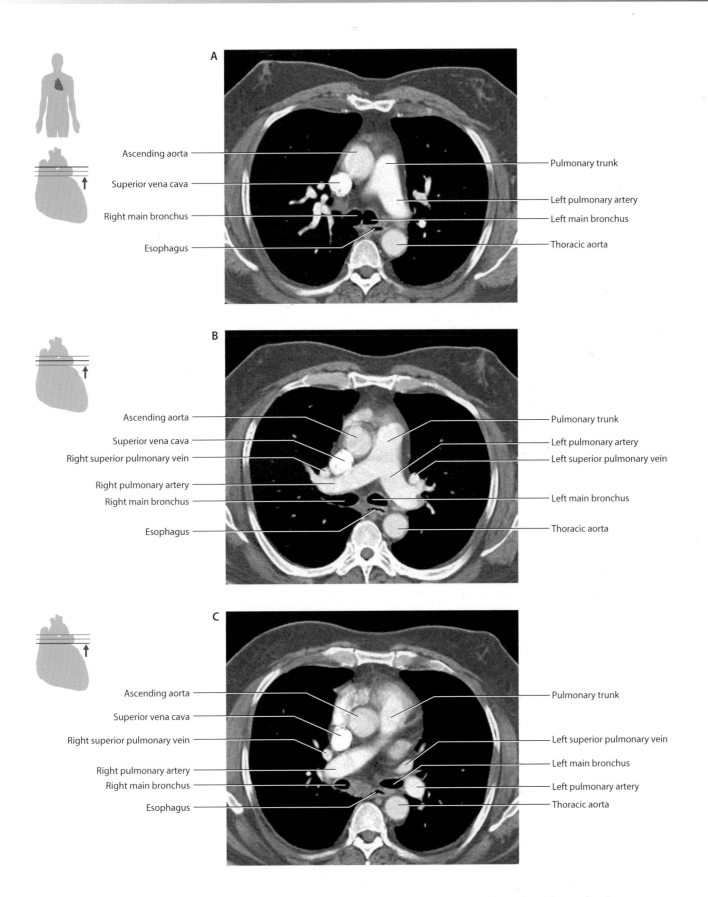

**A through C – Relationships of the pulmonary arteries, pulmonary veins, and bronchi in the mediastinum.**
CT images, with contrast, in axial plane

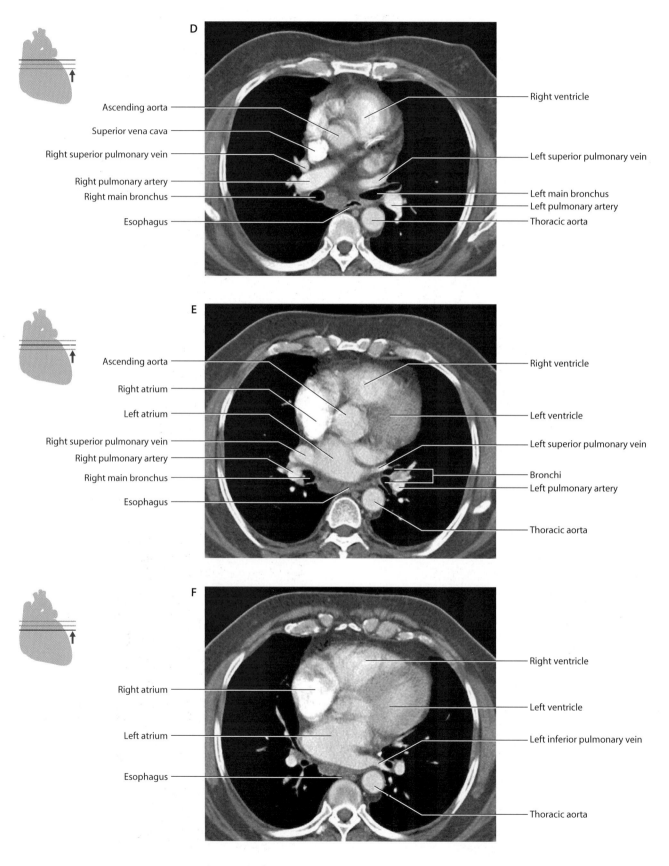

**D** | Ascending aorta | Right ventricle
Superior vena cava
Right superior pulmonary vein | Left superior pulmonary vein
Right pulmonary artery
Right main bronchus | Left main bronchus
Left pulmonary artery
Esophagus | Thoracic aorta

**E** | Ascending aorta | Right ventricle
Right atrium
Left atrium | Left ventricle
Right superior pulmonary vein | Left superior pulmonary vein
Right pulmonary artery
Right main bronchus | Bronchi
Left pulmonary artery
Esophagus | Thoracic aorta

**F** | Right ventricle
Right atrium
Left ventricle
Left atrium | Left inferior pulmonary vein
Esophagus
Thoracic aorta

**D through F – Relationships of the pulmonary arteries, pulmonary veins, and bronchi in the mediastinum.**
CT images, with contrast, in axial plane

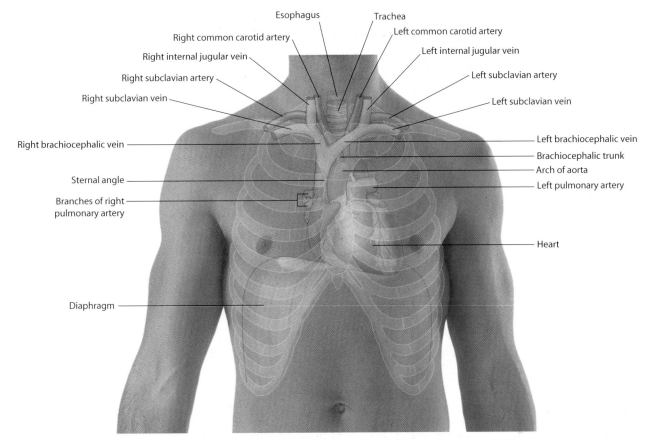

Esophagus
Trachea
Right common carotid artery
Left common carotid artery
Right internal jugular vein
Left internal jugular vein
Right subclavian artery
Left subclavian artery
Right subclavian vein
Left subclavian vein
Right brachiocephalic vein
Left brachiocephalic vein
Brachiocephalic trunk
Arch of aorta
Sternal angle
Left pulmonary artery
Branches of right pulmonary artery
Heart
Diaphragm

**Structures of the mediastinum as they relate to the surface**

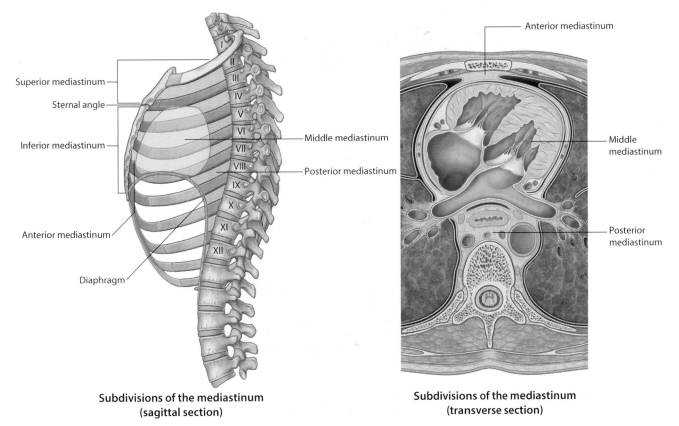

Superior mediastinum
Sternal angle
Inferior mediastinum
Middle mediastinum
Posterior mediastinum
Anterior mediastinum
Diaphragm

**Subdivisions of the mediastinum
(sagittal section)**

Anterior mediastinum
Middle mediastinum
Posterior mediastinum

**Subdivisions of the mediastinum
(transverse section)**

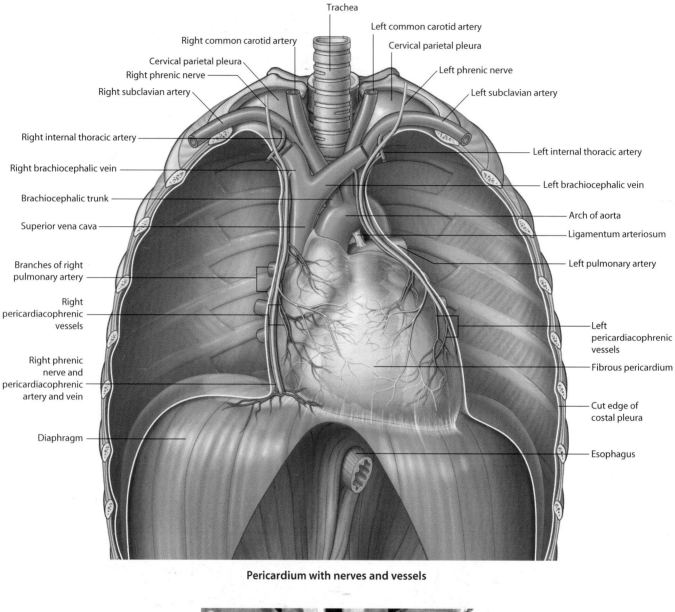

Trachea

Right common carotid artery

Cervical parietal pleura
Right phrenic nerve
Right subclavian artery

Right internal thoracic artery

Right brachiocephalic vein

Brachiocephalic trunk

Superior vena cava

Branches of right
pulmonary artery

Right
pericardiacophrenic
vessels

Right phrenic
nerve and
pericardiacophrenic
artery and vein

Diaphragm

Left common carotid artery

Cervical parietal pleura

Left phrenic nerve

Left subclavian artery

Left internal thoracic artery

Left brachiocephalic vein

Arch of aorta

Ligamentum arteriosum

Left pulmonary artery

Left
pericardiacophrenic
vessels

Fibrous pericardium

Cut edge of
costal pleura

Esophagus

**Pericardium with nerves and vessels**

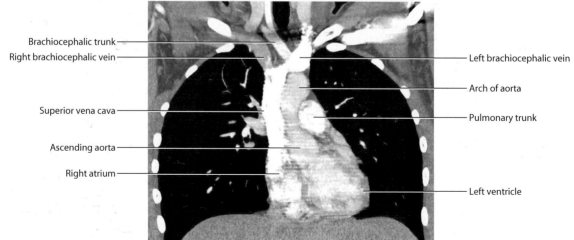

Brachiocephalic trunk

Right brachiocephalic vein

Superior vena cava

Ascending aorta

Right atrium

Left brachiocephalic vein

Arch of aorta

Pulmonary trunk

Left ventricle

**Mediastinal structures and lungs.**
CT image, with contrast, in coronal plane

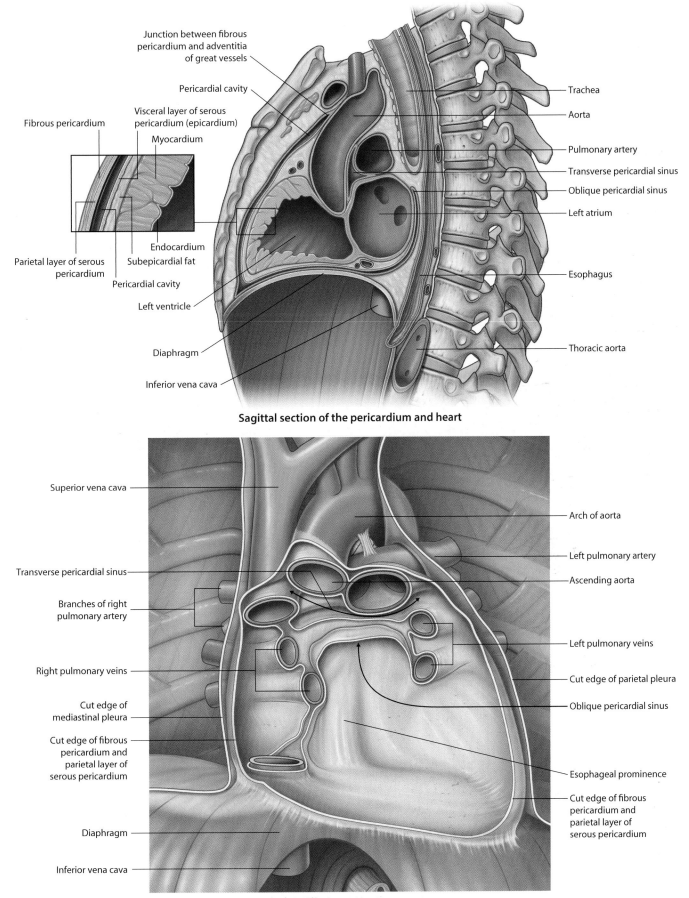

Junction between fibrous pericardium and adventitia of great vessels

Pericardial cavity

Visceral layer of serous pericardium (epicardium)

Myocardium

Fibrous pericardium

Parietal layer of serous pericardium

Subepicardial fat

Pericardial cavity

Endocardium

Left ventricle

Diaphragm

Inferior vena cava

Trachea

Aorta

Pulmonary artery

Transverse pericardial sinus

Oblique pericardial sinus

Left atrium

Esophagus

Thoracic aorta

**Sagittal section of the pericardium and heart**

Superior vena cava

Transverse pericardial sinus

Branches of right pulmonary artery

Right pulmonary veins

Cut edge of mediastinal pleura

Cut edge of fibrous pericardium and parietal layer of serous pericardium

Diaphragm

Inferior vena cava

Arch of aorta

Left pulmonary artery

Ascending aorta

Left pulmonary veins

Cut edge of parietal pleura

Oblique pericardial sinus

Esophageal prominence

Cut edge of fibrous pericardium and parietal layer of serous pericardium

**Pericardial sac with heart removed**

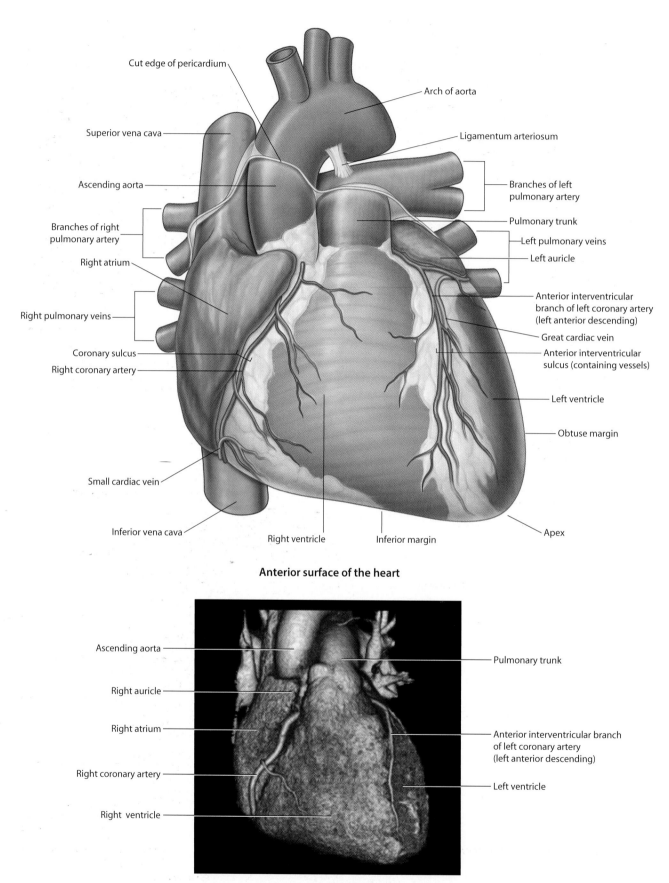

Cut edge of pericardium

Arch of aorta

Superior vena cava

Ligamentum arteriosum

Ascending aorta

Branches of left
pulmonary artery

Pulmonary trunk

Branches of right
pulmonary artery

Left pulmonary veins

Left auricle

Right atrium

Anterior interventricular
branch of left coronary artery
(left anterior descending)

Right pulmonary veins

Great cardiac vein

Coronary sulcus

Anterior interventricular
sulcus (containing vessels)

Right coronary artery

Left ventricle

Obtuse margin

Small cardiac vein

Inferior vena cava

Apex

Right ventricle

Inferior margin

**Anterior surface of the heart**

Ascending aorta

Pulmonary trunk

Right auricle

Right atrium

Anterior interventricular branch
of left coronary artery
(left anterior descending)

Right coronary artery

Left ventricle

Right ventricle

**Anterior view of the heart.**
Volume-rendered anterior view using multidetector computed tomography

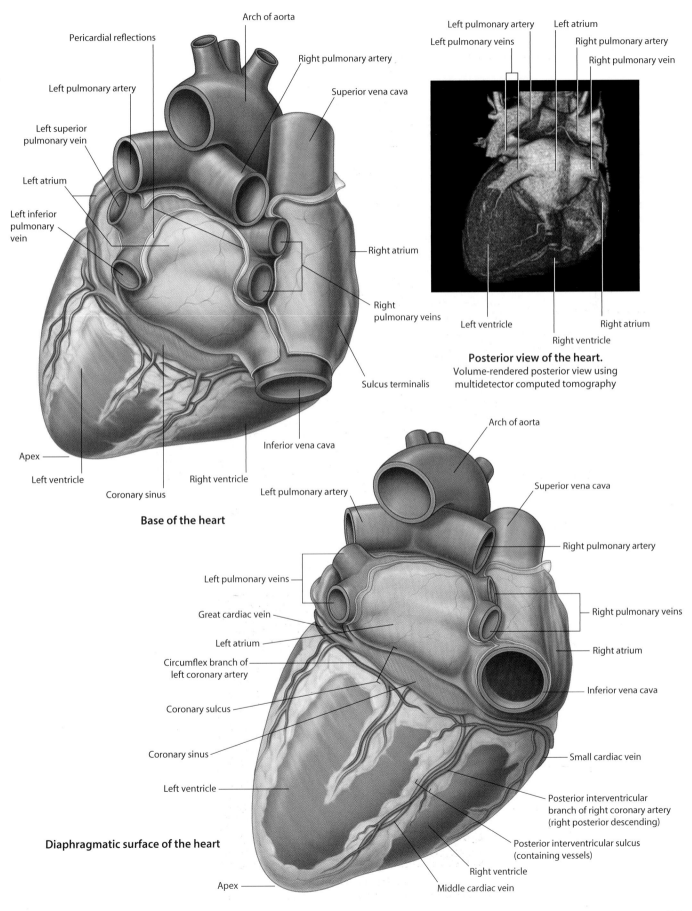

Pericardial reflections

Arch of aorta

Right pulmonary artery

Left pulmonary artery

Superior vena cava

Left superior
pulmonary vein

Left atrium

Left inferior
pulmonary
vein

Right atrium

Right
pulmonary veins

Sulcus terminalis

Apex

Left ventricle

Coronary sinus

Right ventricle

Inferior vena cava

**Base of the heart**

Left pulmonary artery

Left pulmonary veins

Left atrium

Right pulmonary artery

Right pulmonary vein

**Posterior view of the heart.**
Volume-rendered posterior view using
multidetector computed tomography

Left ventricle

Right ventricle

Right atrium

Arch of aorta

Left pulmonary artery

Superior vena cava

Right pulmonary artery

Left pulmonary veins

Great cardiac vein

Left atrium

Circumflex branch of
left coronary artery

Coronary sulcus

Coronary sinus

Left ventricle

Right pulmonary veins

Right atrium

Inferior vena cava

Small cardiac vein

Posterior interventricular
branch of right coronary artery
(right posterior descending)

Posterior interventricular sulcus
(containing vessels)

Right ventricle

**Diaphragmatic surface of the heart**

Apex

Middle cardiac vein

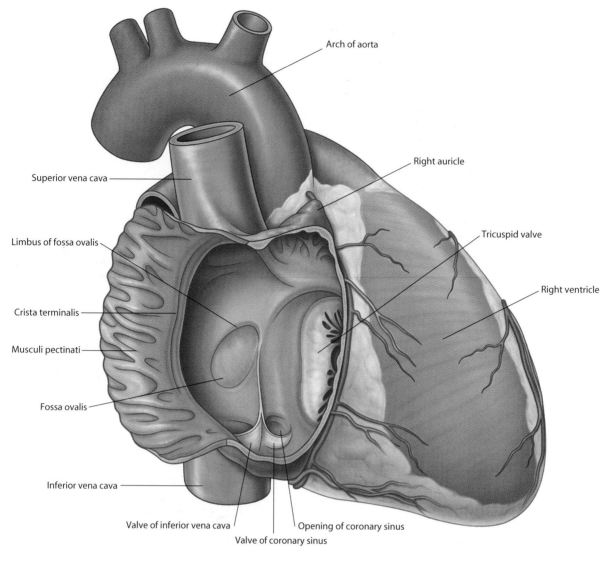

Arch of aorta

Right auricle

Superior vena cava

Tricuspid valve

Limbus of fossa ovalis

Right ventricle

Crista terminalis

Musculi pectinati

Fossa ovalis

Inferior vena cava

Valve of inferior vena cava

Opening of coronary sinus

Valve of coronary sinus

**Internal view of right atrium**

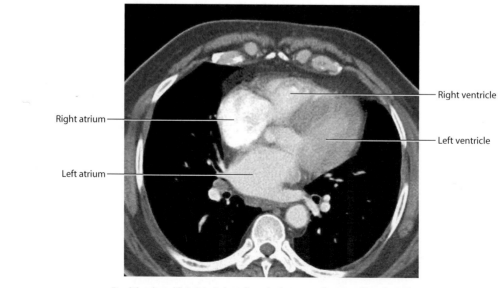

Right ventricle

Right atrium

Left ventricle

Left atrium

**Positioning of right atrium in relation to other cardiac chambers.**
CT image, with contrast, in axial plane

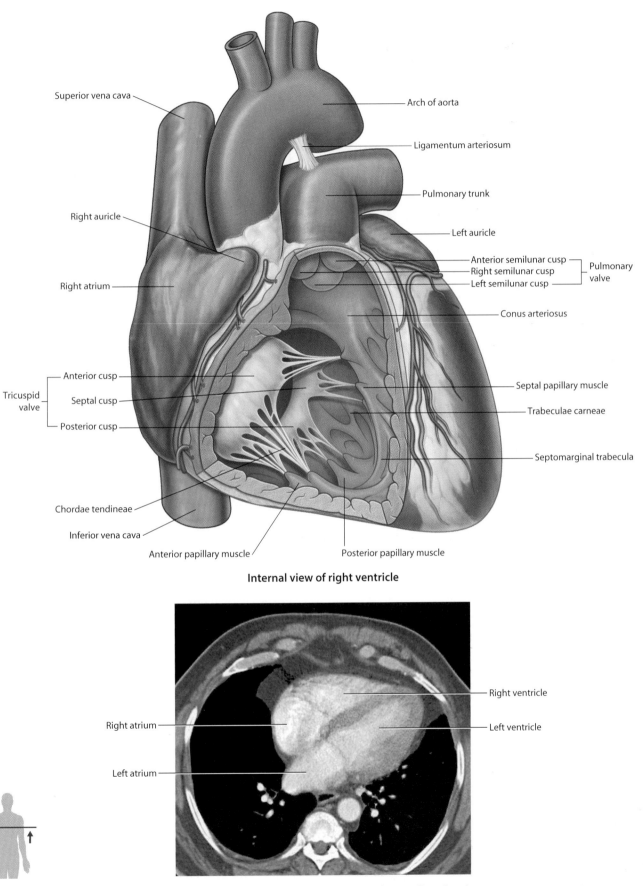

Superior vena cava

Arch of aorta

Ligamentum arteriosum

Pulmonary trunk

Right auricle

Left auricle

Anterior semilunar cusp
Right semilunar cusp — Pulmonary valve
Left semilunar cusp

Right atrium

Conus arteriosus

Anterior cusp

Septal papillary muscle

Tricuspid valve — Septal cusp

Trabeculae carneae

Posterior cusp

Septomarginal trabecula

Chordae tendineae

Inferior vena cava

Anterior papillary muscle

Posterior papillary muscle

**Internal view of right ventricle**

Right ventricle

Right atrium

Left ventricle

Left atrium

**Positioning of right ventricle in relation to other cardiac chambers.**
CT image, with contrast, in axial plane

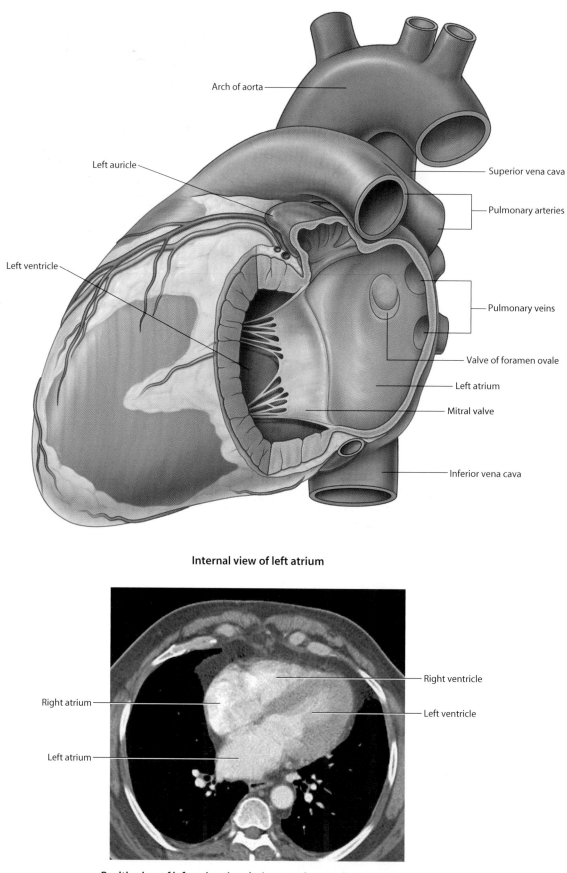

Arch of aorta

Left auricle

Left ventricle

Superior vena cava

Pulmonary arteries

Pulmonary veins

Valve of foramen ovale

Left atrium

Mitral valve

Inferior vena cava

**Internal view of left atrium**

Right ventricle

Right atrium

Left ventricle

Left atrium

**Positioning of left atrium in relation to other cardiac chambers.**
CT image, with contrast, in axial plane

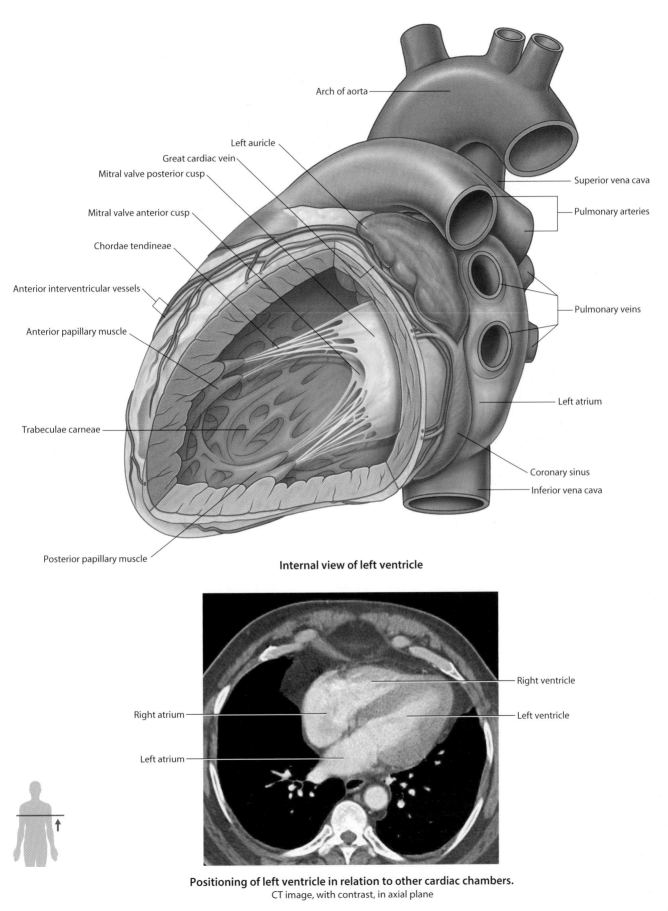

Arch of aorta

Left auricle

Great cardiac vein

Mitral valve posterior cusp

Mitral valve anterior cusp

Chordae tendineae

Anterior interventricular vessels

Anterior papillary muscle

Trabeculae carneae

Posterior papillary muscle

Superior vena cava

Pulmonary arteries

Pulmonary veins

Left atrium

Coronary sinus

Inferior vena cava

**Internal view of left ventricle**

Right atrium

Left atrium

Right ventricle

Left ventricle

**Positioning of left ventricle in relation to other cardiac chambers.**
CT image, with contrast, in axial plane

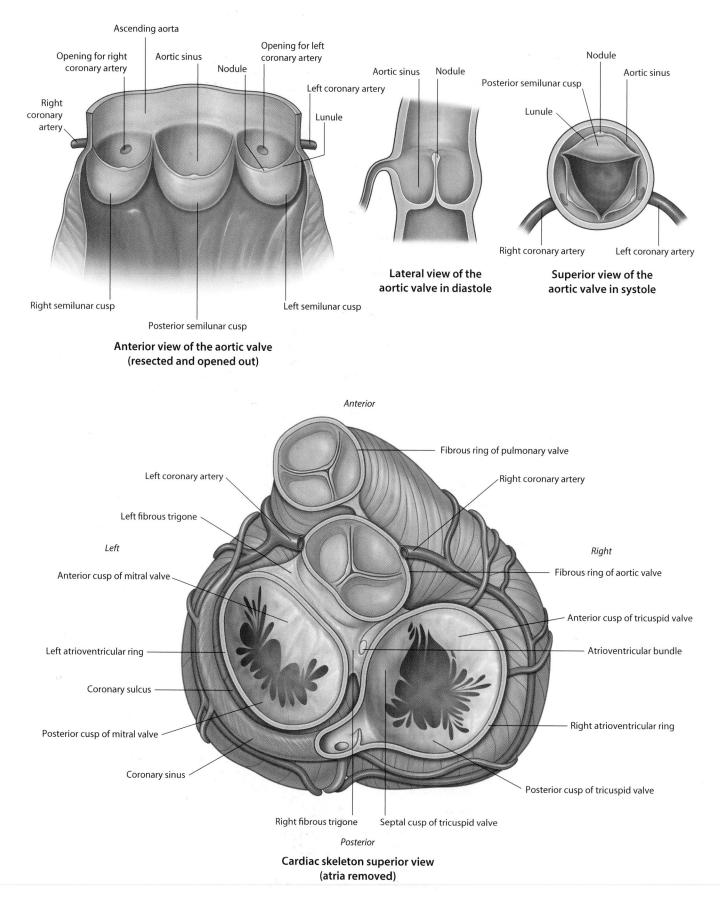

Ascending aorta

Opening for right coronary artery

Aortic sinus

Nodule

Opening for left coronary artery

Left coronary artery

Right coronary artery

Lunule

Right semilunar cusp

Posterior semilunar cusp

Left semilunar cusp

**Anterior view of the aortic valve
(resected and opened out)**

Aortic sinus

Nodule

**Lateral view of the
aortic valve in diastole**

Nodule

Posterior semilunar cusp

Aortic sinus

Lunule

Right coronary artery

Left coronary artery

**Superior view of the
aortic valve in systole**

*Anterior*

Fibrous ring of pulmonary valve

Left coronary artery

Right coronary artery

Left fibrous trigone

*Left*

*Right*

Anterior cusp of mitral valve

Fibrous ring of aortic valve

Left atrioventricular ring

Anterior cusp of tricuspid valve

Coronary sulcus

Atrioventricular bundle

Posterior cusp of mitral valve

Right atrioventricular ring

Coronary sinus

Posterior cusp of tricuspid valve

Right fibrous trigone

Septal cusp of tricuspid valve

*Posterior*

**Cardiac skeleton superior view
(atria removed)**

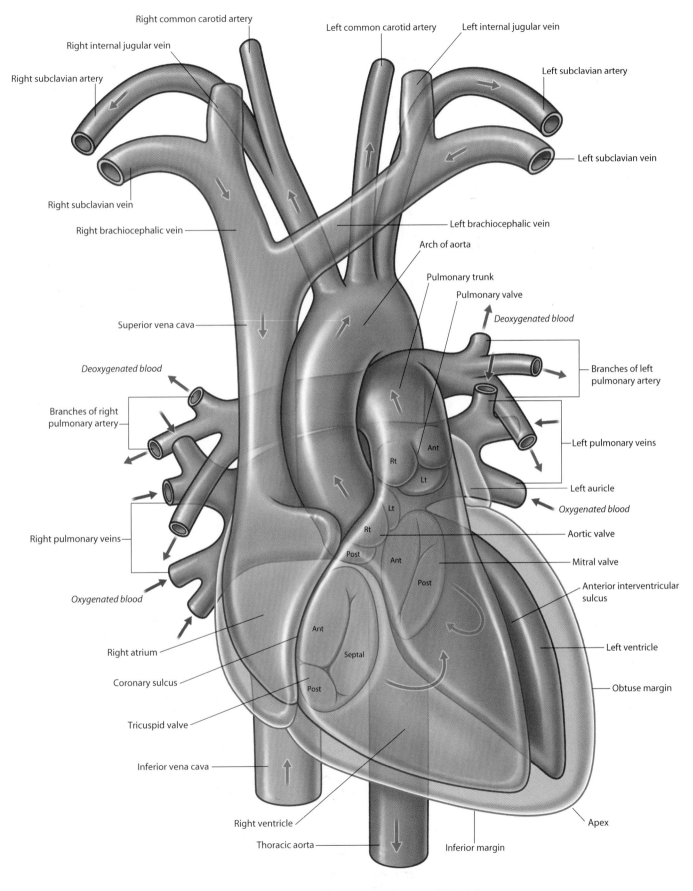

Right common carotid artery

Right internal jugular vein

Right subclavian artery

Left common carotid artery

Left internal jugular vein

Left subclavian artery

Left subclavian vein

Right subclavian vein

Right brachiocephalic vein

Left brachiocephalic vein

Arch of aorta

Pulmonary trunk

Pulmonary valve

Superior vena cava

*Deoxygenated blood*

*Deoxygenated blood*

Branches of left
pulmonary artery

Branches of right
pulmonary artery

Left pulmonary veins

Rt

Ant

Lt

Lt

Right pulmonary veins

Rt

Post

Ant

Post

Left auricle

*Oxygenated blood*

Aortic valve

Mitral valve

Anterior interventricular
sulcus

*Oxygenated blood*

Left ventricle

Right atrium

Ant

Septal

Post

Obtuse margin

Coronary sulcus

Tricuspid valve

Inferior vena cava

Right ventricle

Thoracic aorta

Inferior margin

Apex

**Cardiac chambers and direction of blood flow**

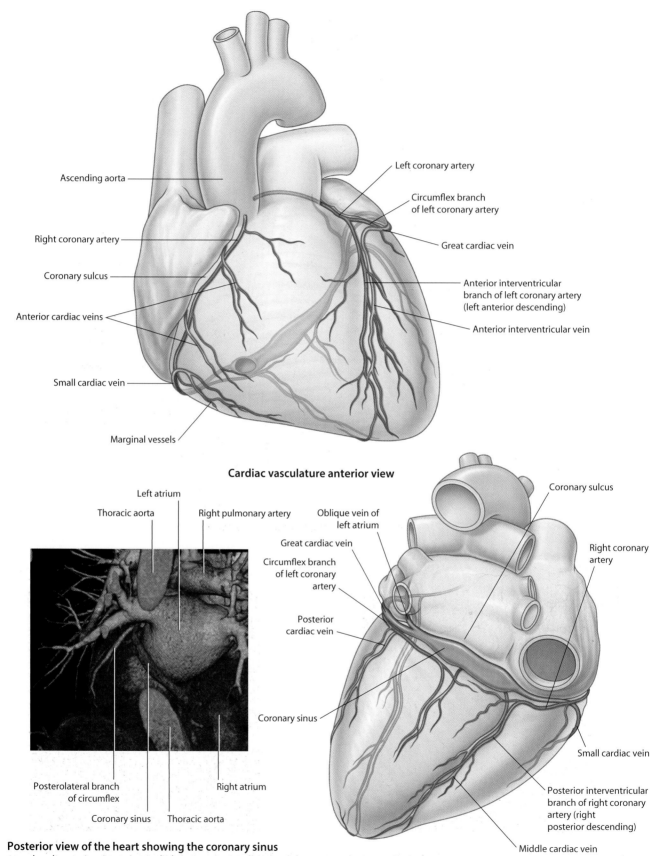

Ascending aorta

Right coronary artery

Coronary sulcus

Anterior cardiac veins

Small cardiac vein

Marginal vessels

Left coronary artery

Circumflex branch
of left coronary artery

Great cardiac vein

Anterior interventricular
branch of left coronary artery
(left anterior descending)

Anterior interventricular vein

**Cardiac vasculature anterior view**

Left atrium

Thoracic aorta

Right pulmonary artery

Posterolateral branch
of circumflex

Coronary sinus

Thoracic aorta

Right atrium

**Posterior view of the heart showing the coronary sinus**
Volume-rendered posterior view using multidetector computed tomography

Oblique vein of
left atrium

Great cardiac vein

Circumflex branch
of left coronary
artery

Posterior
cardiac vein

Coronary sinus

Coronary sulcus

Right coronary
artery

Small cardiac vein

Posterior interventricular
branch of right coronary
artery (right
posterior descending)

Middle cardiac vein

**Posteroinferior view**

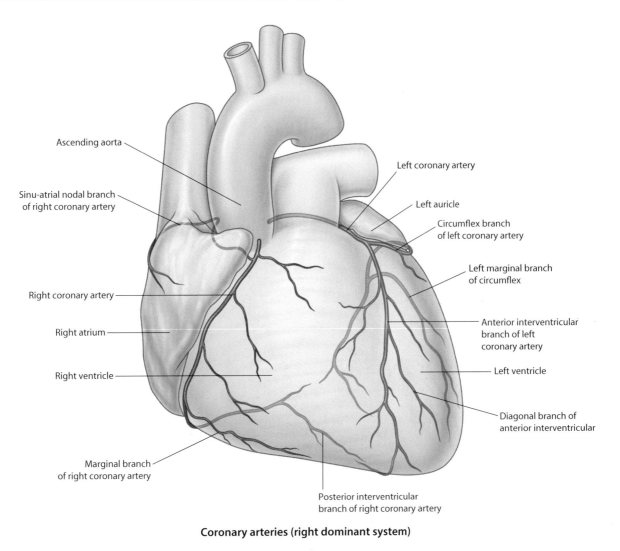

Ascending aorta

Sinu-atrial nodal branch
of right coronary artery

Right coronary artery

Right atrium

Right ventricle

Marginal branch
of right coronary artery

Left coronary artery

Left auricle

Circumflex branch
of left coronary artery

Left marginal branch
of circumflex

Anterior interventricular
branch of left
coronary artery

Left ventricle

Diagonal branch of
anterior interventricular

Posterior interventricular
branch of right coronary artery

**Coronary arteries (right dominant system)**

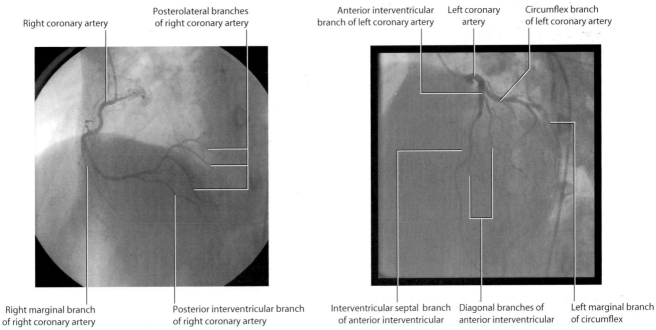

Right coronary artery

Posterolateral branches
of right coronary artery

Anterior interventricular
branch of left coronary artery

Left coronary
artery

Circumflex branch
of left coronary artery

Right marginal branch
of right coronary artery

Posterior interventricular branch
of right coronary artery

Interventricular septal branch
of anterior interventricular

Diagonal branches of
anterior interventricular

Left marginal branch
of circumflex

**Coronary angiography (right dominant system).**
Left anterior oblique projection, cranial angulation, of right coronary artery

**Coronary angiography (right dominant system).**
Left anterior oblique projection, cranial angulation, of left coronary artery

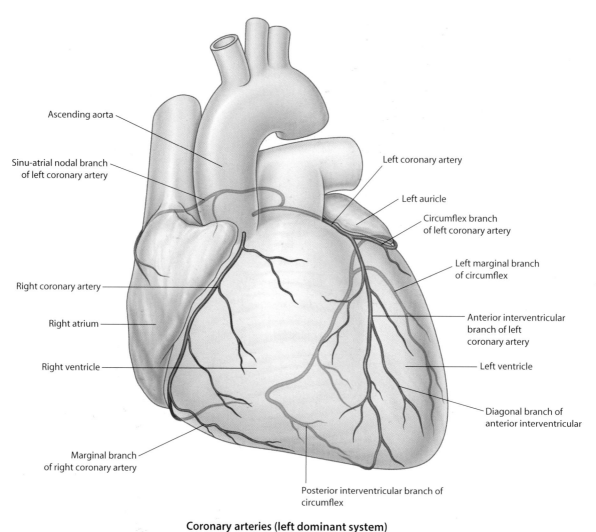

Ascending aorta

Sinu-atrial nodal branch
of left coronary artery

Right coronary artery

Right atrium

Right ventricle

Marginal branch
of right coronary artery

Left coronary artery

Left auricle

Circumflex branch
of left coronary artery

Left marginal branch
of circumflex

Anterior interventricular
branch of left
coronary artery

Left ventricle

Diagonal branch of
anterior interventricular

Posterior interventricular branch of
circumflex

**Coronary arteries (left dominant system)**

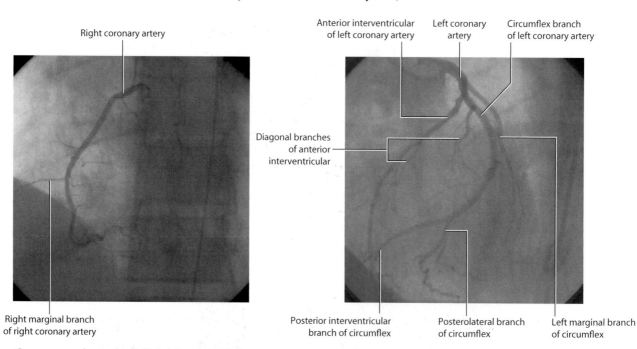

Right coronary artery

Right marginal branch
of right coronary artery

**Coronary angiography (left dominant system).**
Left anterior oblique projection, cranial angulation, of right coronary artery

Anterior interventricular
of left coronary artery

Left coronary
artery

Circumflex branch
of left coronary artery

Diagonal branches
of anterior
interventricular

Posterior interventricular
branch of circumflex

Posterolateral branch
of circumflex

Left marginal branch
of circumflex

**Coronary angiography (left dominant system).**
Left anterior oblique projection, cranial angulation, of left coronary artery

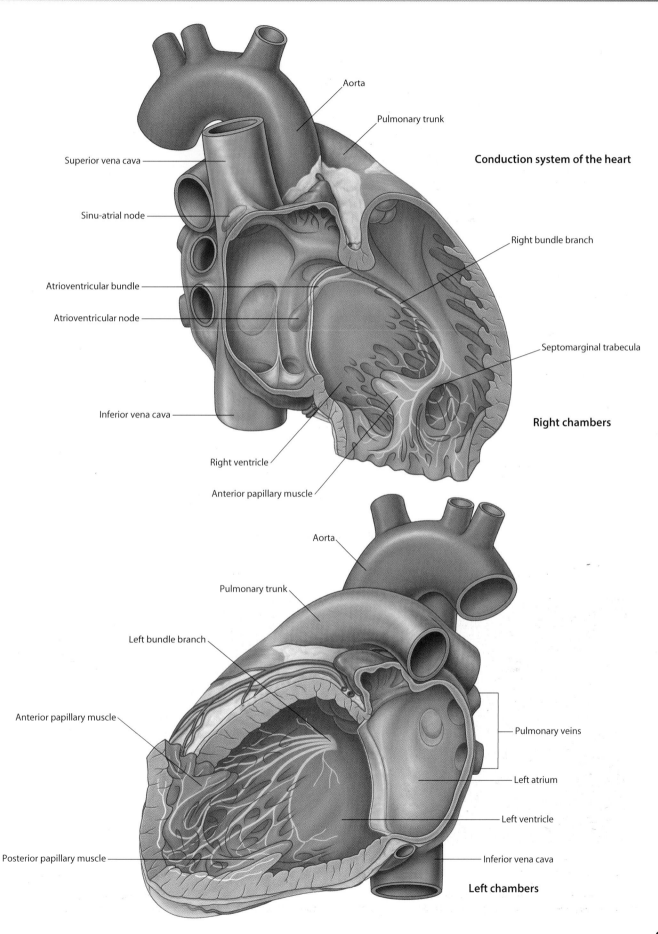

Aorta

Pulmonary trunk

**Conduction system of the heart**

Superior vena cava

Sinu-atrial node

Right bundle branch

Atrioventricular bundle

Atrioventricular node

Septomarginal trabecula

Inferior vena cava

**Right chambers**

Right ventricle

Anterior papillary muscle

Aorta

Pulmonary trunk

Left bundle branch

Anterior papillary muscle

Pulmonary veins

Left atrium

Left ventricle

Posterior papillary muscle

Inferior vena cava

**Left chambers**

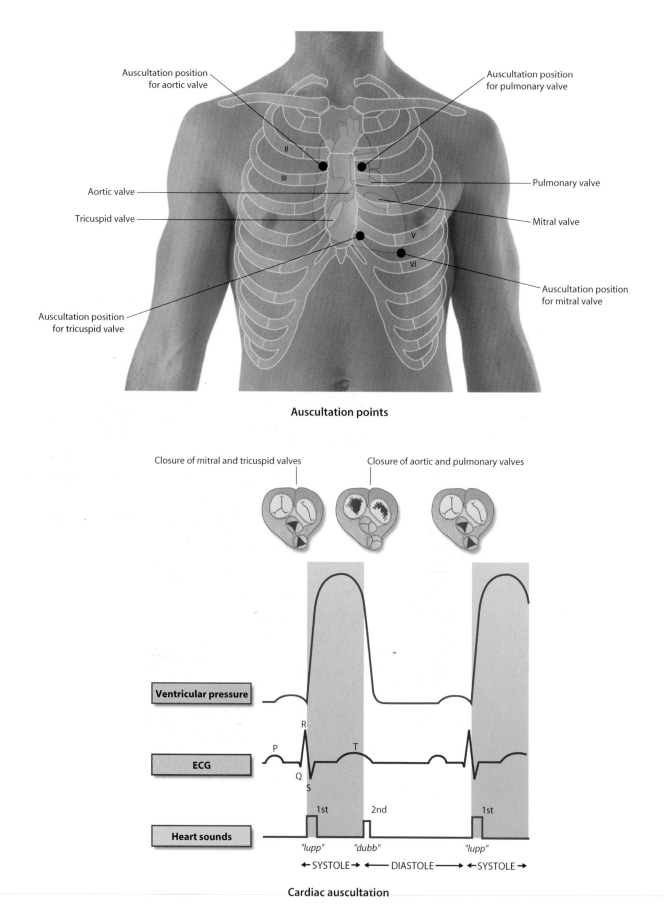

Auscultation position for aortic valve

Auscultation position for pulmonary valve

II

III

Aortic valve

Tricuspid valve

Pulmonary valve

Mitral valve

V

VI

Auscultation position for tricuspid valve

Auscultation position for mitral valve

**Auscultation points**

Closure of mitral and tricuspid valves

Closure of aortic and pulmonary valves

**Ventricular pressure**

R

P

T

**ECG**

Q

S

1st

2nd

1st

**Heart sounds**

*"lupp"*

*"dubb"*

*"lupp"*

← SYSTOLE → ← DIASTOLE → ← SYSTOLE →

**Cardiac auscultation**

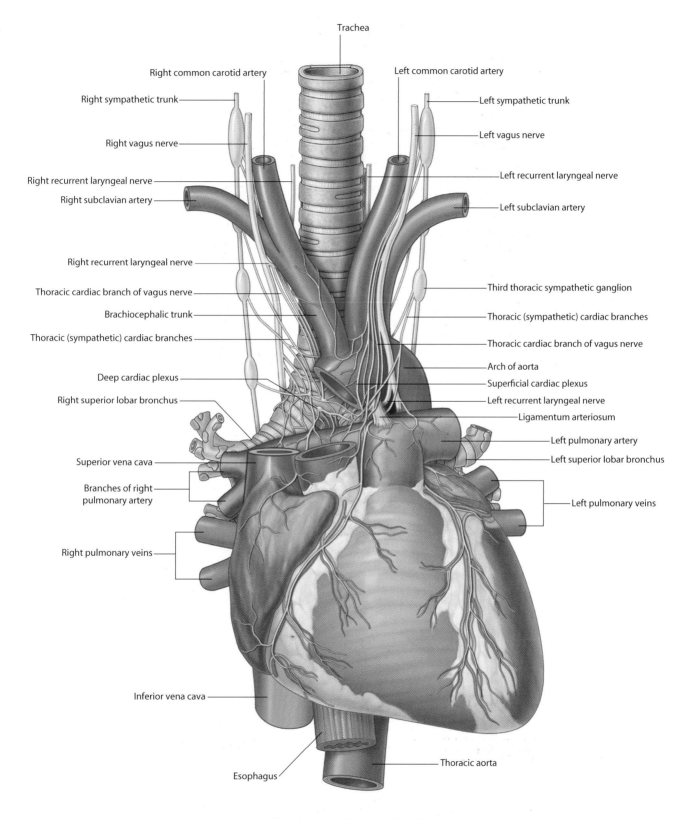

Trachea

Right common carotid artery

Right sympathetic trunk

Right vagus nerve

Right recurrent laryngeal nerve

Right subclavian artery

Right recurrent laryngeal nerve

Thoracic cardiac branch of vagus nerve

Brachiocephalic trunk

Thoracic (sympathetic) cardiac branches

Deep cardiac plexus

Right superior lobar bronchus

Superior vena cava

Branches of right pulmonary artery

Right pulmonary veins

Inferior vena cava

Esophagus

Left common carotid artery

Left sympathetic trunk

Left vagus nerve

Left recurrent laryngeal nerve

Left subclavian artery

Third thoracic sympathetic ganglion

Thoracic (sympathetic) cardiac branches

Thoracic cardiac branch of vagus nerve

Arch of aorta

Superficial cardiac plexus

Left recurrent laryngeal nerve

Ligamentum arteriosum

Left pulmonary artery

Left superior lobar bronchus

Left pulmonary veins

Thoracic aorta

**Cardiac plexus and nerves of the heart**

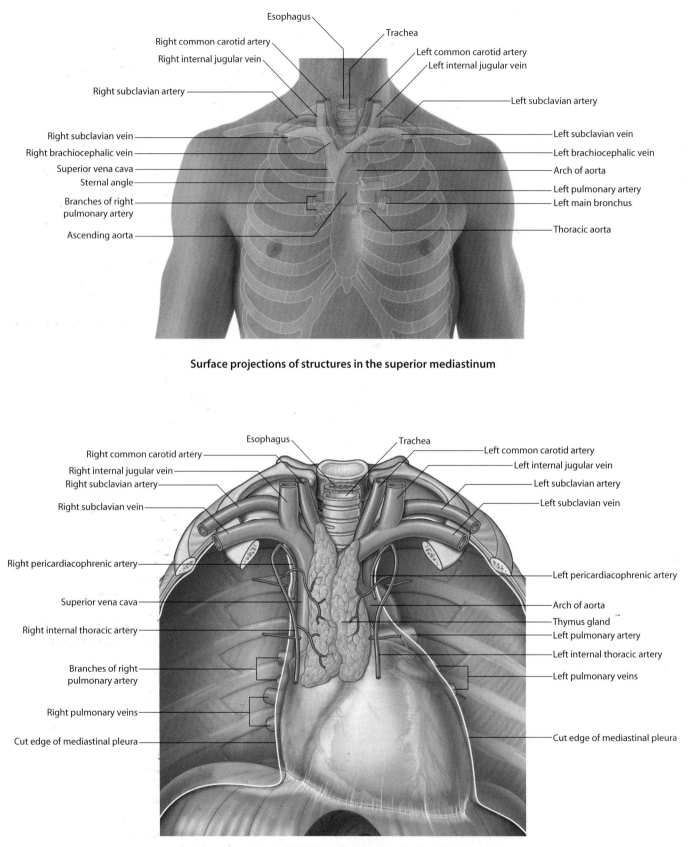

Esophagus

Trachea

Right common carotid artery

Right internal jugular vein

Left common carotid artery

Left internal jugular vein

Right subclavian artery

Left subclavian artery

Right subclavian vein

Left subclavian vein

Right brachiocephalic vein

Left brachiocephalic vein

Superior vena cava

Arch of aorta

Sternal angle

Left pulmonary artery

Branches of right pulmonary artery

Left main bronchus

Ascending aorta

Thoracic aorta

**Surface projections of structures in the superior mediastinum**

Esophagus

Trachea

Right common carotid artery

Left common carotid artery

Right internal jugular vein

Left internal jugular vein

Right subclavian artery

Left subclavian artery

Right subclavian vein

Left subclavian vein

Right pericardiacophrenic artery

Left pericardiacophrenic artery

Superior vena cava

Arch of aorta

Thymus gland

Right internal thoracic artery

Left pulmonary artery

Left internal thoracic artery

Branches of right pulmonary artery

Left pulmonary veins

Right pulmonary veins

Cut edge of mediastinal pleura

Cut edge of mediastinal pleura

**Thymus gland**

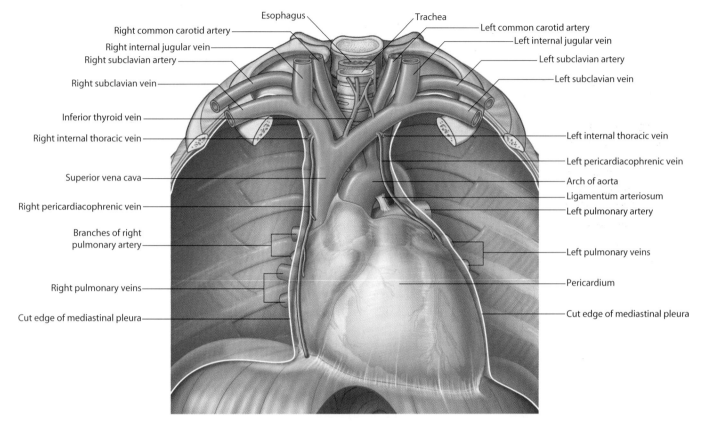

Esophagus
Trachea
Right common carotid artery
Left common carotid artery
Right internal jugular vein
Left internal jugular vein
Right subclavian artery
Left subclavian artery
Right subclavian vein
Left subclavian vein
Inferior thyroid vein
Right internal thoracic vein
Left internal thoracic vein
Left pericardiacophrenic vein
Superior vena cava
Arch of aorta
Right pericardiacophrenic vein
Ligamentum arteriosum
Left pulmonary artery
Branches of right pulmonary artery
Left pulmonary veins
Right pulmonary veins
Pericardium
Cut edge of mediastinal pleura
Cut edge of mediastinal pleura

**Veins of the superior mediastinum**

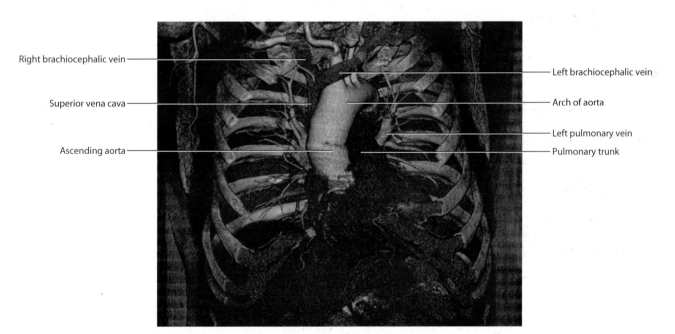

Right brachiocephalic vein
Left brachiocephalic vein
Superior vena cava
Arch of aorta
Left pulmonary vein
Ascending aorta
Pulmonary trunk

**Anterior view of the superior mediastinum showing venous and arterial channels.**
Volume-rendered anterior view using multidetector computed tomography

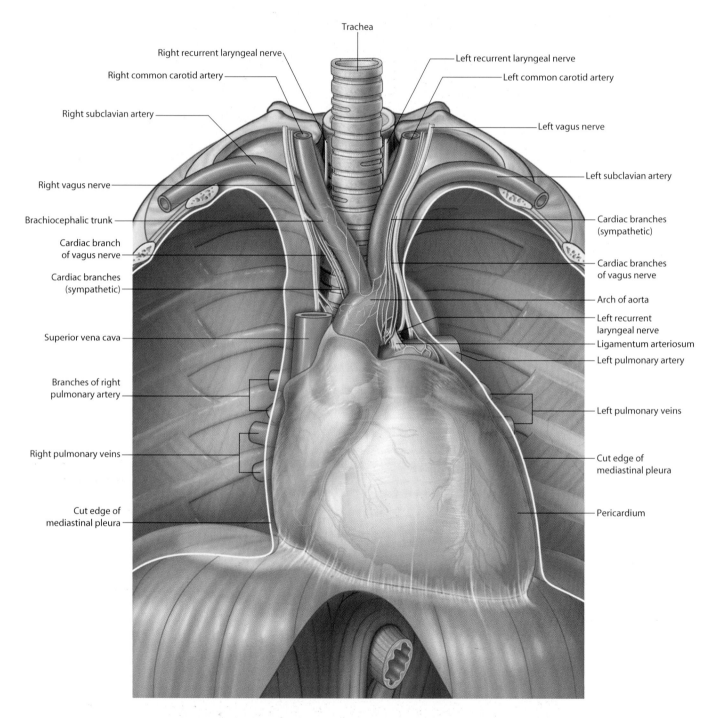

Trachea

Right recurrent laryngeal nerve

Right common carotid artery

Right subclavian artery

Right vagus nerve

Brachiocephalic trunk

Cardiac branch
of vagus nerve

Cardiac branches
(sympathetic)

Superior vena cava

Branches of right
pulmonary artery

Right pulmonary veins

Cut edge of
mediastinal pleura

Left recurrent laryngeal nerve

Left common carotid artery

Left vagus nerve

Left subclavian artery

Cardiac branches
(sympathetic)

Cardiac branches
of vagus nerve

Arch of aorta

Left recurrent
laryngeal nerve

Ligamentum arteriosum

Left pulmonary artery

Left pulmonary veins

Cut edge of
mediastinal pleura

Pericardium

**Arteries and nerves of the superior mediastinum**

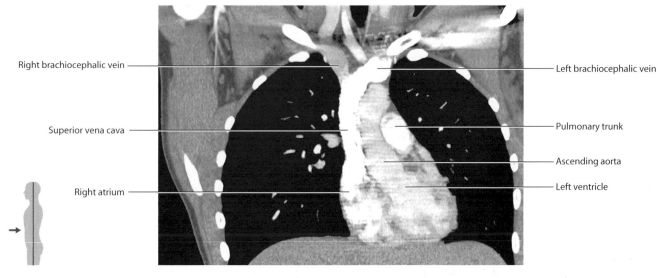

Right brachiocephalic vein

Superior vena cava

Right atrium

Left brachiocephalic vein

Pulmonary trunk

Ascending aorta

Left ventricle

**Positioning of venous channels in the superior mediastinum.**
CT image, with contrast, in coronal plane

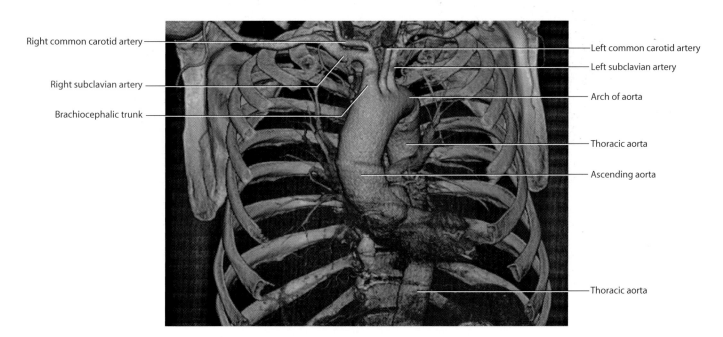

Right common carotid artery

Right subclavian artery

Brachiocephalic trunk

Left common carotid artery

Left subclavian artery

Arch of aorta

Thoracic aorta

Ascending aorta

Thoracic aorta

**Anterior view of the superior mediastinum with the venous
channels, pulmonary trunk, and heart removed.**
Volume-rendered anterior view using multidetector computed tomography

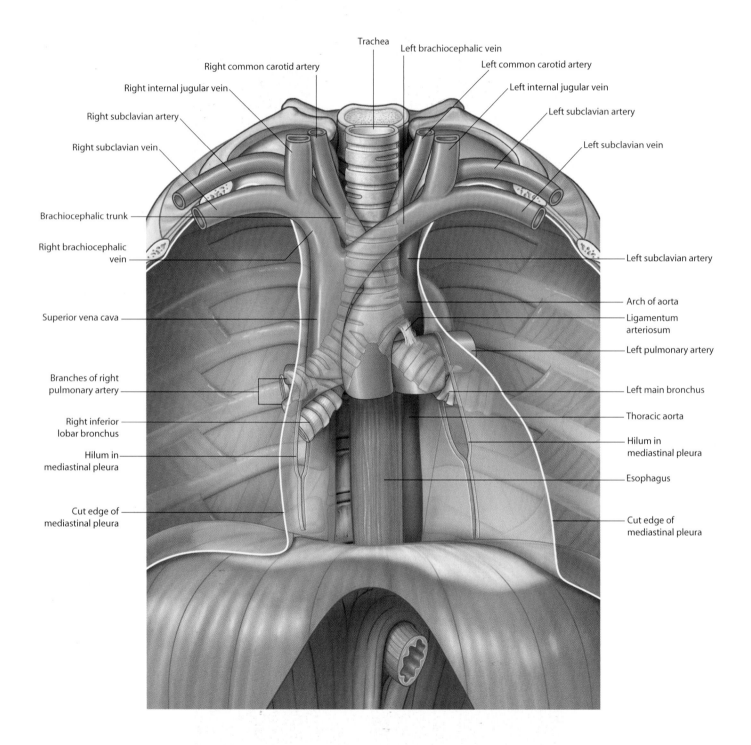

Trachea

Right common carotid artery

Right internal jugular vein

Right subclavian artery

Right subclavian vein

Brachiocephalic trunk

Right brachiocephalic vein

Superior vena cava

Branches of right pulmonary artery

Right inferior lobar bronchus

Hilum in mediastinal pleura

Cut edge of mediastinal pleura

Left brachiocephalic vein

Left common carotid artery

Left internal jugular vein

Left subclavian artery

Left subclavian vein

Left subclavian artery

Arch of aorta

Ligamentum arteriosum

Left pulmonary artery

Left main bronchus

Thoracic aorta

Hilum in mediastinal pleura

Esophagus

Cut edge of mediastinal pleura

**Trachea and structures relating to it in the superior mediastinum**

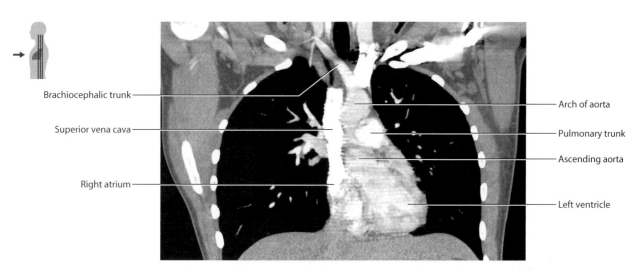

Brachiocephalic trunk

Superior vena cava

Right atrium

Arch of aorta

Pulmonary trunk

Ascending aorta

Left ventricle

**Positioning of brachiocephalic trunk in relation to other structures in the superior mediastinum.**
CT image, with contrast, in coronal plane

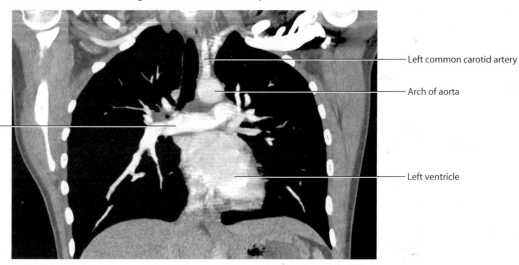

Right pulmonary artery

Left common carotid artery

Arch of aorta

Left ventricle

**Positioning of left common carotid artery in relation to other structures in the superior mediastinum.**
CT image, with contrast, in coronal plane

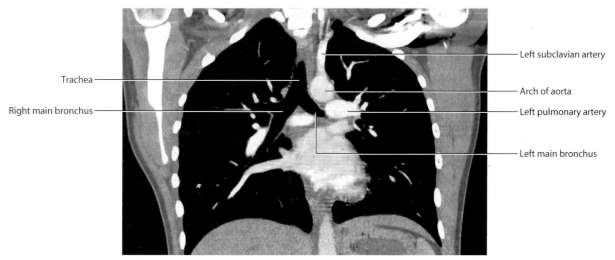

Trachea

Right main bronchus

Left subclavian artery

Arch of aorta

Left pulmonary artery

Left main bronchus

**Positioning of left subclavian artery and the bifurcation of the trachea in relation
to other structures in the superior mediastinum.**
CT image, with contrast, in coronal plane

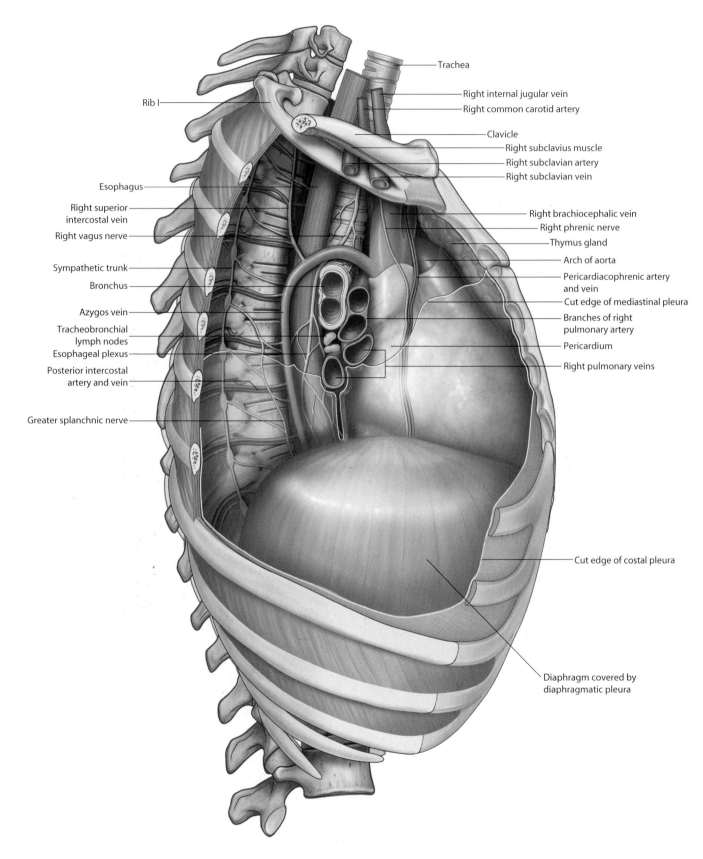

Trachea

Right internal jugular vein

Right common carotid artery

Clavicle

Right subclavius muscle

Right subclavian artery

Right subclavian vein

Right brachiocephalic vein

Right phrenic nerve

Thymus gland

Arch of aorta

Pericardiacophrenic artery and vein

Cut edge of mediastinal pleura

Branches of right pulmonary artery

Pericardium

Right pulmonary veins

Cut edge of costal pleura

Diaphragm covered by diaphragmatic pleura

Rib I

Esophagus

Right superior intercostal vein

Right vagus nerve

Sympathetic trunk

Bronchus

Azygos vein

Tracheobronchial lymph nodes

Esophageal plexus

Posterior intercostal artery and vein

Greater splanchnic nerve

**Right side of mediastinum and right thoracic cavity**

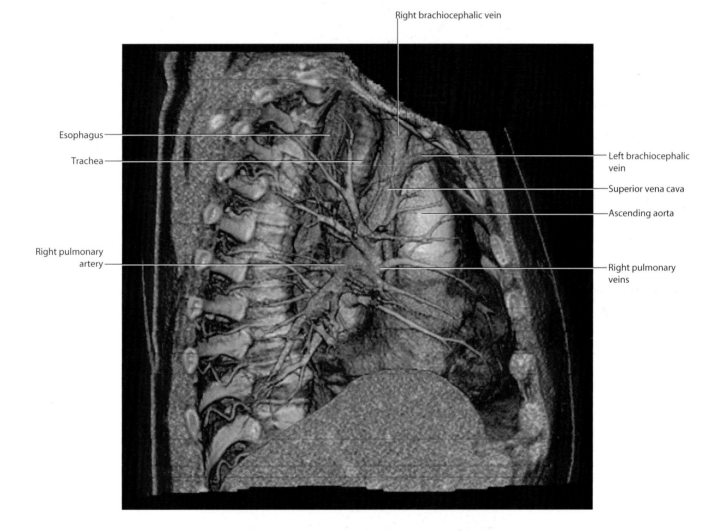

Right brachiocephalic vein

Esophagus

Trachea

Left brachiocephalic vein

Superior vena cava

Ascending aorta

Right pulmonary artery

Right pulmonary veins

**View of mediastinal structures from the right side of the thorax.**
Volume-rendered lateral view from the right side using multidetector computed tomography

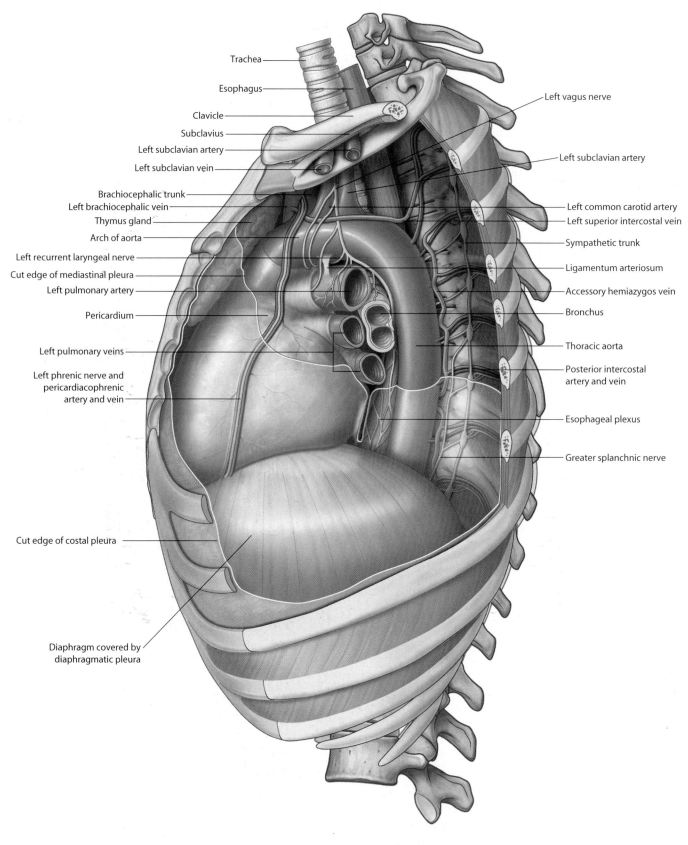

Trachea

Esophagus

Clavicle

Subclavius

Left subclavian artery

Left subclavian vein

Brachiocephalic trunk

Left brachiocephalic vein

Thymus gland

Arch of aorta

Left recurrent laryngeal nerve

Cut edge of mediastinal pleura

Left pulmonary artery

Pericardium

Left pulmonary veins

Left phrenic nerve and
pericardiacophrenic
artery and vein

Cut edge of costal pleura

Diaphragm covered by
diaphragmatic pleura

Left vagus nerve

Left subclavian artery

Left common carotid artery

Left superior intercostal vein

Sympathetic trunk

Ligamentum arteriosum

Accessory hemiazygos vein

Bronchus

Thoracic aorta

Posterior intercostal
artery and vein

Esophageal plexus

Greater splanchnic nerve

**Left side of mediastinum and left thoracic cavity**

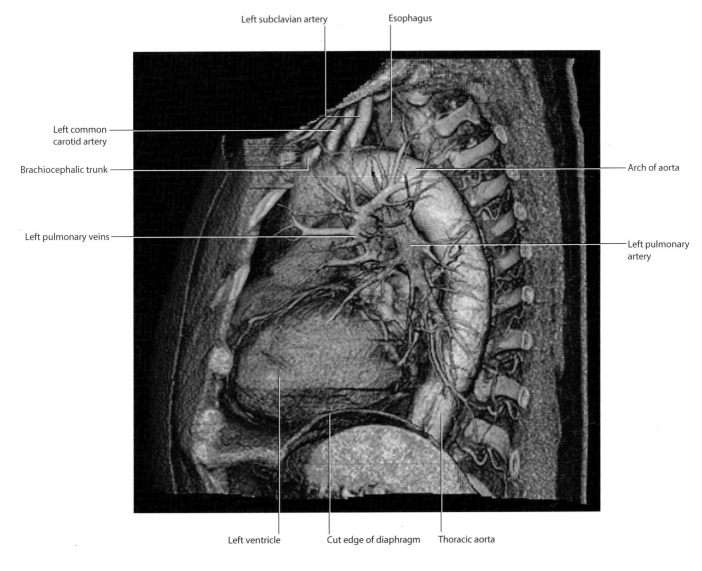

Left subclavian artery

Esophagus

Left common carotid artery

Brachiocephalic trunk

Left pulmonary veins

Arch of aorta

Left pulmonary artery

Left ventricle

Cut edge of diaphragm

Thoracic aorta

**View of mediastinal structures from the left side of the thorax.**
Volume-rendered lateral view from the left side using multidetector computed tomography

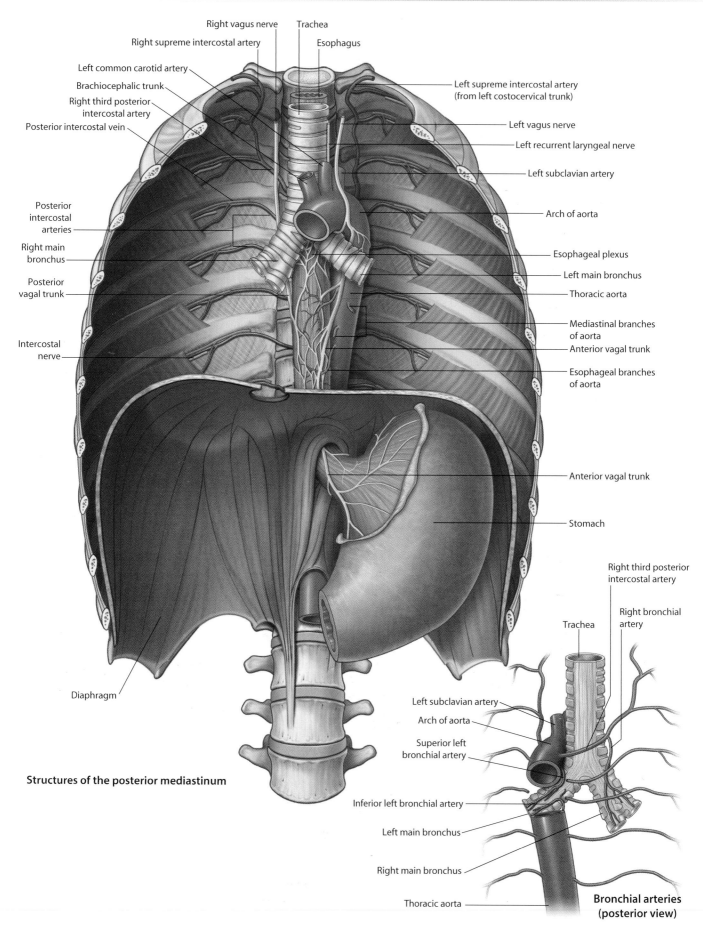

Right vagus nerve

Right supreme intercostal artery

Trachea

Esophagus

Left common carotid artery

Brachiocephalic trunk

Right third posterior intercostal artery

Posterior intercostal vein

Left supreme intercostal artery (from left costocervical trunk)

Left vagus nerve

Left recurrent laryngeal nerve

Left subclavian artery

Posterior intercostal arteries

Right main bronchus

Posterior vagal trunk

Arch of aorta

Esophageal plexus

Left main bronchus

Thoracic aorta

Mediastinal branches of aorta

Anterior vagal trunk

Esophageal branches of aorta

Intercostal nerve

Anterior vagal trunk

Stomach

Diaphragm

**Structures of the posterior mediastinum**

Right third posterior intercostal artery

Right bronchial artery

Trachea

Left subclavian artery

Arch of aorta

Superior left bronchial artery

Inferior left bronchial artery

Left main bronchus

Right main bronchus

Thoracic aorta

**Bronchial arteries (posterior view)**

112

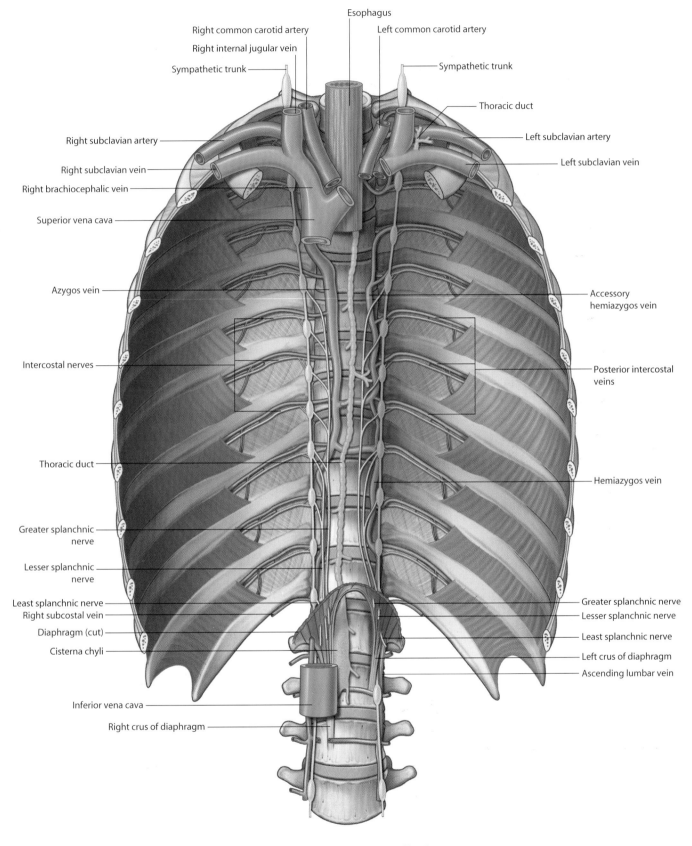

Esophagus

Right common carotid artery

Right internal jugular vein

Sympathetic trunk

Left common carotid artery

Sympathetic trunk

Thoracic duct

Right subclavian artery

Left subclavian artery

Right subclavian vein

Left subclavian vein

Right brachiocephalic vein

Superior vena cava

Azygos vein

Accessory hemiazygos vein

Intercostal nerves

Posterior intercostal veins

Thoracic duct

Hemiazygos vein

Greater splanchnic nerve

Lesser splanchnic nerve

Least splanchnic nerve

Greater splanchnic nerve

Right subcostal vein

Lesser splanchnic nerve

Diaphragm (cut)

Least splanchnic nerve

Cisterna chyli

Left crus of diaphragm

Ascending lumbar vein

Inferior vena cava

Right crus of diaphragm

**Structures of the posterior mediastinum
(thoracic aorta and esophagus removed)**

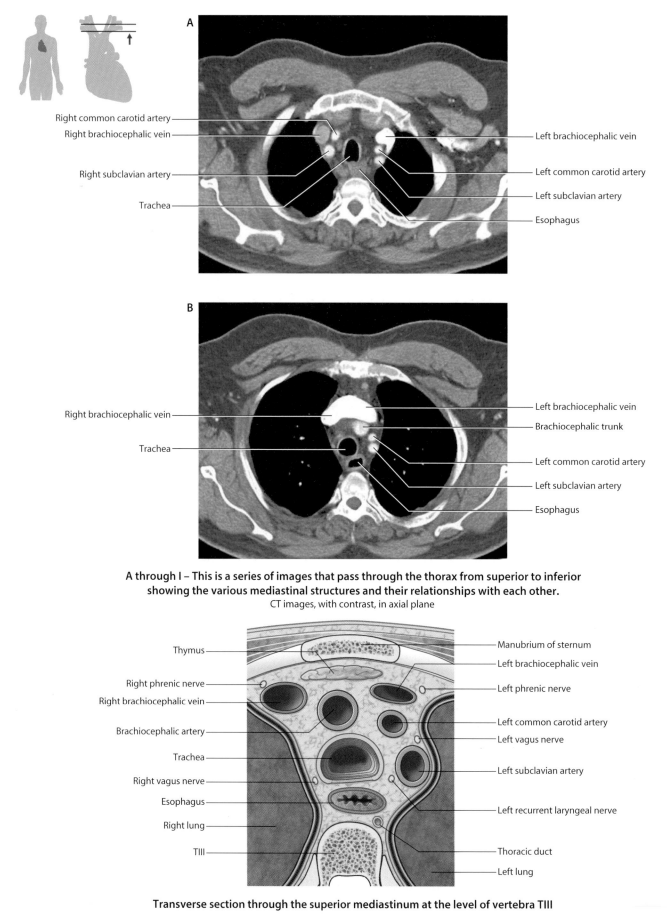

**A** Right common carotid artery
Right brachiocephalic vein
Right subclavian artery
Trachea
Left brachiocephalic vein
Left common carotid artery
Left subclavian artery
Esophagus

**B** Right brachiocephalic vein
Trachea
Left brachiocephalic vein
Brachiocephalic trunk
Left common carotid artery
Left subclavian artery
Esophagus

**A through I** – This is a series of images that pass through the thorax from superior to inferior showing the various mediastinal structures and their relationships with each other.
CT images, with contrast, in axial plane

Thymus
Right phrenic nerve
Right brachiocephalic vein
Brachiocephalic artery
Trachea
Right vagus nerve
Esophagus
Right lung
TIII
Manubrium of sternum
Left brachiocephalic vein
Left phrenic nerve
Left common carotid artery
Left vagus nerve
Left subclavian artery
Left recurrent laryngeal nerve
Thoracic duct
Left lung

**Transverse section through the superior mediastinum at the level of vertebra TIII**

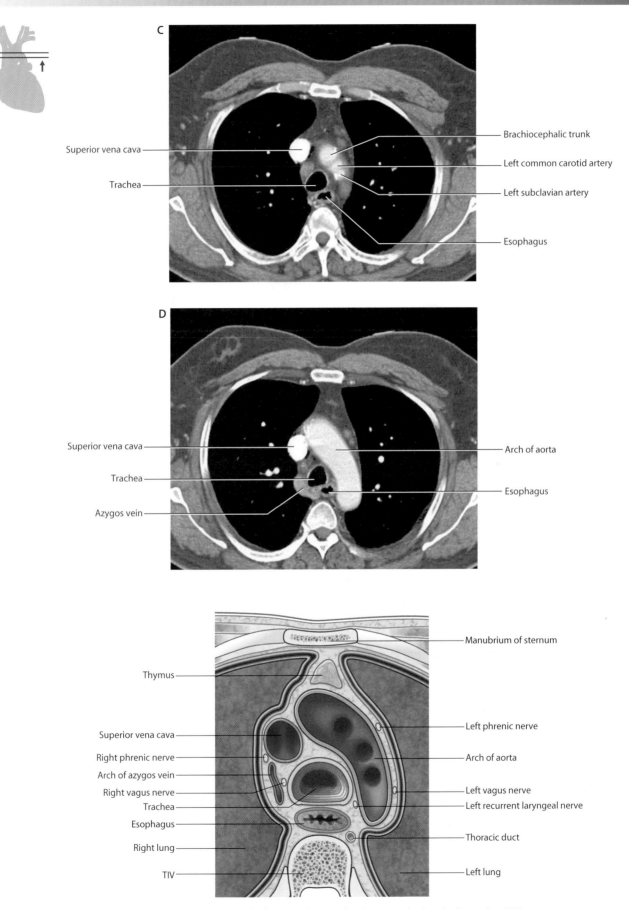

C

Superior vena cava

Trachea

Brachiocephalic trunk

Left common carotid artery

Left subclavian artery

Esophagus

D

Superior vena cava

Trachea

Azygos vein

Arch of aorta

Esophagus

Manubrium of sternum

Thymus

Superior vena cava

Right phrenic nerve

Arch of azygos vein

Right vagus nerve

Trachea

Esophagus

Right lung

TIV

Left phrenic nerve

Arch of aorta

Left vagus nerve

Left recurrent laryngeal nerve

Thoracic duct

Left lung

**Transverse section through the superior mediastinum at the level of vertebra TIV**

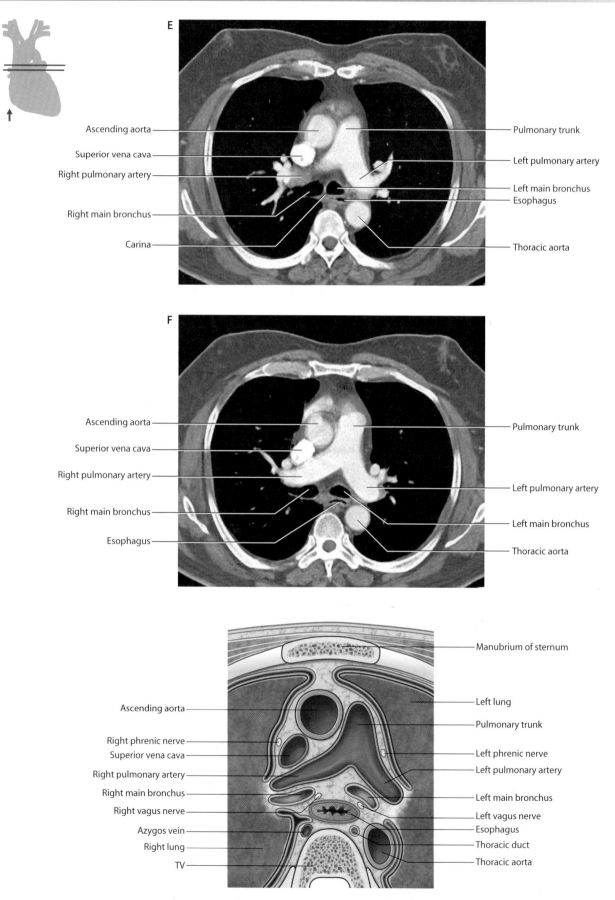

**E**

Ascending aorta
Superior vena cava
Right pulmonary artery

Right main bronchus

Carina

Pulmonary trunk
Left pulmonary artery
Left main bronchus
Esophagus

Thoracic aorta

**F**

Ascending aorta
Superior vena cava
Right pulmonary artery
Right main bronchus
Esophagus

Pulmonary trunk

Left pulmonary artery

Left main bronchus

Thoracic aorta

Manubrium of sternum

Left lung

Pulmonary trunk

Ascending aorta
Right phrenic nerve
Superior vena cava
Right pulmonary artery
Right main bronchus
Right vagus nerve
Azygos vein
Right lung
TV

Left phrenic nerve
Left pulmonary artery
Left main bronchus
Left vagus nerve
Esophagus
Thoracic duct
Thoracic aorta

**Transverse section through the superior mediastinum at the level of vertebra TV**

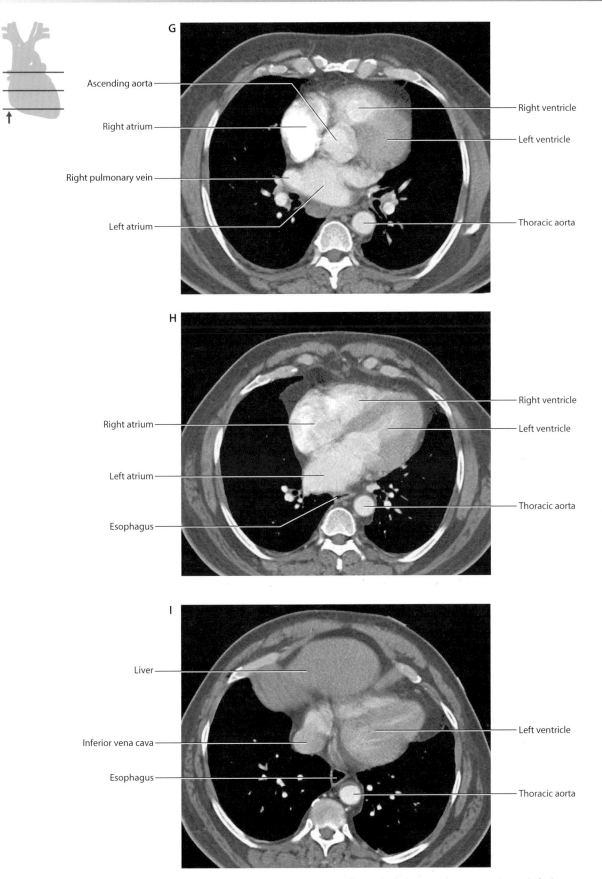

**A through I – This is a series of images that pass through the thorax from superior to inferior showing the various mediastinal structures and their relationships with each other.**

CT images, with contrast, in axial plane

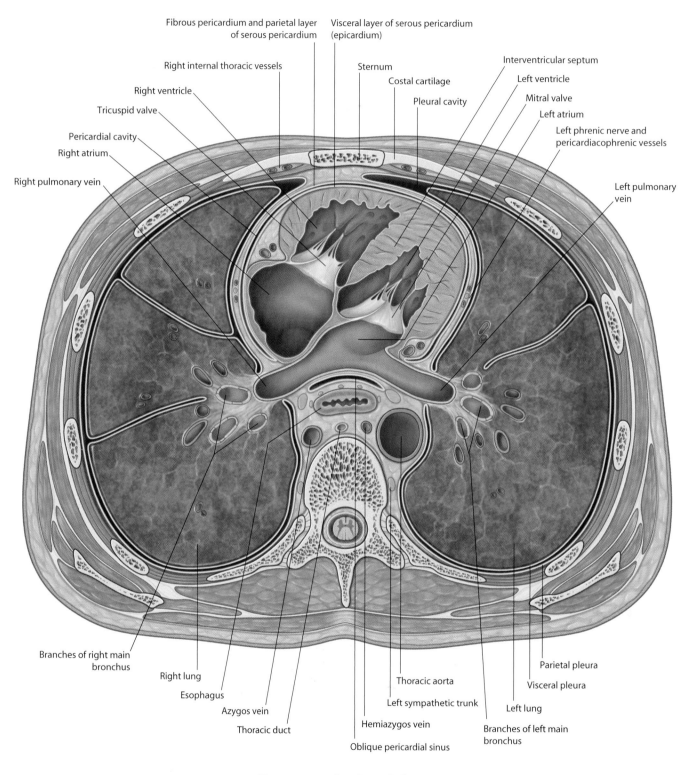

Fibrous pericardium and parietal layer of serous pericardium

Visceral layer of serous pericardium (epicardium)

Right internal thoracic vessels

Sternum

Costal cartilage

Interventricular septum

Left ventricle

Right ventricle

Pleural cavity

Mitral valve

Tricuspid valve

Left atrium

Pericardial cavity

Left phrenic nerve and pericardiacophrenic vessels

Right atrium

Right pulmonary vein

Left pulmonary vein

Branches of right main bronchus

Right lung

Esophagus

Azygos vein

Thoracic duct

Hemiazygos vein

Oblique pericardial sinus

Thoracic aorta

Left sympathetic trunk

Left lung

Branches of left main bronchus

Parietal pleura

Visceral pleura

**Transverse section through thorax
(approximately TVII)**

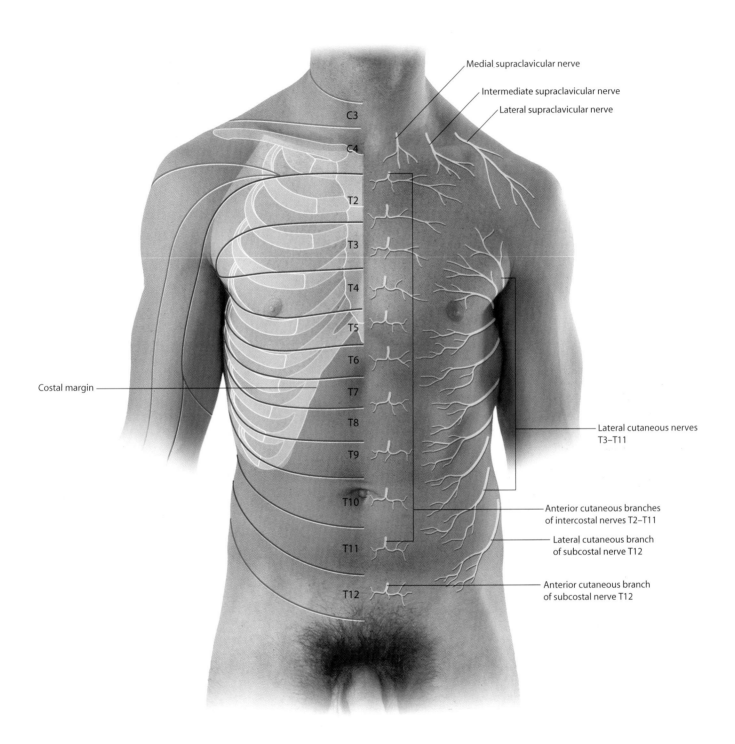

C3
C4
T2
T3
T4
T5
T6
T7
T8
T9
T10
T11
T12

Medial supraclavicular nerve

Intermediate supraclavicular nerve

Lateral supraclavicular nerve

Costal margin

Lateral cutaneous nerves
T3–T11

Anterior cutaneous branches
of intercostal nerves T2–T11

Lateral cutaneous branch
of subcostal nerve T12

Anterior cutaneous branch
of subcostal nerve T12

**Dermatomes and cutaneous nerves of the thoracic region**

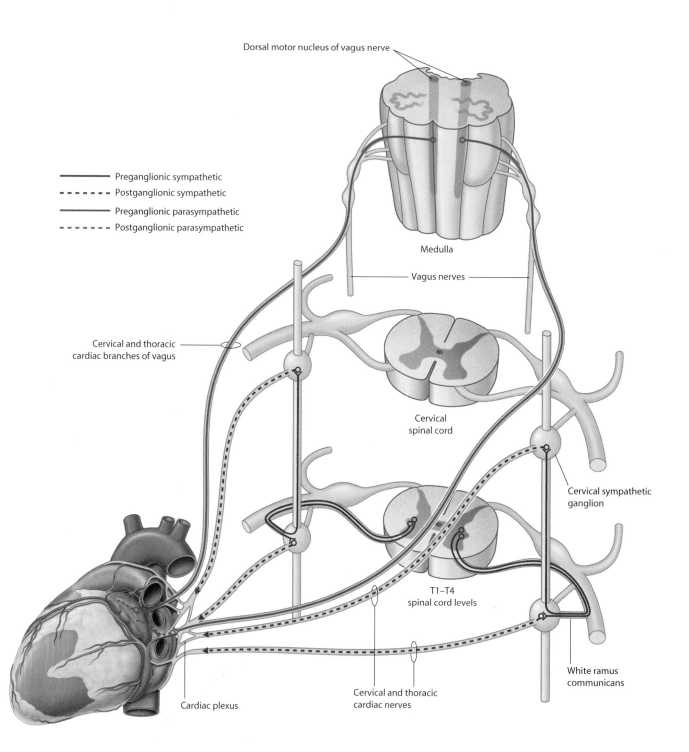

Dorsal motor nucleus of vagus nerve

Preganglionic sympathetic
Postganglionic sympathetic
Preganglionic parasympathetic
Postganglionic parasympathetic

Medulla

Vagus nerves

Cervical and thoracic
cardiac branches of vagus

Cervical
spinal cord

Cervical sympathetic
ganglion

T1–T4
spinal cord levels

White ramus
communicans

Cardiac plexus

Cervical and thoracic
cardiac nerves

**Visceral efferent (motor) innervation of the heart
(sympathetic and parasympathetic)**

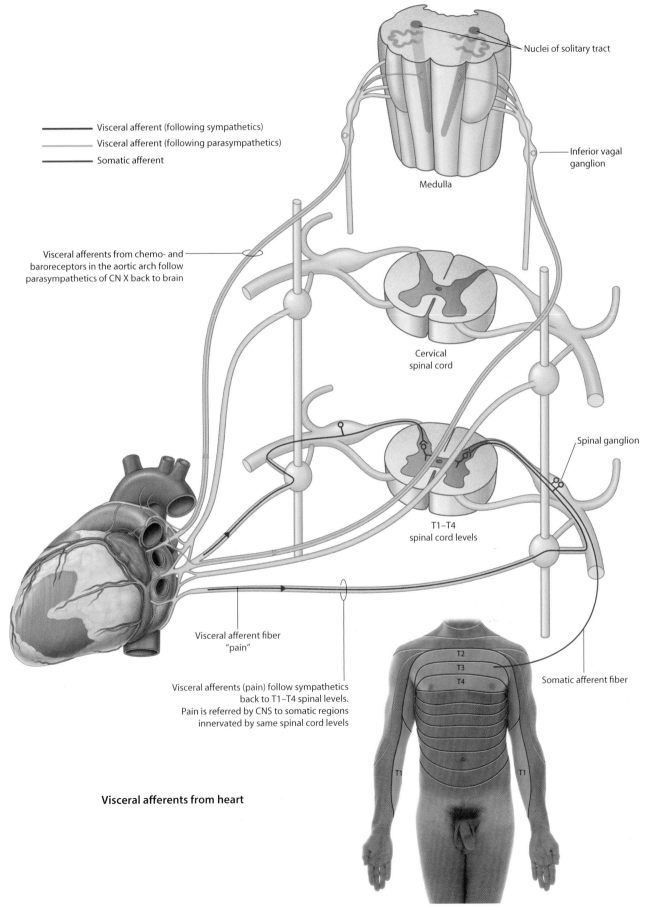

Nuclei of solitary tract

Visceral afferent (following sympathetics)
Visceral afferent (following parasympathetics)
Somatic afferent

Inferior vagal ganglion

Medulla

Visceral afferents from chemo- and baroreceptors in the aortic arch follow parasympathetics of CN X back to brain

Cervical spinal cord

Spinal ganglion

T1–T4 spinal cord levels

Visceral afferent fiber "pain"

T2
T3
T4

T1          T1

Visceral afferents (pain) follow sympathetics back to T1–T4 spinal levels. Pain is referred by CNS to somatic regions innervated by same spinal cord levels

Somatic afferent fiber

**Visceral afferents from heart**

# 4 ABDOMEN

## CONTENTS

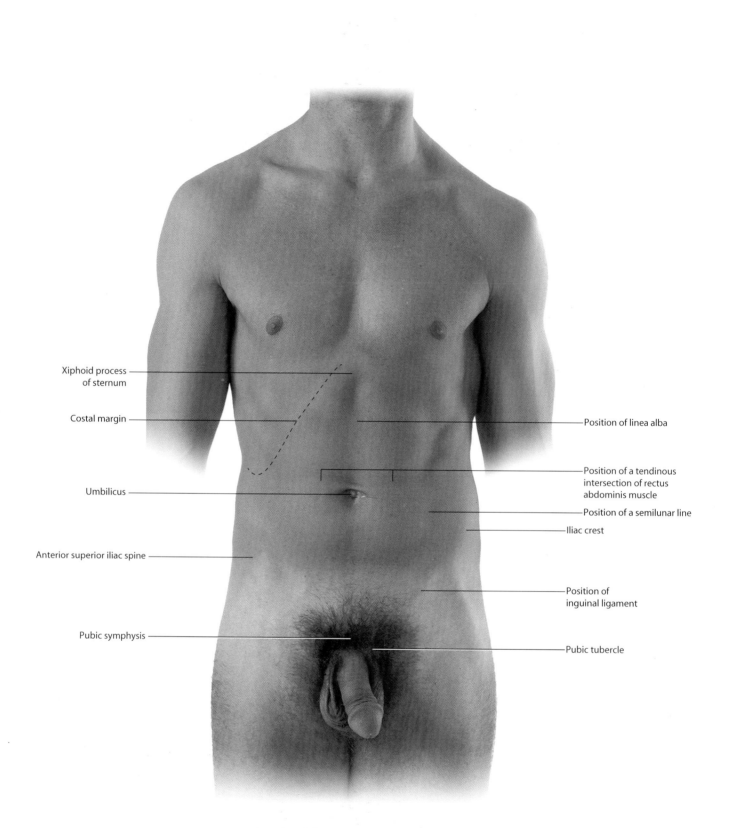

Xiphoid process
of sternum

Costal margin

Umbilicus

Anterior superior iliac spine

Pubic symphysis

Position of linea alba

Position of a tendinous
intersection of rectus
abdominis muscle

Position of a semilunar line

Iliac crest

Position of
inguinal ligament

Pubic tubercle

**Anterior abdominal wall surface anatomy**

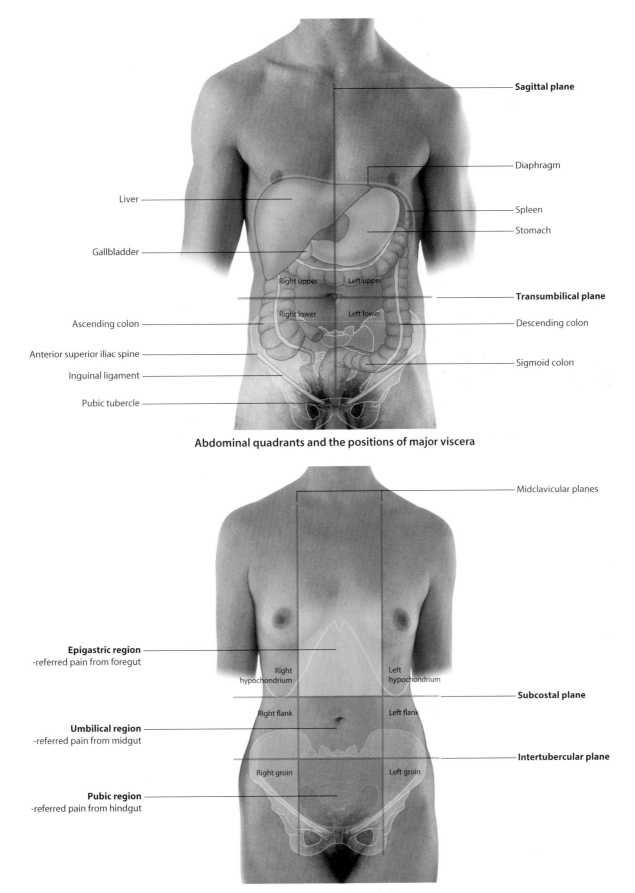

**Sagittal plane**

Diaphragm

Spleen

Stomach

Liver

Gallbladder

Right upper | Left upper

**Transumbilical plane**

Right lower | Left lower

Ascending colon

Descending colon

Anterior superior iliac spine

Inguinal ligament

Sigmoid colon

Pubic tubercle

**Abdominal quadrants and the positions of major viscera**

Midclavicular planes

**Epigastric region**
-referred pain from foregut

Right hypochondrium | Left hypochondrium

**Subcostal plane**

Right flank | Left flank

**Umbilical region**
-referred pain from midgut

**Intertubercular plane**

Right groin | Left groin

**Pubic region**
-referred pain from hindgut

**The nine regions of the abdomen**

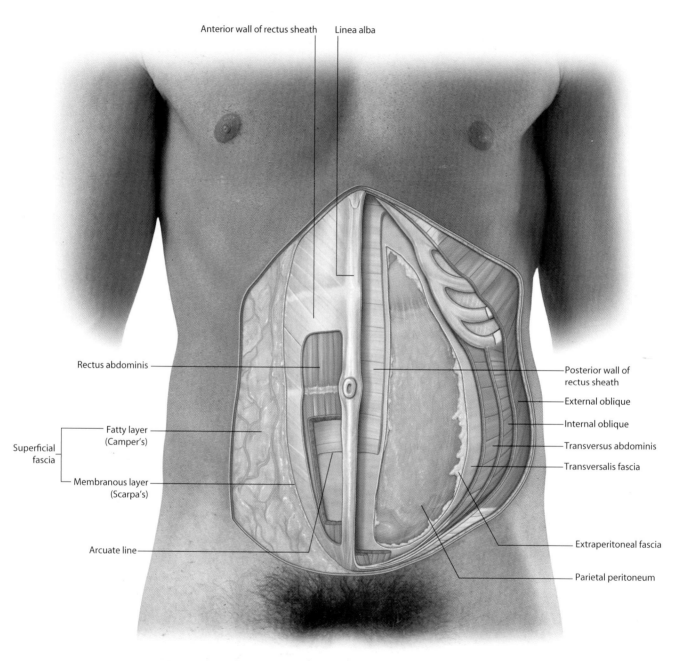

Anterior wall of rectus sheath

Linea alba

Rectus abdominis

Superficial
fascia

Fatty layer
(Camper's)

Membranous layer
(Scarpa's)

Arcuate line

Posterior wall of
rectus sheath

External oblique

Internal oblique

Transversus abdominis

Transversalis fascia

Extraperitoneal fascia

Parietal peritoneum

**Layers of the abdominal wall**

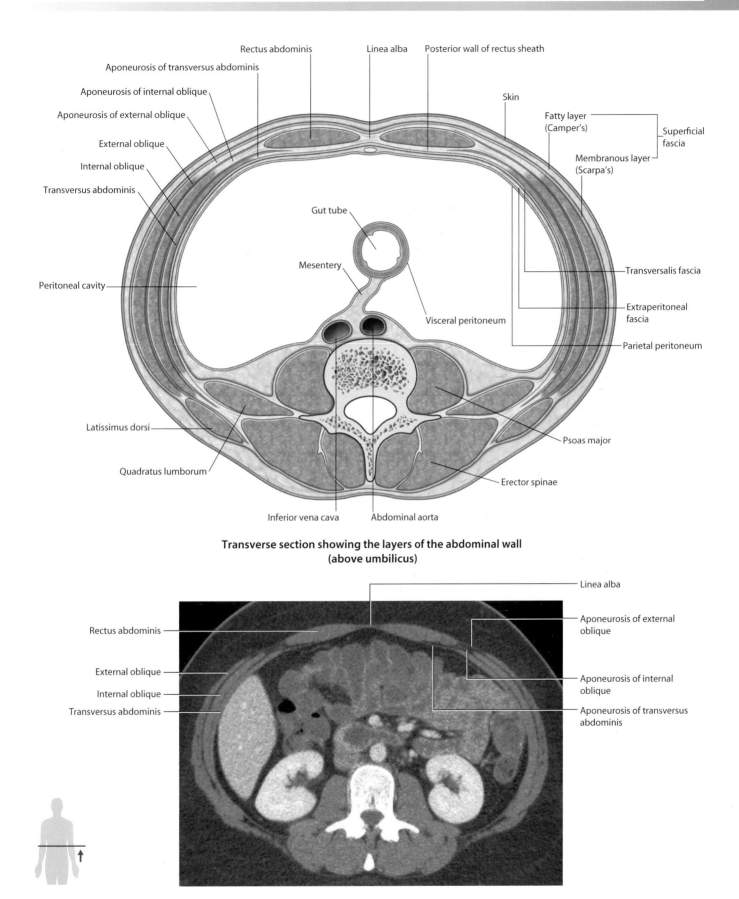

Rectus abdominis

Aponeurosis of transversus abdominis

Aponeurosis of internal oblique

Aponeurosis of external oblique

External oblique

Internal oblique

Transversus abdominis

Peritoneal cavity

Gut tube

Mesentery

Linea alba

Posterior wall of rectus sheath

Skin

Fatty layer (Camper's) ⎤ Superficial
Membranous layer (Scarpa's) ⎦ fascia

Transversalis fascia

Extraperitoneal fascia

Parietal peritoneum

Visceral peritoneum

Latissimus dorsi

Quadratus lumborum

Inferior vena cava

Abdominal aorta

Psoas major

Erector spinae

**Transverse section showing the layers of the abdominal wall
(above umbilicus)**

Linea alba

Rectus abdominis

External oblique

Internal oblique

Transversus abdominis

Aponeurosis of external oblique

Aponeurosis of internal oblique

Aponeurosis of transversus abdominis

**Layers of the abdominal wall.**
CT image, with contrast, in axial plane

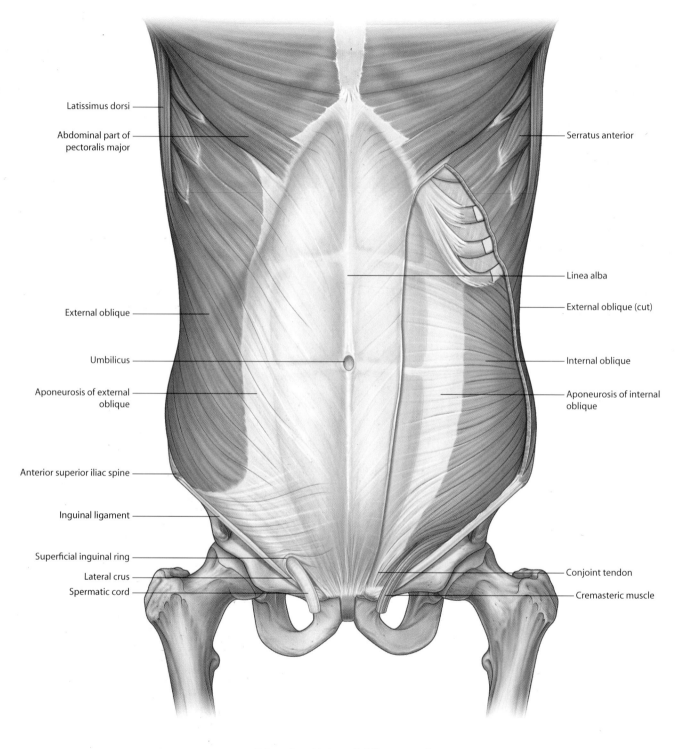

Latissimus dorsi

Abdominal part of
pectoralis major

Serratus anterior

Linea alba

External oblique (cut)

External oblique

Umbilicus

Internal oblique

Aponeurosis of external
oblique

Aponeurosis of internal
oblique

Anterior superior iliac spine

Inguinal ligament

Superficial inguinal ring

Conjoint tendon

Lateral crus

Spermatic cord

Cremasteric muscle

**External and internal oblique muscles**

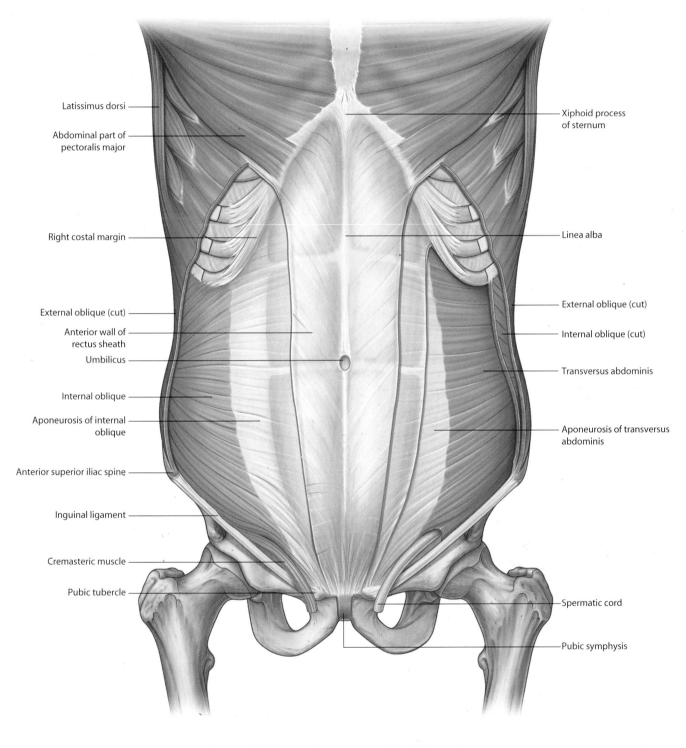

Latissimus dorsi

Abdominal part of
pectoralis major

Right costal margin

External oblique (cut)

Anterior wall of
rectus sheath

Umbilicus

Internal oblique

Aponeurosis of internal
oblique

Anterior superior iliac spine

Inguinal ligament

Cremasteric muscle

Pubic tubercle

Xiphoid process
of sternum

Linea alba

External oblique (cut)

Internal oblique (cut)

Transversus abdominis

Aponeurosis of transversus
abdominis

Spermatic cord

Pubic symphysis

**Internal oblique and transversus abdominis muscles**

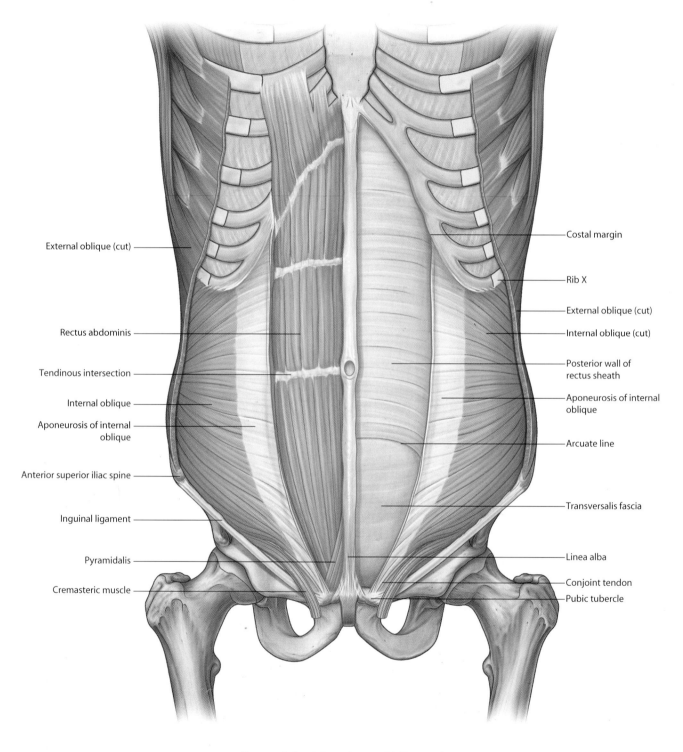

External oblique (cut)

Costal margin

Rib X

External oblique (cut)

Internal oblique (cut)

Rectus abdominis

Posterior wall of
rectus sheath

Tendinous intersection

Aponeurosis of internal
oblique

Internal oblique

Arcuate line

Aponeurosis of internal
oblique

Anterior superior iliac spine

Transversalis fascia

Inguinal ligament

Pyramidalis

Linea alba

Conjoint tendon

Cremasteric muscle

Pubic tubercle

**Rectus abdominis and pyramidalis muscles**

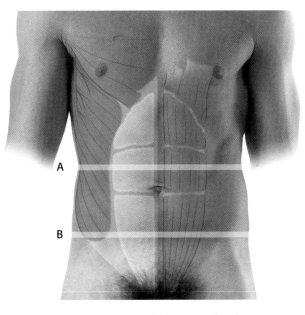

**Organization of the rectus sheath.**
A. Transverse section through the upper three quarters of the rectus sheath
B. Transverse section through the lower one quarter of the rectus sheath

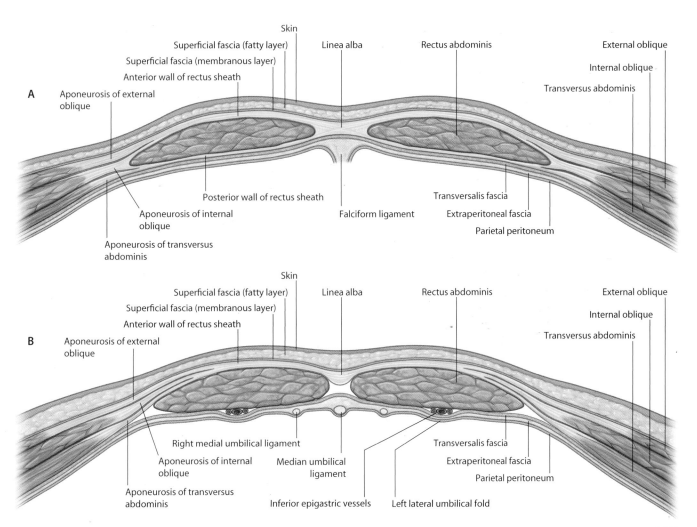

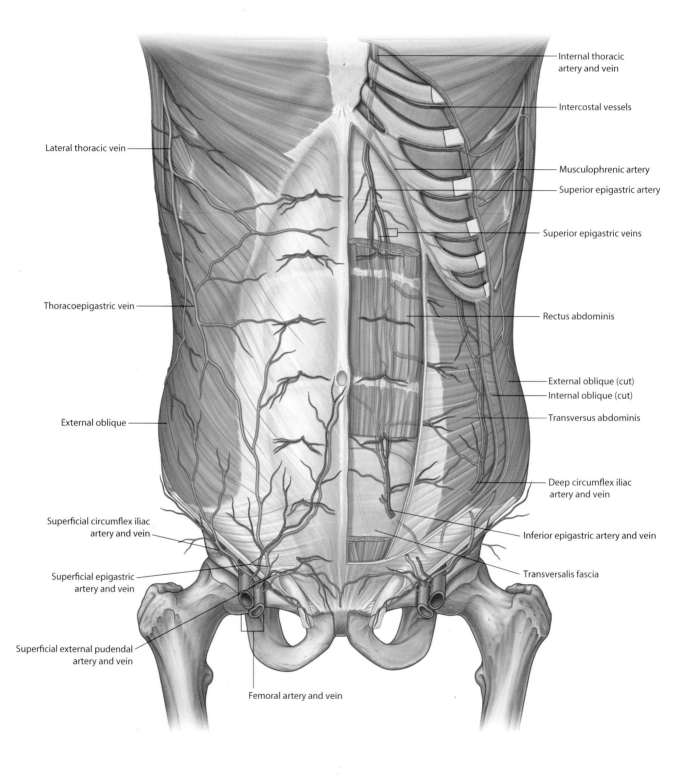

Internal thoracic
artery and vein

Intercostal vessels

Lateral thoracic vein

Musculophrenic artery

Superior epigastric artery

Superior epigastric veins

Thoracoepigastric vein

Rectus abdominis

External oblique (cut)
Internal oblique (cut)

Transversus abdominis

External oblique

Deep circumflex iliac
artery and vein

Superficial circumflex iliac
artery and vein

Inferior epigastric artery and vein

Superficial epigastric
artery and vein

Transversalis fascia

Superficial external pudendal
artery and vein

Femoral artery and vein

**Vasculature of the anterior abdominal wall**

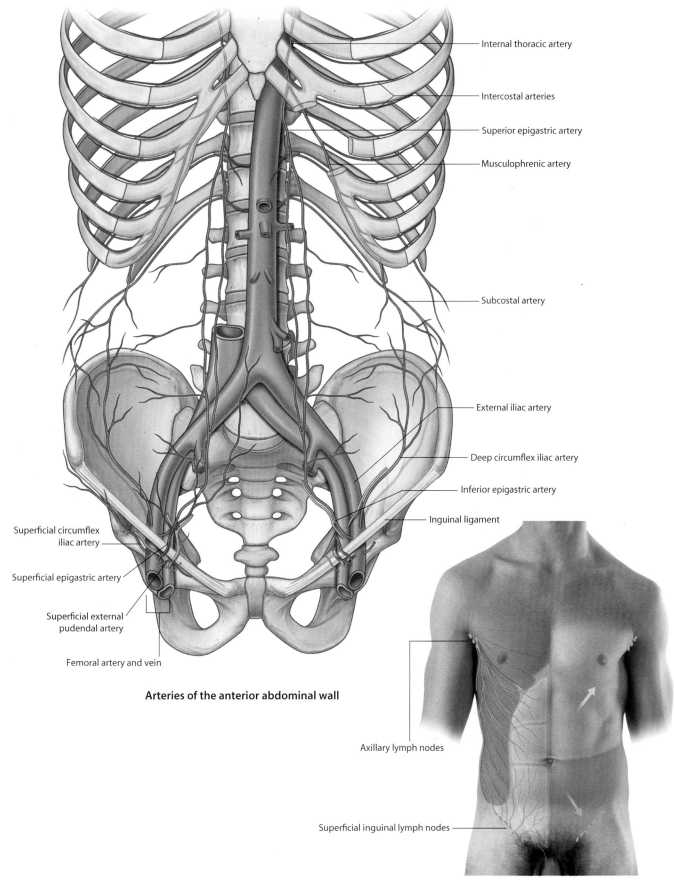

Internal thoracic artery

Intercostal arteries

Superior epigastric artery

Musculophrenic artery

Subcostal artery

External iliac artery

Deep circumflex iliac artery

Inferior epigastric artery

Inguinal ligament

Superficial circumflex
iliac artery

Superficial epigastric artery

Superficial external
pudendal artery

Femoral artery and vein

**Arteries of the anterior abdominal wall**

Axillary lymph nodes

Superficial inguinal lymph nodes

**Superficial lymphatic drainage of the
anterolateral abdominal wall**

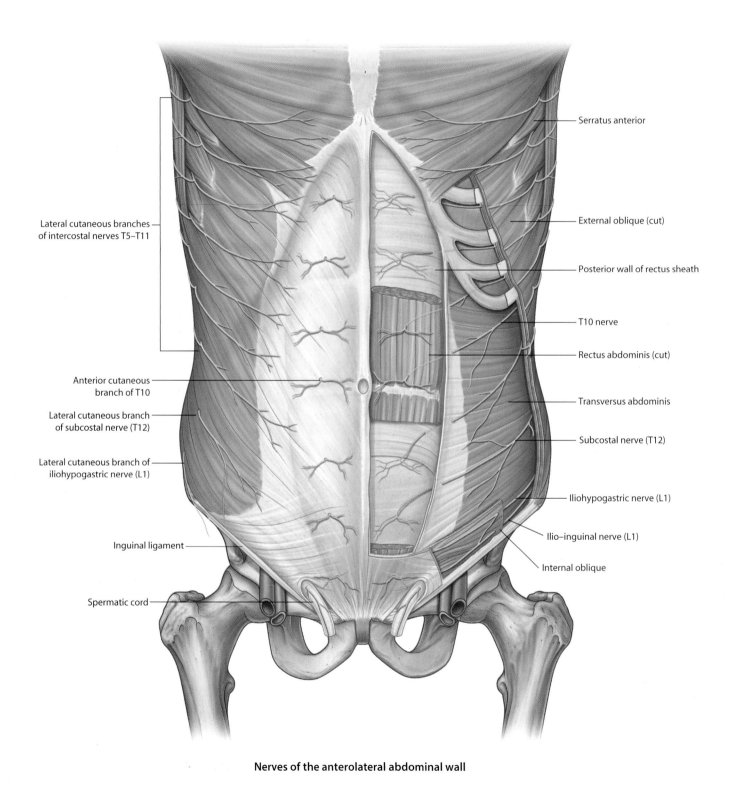

Lateral cutaneous branches of intercostal nerves T5–T11

Anterior cutaneous branch of T10

Lateral cutaneous branch of subcostal nerve (T12)

Lateral cutaneous branch of iliohypogastric nerve (L1)

Inguinal ligament

Spermatic cord

Serratus anterior

External oblique (cut)

Posterior wall of rectus sheath

T10 nerve

Rectus abdominis (cut)

Transversus abdominis

Subcostal nerve (T12)

Iliohypogastric nerve (L1)

Ilio–inguinal nerve (L1)

Internal oblique

**Nerves of the anterolateral abdominal wall**

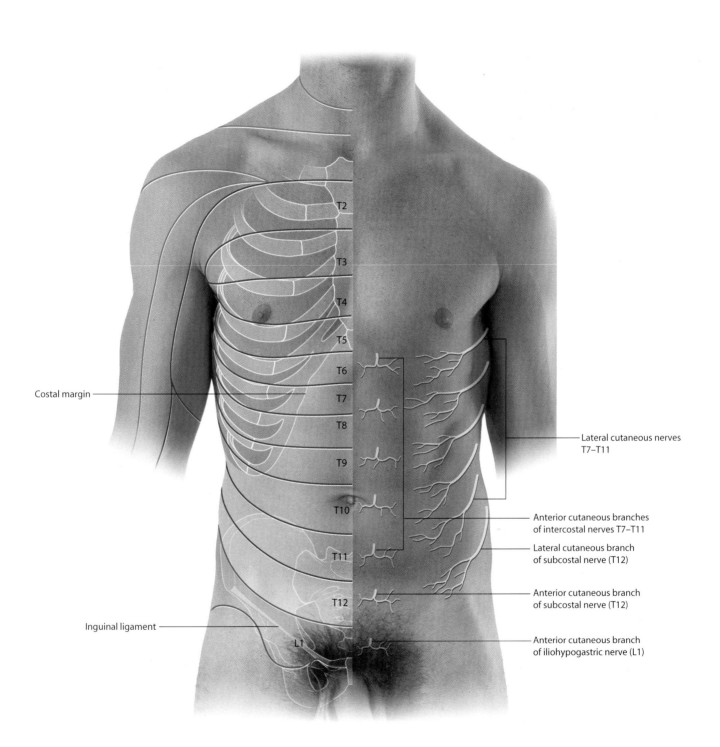

T2
T3
T4
T5
T6
T7
T8
T9
T10
T11
T12
L1

Costal margin

Inguinal ligament

Lateral cutaneous nerves
T7–T11

Anterior cutaneous branches
of intercostal nerves T7–T11

Lateral cutaneous branch
of subcostal nerve (T12)

Anterior cutaneous branch
of subcostal nerve (T12)

Anterior cutaneous branch
of iliohypogastric nerve (L1)

**Dermatomes and cutaneous nerves of the anterolateral abdominal wall**

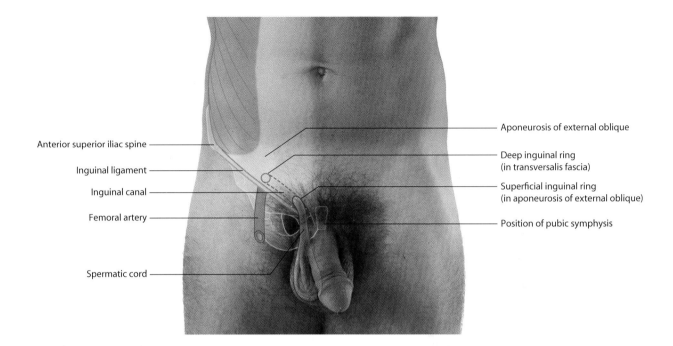

Anterior superior iliac spine

Inguinal ligament

Inguinal canal

Femoral artery

Spermatic cord

Aponeurosis of external oblique

Deep inguinal ring
(in transversalis fascia)

Superficial inguinal ring
(in aponeurosis of external oblique)

Position of pubic symphysis

**Inguinal region in a man**

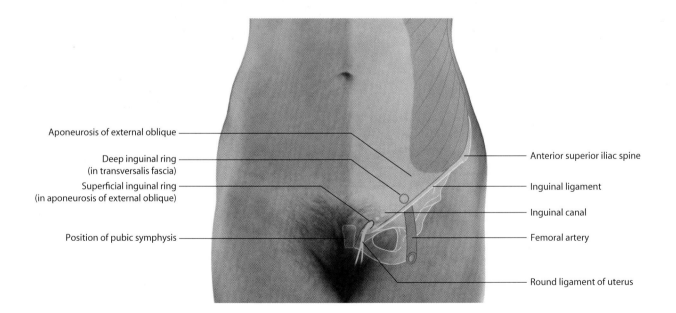

Aponeurosis of external oblique

Deep inguinal ring
(in transversalis fascia)

Superficial inguinal ring
(in aponeurosis of external oblique)

Position of pubic symphysis

Anterior superior iliac spine

Inguinal ligament

Inguinal canal

Femoral artery

Round ligament of uterus

**Inguinal region in a woman**

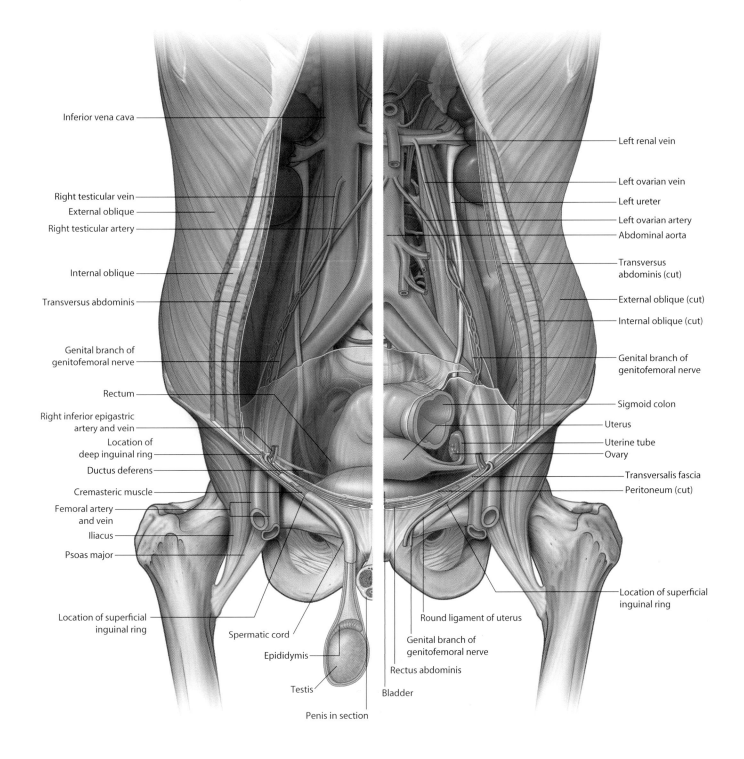

Inferior vena cava

Right testicular vein

External oblique

Right testicular artery

Internal oblique

Transversus abdominis

Genital branch of genitofemoral nerve

Rectum

Right inferior epigastric artery and vein

Location of deep inguinal ring

Ductus deferens

Cremasteric muscle

Femoral artery and vein

Iliacus

Psoas major

Location of superficial inguinal ring

Spermatic cord

Epididymis

Testis

Penis in section

Left renal vein

Left ovarian vein

Left ureter

Left ovarian artery

Abdominal aorta

Transversus abdominis (cut)

External oblique (cut)

Internal oblique (cut)

Genital branch of genitofemoral nerve

Sigmoid colon

Uterus

Uterine tube

Ovary

Transversalis fascia

Peritoneum (cut)

Location of superficial inguinal ring

Round ligament of uterus

Genital branch of genitofemoral nerve

Rectus abdominis

Bladder

**Inguinal region in men**

**Inguinal region in women**

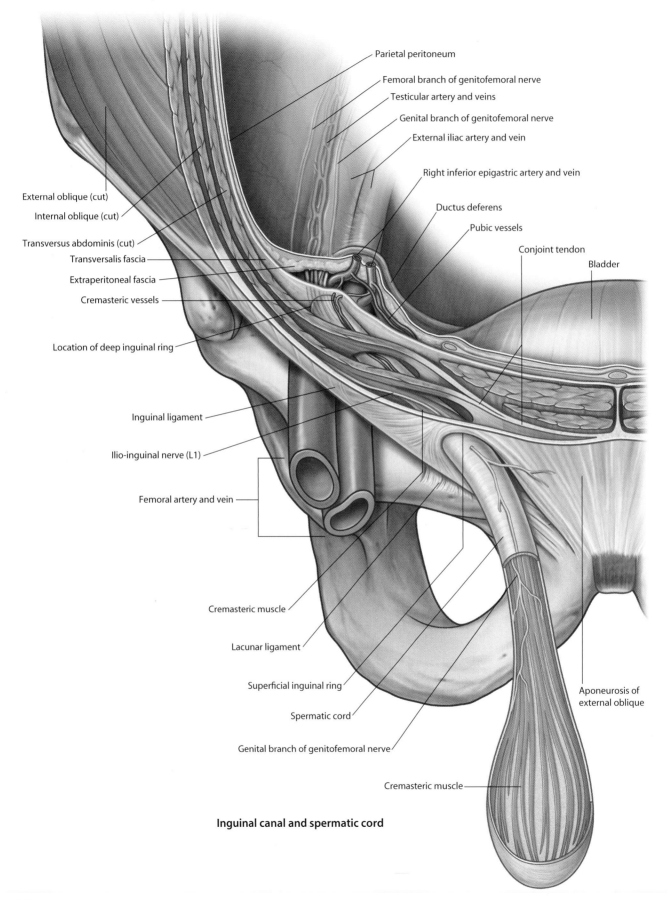

Parietal peritoneum

Femoral branch of genitofemoral nerve

Testicular artery and veins

Genital branch of genitofemoral nerve

External iliac artery and vein

Right inferior epigastric artery and vein

External oblique (cut)

Internal oblique (cut)

Transversus abdominis (cut)

Transversalis fascia

Extraperitoneal fascia

Cremasteric vessels

Ductus deferens

Pubic vessels

Conjoint tendon

Bladder

Location of deep inguinal ring

Inguinal ligament

Ilio-inguinal nerve (L1)

Femoral artery and vein

Cremasteric muscle

Lacunar ligament

Superficial inguinal ring

Spermatic cord

Genital branch of genitofemoral nerve

Aponeurosis of external oblique

Cremasteric muscle

**Inguinal canal and spermatic cord**

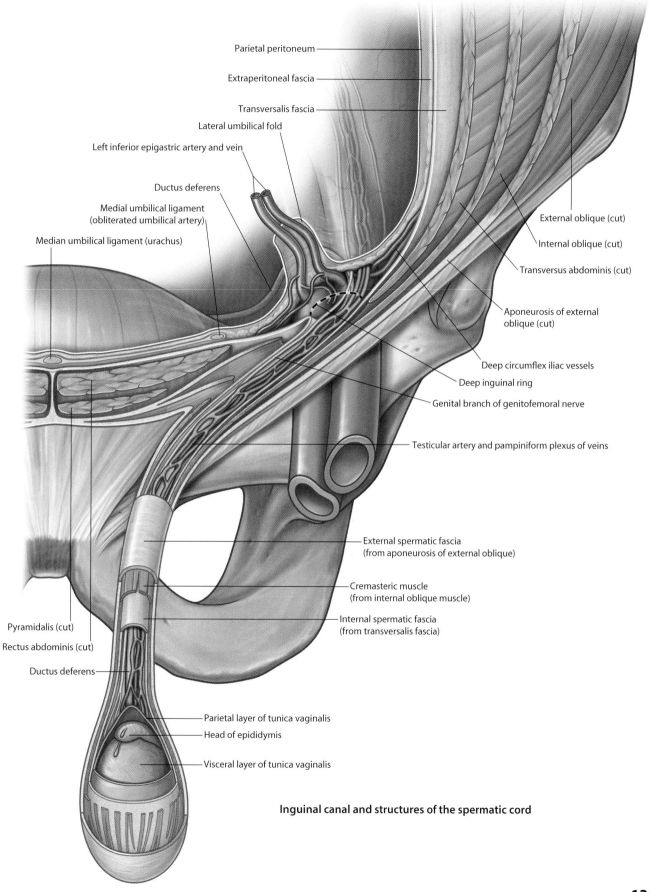

Parietal peritoneum

Extraperitoneal fascia

Transversalis fascia

Lateral umbilical fold

Left inferior epigastric artery and vein

Ductus deferens

Medial umbilical ligament
(obliterated umbilical artery)

Median umbilical ligament (urachus)

External oblique (cut)

Internal oblique (cut)

Transversus abdominis (cut)

Aponeurosis of external
oblique (cut)

Deep circumflex iliac vessels

Deep inguinal ring

Genital branch of genitofemoral nerve

Testicular artery and pampiniform plexus of veins

External spermatic fascia
(from aponeurosis of external oblique)

Cremasteric muscle
(from internal oblique muscle)

Internal spermatic fascia
(from transversalis fascia)

Pyramidalis (cut)

Rectus abdominis (cut)

Ductus deferens

Parietal layer of tunica vaginalis

Head of epididymis

Visceral layer of tunica vaginalis

**Inguinal canal and structures of the spermatic cord**

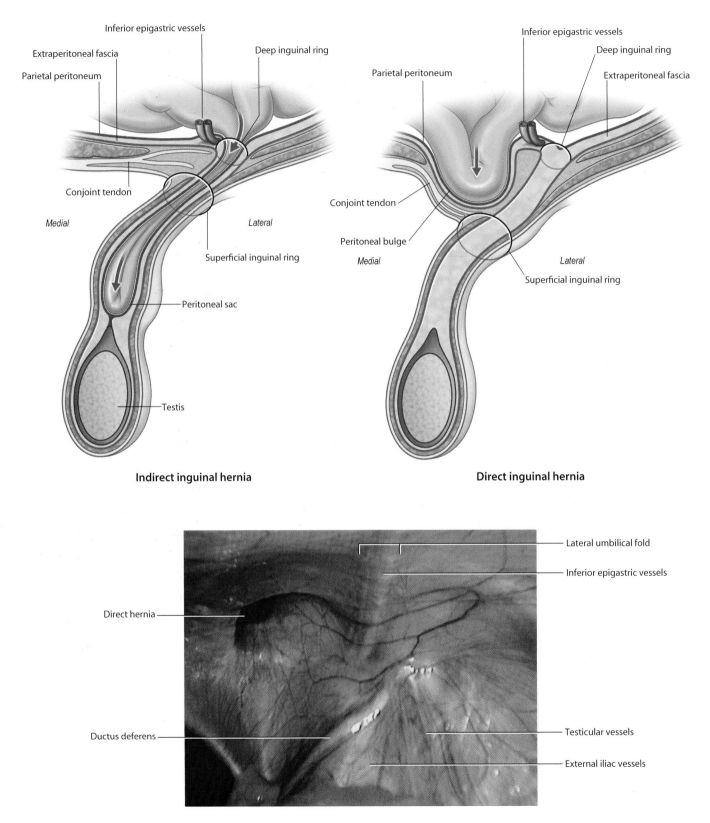

**Indirect inguinal hernia**

**Direct inguinal hernia**

**Right inguinal triangle.**
Laparoscopic view showing the parietal peritoneum still covering the area
(inside the peritoneal cavity looking anteroinferior)

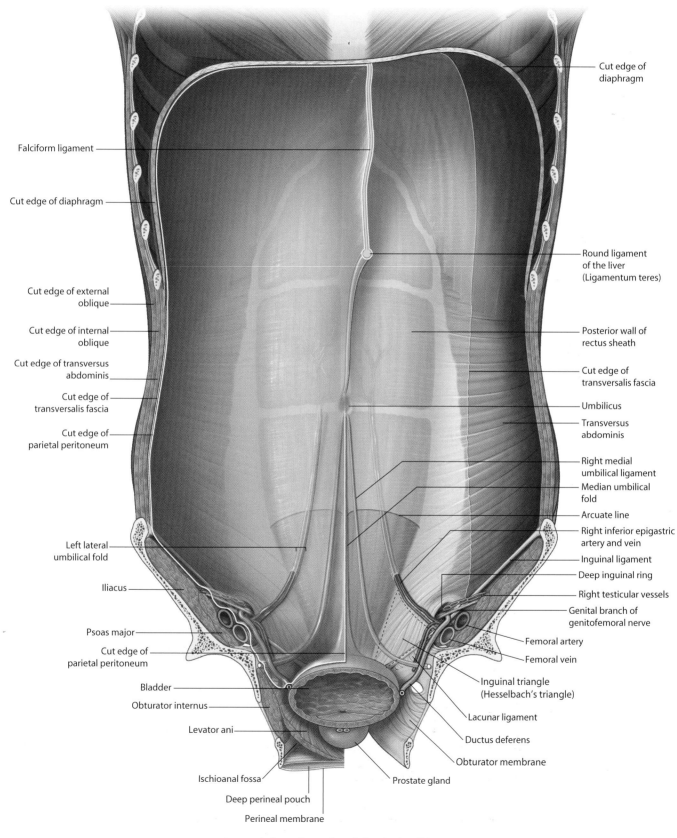

Cut edge of diaphragm

Falciform ligament

Cut edge of diaphragm

Round ligament of the liver (Ligamentum teres)

Cut edge of external oblique

Posterior wall of rectus sheath

Cut edge of internal oblique

Cut edge of transversus abdominis

Cut edge of transversalis fascia

Cut edge of transversalis fascia

Umbilicus

Transversus abdominis

Cut edge of parietal peritoneum

Right medial umbilical ligament

Median umbilical fold

Arcuate line

Right inferior epigastric artery and vein

Left lateral umbilical fold

Inguinal ligament

Deep inguinal ring

Iliacus

Right testicular vessels

Genital branch of genitofemoral nerve

Psoas major

Femoral artery

Cut edge of parietal peritoneum

Femoral vein

Bladder

Inguinal triangle (Hesselbach's triangle)

Obturator internus

Lacunar ligament

Levator ani

Ductus deferens

Obturator membrane

Ischioanal fossa

Prostate gland

Deep perineal pouch

Perineal membrane

**Internal view of anterior abdominal wall in men**

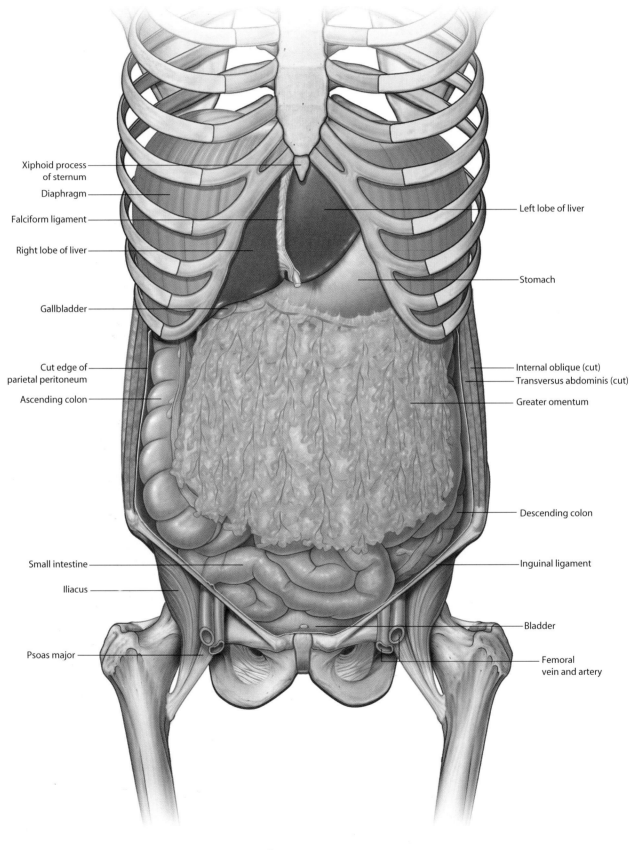

Xiphoid process
of sternum

Diaphragm

Falciform ligament

Right lobe of liver

Gallbladder

Cut edge of
parietal peritoneum

Ascending colon

Small intestine

Iliacus

Psoas major

Left lobe of liver

Stomach

Internal oblique (cut)

Transversus abdominis (cut)

Greater omentum

Descending colon

Inguinal ligament

Bladder

Femoral
vein and artery

**Greater omentum**

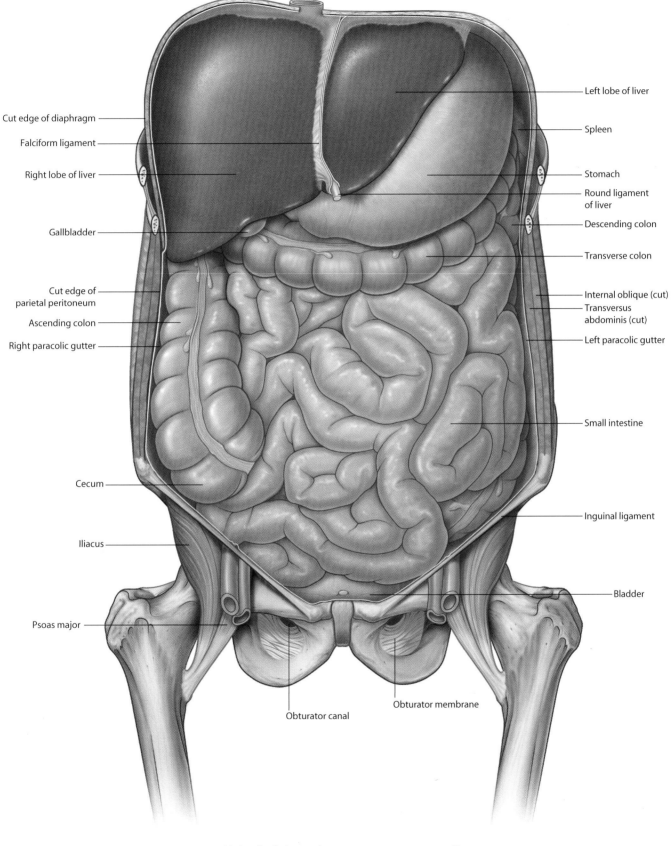

Cut edge of diaphragm

Falciform ligament

Right lobe of liver

Gallbladder

Cut edge of parietal peritoneum

Ascending colon

Right paracolic gutter

Cecum

Iliacus

Psoas major

Left lobe of liver

Spleen

Stomach

Round ligament of liver

Descending colon

Transverse colon

Internal oblique (cut)

Transversus abdominis (cut)

Left paracolic gutter

Small intestine

Inguinal ligament

Bladder

Obturator membrane

Obturator canal

**Abdominal viscera (greater omentum removed)**

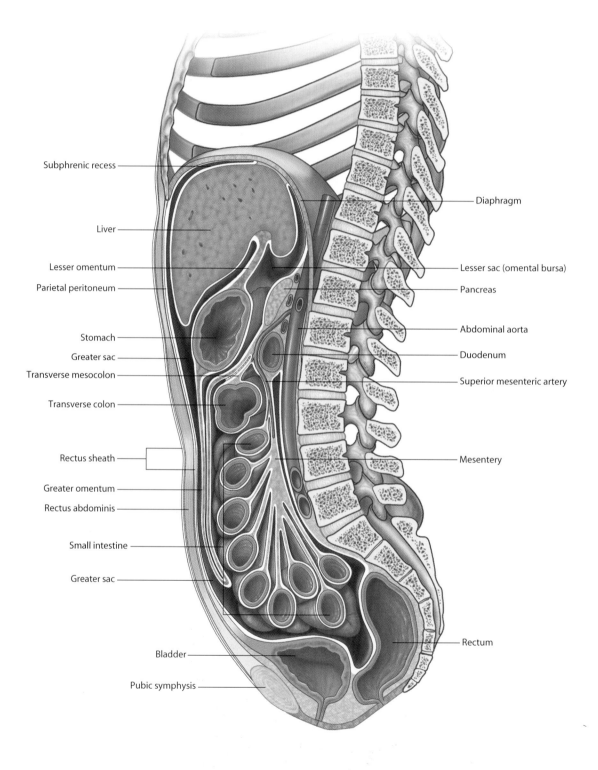

Subphrenic recess

Liver

Lesser omentum

Parietal peritoneum

Stomach

Greater sac

Transverse mesocolon

Transverse colon

Rectus sheath

Greater omentum

Rectus abdominis

Small intestine

Greater sac

Bladder

Pubic symphysis

Diaphragm

Lesser sac (omental bursa)

Pancreas

Abdominal aorta

Duodenum

Superior mesenteric artery

Mesentery

Rectum

**Greater and lesser sacs of the peritoneal cavity**

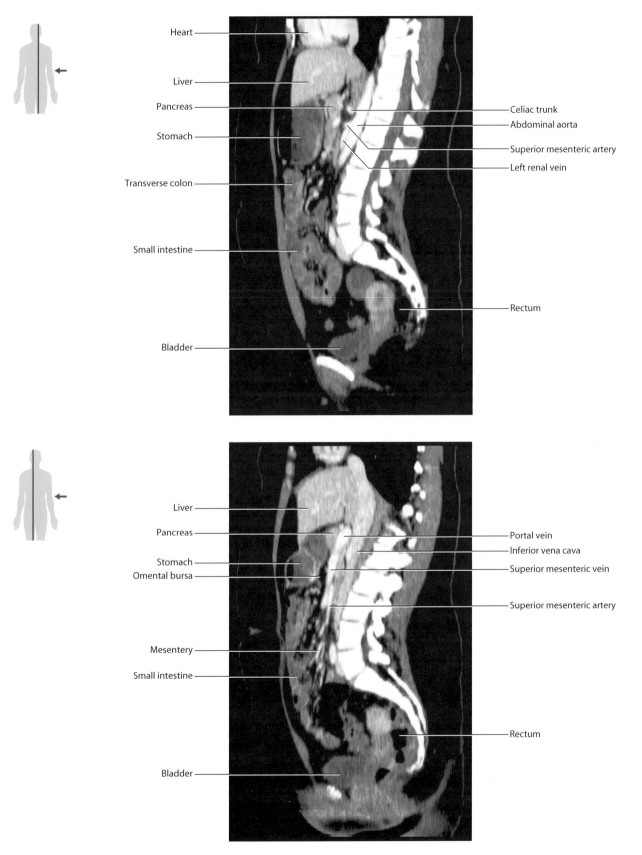

Heart
Liver
Pancreas
Stomach
Transverse colon
Small intestine
Bladder

Celiac trunk
Abdominal aorta
Superior mesenteric artery
Left renal vein

Rectum

Liver
Pancreas
Stomach
Omental bursa
Mesentery
Small intestine
Bladder

Portal vein
Inferior vena cava
Superior mesenteric vein
Superior mesenteric artery

Rectum

**Arrangement of abdominal contents in peritoneal cavity.**
CT images with contrast, in sagittal plane

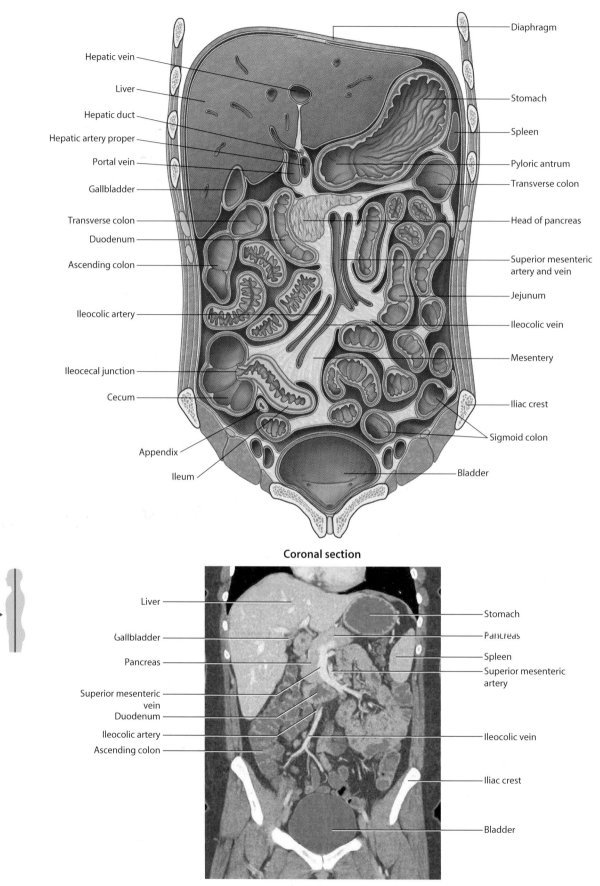

**Coronal section**

**Coronal section.**
CT image with contrast, in coronal plane

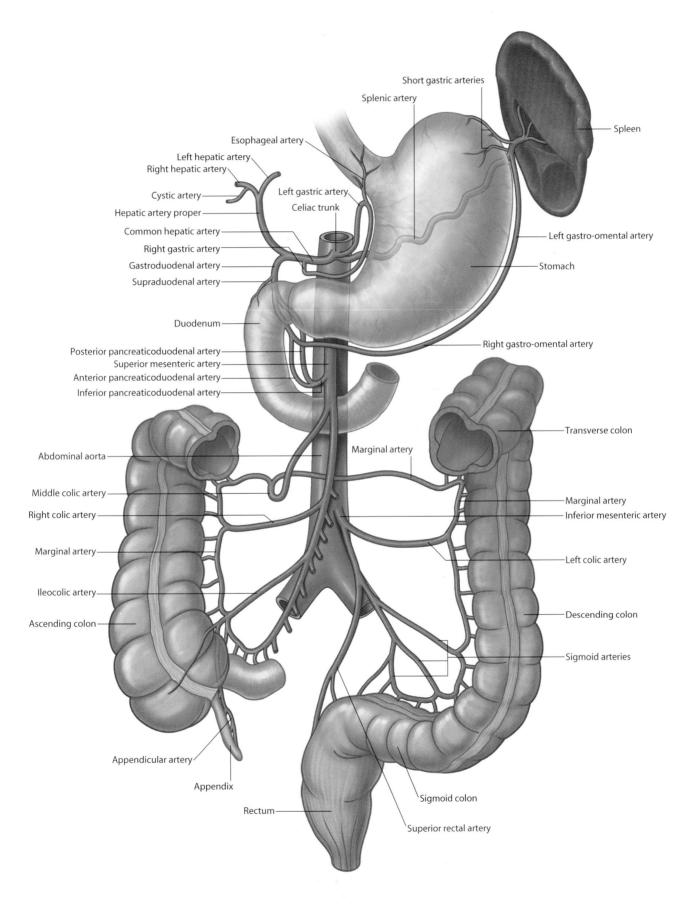

Short gastric arteries

Splenic artery

Esophageal artery

Left hepatic artery

Right hepatic artery

Cystic artery

Left gastric artery

Hepatic artery proper

Celiac trunk

Common hepatic artery

Right gastric artery

Gastroduodenal artery

Supraduodenal artery

Duodenum

Posterior pancreaticoduodenal artery

Superior mesenteric artery

Anterior pancreaticoduodenal artery

Inferior pancreaticoduodenal artery

Abdominal aorta

Middle colic artery

Right colic artery

Marginal artery

Ileocolic artery

Ascending colon

Appendicular artery

Appendix

Rectum

Spleen

Left gastro-omental artery

Stomach

Right gastro-omental artery

Transverse colon

Marginal artery

Marginal artery

Inferior mesenteric artery

Left colic artery

Descending colon

Sigmoid arteries

Sigmoid colon

Superior rectal artery

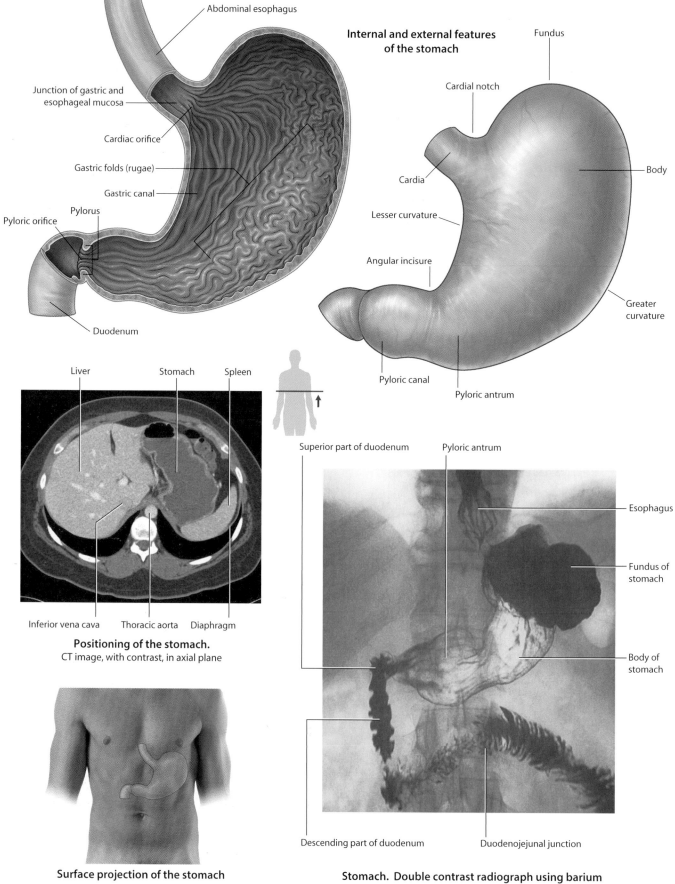

Abdominal esophagus

Junction of gastric and esophageal mucosa

Cardiac orifice

Gastric folds (rugae)

Gastric canal

Pylorus

Pyloric orifice

Duodenum

**Internal and external features of the stomach**

Fundus

Cardial notch

Cardia

Lesser curvature

Angular incisure

Pyloric canal

Pyloric antrum

Body

Greater curvature

Liver    Stomach    Spleen

Inferior vena cava    Thoracic aorta    Diaphragm

**Positioning of the stomach.**
CT image, with contrast, in axial plane

**Surface projection of the stomach**

Superior part of duodenum    Pyloric antrum

Esophagus

Fundus of stomach

Body of stomach

Descending part of duodenum    Duodenojejunal junction

**Stomach. Double contrast radiograph using barium**

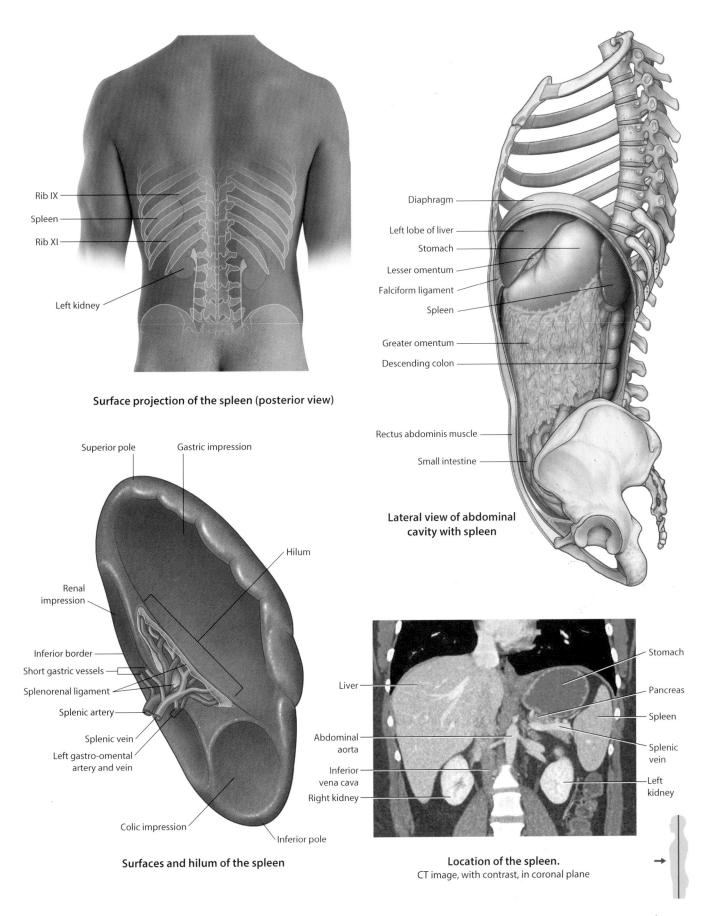

Rib IX
Spleen
Rib XI
Left kidney

**Surface projection of the spleen (posterior view)**

Diaphragm
Left lobe of liver
Stomach
Lesser omentum
Falciform ligament
Spleen
Greater omentum
Descending colon
Rectus abdominis muscle
Small intestine

**Lateral view of abdominal cavity with spleen**

Superior pole
Gastric impression
Hilum
Renal impression
Inferior border
Short gastric vessels
Splenorenal ligament
Splenic artery
Splenic vein
Left gastro-omental artery and vein
Colic impression
Inferior pole

**Surfaces and hilum of the spleen**

Liver
Stomach
Pancreas
Spleen
Abdominal aorta
Splenic vein
Inferior vena cava
Left kidney
Right kidney

**Location of the spleen.**
CT image, with contrast, in coronal plane

**149**

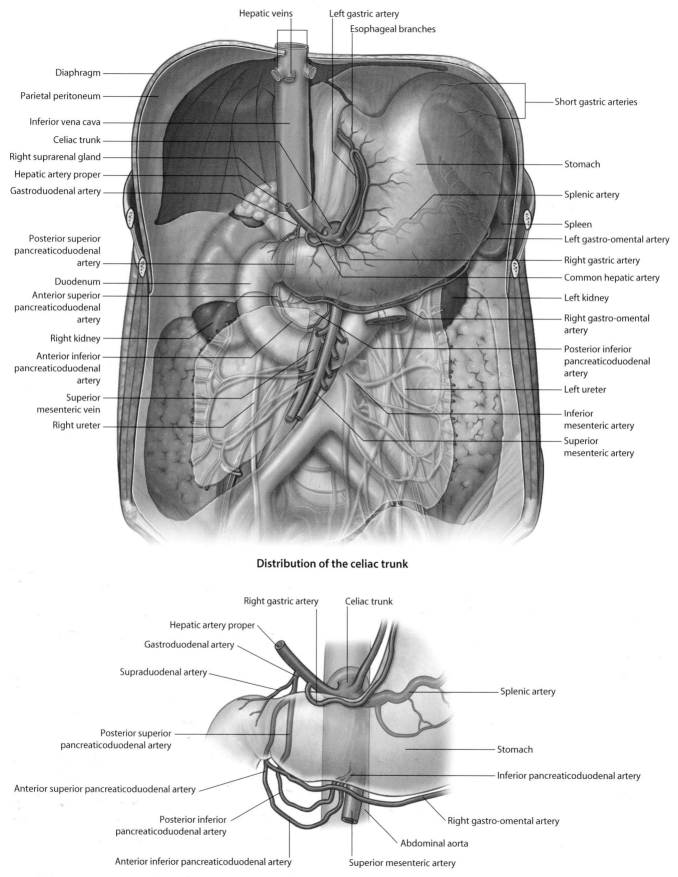

Hepatic veins

Left gastric artery

Esophageal branches

Diaphragm

Parietal peritoneum

Inferior vena cava

Celiac trunk

Right suprarenal gland

Hepatic artery proper

Gastroduodenal artery

Posterior superior pancreaticoduodenal artery

Duodenum

Anterior superior pancreaticoduodenal artery

Right kidney

Anterior inferior pancreaticoduodenal artery

Superior mesenteric vein

Right ureter

Short gastric arteries

Stomach

Splenic artery

Spleen

Left gastro-omental artery

Right gastric artery

Common hepatic artery

Left kidney

Right gastro-omental artery

Posterior inferior pancreaticoduodenal artery

Left ureter

Inferior mesenteric artery

Superior mesenteric artery

**Distribution of the celiac trunk**

Right gastric artery

Celiac trunk

Hepatic artery proper

Gastroduodenal artery

Supraduodenal artery

Splenic artery

Posterior superior pancreaticoduodenal artery

Stomach

Inferior pancreaticoduodenal artery

Anterior superior pancreaticoduodenal artery

Posterior inferior pancreaticoduodenal artery

Right gastro-omental artery

Anterior inferior pancreaticoduodenal artery

Abdominal aorta

Superior mesenteric artery

**Branches of the gastroduodenal artery**

**150**

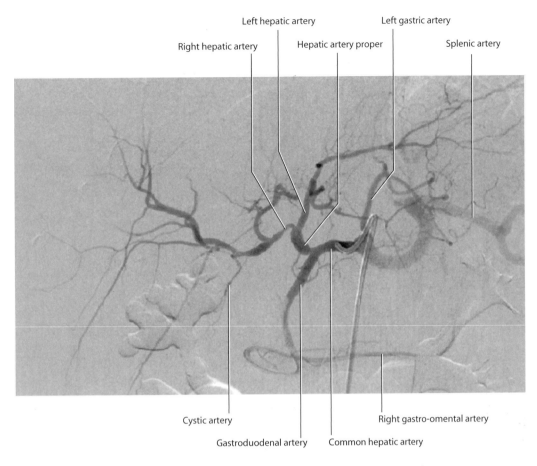

Right hepatic artery    Left hepatic artery    Hepatic artery proper    Left gastric artery    Splenic artery

Cystic artery    Gastroduodenal artery    Common hepatic artery    Right gastro-omental artery

**Digital subtraction angiography of the celiac trunk and its branches**

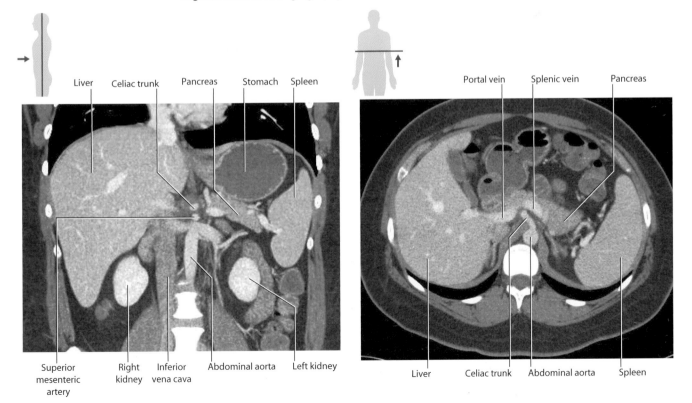

Liver    Celiac trunk    Pancreas    Stomach    Spleen

Superior mesenteric artery    Right kidney    Inferior vena cava    Abdominal aorta    Left kidney

**Positioning of the celiac trunk in relation to other structures.**
CT image, with contrast, in coronal plane

Portal vein    Splenic vein    Pancreas

Liver    Celiac trunk    Abdominal aorta    Spleen

**Branching of the celiac trunk from the abdominal aorta.**
CT image, with contrast, in axial plane

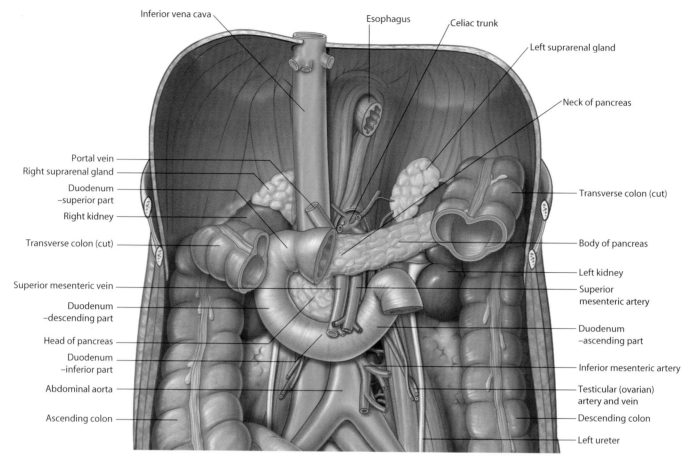

Inferior vena cava

Esophagus

Celiac trunk

Left suprarenal gland

Neck of pancreas

Portal vein

Right suprarenal gland

Duodenum
–superior part

Right kidney

Transverse colon (cut)

Superior mesenteric vein

Duodenum
–descending part

Head of pancreas

Duodenum
–inferior part

Abdominal aorta

Ascending colon

Transverse colon (cut)

Body of pancreas

Left kidney

Superior mesenteric artery

Duodenum
–ascending part

Inferior mesenteric artery

Testicular (ovarian) artery and vein

Descending colon

Left ureter

**Duodenum in situ**

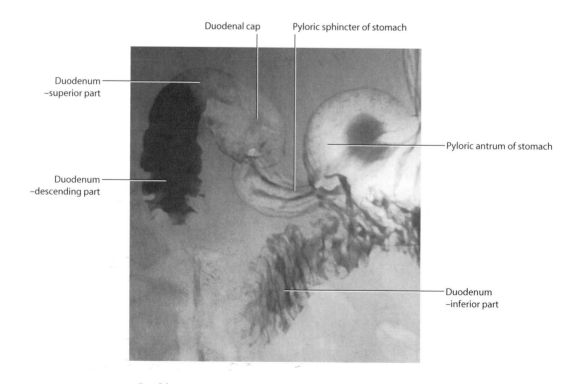

Duodenal cap

Pyloric sphincter of stomach

Duodenum
–superior part

Duodenum
–descending part

Pyloric antrum of stomach

Duodenum
–inferior part

**Double contrast radiograph showing the duodenal cap**

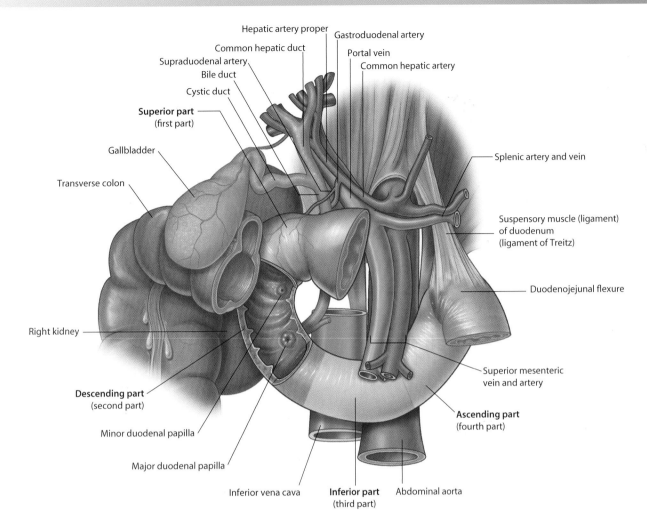

Hepatic artery proper
Common hepatic duct
Supraduodenal artery
Bile duct
Cystic duct
Gastroduodenal artery
Portal vein
Common hepatic artery
**Superior part** (first part)
Gallbladder
Transverse colon
Splenic artery and vein
Suspensory muscle (ligament) of duodenum (ligament of Treitz)
Duodenojejunal flexure
Right kidney
**Descending part** (second part)
Minor duodenal papilla
Major duodenal papilla
Superior mesenteric vein and artery
**Ascending part** (fourth part)
Inferior vena cava
**Inferior part** (third part)
Abdominal aorta

**Parts of the duodenum and related structures**

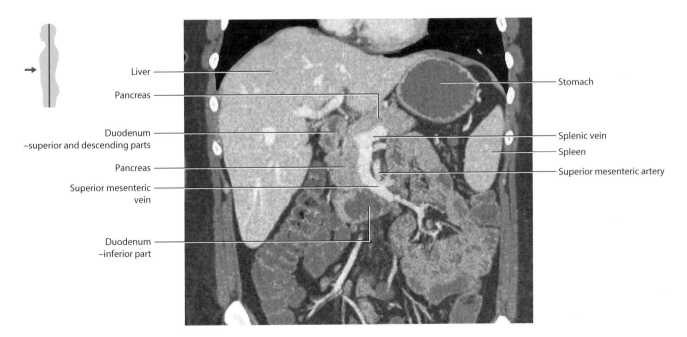

Liver
Pancreas
Duodenum –superior and descending parts
Pancreas
Superior mesenteric vein
Duodenum –inferior part
Stomach
Splenic vein
Spleen
Superior mesenteric artery

**Relationship of duodenum to structures in the vicinity.**
CT image, with contrast, in coronal plane

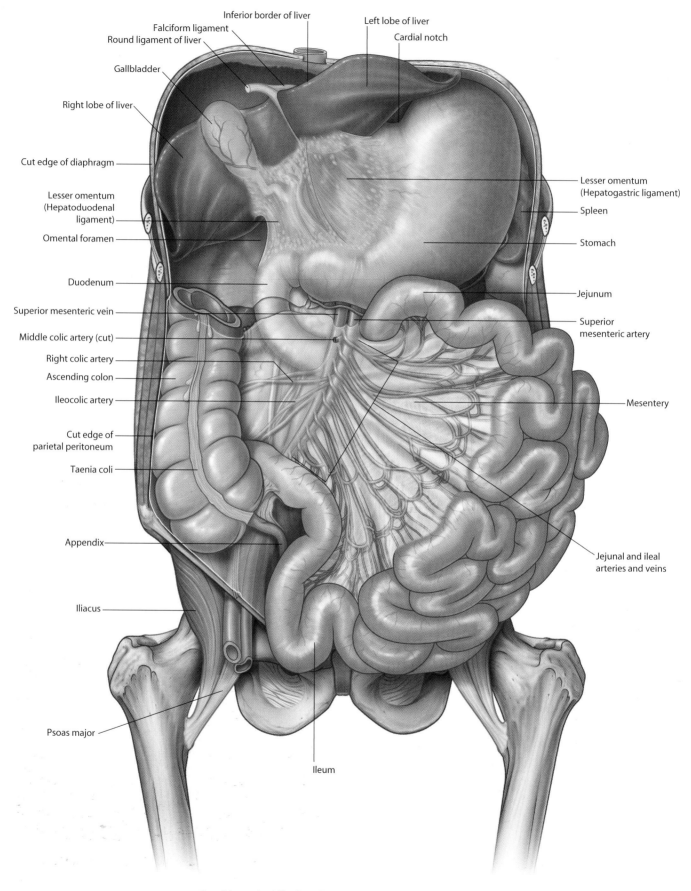

Inferior border of liver

Falciform ligament

Round ligament of liver

Gallbladder

Right lobe of liver

Cut edge of diaphragm

Lesser omentum
(Hepatoduodenal
ligament)

Omental foramen

Duodenum

Superior mesenteric vein

Middle colic artery (cut)

Right colic artery

Ascending colon

Ileocolic artery

Cut edge of
parietal peritoneum

Taenia coli

Appendix

Iliacus

Psoas major

Left lobe of liver

Cardial notch

Lesser omentum
(Hepatogastric ligament)

Spleen

Stomach

Jejunum

Superior
mesenteric artery

Mesentery

Jejunal and ileal
arteries and veins

Ileum

**Small intestine displaced to show superior mesenteric vessels**

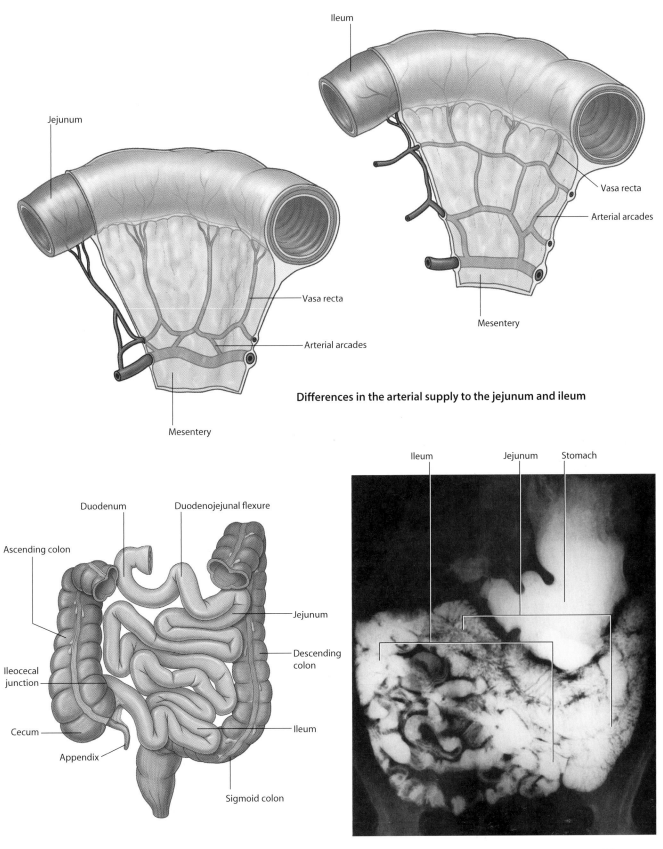

Jejunum

Ileum

Vasa recta

Arterial arcades

Mesentery

Vasa recta

Arterial arcades

Mesentery

**Differences in the arterial supply to the jejunum and ileum**

Duodenum

Duodenojejunal flexure

Ascending colon

Jejunum

Descending colon

Ileocecal junction

Cecum

Ileum

Appendix

Sigmoid colon

**Jejunum and ileum**

Ileum

Jejunum

Stomach

**Radiograph using barium, showing jejunum and ileum**

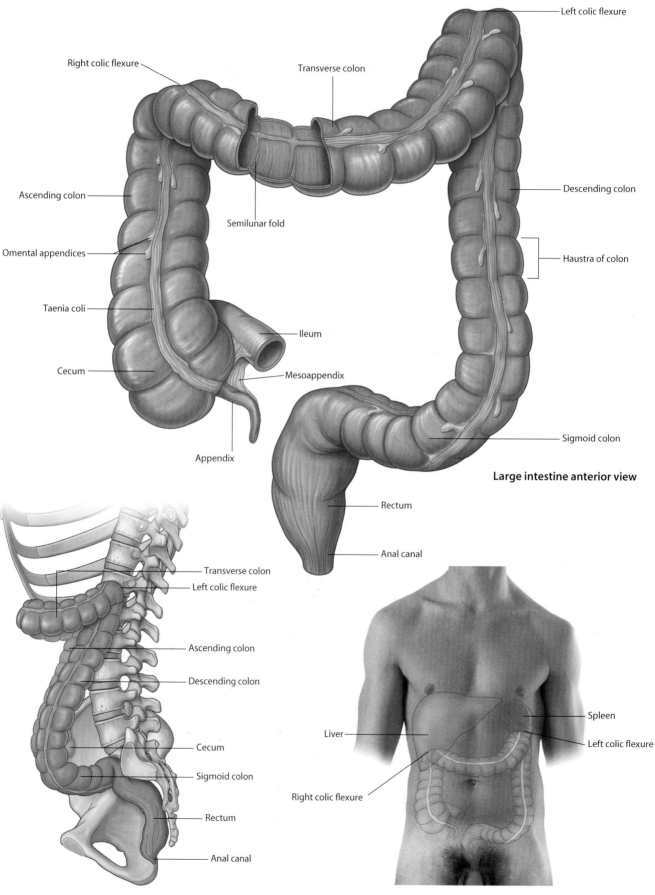

Large intestine anterior view

- Left colic flexure
- Right colic flexure
- Transverse colon
- Ascending colon
- Descending colon
- Semilunar fold
- Omental appendices
- Haustra of colon
- Taenia coli
- Ileum
- Cecum
- Mesoappendix
- Appendix
- Sigmoid colon
- Rectum
- Anal canal

**Large intestine left lateral view**

- Transverse colon
- Left colic flexure
- Ascending colon
- Descending colon
- Cecum
- Sigmoid colon
- Rectum
- Anal canal

**Surface projection of the large intestine**

- Spleen
- Liver
- Left colic flexure
- Right colic flexure

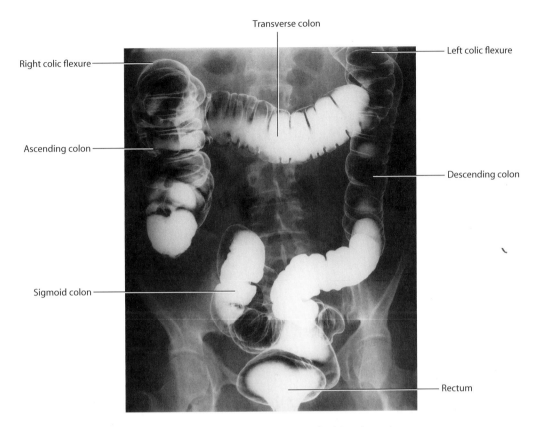

Transverse colon

Right colic flexure

Left colic flexure

Ascending colon

Descending colon

Sigmoid colon

Rectum

**Radiograph using barium showing the large intestine**

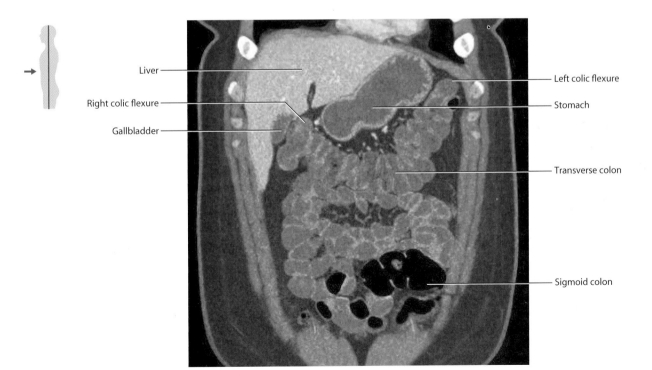

Liver

Left colic flexure

Right colic flexure

Stomach

Gallbladder

Transverse colon

Sigmoid colon

**Transverse colon showing right and left colic flexures.**
CT image, with contrast, in coronal plane

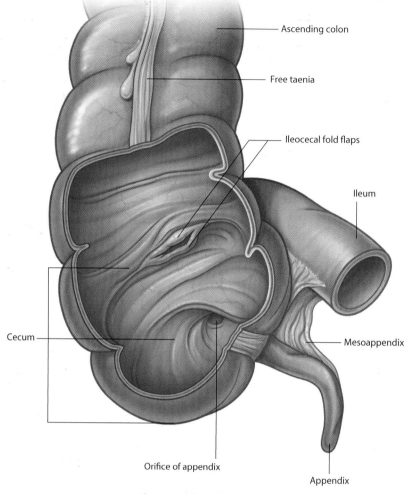

Ascending colon

Free taenia

Ileocecal fold flaps

Ileum

Cecum

Mesoappendix

Orifice of appendix

Appendix

**Ileocecal junction**

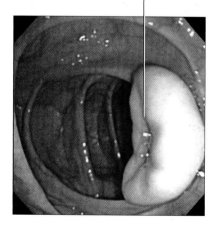

Ileocecal fold

**Colonoscopy showing ileocecal fold**

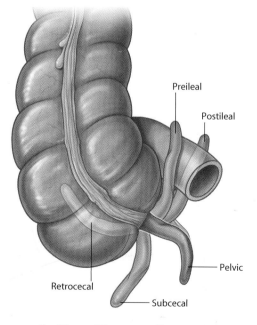

Preileal

Postileal

Retrocecal

Subcecal

Pelvic

**Positions of the appendix**

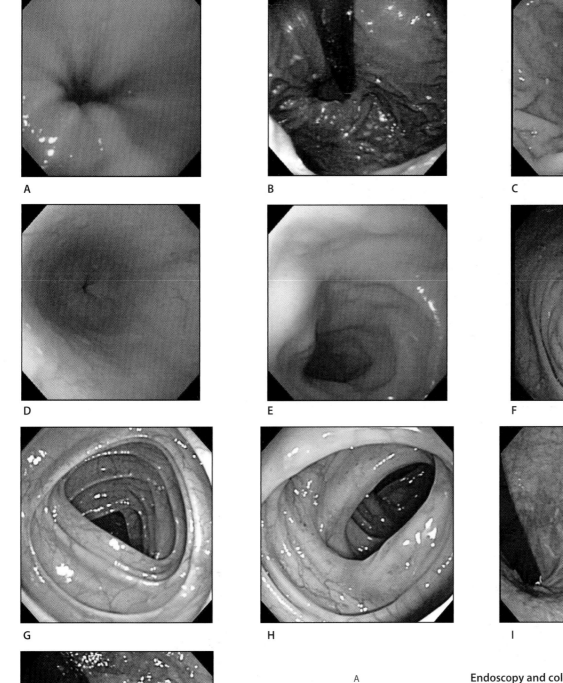

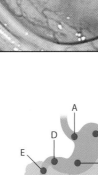

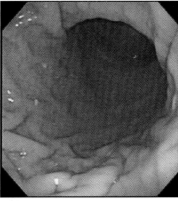

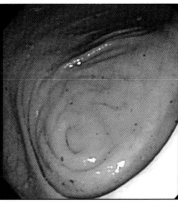

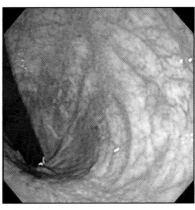

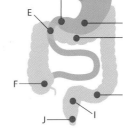

**Endoscopy and colonoscopy showing different parts of the gastrointestinal tract.**

A. Gastroesophageal junction
B. Cardiac orifice and fundus of stomach-retroflexed view
C. Body of stomach
D. Pylorus of stomach and pyloric sphincter
E. Duodenum
F. Cecum showing appendiceal opening.
G. Transverse colon
H. Sigmoid colon
I. Rectum-retroflexed view
J. Pectinate line

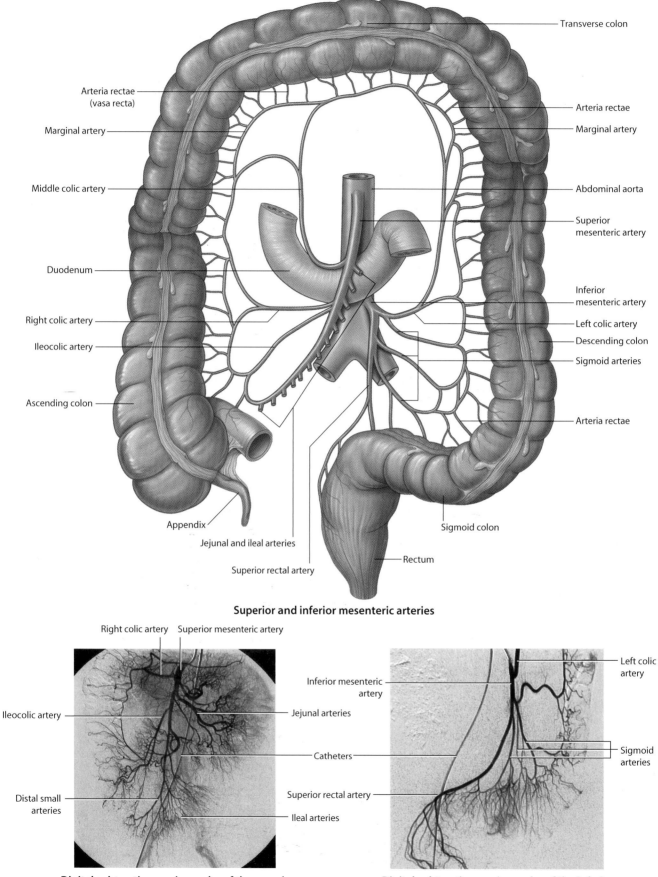

Transverse colon

Arteria rectae
(vasa recta)

Arteria rectae

Marginal artery

Marginal artery

Middle colic artery

Abdominal aorta

Superior
mesenteric artery

Duodenum

Inferior
mesenteric artery

Right colic artery

Left colic artery

Ileocolic artery

Descending colon

Sigmoid arteries

Ascending colon

Arteria rectae

Appendix

Sigmoid colon

Jejunal and ileal arteries

Rectum

Superior rectal artery

**Superior and inferior mesenteric arteries**

Right colic artery   Superior mesenteric artery

Left colic
artery

Inferior mesenteric
artery

Ileocolic artery

Jejunal arteries

Sigmoid
arteries

Catheters

Distal small
arteries

Superior rectal artery

Ileal arteries

**Digital subtraction angiography of the superior
mesenteric artery and its branches**

**Digital subtraction angiography of the inferior
mesenteric artery and its branches**

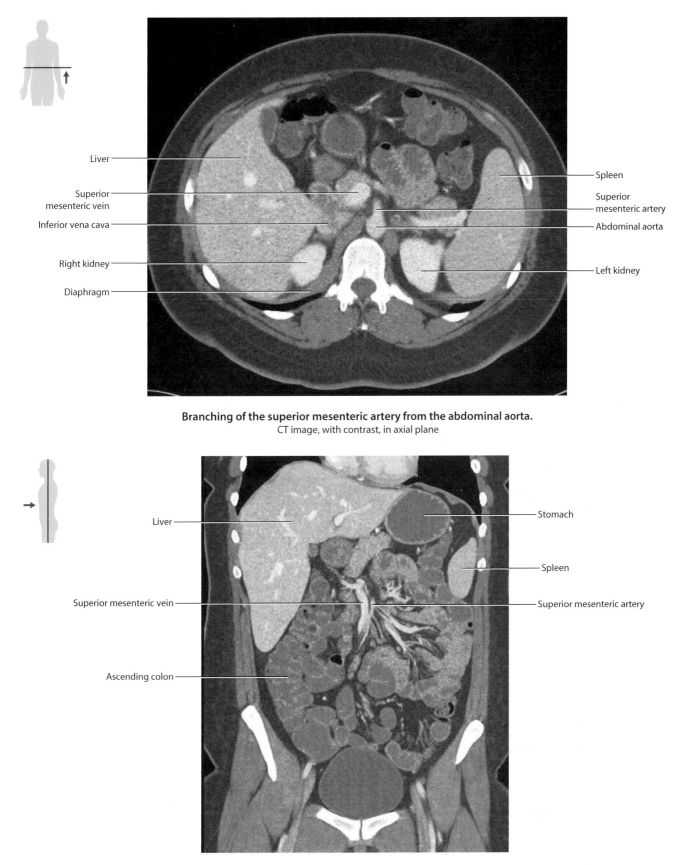

**Branching of the superior mesenteric artery from the abdominal aorta.**
CT image, with contrast, in axial plane

**Positioning of the superior mesenteric artery in relation to other structures.**
CT image, with contrast, in coronal plane

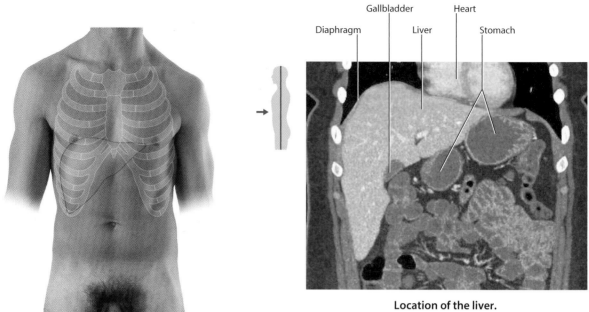

**Surface projection of the liver anterior view**

**Location of the liver.**
CT image, with contrast, in coronal plane

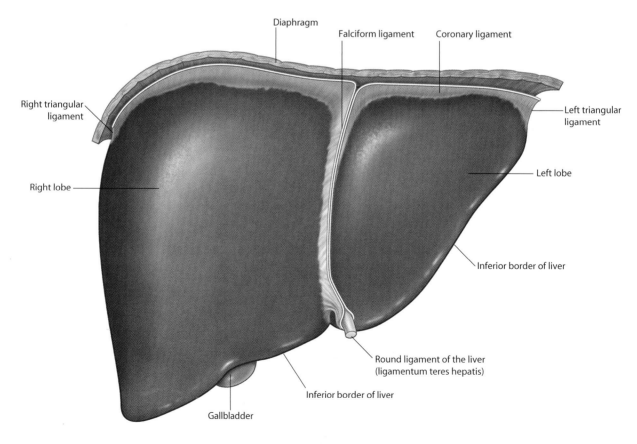

**Anterior surface of liver**

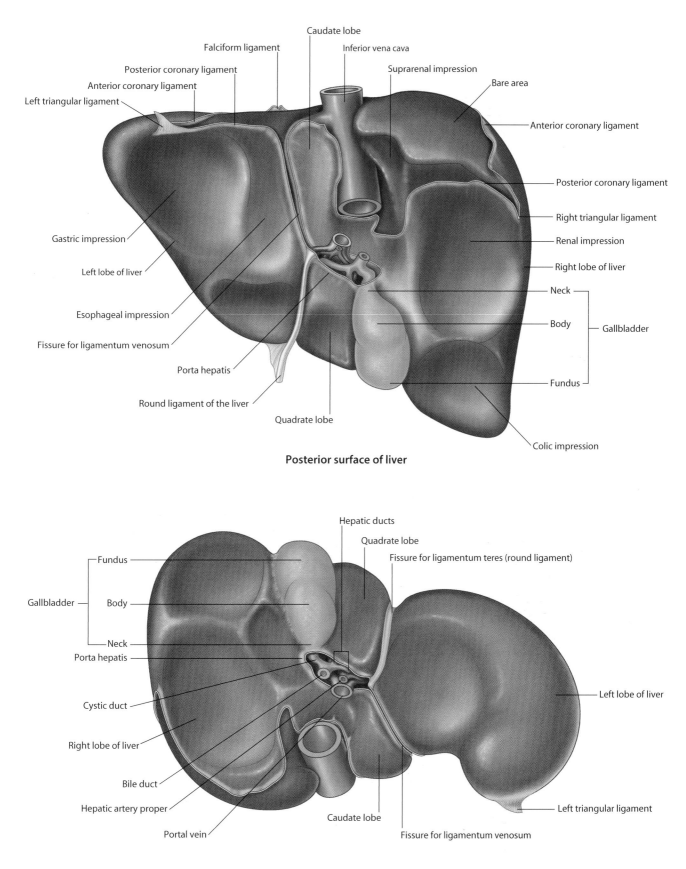

**Posterior surface of liver**

Caudate lobe
Falciform ligament
Inferior vena cava
Posterior coronary ligament
Suprarenal impression
Anterior coronary ligament
Bare area
Left triangular ligament
Anterior coronary ligament
Posterior coronary ligament
Right triangular ligament
Gastric impression
Renal impression
Left lobe of liver
Right lobe of liver
Neck
Esophageal impression
Body ⎤ Gallblabber
Fissure for ligamentum venosum
Porta hepatis
Fundus ⎦
Round ligament of the liver
Quadrate lobe
Colic impression

**Visceral surface of liver**

Hepatic ducts
Quadrate lobe
Fundus ⎤
Fissure for ligamentum teres (round ligament)
Gallbladder ⎱ Body
Neck ⎦
Porta hepatis
Left lobe of liver
Cystic duct
Right lobe of liver
Bile duct
Left triangular ligament
Hepatic artery proper
Caudate lobe
Portal vein
Fissure for ligamentum venosum

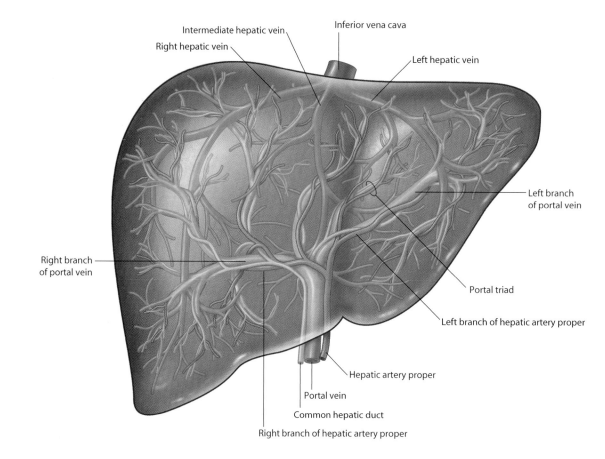

Anterior surface of liver with hepatic veins, portal vein, and associated vessels

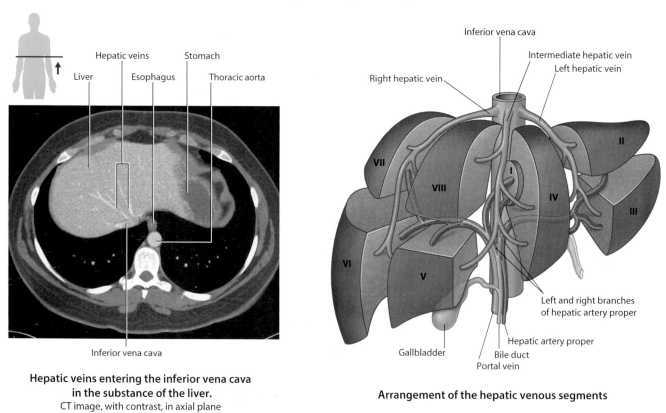

**Hepatic veins entering the inferior vena cava in the substance of the liver.**
CT image, with contrast, in axial plane

**Arrangement of the hepatic venous segments**

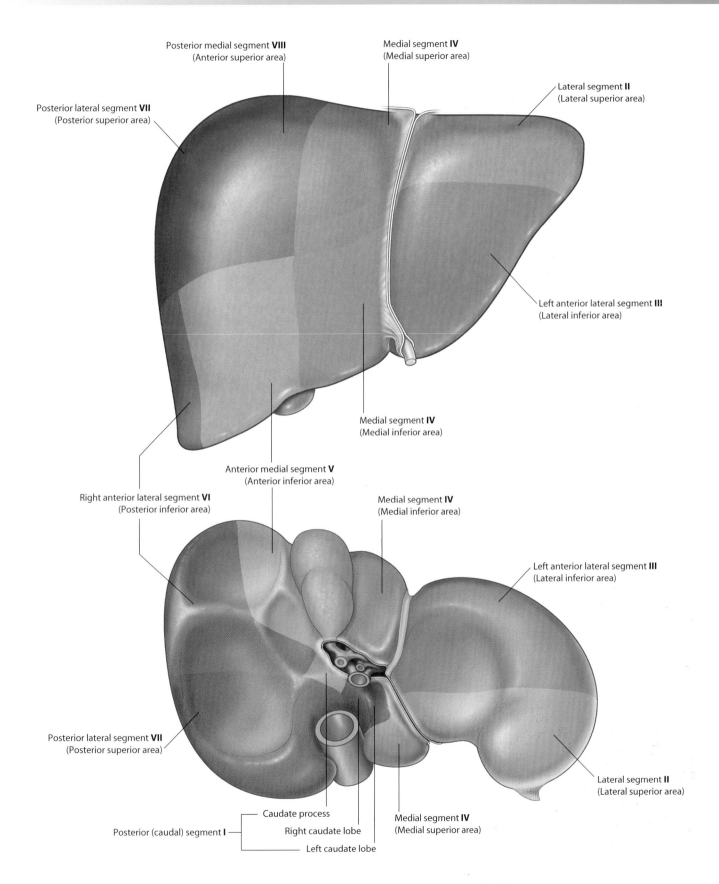

Posterior medial segment **VIII**
(Anterior superior area)

Medial segment **IV**
(Medial superior area)

Lateral segment **II**
(Lateral superior area)

Posterior lateral segment **VII**
(Posterior superior area)

Left anterior lateral segment **III**
(Lateral inferior area)

Medial segment **IV**
(Medial inferior area)

Anterior medial segment **V**
(Anterior inferior area)

Right anterior lateral segment **VI**
(Posterior inferior area)

Medial segment **IV**
(Medial inferior area)

Left anterior lateral segment **III**
(Lateral inferior area)

Posterior lateral segment **VII**
(Posterior superior area)

Lateral segment **II**
(Lateral superior area)

Caudate process

Posterior (caudal) segment **I**

Right caudate lobe

Left caudate lobe

Medial segment **IV**
(Medial superior area)

**Segments of the liver shown on anterior and visceral surfaces**

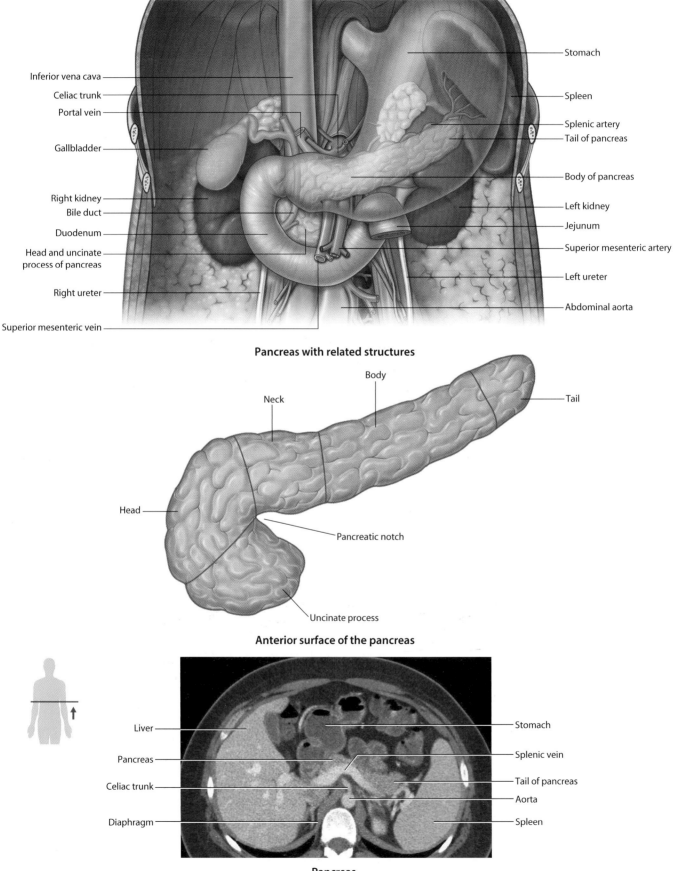

**Pancreas with related structures**

**Anterior surface of the pancreas**

**Pancreas.**
CT image, with contrast, in axial plane

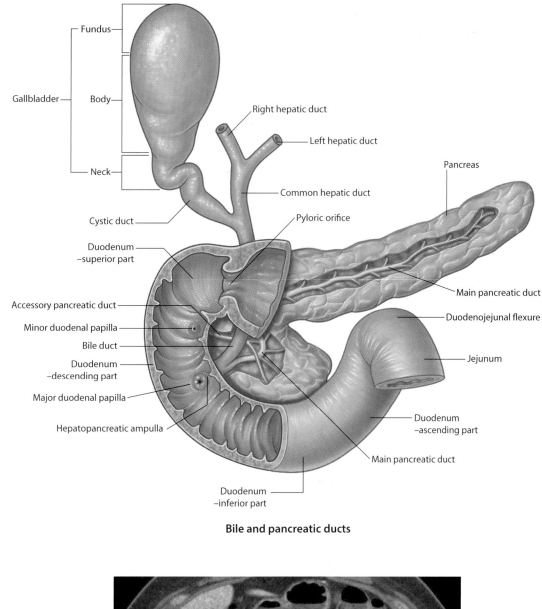

- Fundus
- Gallbladder
  - Body
  - Neck
- Right hepatic duct
- Left hepatic duct
- Pancreas
- Common hepatic duct
- Cystic duct
- Pyloric orifice
- Duodenum –superior part
- Accessory pancreatic duct
- Minor duodenal papilla
- Bile duct
- Duodenum –descending part
- Major duodenal papilla
- Hepatopancreatic ampulla
- Main pancreatic duct
- Duodenojejunal flexure
- Jejunum
- Duodenum –ascending part
- Main pancreatic duct
- Duodenum –inferior part

**Bile and pancreatic ducts**

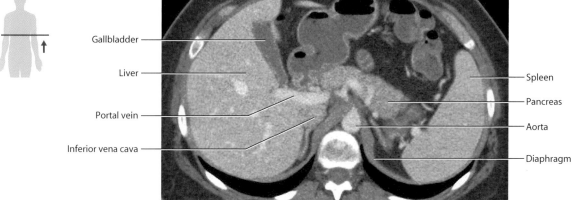

- Gallbladder
- Liver
- Portal vein
- Inferior vena cava
- Spleen
- Pancreas
- Aorta
- Diaphragm

**Positioning of the gallbladder in relation to other structures.**
CT image, with contrast, in axial plane

**167**

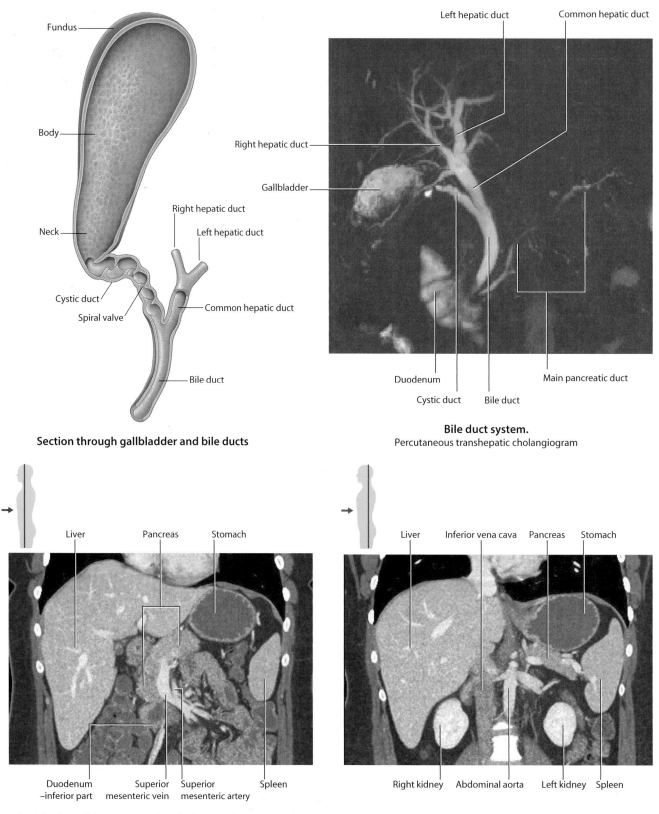

Fundus

Body

Neck

Cystic duct

Spiral valve

Right hepatic duct

Left hepatic duct

Common hepatic duct

Bile duct

**Section through gallbladder and bile ducts**

Left hepatic duct

Common hepatic duct

Right hepatic duct

Gallbladder

Duodenum

Cystic duct

Bile duct

Main pancreatic duct

**Bile duct system.**
Percutaneous transhepatic cholangiogram

Liver

Pancreas

Stomach

Duodenum
–inferior part

Superior mesenteric vein

Superior mesenteric artery

Spleen

**Positioning of the pancreas in relation to other structures.**
CT image, with contrast, in coronal plane

Liver

Inferior vena cava

Pancreas

Stomach

Right kidney

Abdominal aorta

Left kidney

Spleen

**Relationship of pancreas to the stomach and spleen.**
CT image, with contrast, in coronal plane

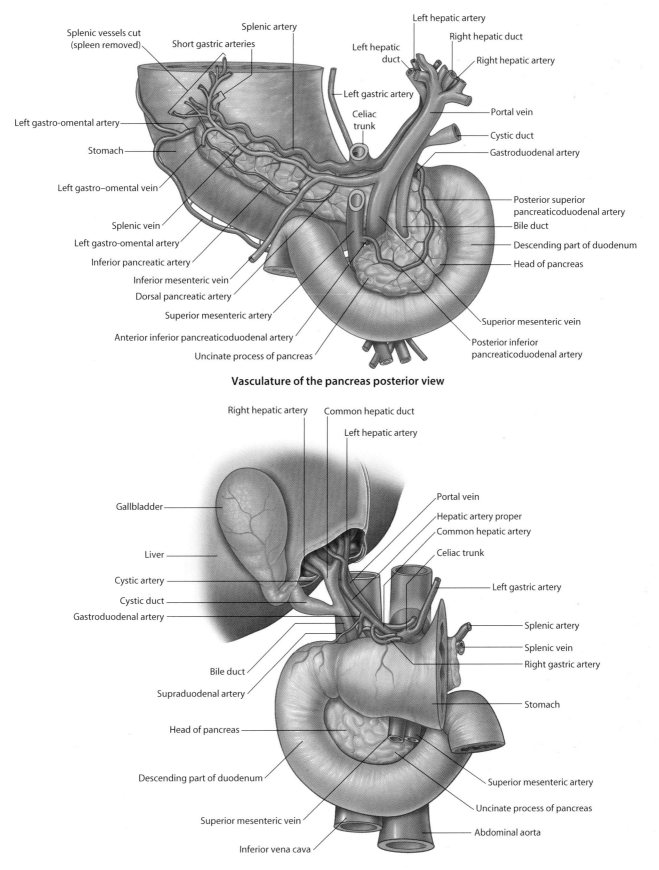

Splenic vessels cut
(spleen removed)

Short gastric arteries

Splenic artery

Left hepatic artery

Right hepatic duct

Left hepatic
duct

Right hepatic artery

Left gastric artery

Celiac
trunk

Portal vein

Cystic duct

Gastroduodenal artery

Left gastro-omental artery

Stomach

Left gastro–omental vein

Splenic vein

Left gastro-omental artery

Inferior pancreatic artery

Inferior mesenteric vein

Dorsal pancreatic artery

Superior mesenteric artery

Anterior inferior pancreaticoduodenal artery

Uncinate process of pancreas

Posterior superior
pancreaticoduodenal artery

Bile duct

Descending part of duodenum

Head of pancreas

Superior mesenteric vein

Posterior inferior
pancreaticoduodenal artery

**Vasculature of the pancreas posterior view**

Right hepatic artery

Common hepatic duct

Left hepatic artery

Gallbladder

Liver

Cystic artery

Cystic duct

Gastroduodenal artery

Bile duct

Supraduodenal artery

Head of pancreas

Descending part of duodenum

Superior mesenteric vein

Inferior vena cava

Portal vein

Hepatic artery proper

Common hepatic artery

Celiac trunk

Left gastric artery

Splenic artery

Splenic vein

Right gastric artery

Stomach

Superior mesenteric artery

Uncinate process of pancreas

Abdominal aorta

**Distribution of the common hepatic artery**

**169**

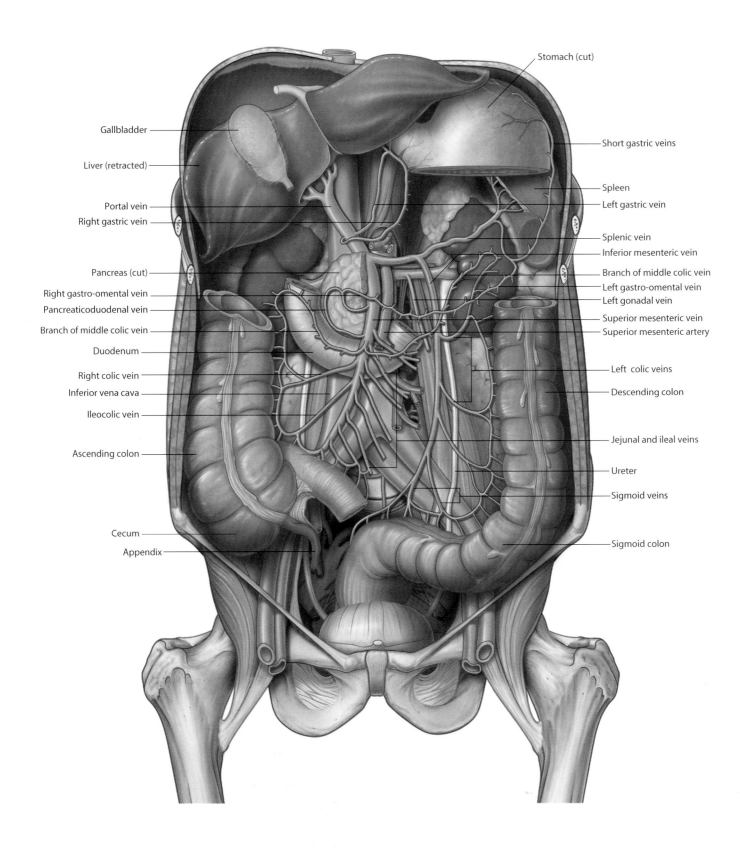

Gallbladder

Liver (retracted)

Portal vein

Right gastric vein

Pancreas (cut)

Right gastro-omental vein

Pancreaticoduodenal vein

Branch of middle colic vein

Duodenum

Right colic vein

Inferior vena cava

Ileocolic vein

Ascending colon

Cecum

Appendix

Stomach (cut)

Short gastric veins

Spleen

Left gastric vein

Splenic vein

Inferior mesenteric vein

Branch of middle colic vein

Left gastro-omental vein

Left gonadal vein

Superior mesenteric vein

Superior mesenteric artery

Left colic veins

Descending colon

Jejunal and ileal veins

Ureter

Sigmoid veins

Sigmoid colon

**Venous drainage of the abdominal portion of the gastrointestinal tract in situ**

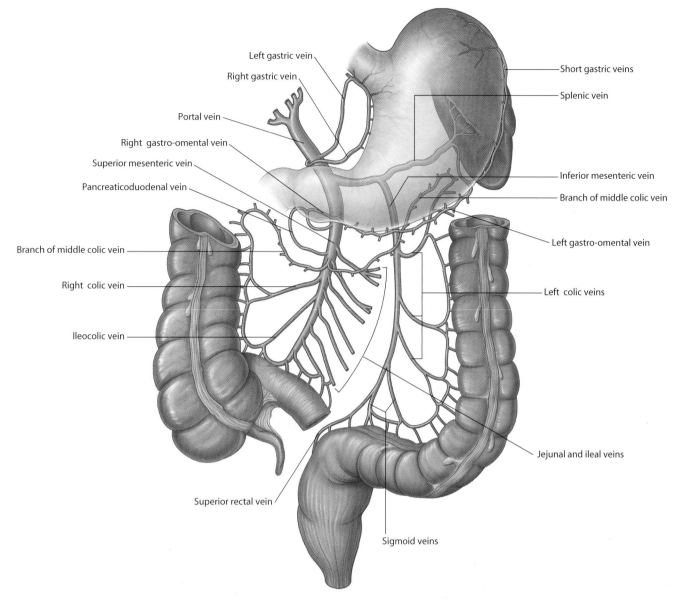

Left gastric vein

Right gastric vein

Portal vein

Right gastro-omental vein

Superior mesenteric vein

Pancreaticoduodenal vein

Branch of middle colic vein

Right colic vein

Ileocolic vein

Superior rectal vein

Short gastric veins

Splenic vein

Inferior mesenteric vein

Branch of middle colic vein

Left gastro-omental vein

Left colic veins

Jejunal and ileal veins

Sigmoid veins

**Venous drainage of the abdominal portion of the gastrointestinal tract**

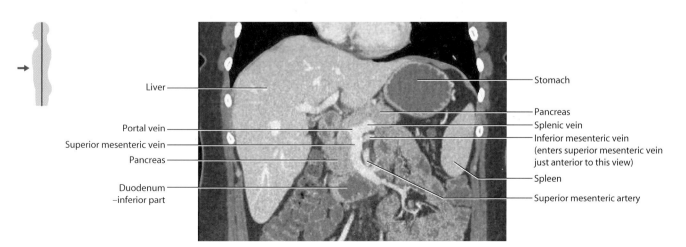

Liver

Portal vein

Superior mesenteric vein

Pancreas

Duodenum
–inferior part

Stomach

Pancreas

Splenic vein

Inferior mesenteric vein
(enters superior mesenteric vein
just anterior to this view)

Spleen

Superior mesenteric artery

**Formation of the portal vein.**
CT image, with contrast, in coronal plane

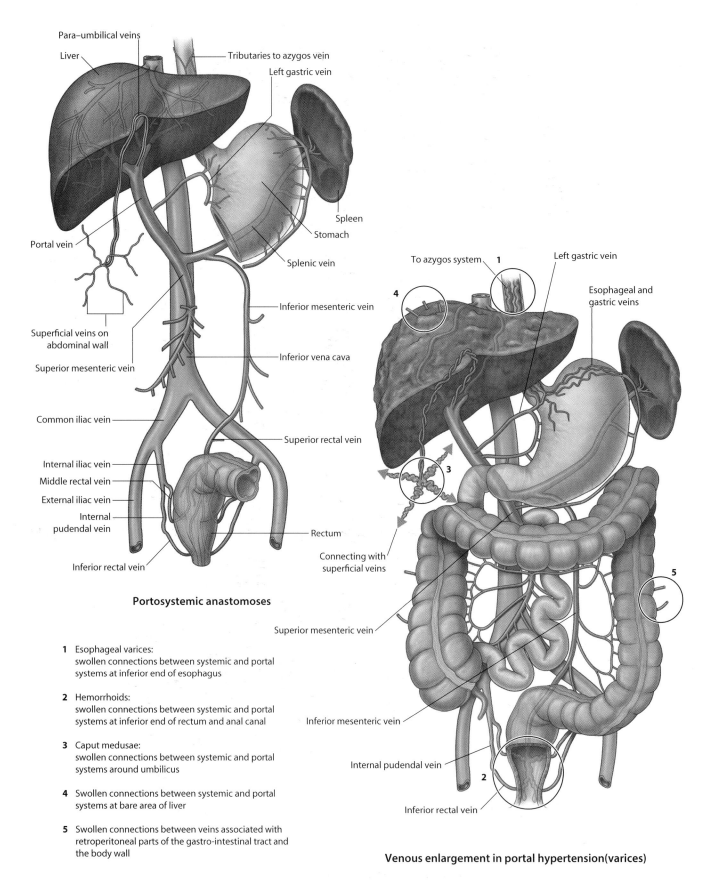

Para–umbilical veins

Liver

Tributaries to azygos vein

Left gastric vein

Spleen

Stomach

Portal vein

Splenic vein

Superficial veins on abdominal wall

Inferior mesenteric vein

Superior mesenteric vein

Inferior vena cava

Common iliac vein

Superior rectal vein

Internal iliac vein

Middle rectal vein

External iliac vein

Internal pudendal vein

Rectum

Inferior rectal vein

**Portosystemic anastomoses**

To azygos system  1

Left gastric vein

4

Esophageal and gastric veins

3

Connecting with superficial veins

5

Superior mesenteric vein

Inferior mesenteric vein

Internal pudendal vein

2

Inferior rectal vein

**1** Esophageal varices:
swollen connections between systemic and portal systems at inferior end of esophagus

**2** Hemorrhoids:
swollen connections between systemic and portal systems at inferior end of rectum and anal canal

**3** Caput medusae:
swollen connections between systemic and portal systems around umbilicus

**4** Swollen connections between systemic and portal systems at bare area of liver

**5** Swollen connections between veins associated with retroperitoneal parts of the gastro-intestinal tract and the body wall

**Venous enlargement in portal hypertension(varices)**

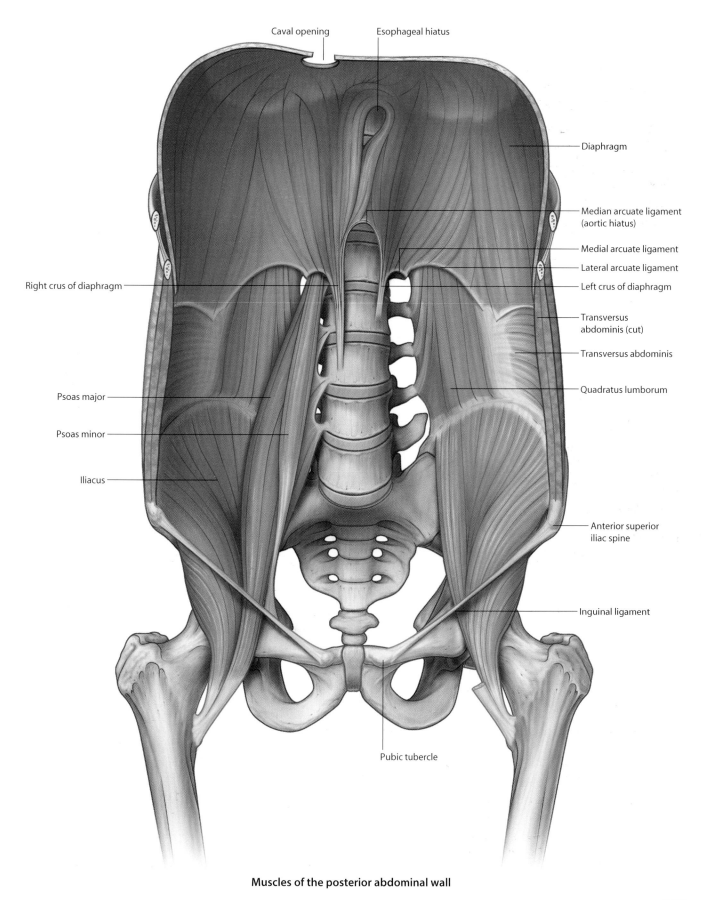

Caval opening

Esophageal hiatus

Diaphragm

Median arcuate ligament
(aortic hiatus)

Medial arcuate ligament

Lateral arcuate ligament

Right crus of diaphragm

Left crus of diaphragm

Transversus
abdominis (cut)

Transversus abdominis

Psoas major

Quadratus lumborum

Psoas minor

Iliacus

Anterior superior
iliac spine

Inguinal ligament

Pubic tubercle

**Muscles of the posterior abdominal wall**

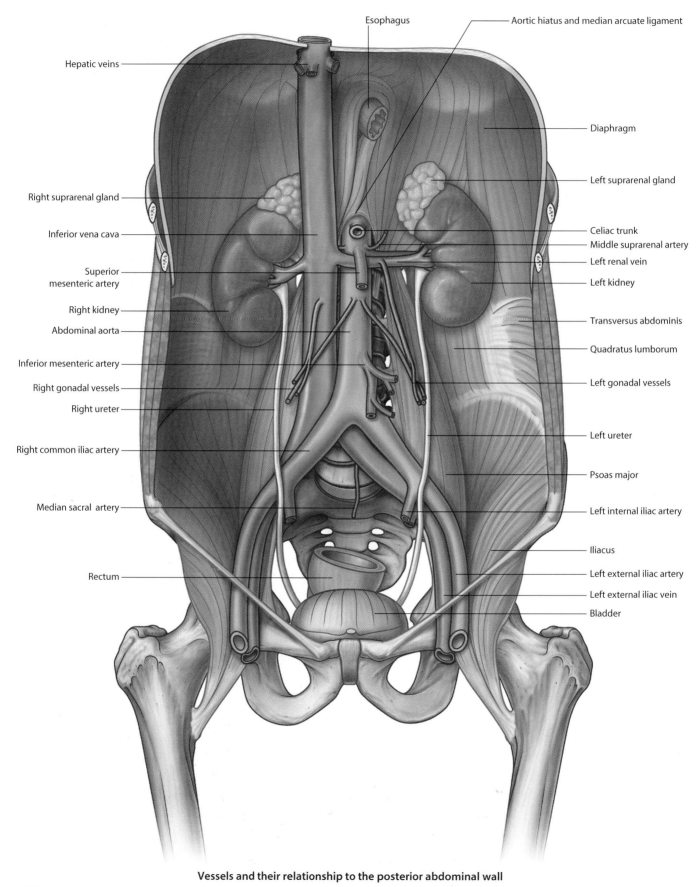

Esophagus

Aortic hiatus and median arcuate ligament

Hepatic veins

Diaphragm

Right suprarenal gland

Left suprarenal gland

Inferior vena cava

Celiac trunk

Middle suprarenal artery

Left renal vein

Superior mesenteric artery

Left kidney

Right kidney

Transversus abdominis

Abdominal aorta

Quadratus lumborum

Inferior mesenteric artery

Right gonadal vessels

Left gonadal vessels

Right ureter

Right common iliac artery

Left ureter

Psoas major

Median sacral artery

Left internal iliac artery

Iliacus

Left external iliac artery

Left external iliac vein

Rectum

Bladder

**Vessels and their relationship to the posterior abdominal wall**

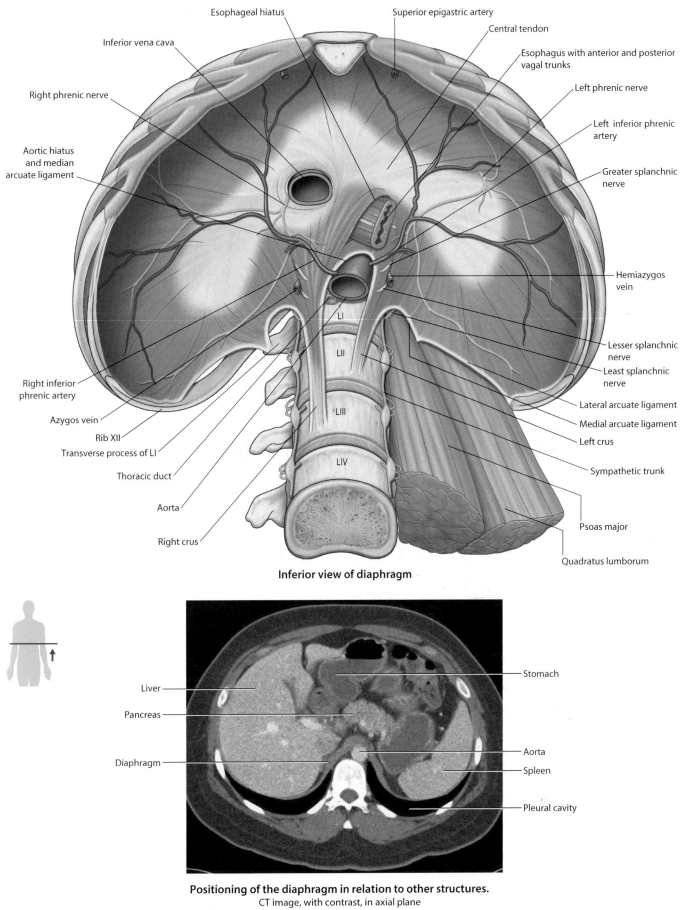

**Inferior view of diaphragm**

Esophageal hiatus
Superior epigastric artery
Central tendon
Inferior vena cava
Esophagus with anterior and posterior vagal trunks
Right phrenic nerve
Left phrenic nerve
Left inferior phrenic artery
Aortic hiatus and median arcuate ligament
Greater splanchnic nerve
Hemiazygos vein
Lesser splanchnic nerve
Least splanchnic nerve
Right inferior phrenic artery
Lateral arcuate ligament
Medial arcuate ligament
Azygos vein
Left crus
Rib XII
Sympathetic trunk
Transverse process of LI
Thoracic duct
Psoas major
Aorta
Right crus
Quadratus lumborum

LI
LII
LIII
LIV

**Positioning of the diaphragm in relation to other structures.**
CT image, with contrast, in axial plane

Liver
Stomach
Pancreas
Diaphragm
Aorta
Spleen
Pleural cavity

**175**

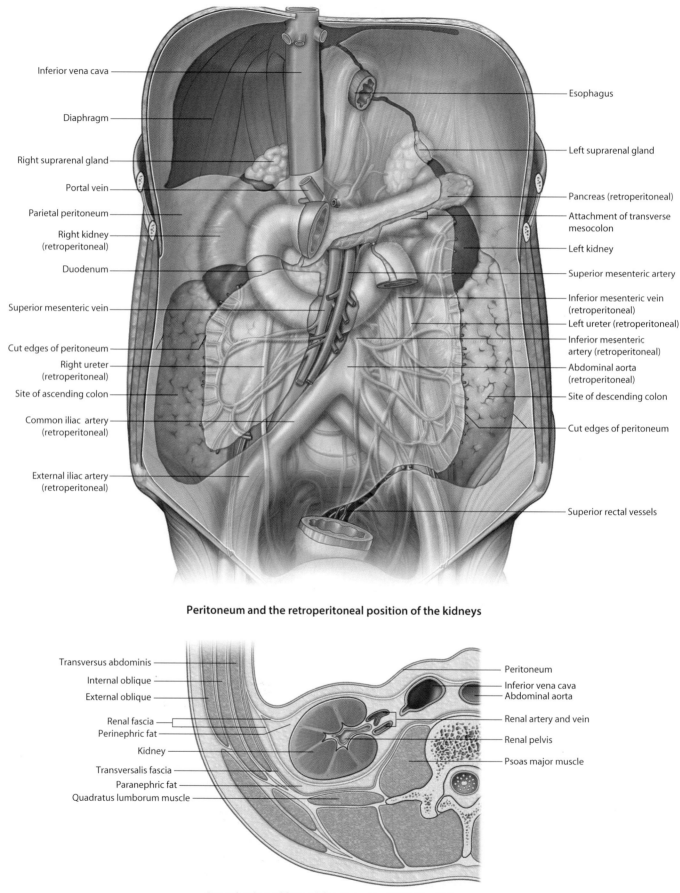

Inferior vena cava

Diaphragm

Right suprarenal gland

Portal vein

Parietal peritoneum

Right kidney (retroperitoneal)

Duodenum

Superior mesenteric vein

Cut edges of peritoneum

Right ureter (retroperitoneal)

Site of ascending colon

Common iliac artery (retroperitoneal)

External iliac artery (retroperitoneal)

Esophagus

Left suprarenal gland

Pancreas (retroperitoneal)

Attachment of transverse mesocolon

Left kidney

Superior mesenteric artery

Inferior mesenteric vein (retroperitoneal)

Left ureter (retroperitoneal)

Inferior mesenteric artery (retroperitoneal)

Abdominal aorta (retroperitoneal)

Site of descending colon

Cut edges of peritoneum

Superior rectal vessels

**Peritoneum and the retroperitoneal position of the kidneys**

Transversus abdominis

Internal oblique

External oblique

Renal fascia

Perinephric fat

Kidney

Transversalis fascia

Paranephric fat

Quadratus lumborum muscle

Peritoneum

Inferior vena cava

Abdominal aorta

Renal artery and vein

Renal pelvis

Psoas major muscle

**Organization of fat and fascia surrounding the kidneys**

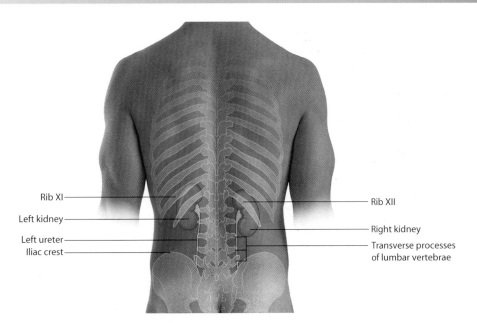

**Surface projection of the kidneys and ureters (posterior view)**

Rib XI
Left kidney
Left ureter
Iliac crest
Rib XII
Right kidney
Transverse processes of lumbar vertebrae

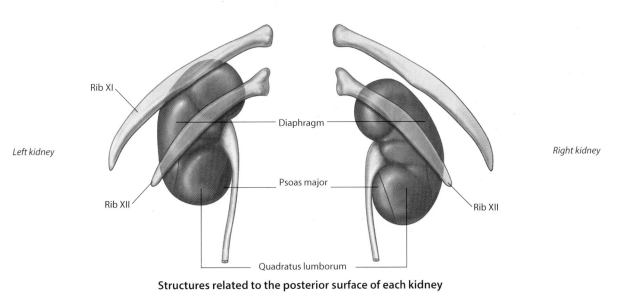

Rib XI
*Left kidney*
Rib XII
Diaphragm
Psoas major
Quadratus lumborum
*Right kidney*
Rib XII

**Structures related to the posterior surface of each kidney**

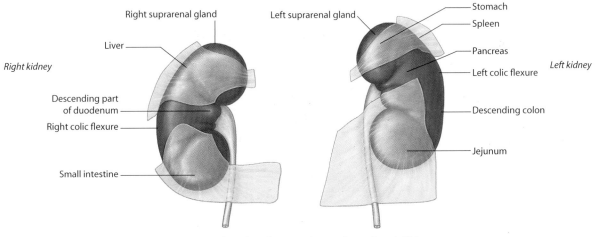

Right suprarenal gland
Liver
*Right kidney*
Descending part of duodenum
Right colic flexure
Small intestine
Left suprarenal gland
Stomach
Spleen
Pancreas
Left colic flexure
*Left kidney*
Descending colon
Jejunum

**Structures related to the anterior surface of each kidney**

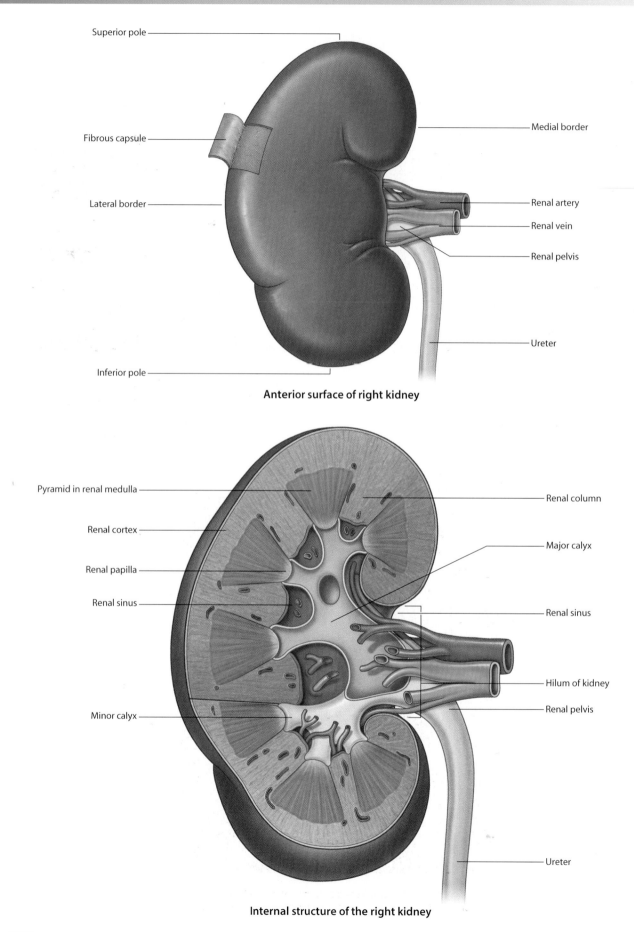

Superior pole

Fibrous capsule

Lateral border

Inferior pole

Medial border

Renal artery

Renal vein

Renal pelvis

Ureter

**Anterior surface of right kidney**

Pyramid in renal medulla

Renal cortex

Renal papilla

Renal sinus

Minor calyx

Renal column

Major calyx

Renal sinus

Hilum of kidney

Renal pelvis

Ureter

**Internal structure of the right kidney**

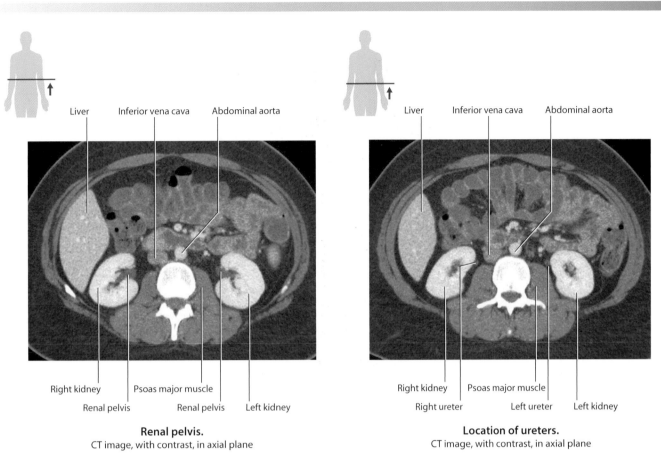

Liver    Inferior vena cava    Abdominal aorta

Right kidney    Psoas major muscle

Renal pelvis    Renal pelvis    Left kidney

**Renal pelvis.**
CT image, with contrast, in axial plane

Liver    Inferior vena cava    Abdominal aorta

Right kidney    Psoas major muscle

Right ureter    Left ureter    Left kidney

**Location of ureters.**
CT image, with contrast, in axial plane

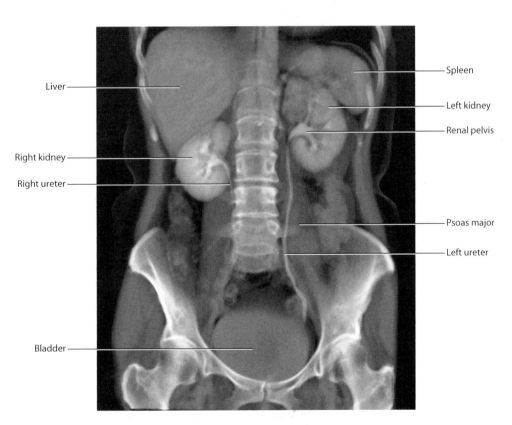

Liver

Right kidney

Right ureter

Bladder

Spleen

Left kidney

Renal pelvis

Psoas major

Left ureter

**Pathway of ureter in relation to other structures.**
Coronal view of 3-D urogram using multidetector computed tomography

**179**

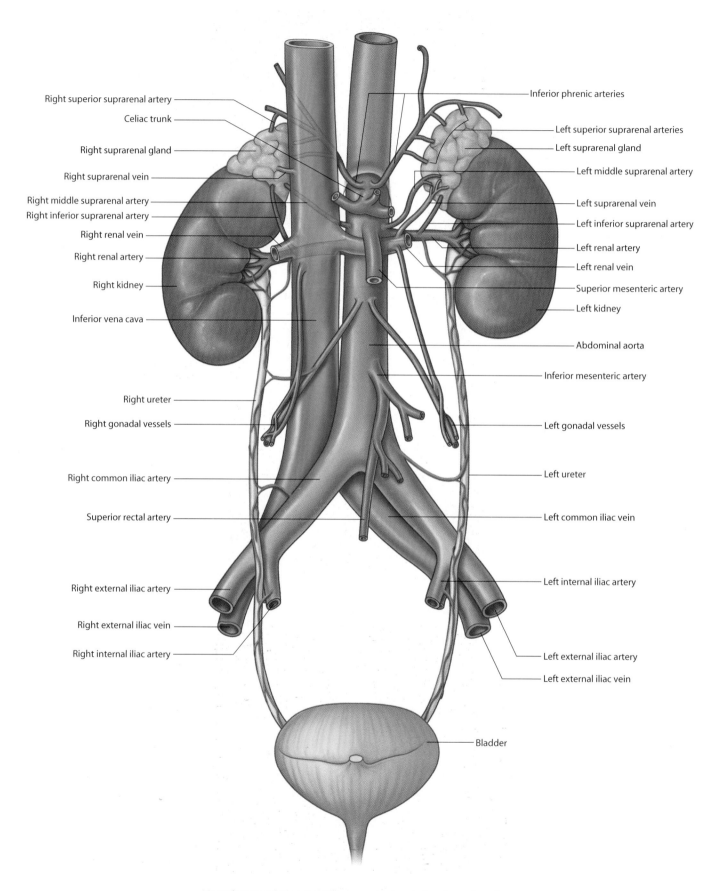

Right superior suprarenal artery

Celiac trunk

Right suprarenal gland

Right suprarenal vein

Right middle suprarenal artery

Right inferior suprarenal artery

Right renal vein

Right renal artery

Right kidney

Inferior vena cava

Right ureter

Right gonadal vessels

Right common iliac artery

Superior rectal artery

Right external iliac artery

Right external iliac vein

Right internal iliac artery

Inferior phrenic arteries

Left superior suprarenal arteries

Left suprarenal gland

Left middle suprarenal artery

Left suprarenal vein

Left inferior suprarenal artery

Left renal artery

Left renal vein

Superior mesenteric artery

Left kidney

Abdominal aorta

Inferior mesenteric artery

Left gonadal vessels

Left ureter

Left common iliac vein

Left internal iliac artery

Left external iliac artery

Left external iliac vein

Bladder

**Vasculature relating to kidneys, suprarenal glands, and ureters**

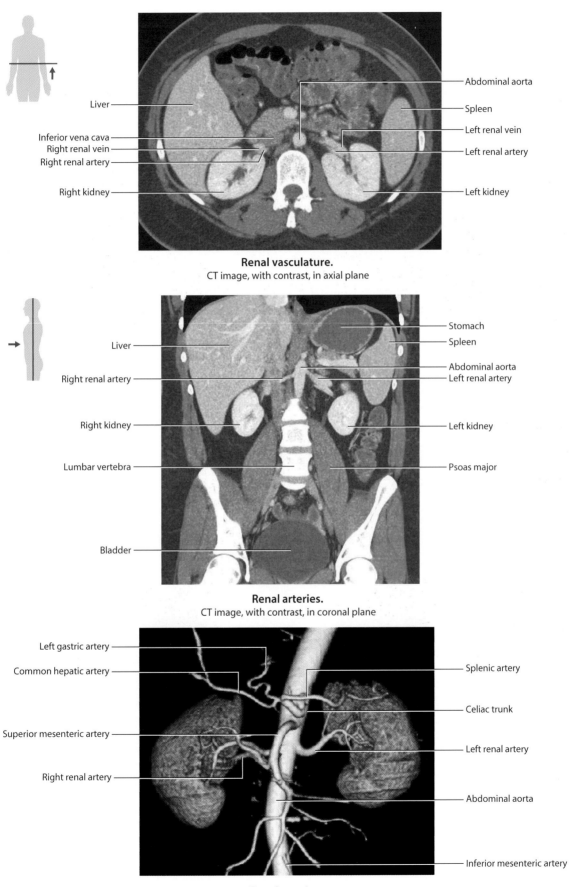

**Renal vasculature.**
CT image, with contrast, in axial plane

Liver
Inferior vena cava
Right renal vein
Right renal artery
Right kidney

Abdominal aorta
Spleen
Left renal vein
Left renal artery
Left kidney

**Renal arteries.**
CT image, with contrast, in coronal plane

Liver
Right renal artery
Right kidney
Lumbar vertebra
Bladder

Stomach
Spleen
Abdominal aorta
Left renal artery
Left kidney
Psoas major

**Renal arteries.**
Volume-rendered anterior view using multidetector computer tomography

Left gastric artery
Common hepatic artery
Superior mesenteric artery
Right renal artery

Splenic artery
Celiac trunk
Left renal artery
Abdominal aorta
Inferior mesenteric artery

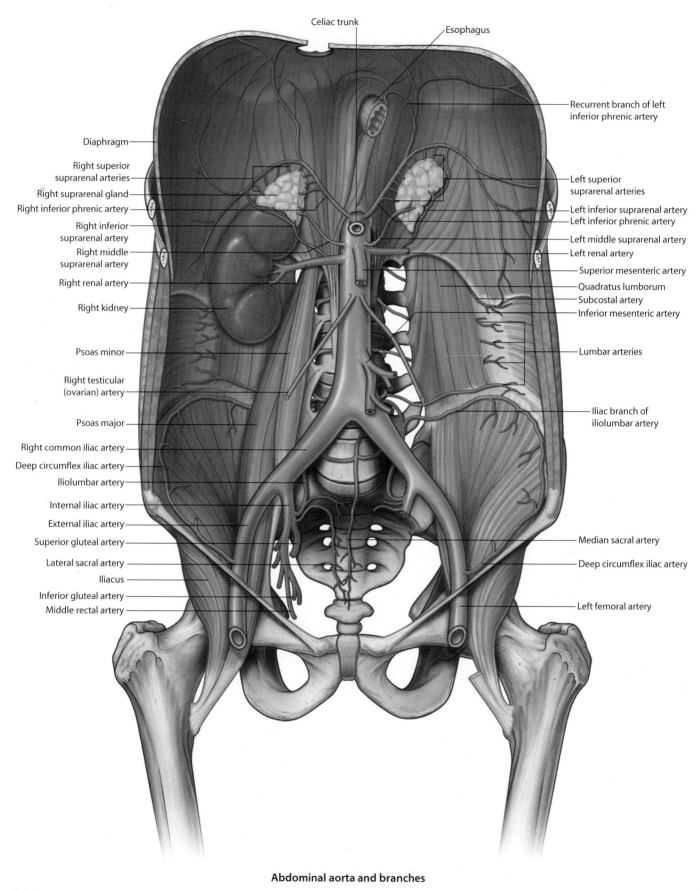

Celiac trunk

Esophagus

Recurrent branch of left
inferior phrenic artery

Diaphragm

Right superior
suprarenal arteries

Right suprarenal gland

Right inferior phrenic artery

Right inferior
suprarenal artery

Right middle
suprarenal artery

Right renal artery

Right kidney

Psoas minor

Right testicular
(ovarian) artery

Psoas major

Right common iliac artery

Deep circumflex iliac artery

Iliolumbar artery

Internal iliac artery

External iliac artery

Superior gluteal artery

Lateral sacral artery

Iliacus

Inferior gluteal artery

Middle rectal artery

Left superior
suprarenal arteries

Left inferior suprarenal artery

Left inferior phrenic artery

Left middle suprarenal artery

Left renal artery

Superior mesenteric artery

Quadratus lumborum

Subcostal artery

Inferior mesenteric artery

Lumbar arteries

Iliac branch of
iliolumbar artery

Median sacral artery

Deep circumflex iliac artery

Left femoral artery

**Abdominal aorta and branches**

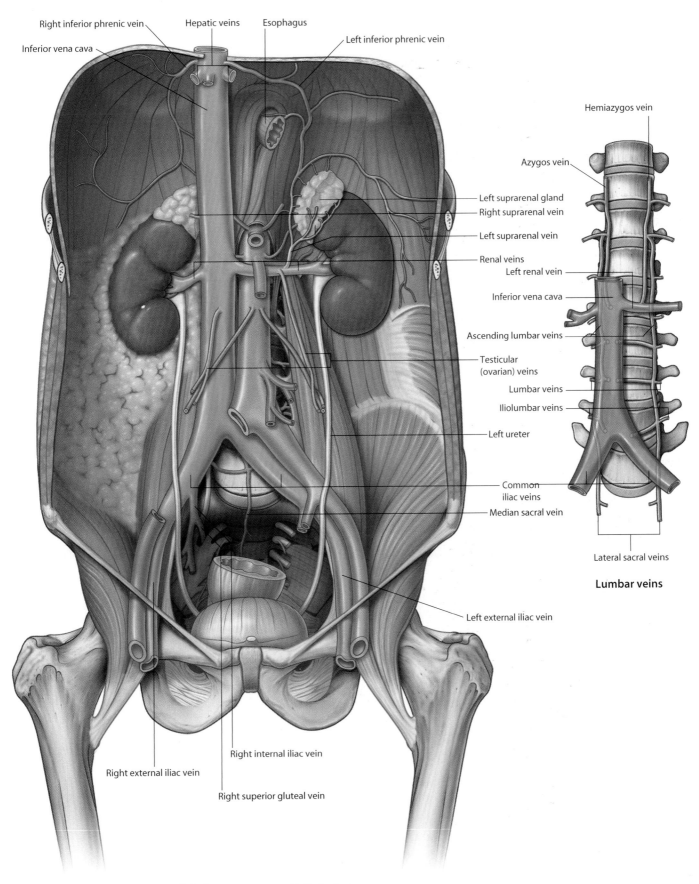

Right inferior phrenic vein

Inferior vena cava

Hepatic veins

Esophagus

Left inferior phrenic vein

Hemiazygos vein

Azygos vein

Left suprarenal gland

Right suprarenal vein

Left suprarenal vein

Renal veins

Left renal vein

Inferior vena cava

Ascending lumbar veins

Testicular
(ovarian) veins

Lumbar veins

Iliolumbar veins

Left ureter

Common
iliac veins

Median sacral vein

Lateral sacral veins

**Lumbar veins**

Left external iliac vein

Right internal iliac vein

Right external iliac vein

Right superior gluteal vein

**Inferior vena cava and tributaries**

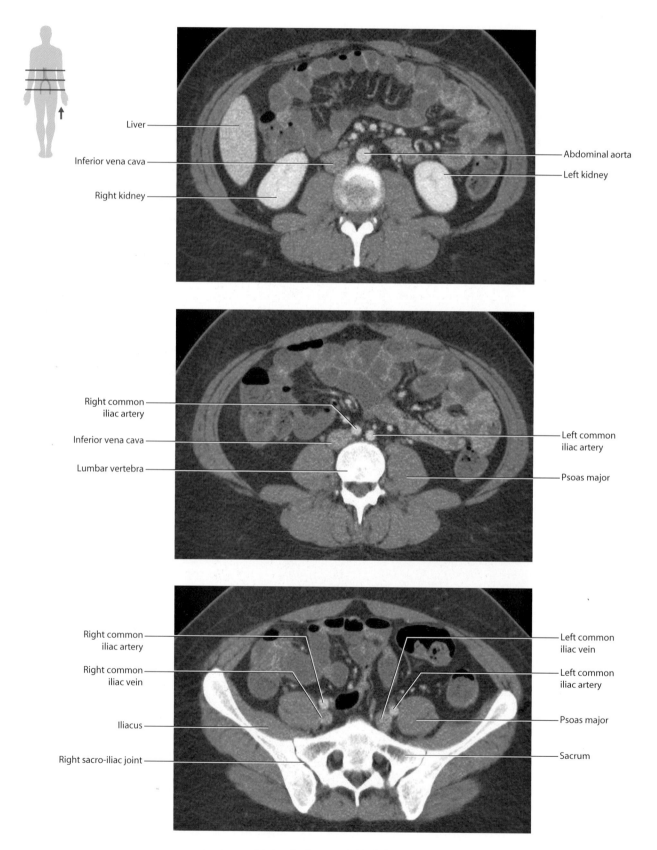

**Abdominal aorta and inferior vena cava.**
CT images, with contrast, in axial plane

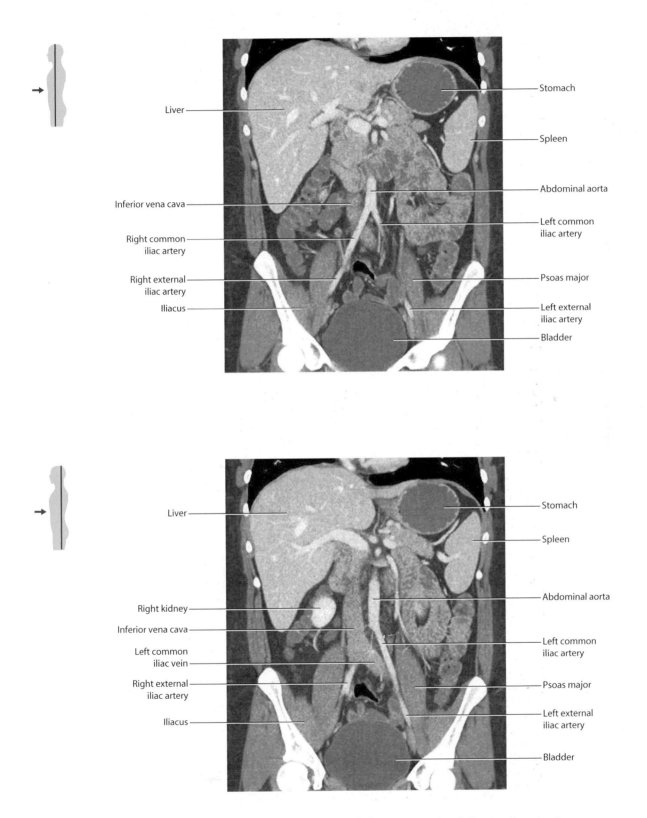

Liver

Stomach

Spleen

Abdominal aorta

Inferior vena cava

Left common iliac artery

Right common iliac artery

Right external iliac artery

Psoas major

Iliacus

Left external iliac artery

Bladder

Liver

Stomach

Spleen

Abdominal aorta

Right kidney

Inferior vena cava

Left common iliac vein

Left common iliac artery

Right external iliac artery

Psoas major

Iliacus

Left external iliac artery

Bladder

**Positioning of the abdominal aorta and inferior vena cava in relation to other structures.**
CT images, with contrast, in coronal plane

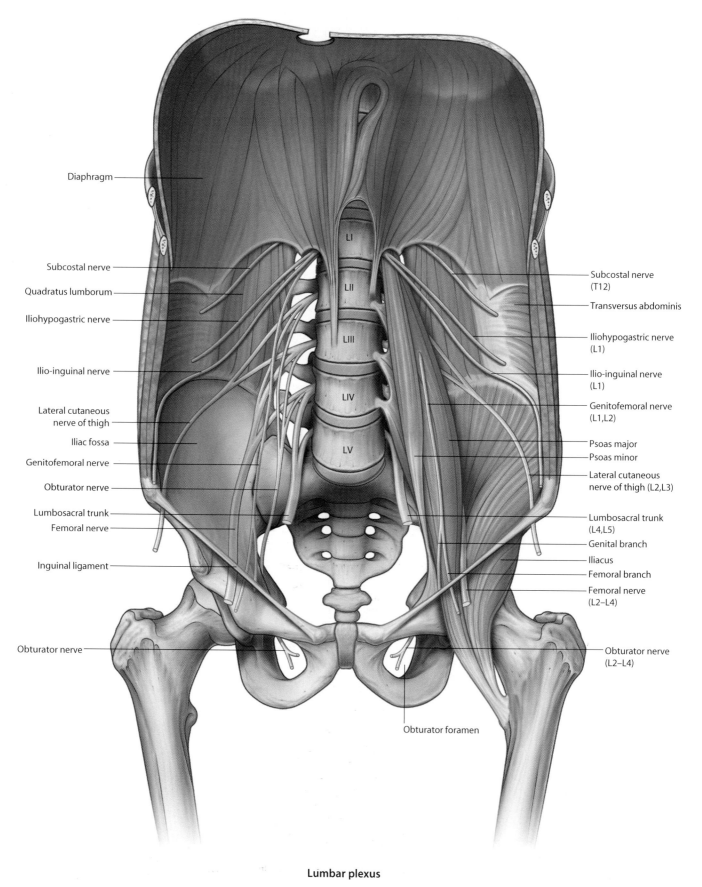

Diaphragm

Subcostal nerve

Quadratus lumborum

Iliohypogastric nerve

Ilio-inguinal nerve

Lateral cutaneous
nerve of thigh

Iliac fossa

Genitofemoral nerve

Obturator nerve

Lumbosacral trunk

Femoral nerve

Inguinal ligament

Obturator nerve

LI

LII

LIII

LIV

LV

Subcostal nerve
(T12)

Transversus abdominis

Iliohypogastric nerve
(L1)

Ilio-inguinal nerve
(L1)

Genitofemoral nerve
(L1,L2)

Psoas major

Psoas minor

Lateral cutaneous
nerve of thigh (L2,L3)

Lumbosacral trunk
(L4,L5)

Genital branch

Iliacus

Femoral branch

Femoral nerve
(L2–L4)

Obturator nerve
(L2–L4)

Obturator foramen

**Lumbar plexus**

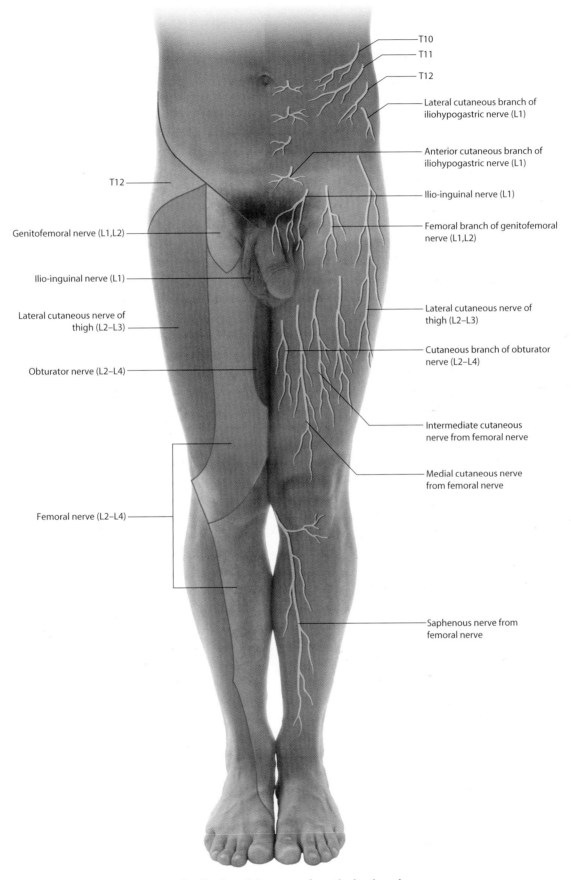

T10
T11
T12
Lateral cutaneous branch of
iliohypogastric nerve (L1)

Anterior cutaneous branch of
iliohypogastric nerve (L1)

Ilio-inguinal nerve (L1)

Femoral branch of genitofemoral
nerve (L1,L2)

Lateral cutaneous nerve of
thigh (L2–L3)

Cutaneous branch of obturator
nerve (L2–L4)

Intermediate cutaneous
nerve from femoral nerve

Medial cutaneous nerve
from femoral nerve

Saphenous nerve from
femoral nerve

T12

Genitofemoral nerve (L1,L2)

Ilio-inguinal nerve (L1)

Lateral cutaneous nerve of
thigh (L2–L3)

Obturator nerve (L2–L4)

Femoral nerve (L2–L4)

**Cutaneous distribution of the nerves from the lumbar plexus**

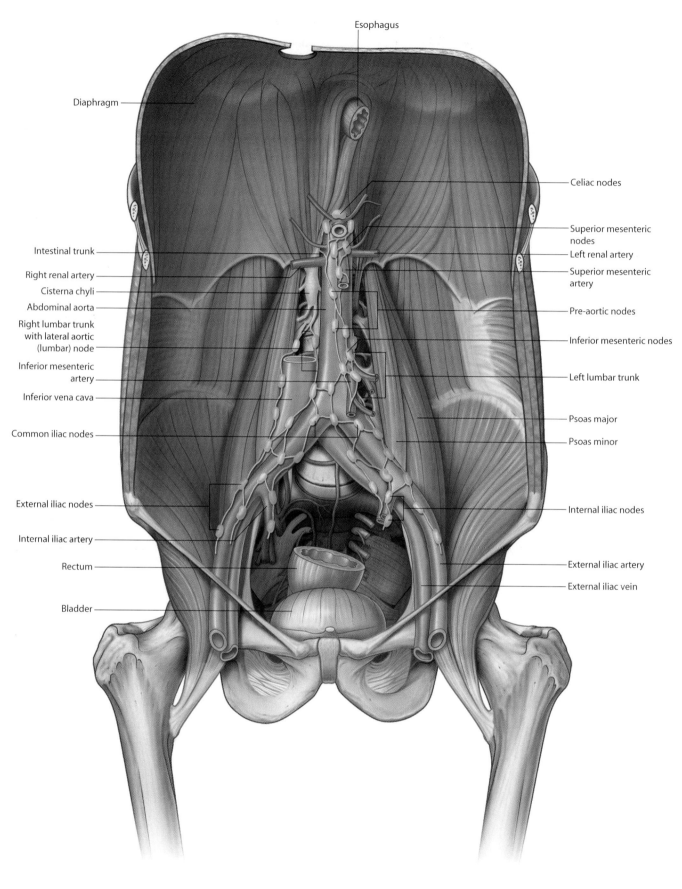

Esophagus

Diaphragm

Celiac nodes

Superior mesenteric nodes

Left renal artery

Superior mesenteric artery

Intestinal trunk

Right renal artery

Cisterna chyli

Abdominal aorta

Right lumbar trunk with lateral aortic (lumbar) node

Pre-aortic nodes

Inferior mesenteric nodes

Inferior mesenteric artery

Left lumbar trunk

Inferior vena cava

Common iliac nodes

Psoas major

Psoas minor

External iliac nodes

Internal iliac artery

Internal iliac nodes

Rectum

External iliac artery

External iliac vein

Bladder

**Abdominal lymphatics**

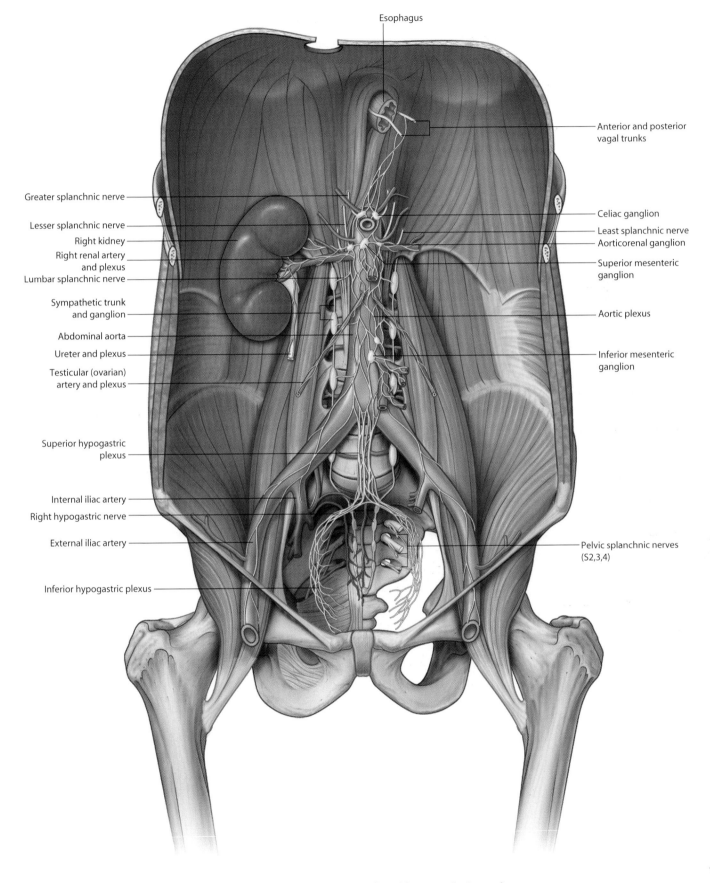

Esophagus

Anterior and posterior vagal trunks

Greater splanchnic nerve

Lesser splanchnic nerve

Right kidney

Right renal artery and plexus

Lumbar splanchnic nerve

Sympathetic trunk and ganglion

Abdominal aorta

Ureter and plexus

Testicular (ovarian) artery and plexus

Superior hypogastric plexus

Internal iliac artery

Right hypogastric nerve

External iliac artery

Inferior hypogastric plexus

Celiac ganglion

Least splanchnic nerve

Aorticorenal ganglion

Superior mesenteric ganglion

Aortic plexus

Inferior mesenteric ganglion

Pelvic splanchnic nerves (S2,3,4)

**Prevertebral plexuses and ganglia with sympathetic trunks**

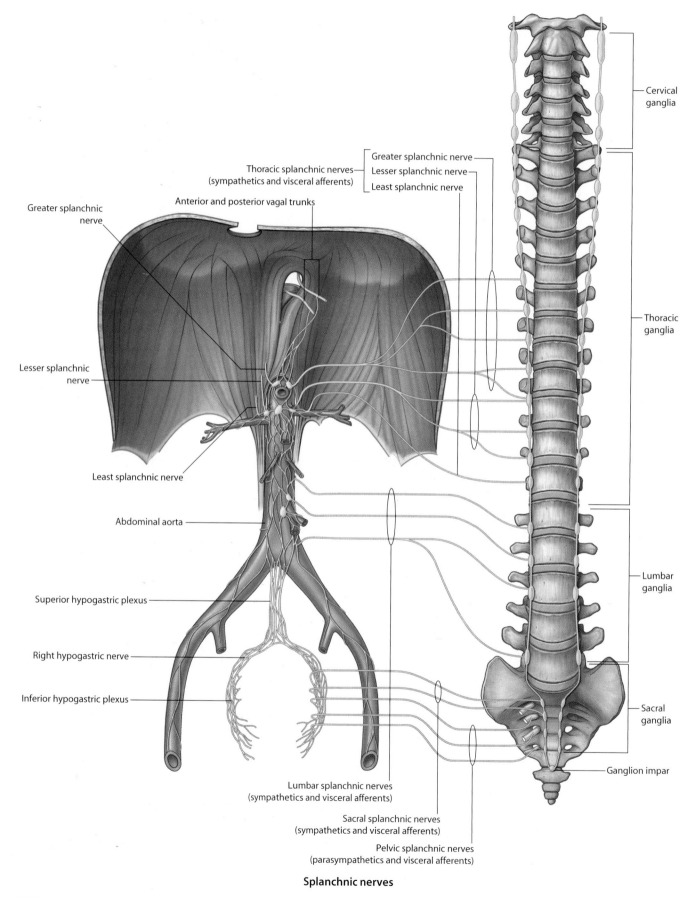

Cervical
ganglia

Greater splanchnic nerve
Lesser splanchnic nerve
Least splanchnic nerve

Thoracic splanchnic nerves
(sympathetics and visceral afferents)

Anterior and posterior vagal trunks

Greater splanchnic
nerve

Thoracic
ganglia

Lesser splanchnic
nerve

Least splanchnic nerve

Abdominal aorta

Lumbar
ganglia

Superior hypogastric plexus

Right hypogastric nerve

Inferior hypogastric plexus

Sacral
ganglia

Ganglion impar

Lumbar splanchnic nerves
(sympathetics and visceral afferents)

Sacral splanchnic nerves
(sympathetics and visceral afferents)

Pelvic splanchnic nerves
(parasympathetics and visceral afferents)

**Splanchnic nerves**

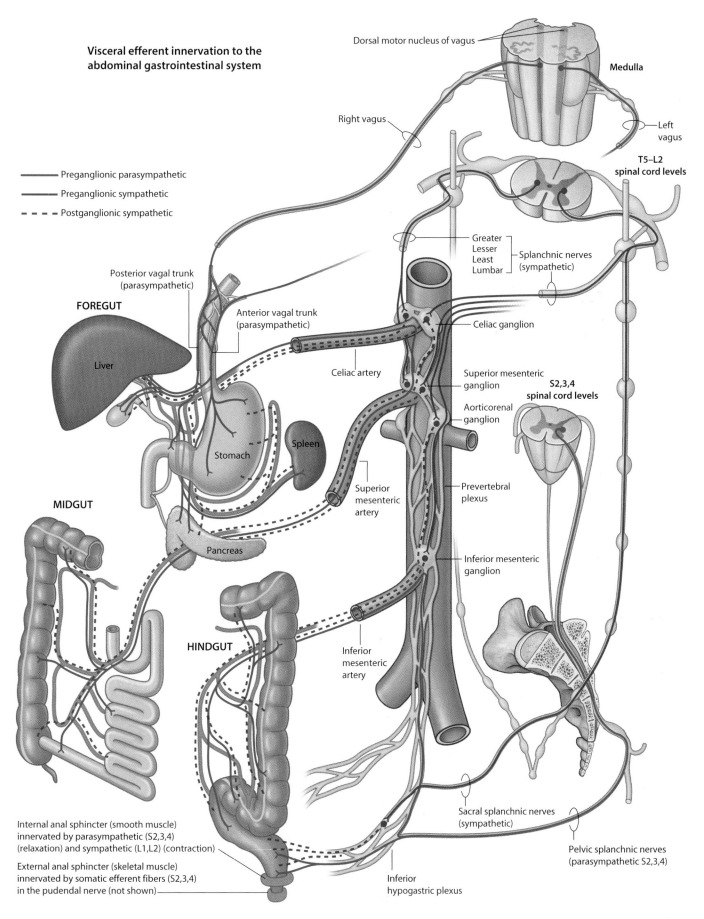

Visceral efferent innervation to the
abdominal gastrointestinal system

Dorsal motor nucleus of vagus

Medulla

Right vagus

Left vagus

T5–L2
spinal cord levels

——— Preganglionic parasympathetic

——— Preganglionic sympathetic

– – – Postganglionic sympathetic

Greater
Lesser
Least
Lumbar — Splanchnic nerves
(sympathetic)

Posterior vagal trunk
(parasympathetic)

FOREGUT

Anterior vagal trunk
(parasympathetic)

Liver

Celiac artery

Celiac ganglion

Superior mesenteric
ganglion

S2,3,4
spinal cord levels

Aorticorenal
ganglion

Spleen

Stomach

Superior
mesenteric
artery

Prevertebral
plexus

MIDGUT

Pancreas

Inferior mesenteric
ganglion

HINDGUT

Inferior
mesenteric
artery

Sacral splanchnic nerves
(sympathetic)

Internal anal sphincter (smooth muscle)
innervated by parasympathetic (S2,3,4)
(relaxation) and sympathetic (L1,L2) (contraction)

External anal sphincter (skeletal muscle)
innervated by somatic efferent fibers (S2,3,4)
in the pudendal nerve (not shown)

Pelvic splanchnic nerves
(parasympathetic S2,3,4)

Inferior
hypogastric plexus

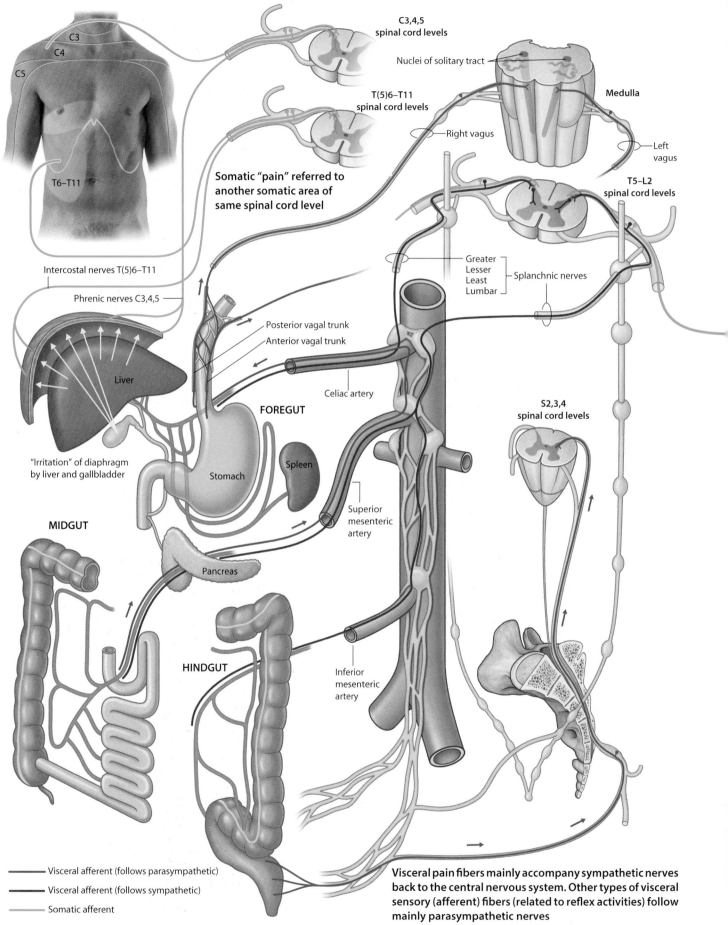

C3
C4
C5

T6–T11

C3,4,5
spinal cord levels

Nuclei of solitary tract

T(5)6–T11
spinal cord levels

Medulla

Right vagus

Left vagus

Somatic "pain" referred to
another somatic area of
same spinal cord level

T5–L2
spinal cord levels

Intercostal nerves T(5)6–T11

Phrenic nerves C3,4,5

Greater
Lesser
Least
Lumbar
Splanchnic nerves

Posterior vagal trunk

Anterior vagal trunk

Celiac artery

FOREGUT

Liver

S2,3,4
spinal cord levels

"Irritation" of diaphragm
by liver and gallbladder

Stomach

Spleen

MIDGUT

Superior
mesenteric
artery

Pancreas

HINDGUT

Inferior
mesenteric
artery

— Visceral afferent (follows parasympathetic)

— Visceral afferent (follows sympathetic)

— Somatic afferent

Visceral pain fibers mainly accompany sympathetic nerves
back to the central nervous system. Other types of visceral
sensory (afferent) fibers (related to reflex activities) follow
mainly parasympathetic nerves

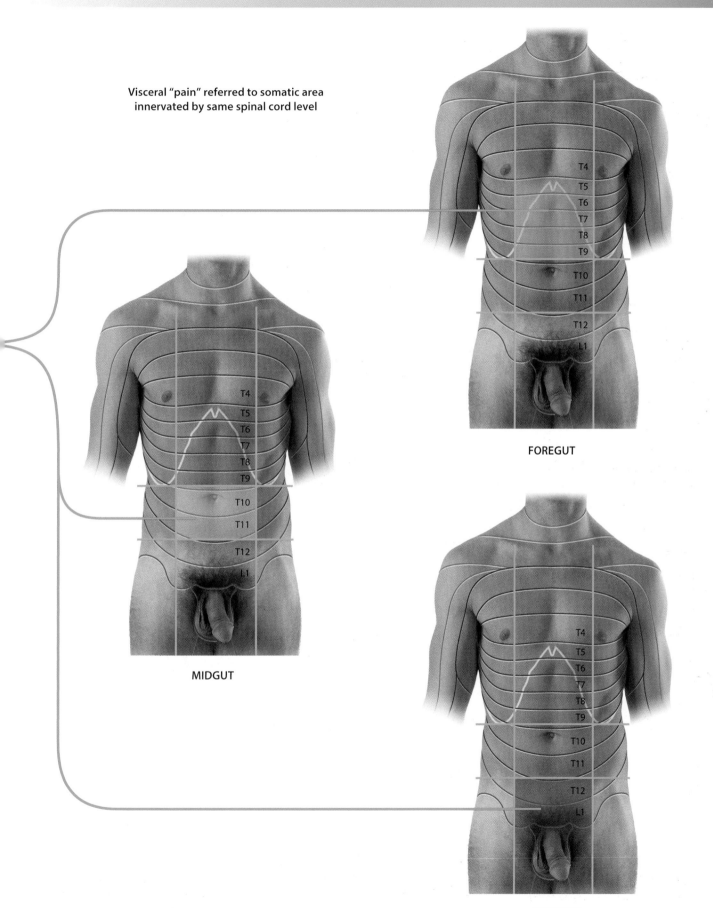

Visceral "pain" referred to somatic area
innervated by same spinal cord level

FOREGUT

MIDGUT

HINDGUT

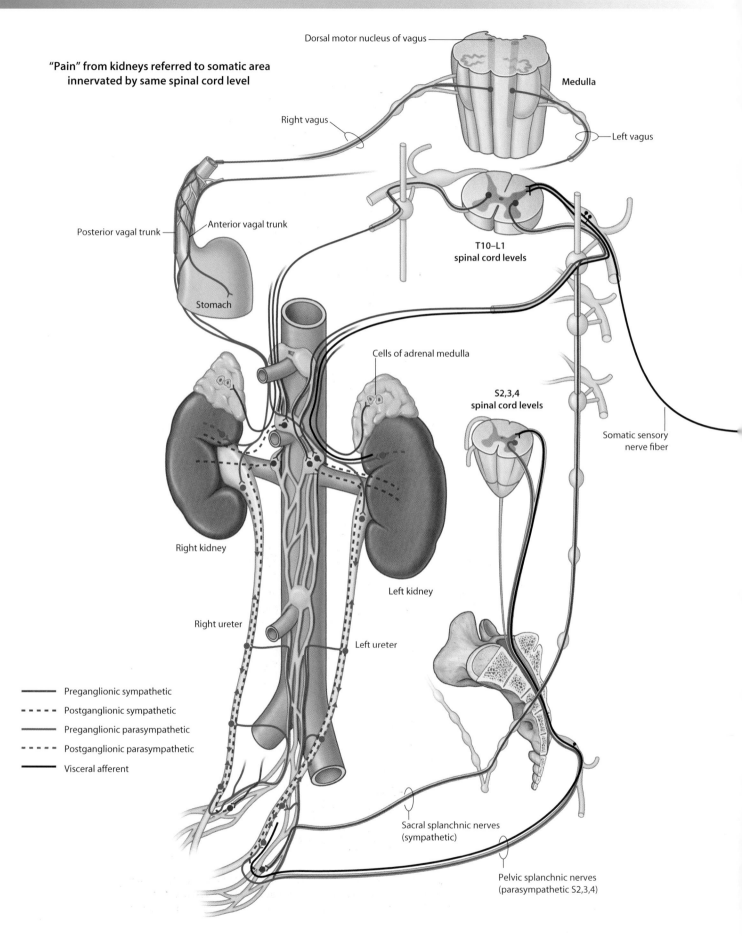

Dorsal motor nucleus of vagus

Medulla

"Pain" from kidneys referred to somatic area
innervated by same spinal cord level

Right vagus

Left vagus

Posterior vagal trunk

Anterior vagal trunk

T10–L1
spinal cord levels

Stomach

Cells of adrenal medulla

S2,3,4
spinal cord levels

Somatic sensory
nerve fiber

Right kidney

Left kidney

Right ureter

Left ureter

Preganglionic sympathetic

Postganglionic sympathetic

Preganglionic parasympathetic

Postganglionic parasympathetic

Visceral afferent

Sacral splanchnic nerves
(sympathetic)

Pelvic splanchnic nerves
(parasympathetic S2,3,4)

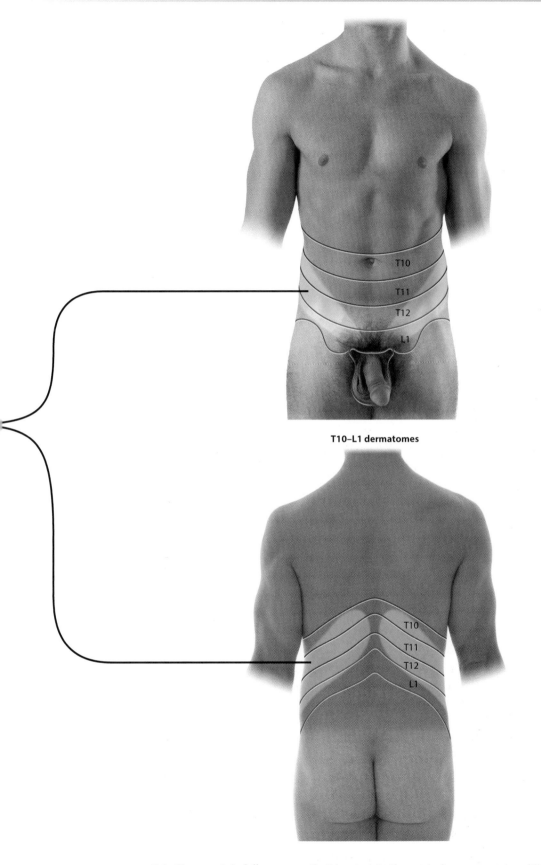

**T10–L1 dermatomes**

Pain fibers mainly follow sympathetic nerves to the central nervous system (CNS). This pain is 'referred' by the CNS to the somatic area innervated by the same spinal levels. Other types of visceral afferent (sensory) fibers (related to reflex activities) follow mainly parasympathetic nerves

# 5

# PELVIS AND PERINEUM

## CONTENTS

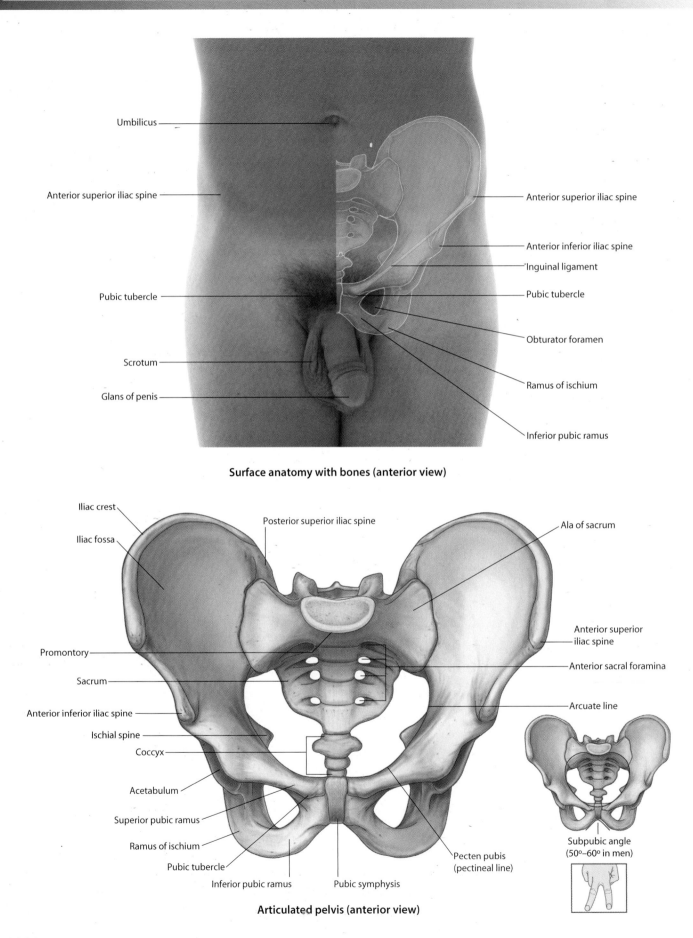

Umbilicus

Anterior superior iliac spine

Anterior superior iliac spine

Anterior inferior iliac spine

Inguinal ligament

Pubic tubercle

Pubic tubercle

Obturator foramen

Scrotum

Ramus of ischium

Glans of penis

Inferior pubic ramus

**Surface anatomy with bones (anterior view)**

Iliac crest

Posterior superior iliac spine

Ala of sacrum

Iliac fossa

Promontory

Anterior superior iliac spine

Anterior sacral foramina

Sacrum

Anterior inferior iliac spine

Arcuate line

Ischial spine

Coccyx

Acetabulum

Superior pubic ramus

Ramus of ischium

Pubic tubercle

Pecten pubis (pectineal line)

Subpubic angle (50°–60° in men)

Inferior pubic ramus

Pubic symphysis

**Articulated pelvis (anterior view)**

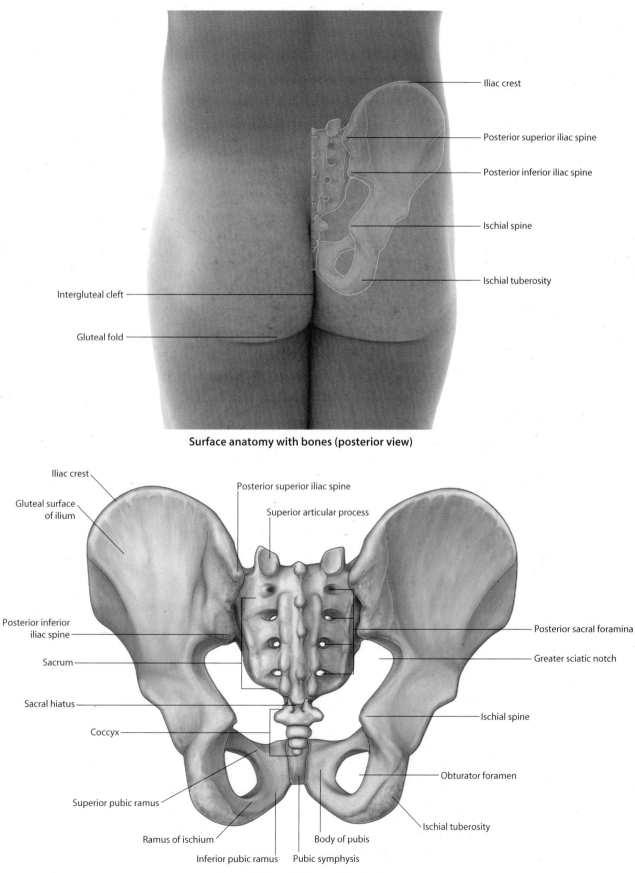

**Surface anatomy with bones (posterior view)**

Iliac crest

Posterior superior iliac spine

Posterior inferior iliac spine

Ischial spine

Ischial tuberosity

Intergluteal cleft

Gluteal fold

Iliac crest

Gluteal surface
of ilium

Posterior superior iliac spine

Superior articular process

Posterior inferior
iliac spine

Sacrum

Sacral hiatus

Coccyx

Superior pubic ramus

Ramus of ischium

Inferior pubic ramus

Pubic symphysis

Body of pubis

Posterior sacral foramina

Greater sciatic notch

Ischial spine

Obturator foramen

Ischial tuberosity

**Articulated pelvis (posterior view)**

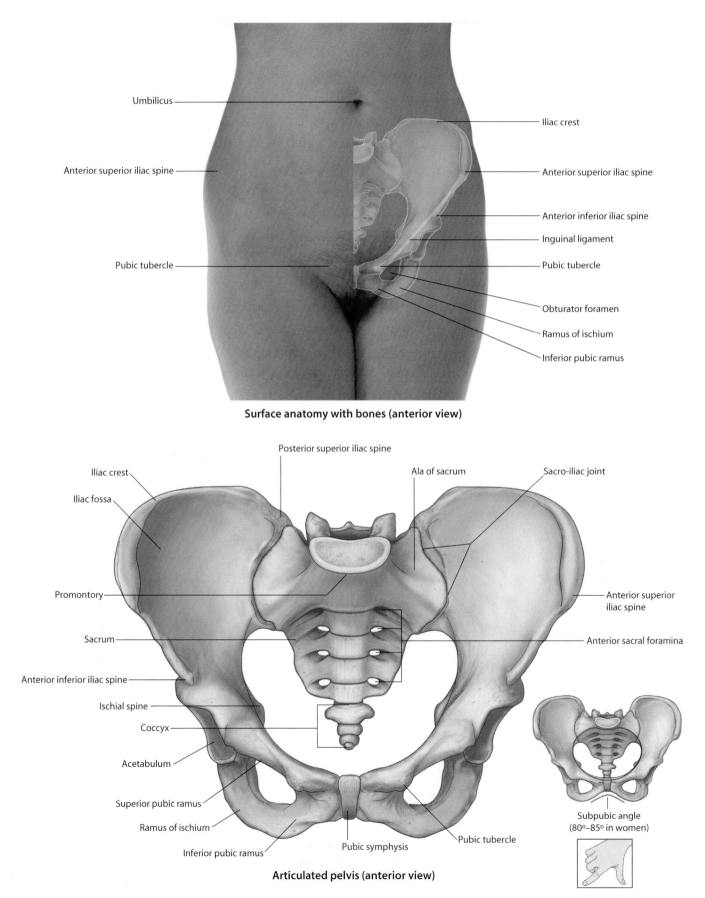

Umbilicus

Anterior superior iliac spine

Pubic tubercle

Iliac crest

Anterior superior iliac spine

Anterior inferior iliac spine

Inguinal ligament

Pubic tubercle

Obturator foramen

Ramus of ischium

Inferior pubic ramus

**Surface anatomy with bones (anterior view)**

Posterior superior iliac spine

Ala of sacrum

Sacro-iliac joint

Iliac crest

Iliac fossa

Promontory

Sacrum

Anterior inferior iliac spine

Ischial spine

Coccyx

Acetabulum

Superior pubic ramus

Ramus of ischium

Inferior pubic ramus

Anterior superior iliac spine

Anterior sacral foramina

Pubic symphysis

Pubic tubercle

**Articulated pelvis (anterior view)**

Subpubic angle
(80°–85° in women)

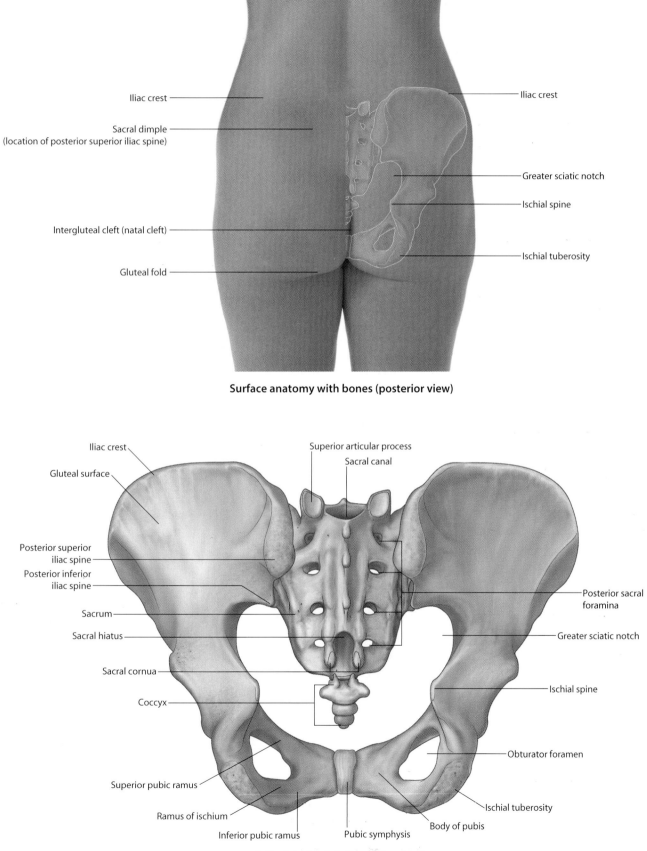

Iliac crest

Sacral dimple
(location of posterior superior iliac spine)

Intergluteal cleft (natal cleft)

Gluteal fold

Iliac crest

Greater sciatic notch

Ischial spine

Ischial tuberosity

**Surface anatomy with bones (posterior view)**

Iliac crest

Gluteal surface

Posterior superior
iliac spine

Posterior inferior
iliac spine

Sacrum

Sacral hiatus

Sacral cornua

Coccyx

Superior pubic ramus

Ramus of ischium

Inferior pubic ramus

Superior articular process

Sacral canal

Posterior sacral
foramina

Greater sciatic notch

Ischial spine

Obturator foramen

Ischial tuberosity

Body of pubis

Pubic symphysis

**Articulated pelvis (posterior view)**

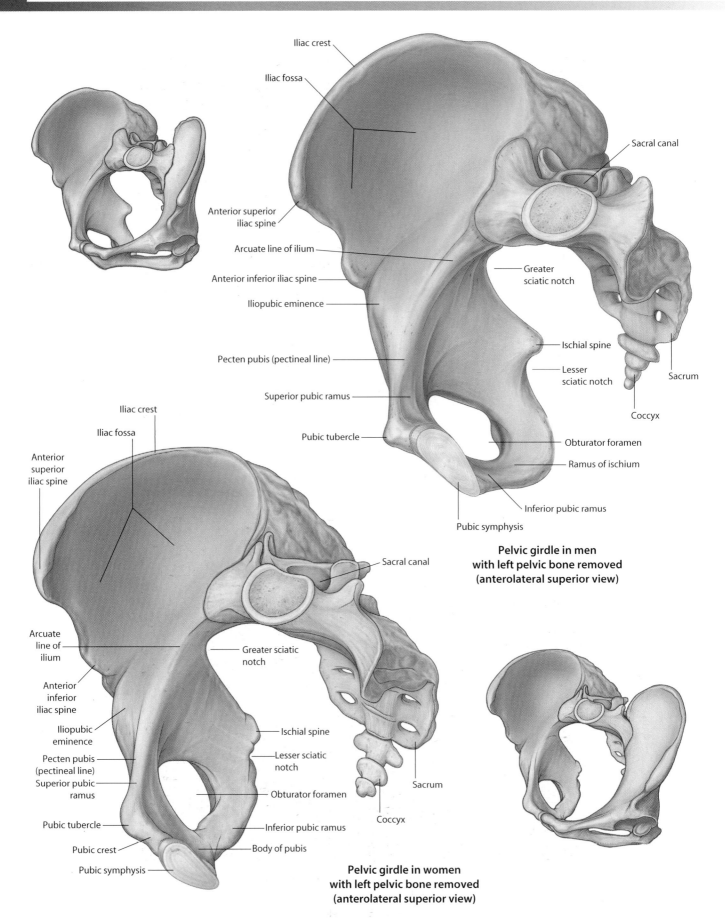

Iliac crest

Iliac fossa

Anterior superior iliac spine

Arcuate line of ilium

Anterior inferior iliac spine

Iliopubic eminence

Pecten pubis (pectineal line)

Superior pubic ramus

Pubic tubercle

Pubic symphysis

Sacral canal

Greater sciatic notch

Ischial spine

Lesser sciatic notch

Sacrum

Coccyx

Obturator foramen

Ramus of ischium

Inferior pubic ramus

**Pelvic girdle in men
with left pelvic bone removed
(anterolateral superior view)**

Iliac crest

Iliac fossa

Anterior superior iliac spine

Arcuate line of ilium

Anterior inferior iliac spine

Iliopubic eminence

Pecten pubis (pectineal line)

Superior pubic ramus

Pubic tubercle

Pubic crest

Pubic symphysis

Sacral canal

Greater sciatic notch

Ischial spine

Lesser sciatic notch

Obturator foramen

Inferior pubic ramus

Body of pubis

Sacrum

Coccyx

**Pelvic girdle in women
with left pelvic bone removed
(anterolateral superior view)**

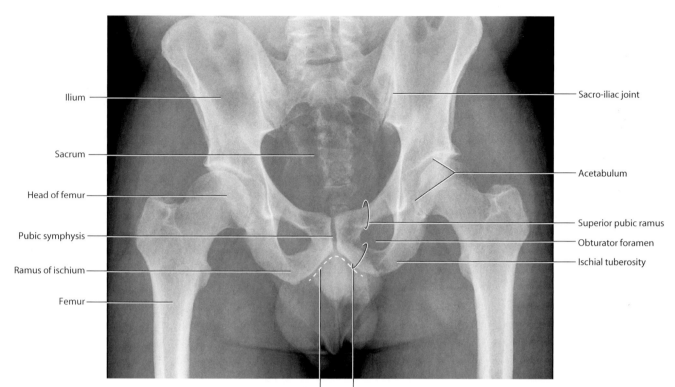

Ilium

Sacrum

Head of femur

Pubic symphysis

Ramus of ischium

Femur

Sacro-iliac joint

Acetabulum

Superior pubic ramus

Obturator foramen

Ischial tuberosity

Subpubic angle
(smaller in men than in women)

Inferior pubic ramus

**Male bony pelvis.**
Radiograph, anterior-posterior view

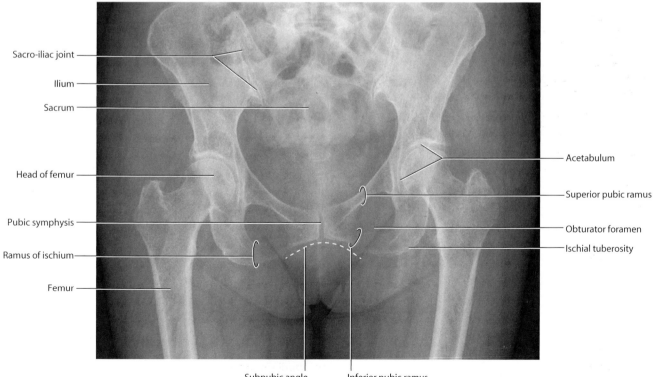

Sacro-iliac joint

Ilium

Sacrum

Head of femur

Pubic symphysis

Ramus of ischium

Femur

Acetabulum

Superior pubic ramus

Obturator foramen

Ischial tuberosity

Subpubic angle
(larger in women than in men)

Inferior pubic ramus

**Female bony pelvis.**
Radiograph, anterior-posterior view

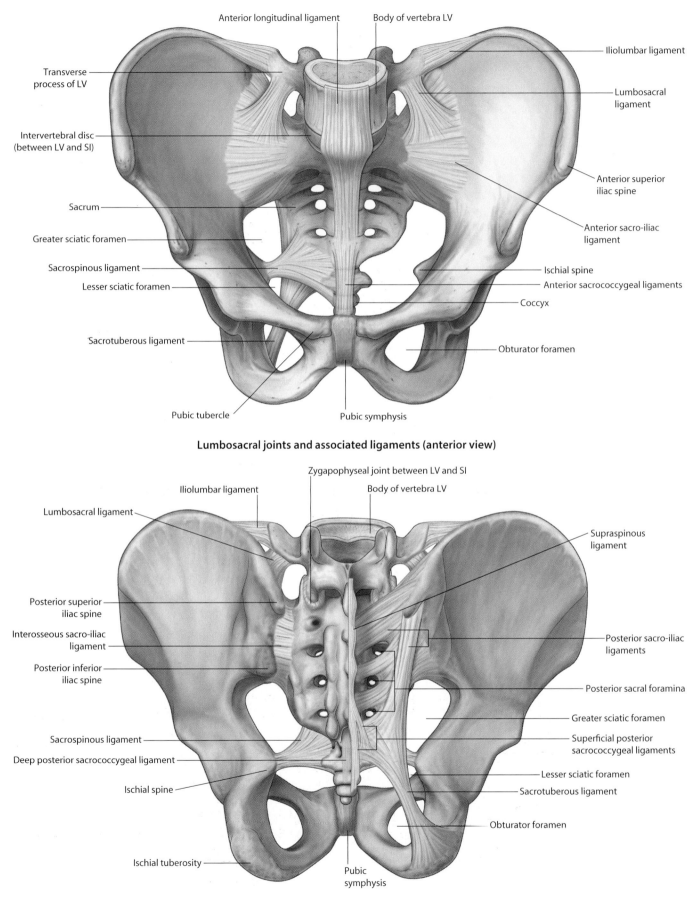

Lumbosacral joints and associated ligaments (anterior view)

Lumbosacral joints and associated ligaments (posterior view)

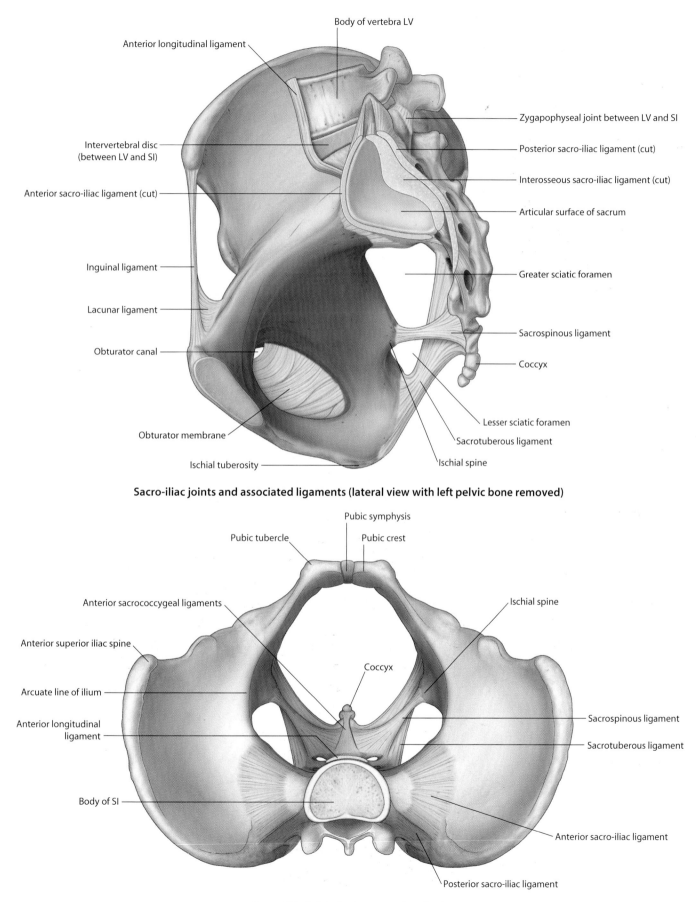

Body of vertebra LV

Anterior longitudinal ligament

Zygapophyseal joint between LV and SI

Intervertebral disc (between LV and SI)

Posterior sacro-iliac ligament (cut)

Interosseous sacro-iliac ligament (cut)

Anterior sacro-iliac ligament (cut)

Articular surface of sacrum

Inguinal ligament

Greater sciatic foramen

Lacunar ligament

Sacrospinous ligament

Obturator canal

Coccyx

Obturator membrane

Lesser sciatic foramen

Ischial tuberosity

Sacrotuberous ligament

Ischial spine

**Sacro-iliac joints and associated ligaments (lateral view with left pelvic bone removed)**

Pubic symphysis

Pubic tubercle

Pubic crest

Anterior sacrococcygeal ligaments

Ischial spine

Anterior superior iliac spine

Coccyx

Arcuate line of ilium

Anterior longitudinal ligament

Sacrospinous ligament

Sacrotuberous ligament

Body of SI

Anterior sacro-iliac ligament

Posterior sacro-iliac ligament

**Sacro-iliac joints (anterosuperior view)**

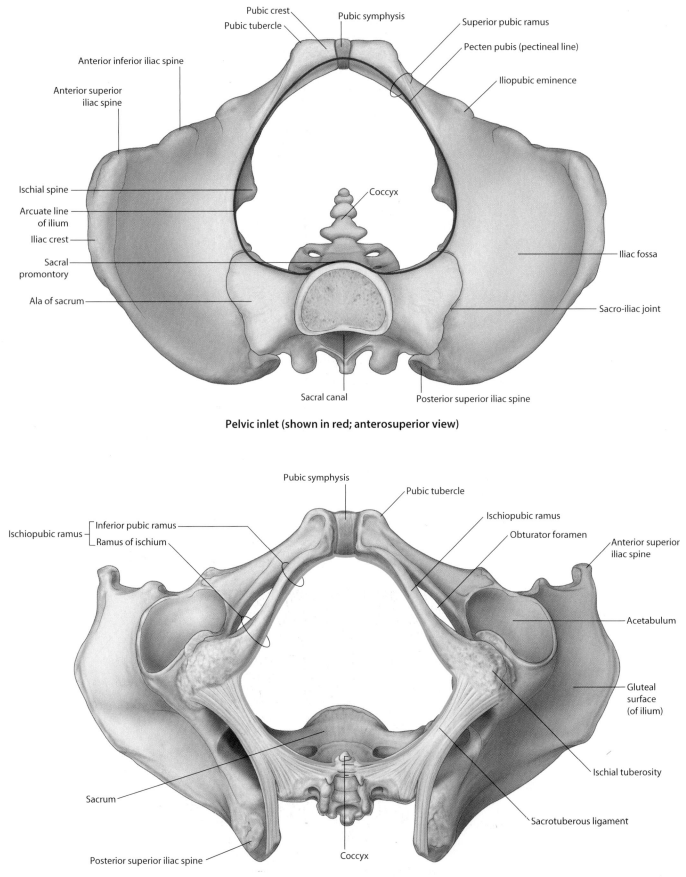

**Pelvic inlet (shown in red; anterosuperior view)**

Pubic crest
Pubic tubercle
Pubic symphysis
Superior pubic ramus
Pecten pubis (pectineal line)
Iliopubic eminence
Anterior inferior iliac spine
Anterior superior iliac spine
Ischial spine
Arcuate line of ilium
Iliac crest
Sacral promontory
Ala of sacrum
Coccyx
Iliac fossa
Sacro-iliac joint
Sacral canal
Posterior superior iliac spine

**Pelvic outlet (shown in green; anteroinferior view)**

Pubic symphysis
Pubic tubercle
Ischiopubic ramus
Obturator foramen
Anterior superior iliac spine
Ischiopubic ramus
Inferior pubic ramus
Ramus of ischium
Acetabulum
Gluteal surface (of ilium)
Ischial tuberosity
Sacrum
Sacrotuberous ligament
Posterior superior iliac spine
Coccyx

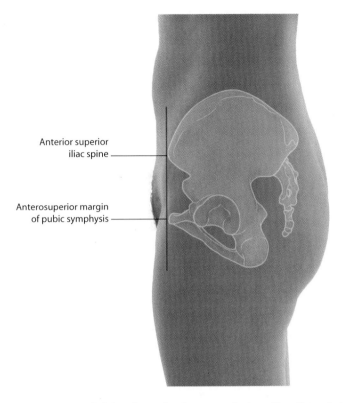

Anterior superior
iliac spine

Anterosuperior margin
of pubic symphysis

**Pelvic orientation in anatomical position (lateral view)**

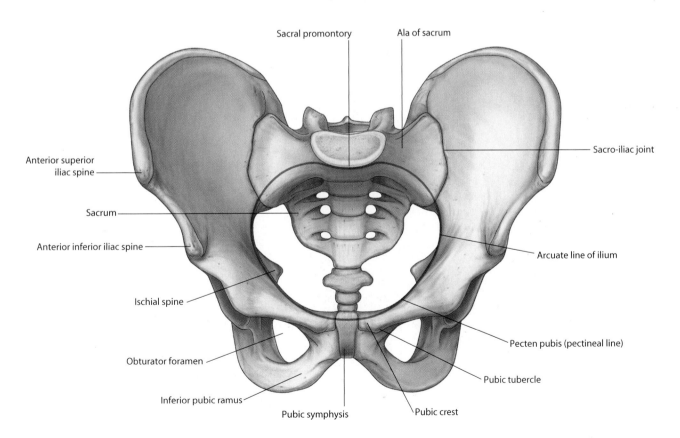

Sacral promontory

Ala of sacrum

Anterior superior
iliac spine

Sacro-iliac joint

Sacrum

Anterior inferior iliac spine

Arcuate line of ilium

Ischial spine

Obturator foramen

Pecten pubis (pectineal line)

Pubic tubercle

Inferior pubic ramus

Pubic symphysis

Pubic crest

**Pelvic brim (shown in red; anterior view)**

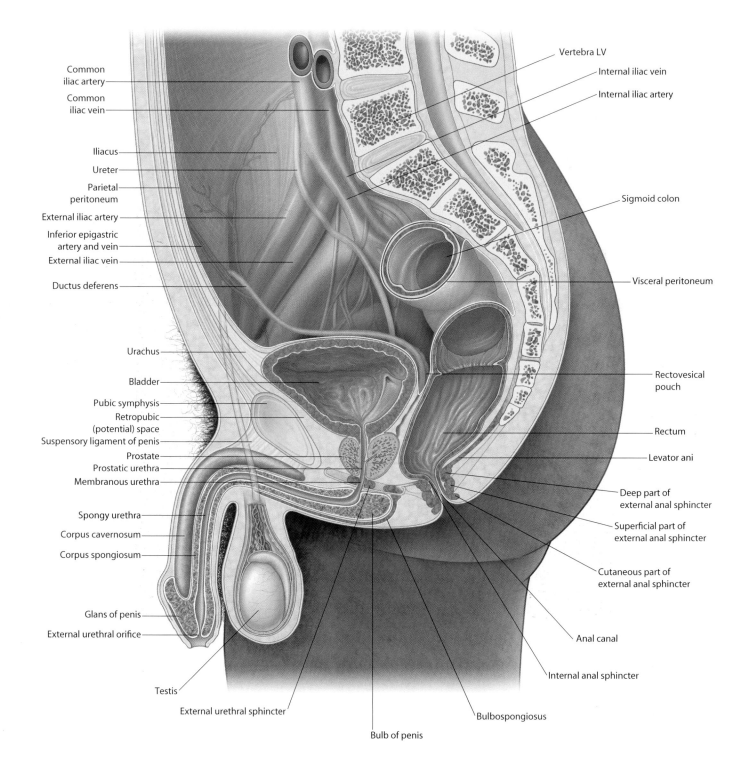

Common iliac artery

Common iliac vein

Iliacus

Ureter

Parietal peritoneum

External iliac artery

Inferior epigastric artery and vein

External iliac vein

Ductus deferens

Urachus

Bladder

Pubic symphysis

Retropubic (potential) space

Suspensory ligament of penis

Prostate

Prostatic urethra

Membranous urethra

Spongy urethra

Corpus cavernosum

Corpus spongiosum

Glans of penis

External urethral orifice

Testis

External urethral sphincter

Bulb of penis

Vertebra LV

Internal iliac vein

Internal iliac artery

Sigmoid colon

Visceral peritoneum

Rectovesical pouch

Rectum

Levator ani

Deep part of external anal sphincter

Superficial part of external anal sphincter

Cutaneous part of external anal sphincter

Anal canal

Internal anal sphincter

Bulbospongiosus

**Pelvic viscera and perineum in men *in situ* (sagittal section)**

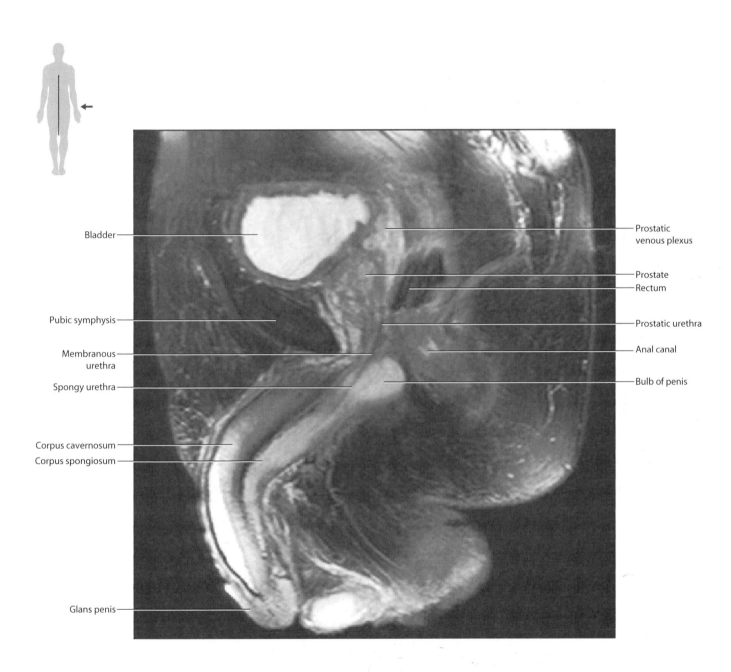

Bladder

Pubic symphysis

Membranous urethra

Spongy urethra

Corpus cavernosum

Corpus spongiosum

Glans penis

Prostatic venous plexus

Prostate

Rectum

Prostatic urethra

Anal canal

Bulb of penis

**Pelvic viscera in men.**
T2-weighted MR image in sagittal plane

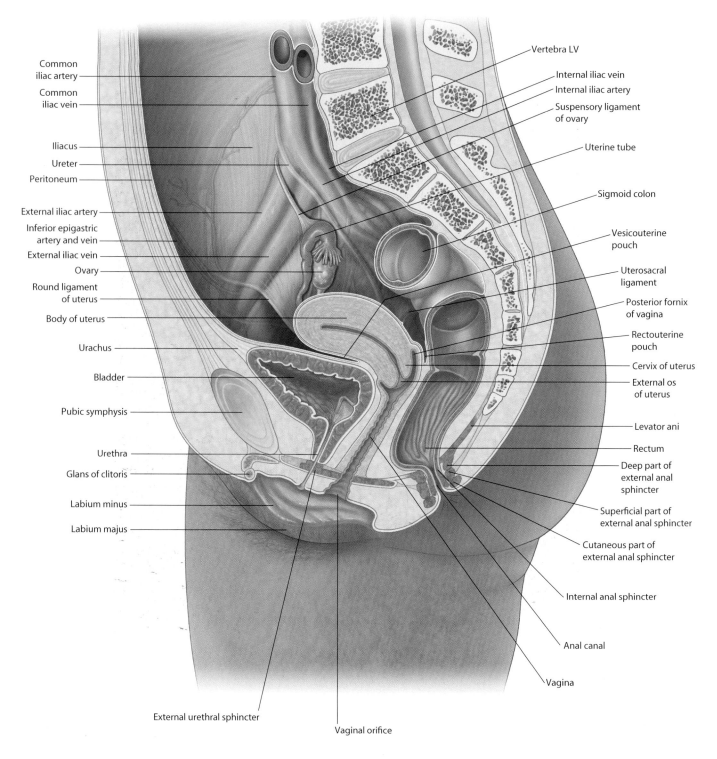

Common iliac artery

Common iliac vein

Iliacus

Ureter

Peritoneum

External iliac artery

Inferior epigastric artery and vein

External iliac vein

Ovary

Round ligament of uterus

Body of uterus

Urachus

Bladder

Pubic symphysis

Urethra

Glans of clitoris

Labium minus

Labium majus

External urethral sphincter

Vaginal orifice

Vertebra LV

Internal iliac vein

Internal iliac artery

Suspensory ligament of ovary

Uterine tube

Sigmoid colon

Vesicouterine pouch

Uterosacral ligament

Posterior fornix of vagina

Rectouterine pouch

Cervix of uterus

External os of uterus

Levator ani

Rectum

Deep part of external anal sphincter

Superficial part of external anal sphincter

Cutaneous part of external anal sphincter

Internal anal sphincter

Anal canal

Vagina

Pelvic viscera and perineum in women *in situ* (sagittal section)

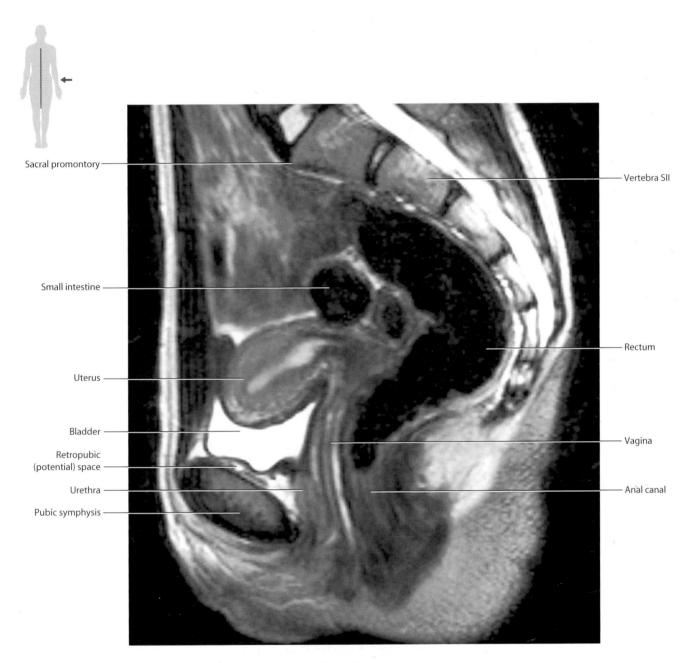

Sacral promontory

Small intestine

Uterus

Bladder

Retropubic (potential) space

Urethra

Pubic symphysis

Vertebra SII

Rectum

Vagina

Anal canal

**Pelvic viscera in women.**
T2-weighted MR image in sagittal plane

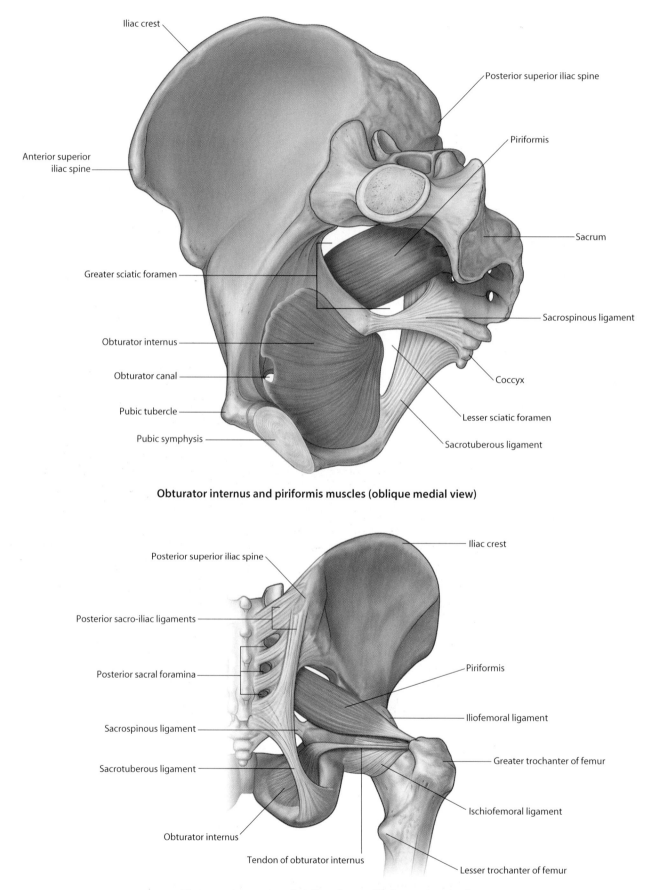

Iliac crest

Posterior superior iliac spine

Anterior superior iliac spine

Piriformis

Greater sciatic foramen

Sacrum

Obturator internus

Obturator canal

Sacrospinous ligament

Pubic tubercle

Coccyx

Pubic symphysis

Lesser sciatic foramen

Sacrotuberous ligament

**Obturator internus and piriformis muscles (oblique medial view)**

Iliac crest

Posterior superior iliac spine

Posterior sacro-iliac ligaments

Posterior sacral foramina

Piriformis

Iliofemoral ligament

Sacrospinous ligament

Sacrotuberous ligament

Greater trochanter of femur

Ischiofemoral ligament

Obturator internus

Tendon of obturator internus

Lesser trochanter of femur

**Obturator internus and piriformis muscles (posterior view)**

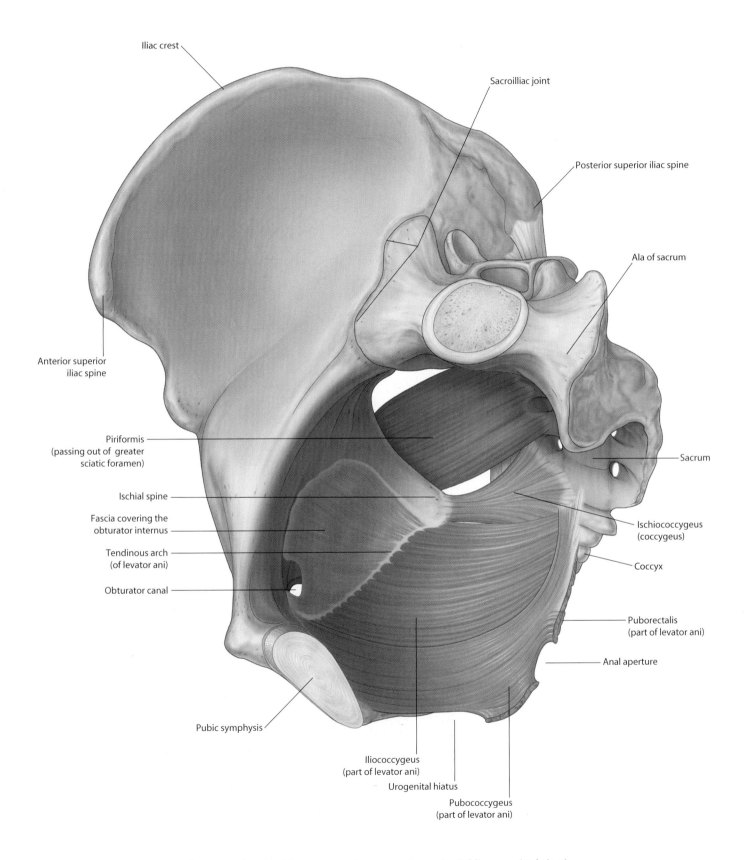

Iliac crest

Sacroilliac joint

Posterior superior iliac spine

Ala of sacrum

Anterior superior
iliac spine

Piriformis
(passing out of greater
sciatic foramen)

Sacrum

Ischial spine

Fascia covering the
obturator internus

Ischiococcygeus
(coccygeus)

Tendinous arch
(of levator ani)

Coccyx

Obturator canal

Puborectalis
(part of levator ani)

Anal aperture

Pubic symphysis

Iliococcygeus
(part of levator ani)

Urogenital hiatus

Pubococcygeus
(part of levator ani)

**Levator ani and ischiococcygeus (coccygeus) muscles (oblique sagittal view)**

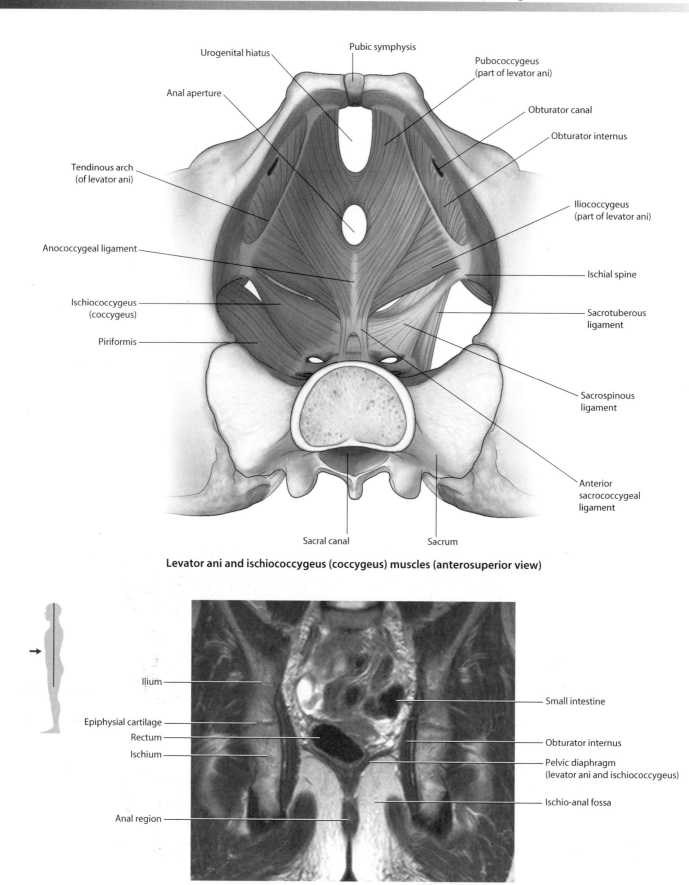

**Levator ani and ischiococcygeus (coccygeus) muscles (anterosuperior view)**

**Pelvic diaphragm in relation to other structures in the pelvic cavity and perineum.**
T2-weighted MR image in coronal plane

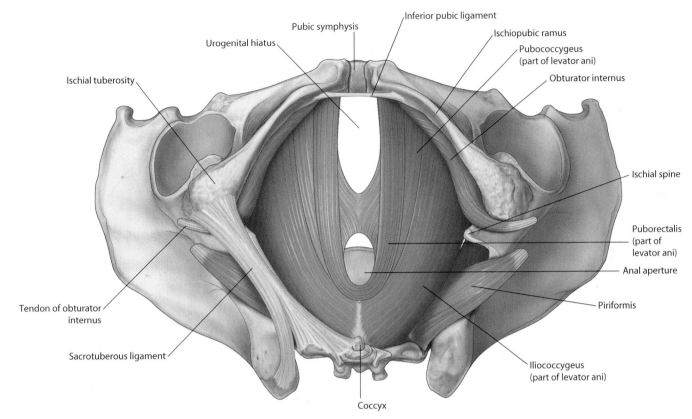

Inferior pubic ligament

Pubic symphysis

Urogenital hiatus

Ischiopubic ramus

Pubococcygeus
(part of levator ani)

Obturator internus

Ischial tuberosity

Ischial spine

Puborectalis
(part of
levator ani)

Anal aperture

Piriformis

Tendon of obturator
internus

Sacrotuberous ligament

Iliococcygeus
(part of levator ani)

Coccyx

**Levator ani muscle (inferior view)**

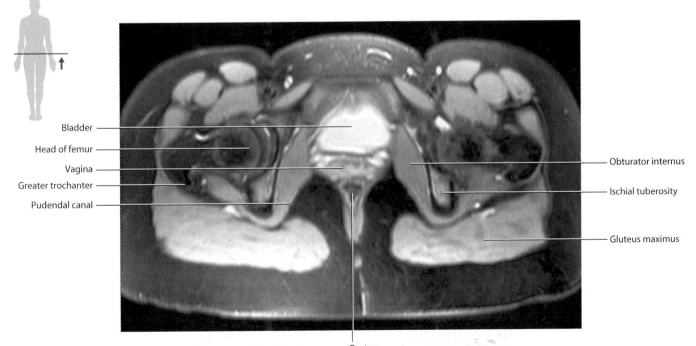

Bladder

Head of femur

Vagina

Greater trochanter

Pudendal canal

Obturator internus

Ischial tuberosity

Gluteus maximus

Rectum

**Obturator internus muscle and its relationship to other pelvic structures.**
T2-weighted MR image in axial plane

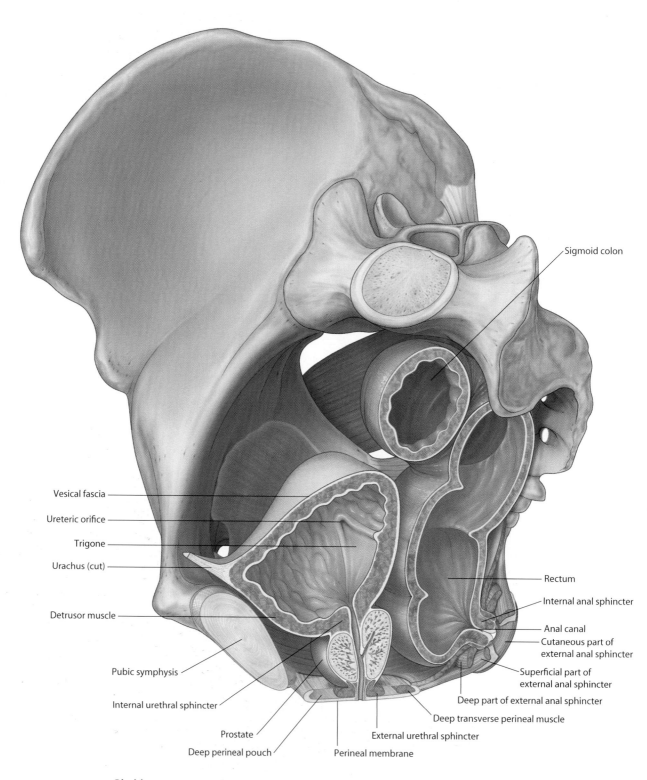

Sigmoid colon

Vesical fascia

Ureteric orifice

Trigone

Urachus (cut)

Detrusor muscle

Pubic symphysis

Internal urethral sphincter

Prostate

Deep perineal pouch

Perineal membrane

External urethral sphincter

Deep transverse perineal muscle

Deep part of external anal sphincter

Superficial part of external anal sphincter

Cutaneous part of external anal sphincter

Anal canal

Internal anal sphincter

Rectum

**Bladder, prostate, and rectum within pelvic cavity in men (oblique sagittal view)**

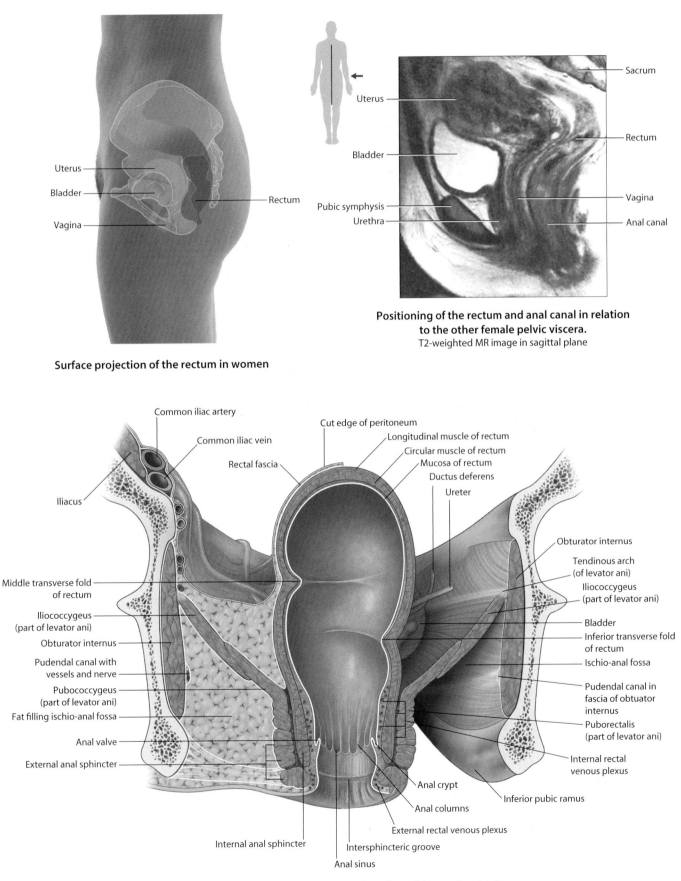

**Surface projection of the rectum in women**

Uterus
Bladder
Vagina
Rectum

**Positioning of the rectum and anal canal in relation to the other female pelvic viscera.**
T2-weighted MR image in sagittal plane

Uterus
Bladder
Pubic symphysis
Urethra
Sacrum
Rectum
Vagina
Anal canal

Common iliac artery
Common iliac vein
Cut edge of peritoneum
Longitudinal muscle of rectum
Circular muscle of rectum
Mucosa of rectum
Ductus deferens
Ureter
Rectal fascia
Iliacus
Obturator internus
Tendinous arch (of levator ani)
Iliococcygeus (part of levator ani)
Middle transverse fold of rectum
Iliococcygeus (part of levator ani)
Obturator internus
Pudendal canal with vessels and nerve
Pubococcygeus (part of levator ani)
Fat filling ischio-anal fossa
Anal valve
External anal sphincter
Bladder
Inferior transverse fold of rectum
Ischio-anal fossa
Pudendal canal in fascia of obturator internus
Puborectalis (part of levator ani)
Internal rectal venous plexus
Inferior pubic ramus
External rectal venous plexus
Internal anal sphincter
Intersphincteric groove
Anal sinus
Anal crypt
Anal columns

**Coronal section through rectum and anal canal (posterior view)**

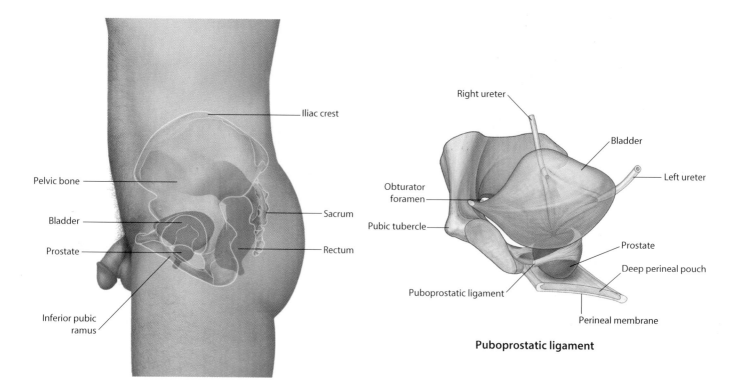

**Surface projection of the bladder in men (lateral view)**

Iliac crest

Pelvic bone

Bladder

Prostate

Inferior pubic ramus

Sacrum

Rectum

Right ureter

Bladder

Obturator foramen

Pubic tubercle

Left ureter

Prostate

Deep perineal pouch

Puboprostatic ligament

Perineal membrane

**Puboprostatic ligament**

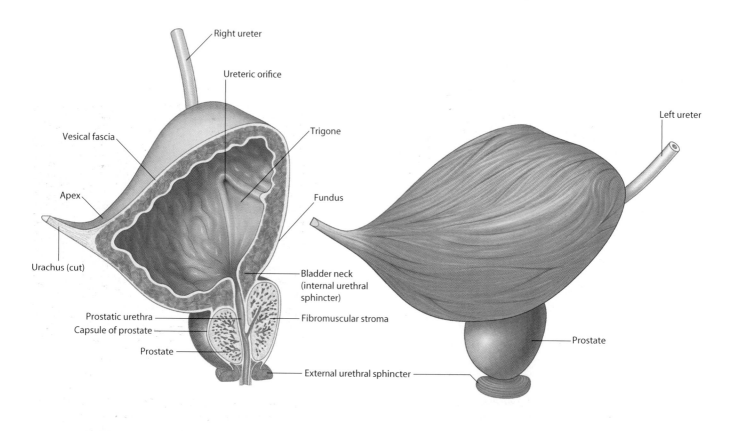

Right ureter

Ureteric orifice

Vesical fascia

Trigone

Apex

Fundus

Urachus (cut)

Left ureter

Bladder neck (internal urethral sphincter)

Prostatic urethra

Capsule of prostate

Prostate

Fibromuscular stroma

Prostate

External urethral sphincter

**Urinary bladder in men**

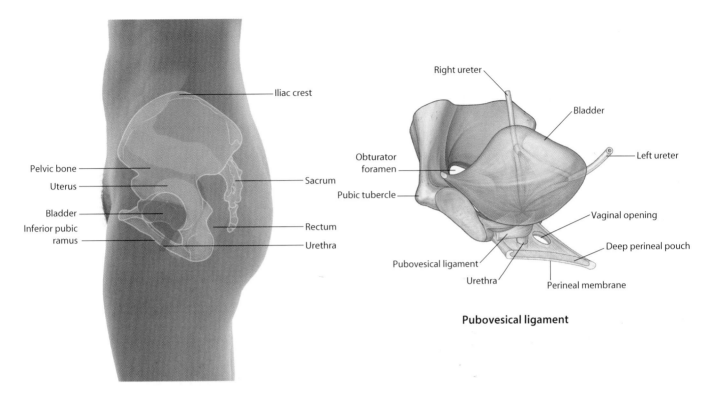

Iliac crest

Pelvic bone

Uterus

Bladder

Inferior pubic ramus

Sacrum

Rectum

Urethra

**Surface projection of the bladder in women (lateral view)**

Right ureter

Bladder

Obturator foramen

Pubic tubercle

Left ureter

Vaginal opening

Deep perineal pouch

Pubovesical ligament

Urethra

Perineal membrane

**Pubovesical ligament**

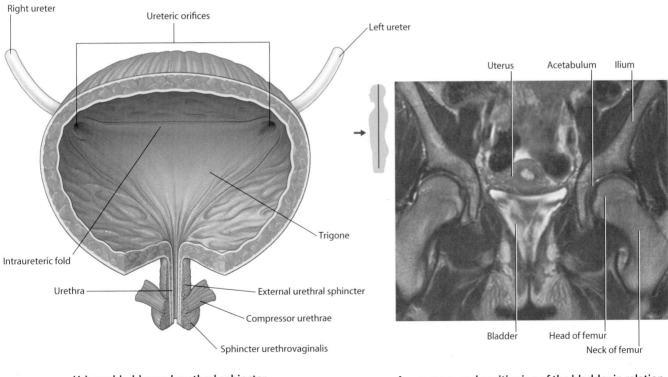

Right ureter

Ureteric orifices

Left ureter

Intraureteric fold

Trigone

Urethra

External urethral sphincter

Compressor urethrae

Sphincter urethrovaginalis

**Urinary bladder and urethral sphincter muscles in women (anterior view of posterior wall)**

Uterus

Acetabulum

Ilium

Bladder

Head of femur

Neck of femur

**Appearance and positioning of the bladder in relation to other structures in the female pelvic cavity.**
T2-weighted MR image in coronal plane

**219**

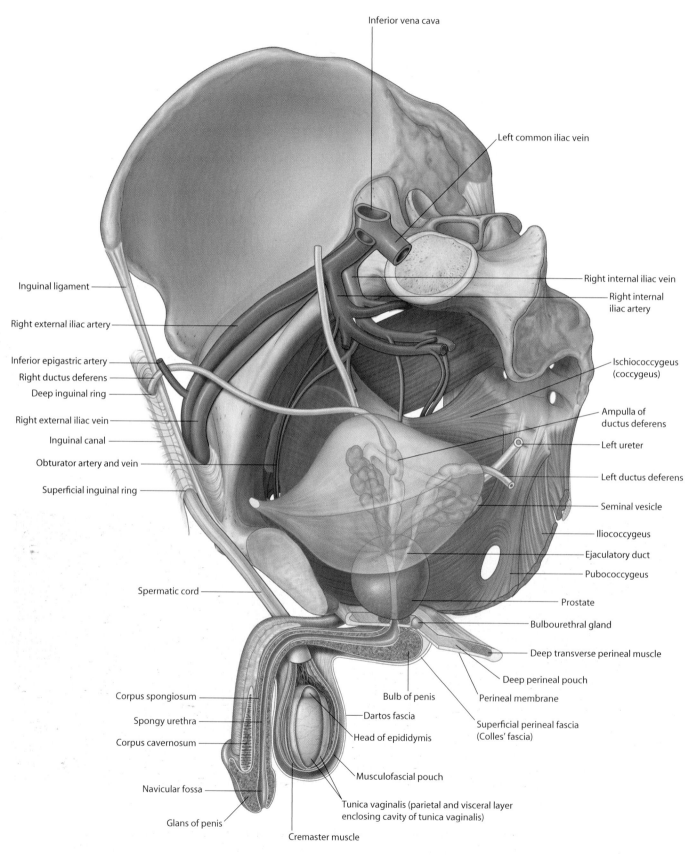

Inferior vena cava

Left common iliac vein

Right internal iliac vein

Right internal iliac artery

Inguinal ligament

Right external iliac artery

Inferior epigastric artery

Right ductus deferens

Deep inguinal ring

Right external iliac vein

Inguinal canal

Obturator artery and vein

Superficial inguinal ring

Ischiococcygeus (coccygeus)

Ampulla of ductus deferens

Left ureter

Left ductus deferens

Seminal vesicle

Iliococcygeus

Ejaculatory duct

Pubococcygeus

Prostate

Bulbourethral gland

Deep transverse perineal muscle

Deep perineal pouch

Perineal membrane

Superficial perineal fascia (Colles' fascia)

Spermatic cord

Corpus spongiosum

Spongy urethra

Corpus cavernosum

Navicular fossa

Glans of penis

Bulb of penis

Dartos fascia

Head of epididymis

Musculofascial pouch

Tunica vaginalis (parietal and visceral layer enclosing cavity of tunica vaginalis)

Cremaster muscle

**Reproductive system in men (oblique sagittal view)**

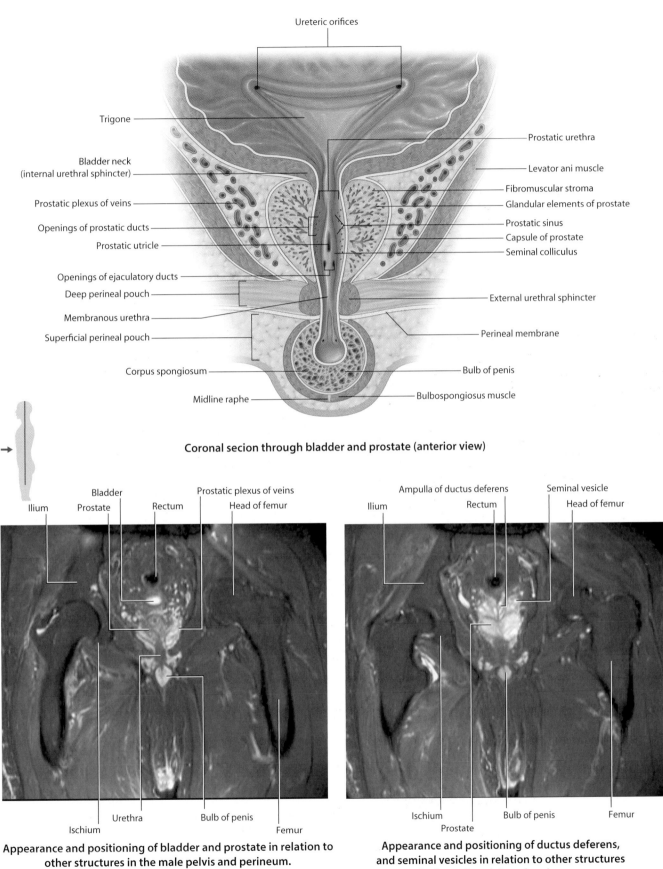

Ureteric orifices

Trigone

Bladder neck
(internal urethral sphincter)

Prostatic plexus of veins

Openings of prostatic ducts

Prostatic utricle

Openings of ejaculatory ducts

Deep perineal pouch

Membranous urethra

Superficial perineal pouch

Corpus spongiosum

Midline raphe

Prostatic urethra

Levator ani muscle

Fibromuscular stroma

Glandular elements of prostate

Prostatic sinus

Capsule of prostate

Seminal colliculus

External urethral sphincter

Perineal membrane

Bulb of penis

Bulbospongiosus muscle

**Coronal secion through bladder and prostate (anterior view)**

Bladder

Ilium  Prostate  Rectum

Prostatic plexus of veins
Head of femur

Urethra  Bulb of penis

Ischium  Femur

**Appearance and positioning of bladder and prostate in relation to
other structures in the male pelvis and perineum.**
T2-weighted MR image in coronal plane

Ampulla of ductus deferens
Rectum

Seminal vesicle
Head of femur

Ilium

Ischium  Bulb of penis  Femur
Prostate

**Appearance and positioning of ductus deferens,
and seminal vesicles in relation to other structures
in the male pelvis and perineum.**
T2-weighted MR image in coronal plane

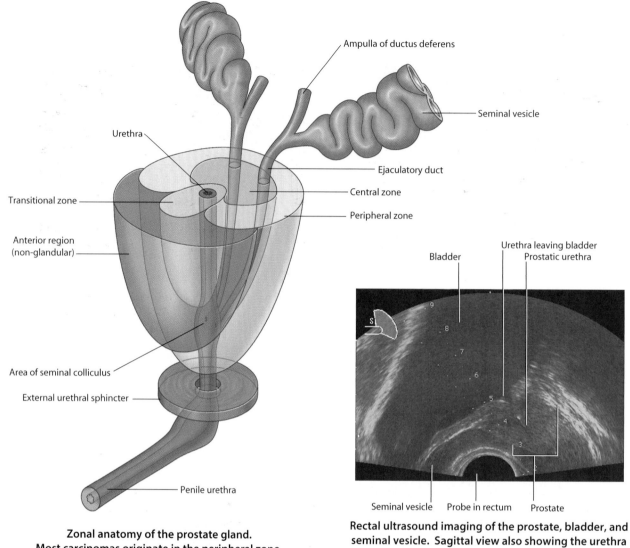

Urethra

Transitional zone

Anterior region
(non-glandular)

Area of seminal colliculus

External urethral sphincter

Ampulla of ductus deferens

Seminal vesicle

Ejaculatory duct

Central zone

Peripheral zone

Penile urethra

**Zonal anatomy of the prostate gland.
Most carcinomas originate in the peripheral zone.
Benign prostatic hypertrophy (BPH)
affects mainly the transitional zone**

Bladder

Urethra leaving bladder
Prostatic urethra

Seminal vesicle      Probe in rectum      Prostate

**Rectal ultrasound imaging of the prostate, bladder, and
seminal vesicle. Sagittal view also showing the urethra**

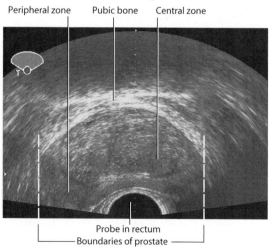

Peripheral zone      Pubic bone      Central zone

Probe in rectum
Boundaries of prostate

**Rectal ultrasound imaging of the prostate.
Axial view showing the central and peripheral zones**

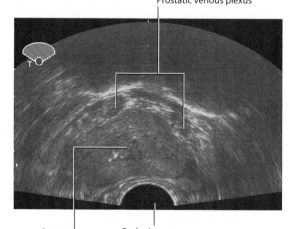

Prostatic venous plexus

Prostate      Probe in rectum

**Rectal ultrasound imaging of the prostate.
Axial view showing the surrounding plexus of veins**

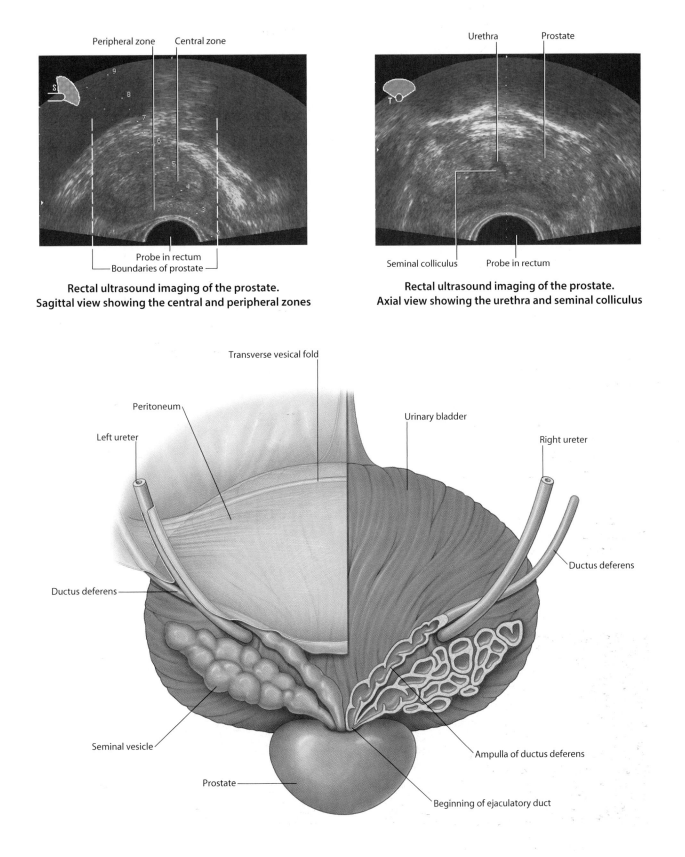

Peripheral zone    Central zone

Probe in rectum
Boundaries of prostate

**Rectal ultrasound imaging of the prostate.
Sagittal view showing the central and peripheral zones**

Urethra    Prostate

Seminal colliculus    Probe in rectum

**Rectal ultrasound imaging of the prostate.
Axial view showing the urethra and seminal colliculus**

Transverse vesical fold

Peritoneum

Left ureter

Urinary bladder

Right ureter

Ductus deferens

Ductus deferens

Seminal vesicle

Ampulla of ductus deferens

Prostate

Beginning of ejaculatory duct

**Bladder and prostate (posterior view)**

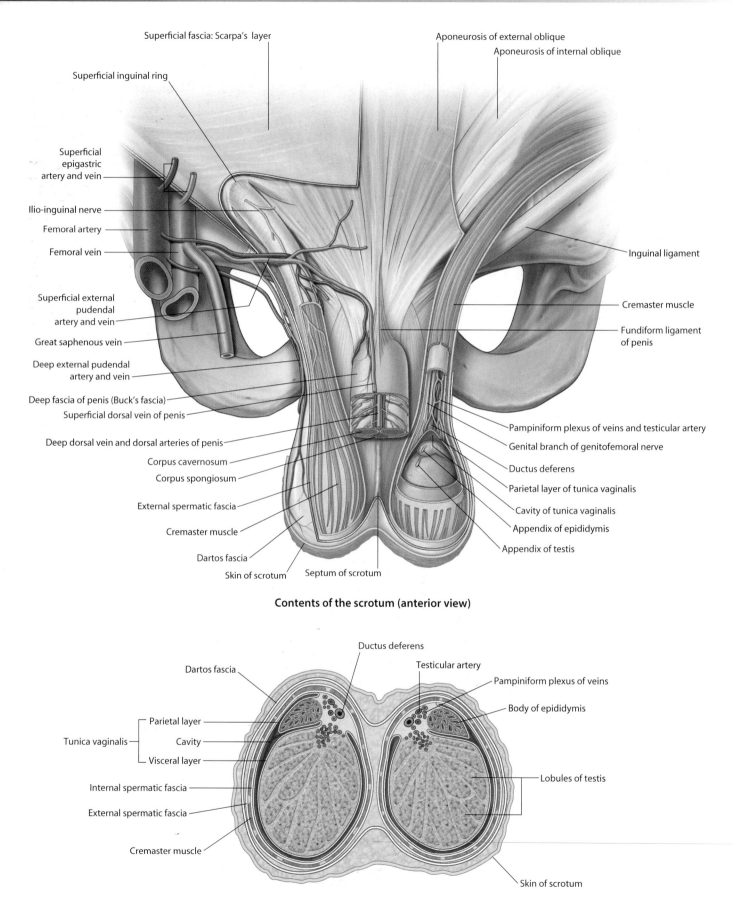

Superficial fascia: Scarpa's layer

Superficial inguinal ring

Superficial epigastric artery and vein

Ilio-inguinal nerve

Femoral artery

Femoral vein

Superficial external pudendal artery and vein

Great saphenous vein

Deep external pudendal artery and vein

Deep fascia of penis (Buck's fascia)

Superficial dorsal vein of penis

Deep dorsal vein and dorsal arteries of penis

Corpus cavernosum

Corpus spongiosum

External spermatic fascia

Cremaster muscle

Dartos fascia

Skin of scrotum

Septum of scrotum

Aponeurosis of external oblique

Aponeurosis of internal oblique

Inguinal ligament

Cremaster muscle

Fundiform ligament of penis

Pampiniform plexus of veins and testicular artery

Genital branch of genitofemoral nerve

Ductus deferens

Parietal layer of tunica vaginalis

Cavity of tunica vaginalis

Appendix of epididymis

Appendix of testis

**Contents of the scrotum (anterior view)**

Ductus deferens

Testicular artery

Dartos fascia

Pampiniform plexus of veins

Body of epididymis

Parietal layer

Tunica vaginalis — Cavity

Visceral layer

Internal spermatic fascia

External spermatic fascia

Cremaster muscle

Lobules of testis

Skin of scrotum

**Transverse section through the scrotum and testes**

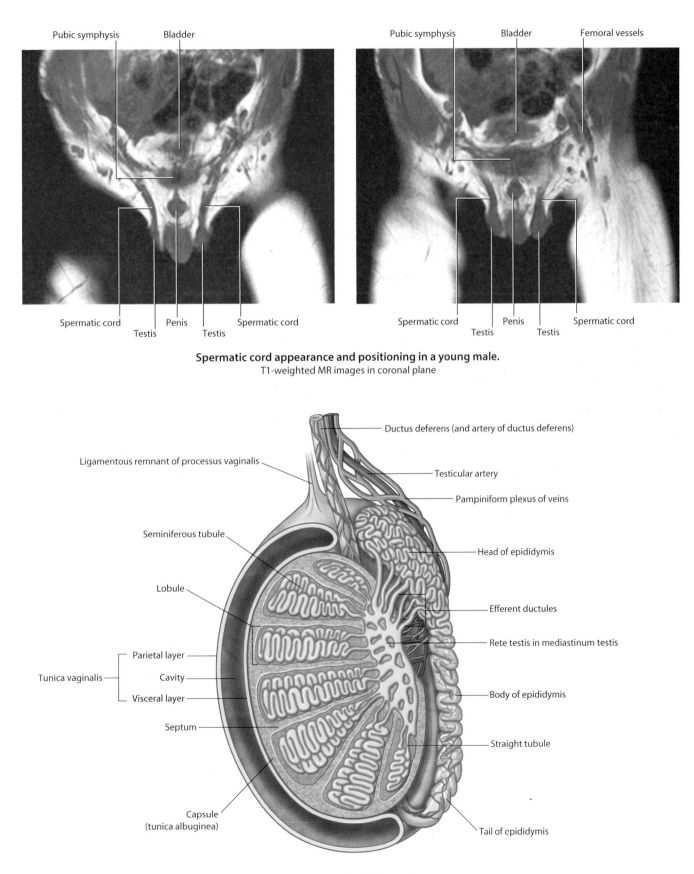

**Spermatic cord appearance and positioning in a young male.**
T1-weighted MR images in coronal plane

Pubic symphysis    Bladder

Spermatic cord    Penis    Spermatic cord
Testis    Testis

Pubic symphysis    Bladder    Femoral vessels

Spermatic cord    Penis    Spermatic cord
Testis    Testis

Ductus deferens (and artery of ductus deferens)

Ligamentous remnant of processus vaginalis

Testicular artery

Pampiniform plexus of veins

Seminiferous tubule

Head of epididymis

Lobule

Efferent ductules

Rete testis in mediastinum testis

Parietal layer
Tunica vaginalis    Cavity
Visceral layer

Body of epididymis

Septum

Straight tubule

Capsule
(tunica albuginea)

Tail of epididymis

**Testis and surrounding structures**

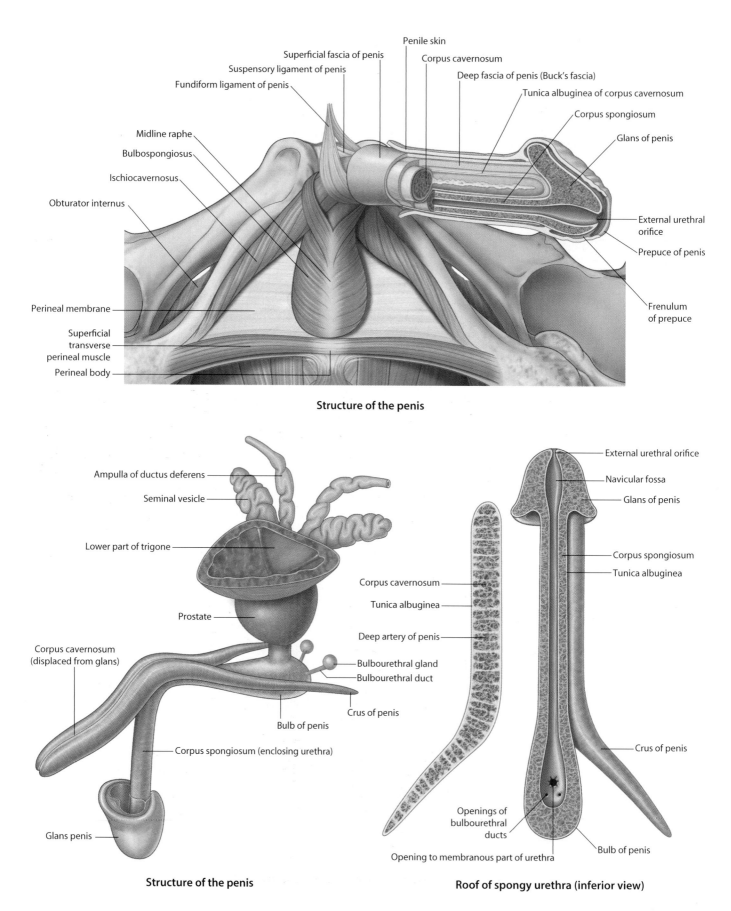

**Structure of the penis**

**Structure of the penis**

**Roof of spongy urethra (inferior view)**

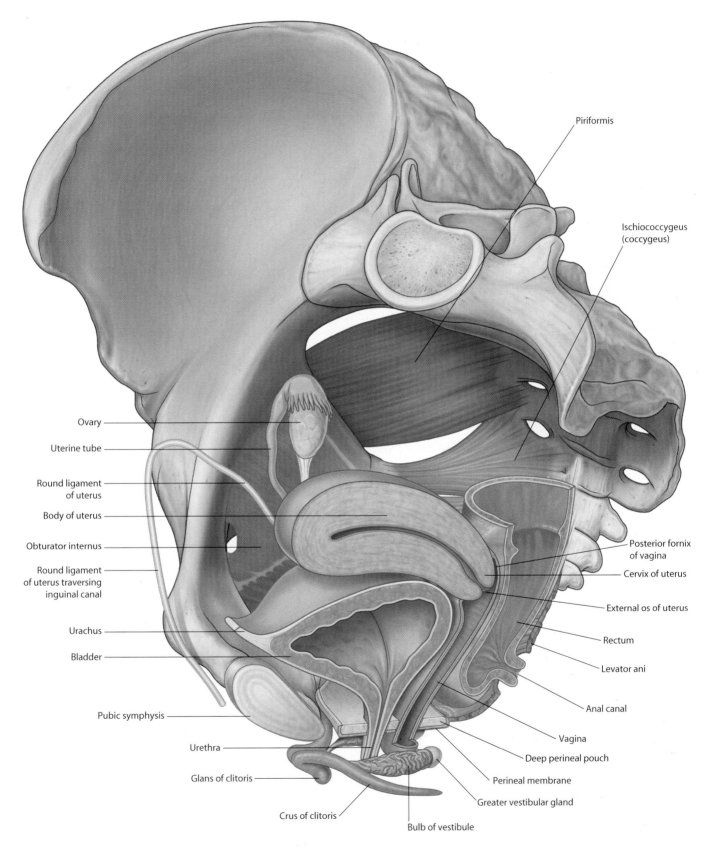

Piriformis

Ischiococcygeus (coccygeus)

Ovary

Uterine tube

Round ligament of uterus

Body of uterus

Obturator internus

Round ligament of uterus traversing inguinal canal

Urachus

Bladder

Pubic symphysis

Urethra

Glans of clitoris

Crus of clitoris

Bulb of vestibule

Posterior fornix of vagina

Cervix of uterus

External os of uterus

Rectum

Levator ani

Anal canal

Vagina

Deep perineal pouch

Perineal membrane

Greater vestibular gland

**Reproductive system in women (oblique sagittal view)**

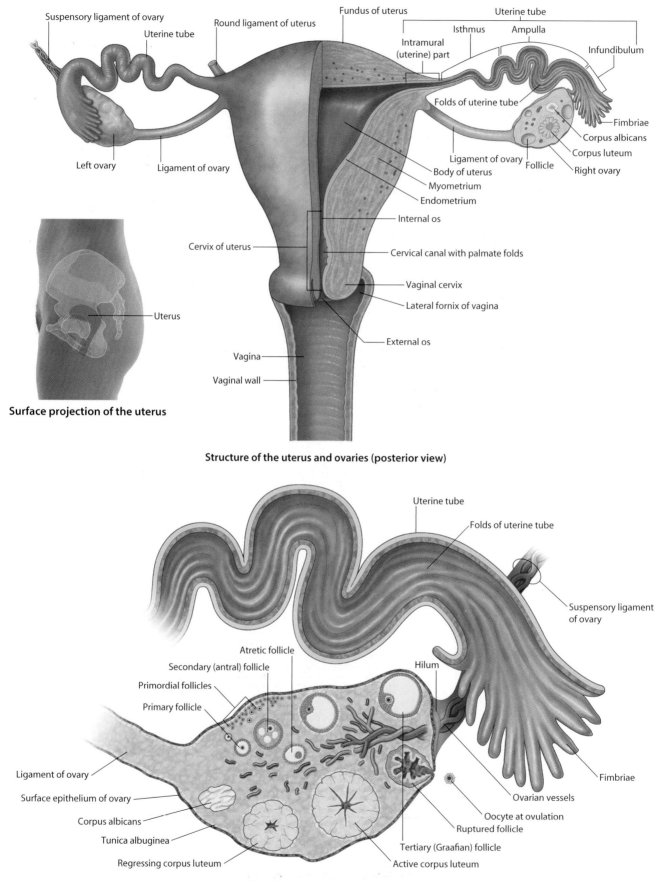

Suspensory ligament of ovary

Uterine tube

Round ligament of uterus

Fundus of uterus

Uterine tube

Isthmus    Ampulla

Intramural (uterine) part

Infundibulum

Folds of uterine tube

Fimbriae

Corpus albicans

Corpus luteum

Left ovary

Ligament of ovary

Ligament of ovary    Follicle    Right ovary

Body of uterus

Myometrium

Endometrium

Internal os

Cervix of uterus

Cervical canal with palmate folds

Vaginal cervix

Lateral fornix of vagina

External os

Vagina

Vaginal wall

Uterus

**Surface projection of the uterus**

**Structure of the uterus and ovaries (posterior view)**

Uterine tube

Folds of uterine tube

Suspensory ligament of ovary

Atretic follicle

Secondary (antral) follicle

Primordial follicles

Primary follicle

Hilum

Ligament of ovary

Surface epithelium of ovary

Corpus albicans

Tunica albuginea

Regressing corpus luteum

Fimbriae

Ovarian vessels

Oocyte at ovulation

Ruptured follicle

Tertiary (Graafian) follicle

Active corpus luteum

**Structure of the uterine tube and ovary (posterior view)**

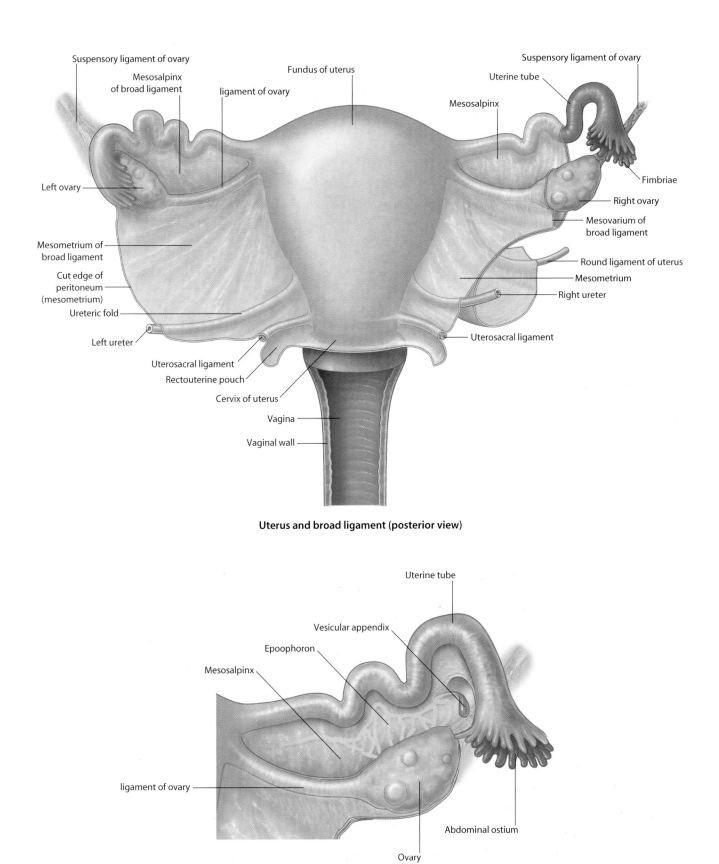

Suspensory ligament of ovary

Mesosalpinx of broad ligament

ligament of ovary

Fundus of uterus

Suspensory ligament of ovary

Uterine tube

Mesosalpinx

Left ovary

Fimbriae

Right ovary

Mesovarium of broad ligament

Mesometrium of broad ligament

Round ligament of uterus

Mesometrium

Cut edge of peritoneum (mesometrium)

Right ureter

Ureteric fold

Left ureter

Uterosacral ligament

Uterosacral ligament

Rectouterine pouch

Cervix of uterus

Vagina

Vaginal wall

**Uterus and broad ligament (posterior view)**

Uterine tube

Vesicular appendix

Epoophoron

Mesosalpinx

ligament of ovary

Abdominal ostium

Ovary

**Uterine tube and ovary (posterior view)**

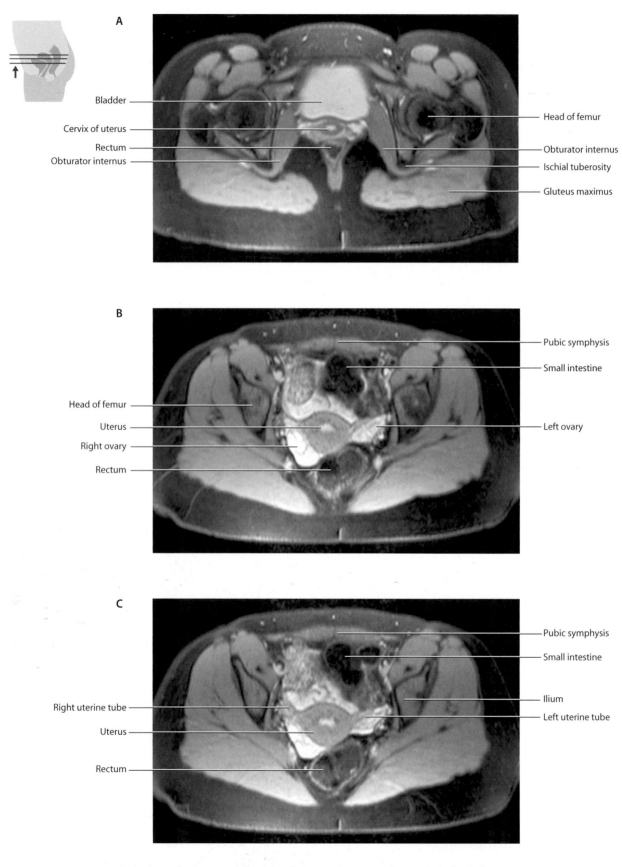

**A**

Bladder

Cervix of uterus

Rectum

Obturator internus

Head of femur

Obturator internus

Ischial tuberosity

Gluteus maximus

**B**

Head of femur

Uterus

Right ovary

Rectum

Pubic symphysis

Small intestine

Left ovary

**C**

Right uterine tube

Uterus

Rectum

Pubic symphysis

Small intestine

Ilium

Left uterine tube

**Appearance of cervix of uterus, uterus, ovaries, and uterine tubes
in relation to other pelvic structures.**
T2-weighted MR images in axial plane

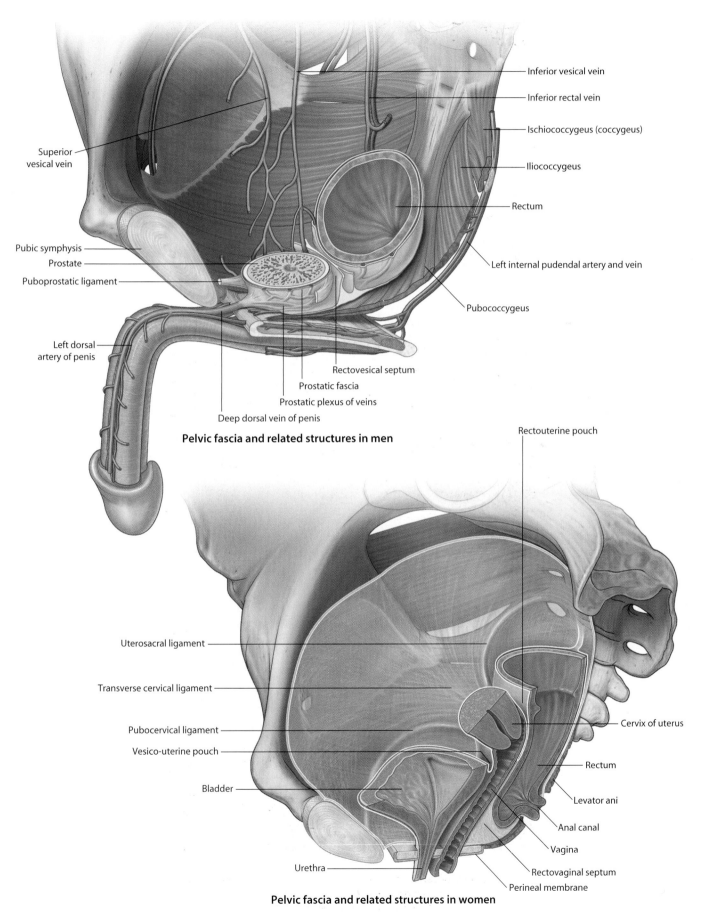

**Pelvic fascia and related structures in men**

Inferior vesical vein

Inferior rectal vein

Ischiococcygeus (coccygeus)

Iliococcygeus

Rectum

Left internal pudendal artery and vein

Pubococcygeus

Superior vesical vein

Pubic symphysis

Prostate

Puboprostatic ligament

Left dorsal artery of penis

Rectovesical septum

Prostatic fascia

Prostatic plexus of veins

Deep dorsal vein of penis

**Pelvic fascia and related structures in women**

Rectouterine pouch

Uterosacral ligament

Transverse cervical ligament

Pubocervical ligament

Vesico-uterine pouch

Bladder

Urethra

Cervix of uterus

Rectum

Levator ani

Anal canal

Vagina

Rectovaginal septum

Perineal membrane

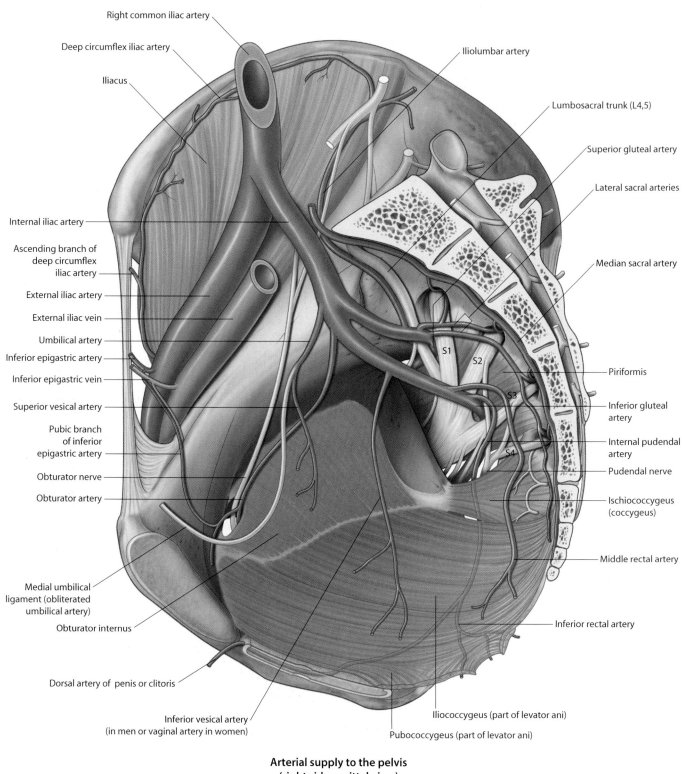

Right common iliac artery

Deep circumflex iliac artery

Iliacus

Iliolumbar artery

Lumbosacral trunk (L4,5)

Superior gluteal artery

Lateral sacral arteries

Internal iliac artery

Ascending branch of deep circumflex iliac artery

External iliac artery

External iliac vein

Umbilical artery

Inferior epigastric artery

Inferior epigastric vein

Superior vesical artery

Pubic branch of inferior epigastric artery

Obturator nerve

Obturator artery

Median sacral artery

Piriformis

Inferior gluteal artery

Internal pudendal artery

Pudendal nerve

Ischiococcygeus (coccygeus)

Middle rectal artery

Medial umbilical ligament (obliterated umbilical artery)

Obturator internus

Dorsal artery of penis or clitoris

Inferior vesical artery (in men or vaginal artery in women)

Inferior rectal artery

Iliococcygeus (part of levator ani)

Pubococcygeus (part of levator ani)

S1

S2

S3

S4

**Arterial supply to the pelvis (right side sagittal view)**

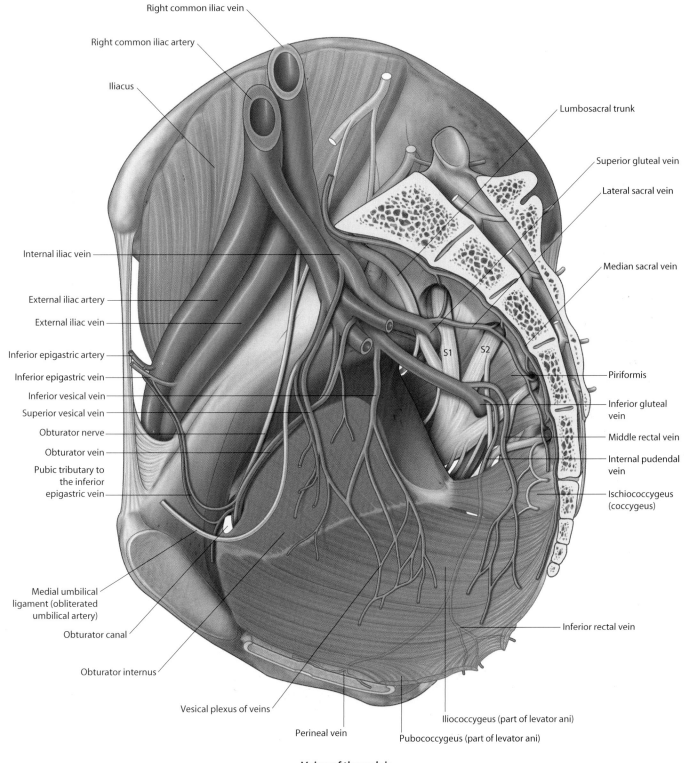

Right common iliac vein

Right common iliac artery

Iliacus

Lumbosacral trunk

Superior gluteal vein

Lateral sacral vein

Internal iliac vein

Median sacral vein

External iliac artery

External iliac vein

S1

S2

Inferior epigastric artery

Inferior epigastric vein

Piriformis

Inferior vesical vein

Superior vesical vein

Inferior gluteal vein

Obturator nerve

Obturator vein

Middle rectal vein

Pubic tributary to the inferior epigastric vein

Internal pudendal vein

Ischiococcygeus (coccygeus)

Medial umbilical ligament (obliterated umbilical artery)

Obturator canal

Inferior rectal vein

Obturator internus

Vesical plexus of veins

Iliococcygeus (part of levator ani)

Perineal vein

Pubococcygeus (part of levator ani)

**Veins of the pelvis
(right side sagittal view)**

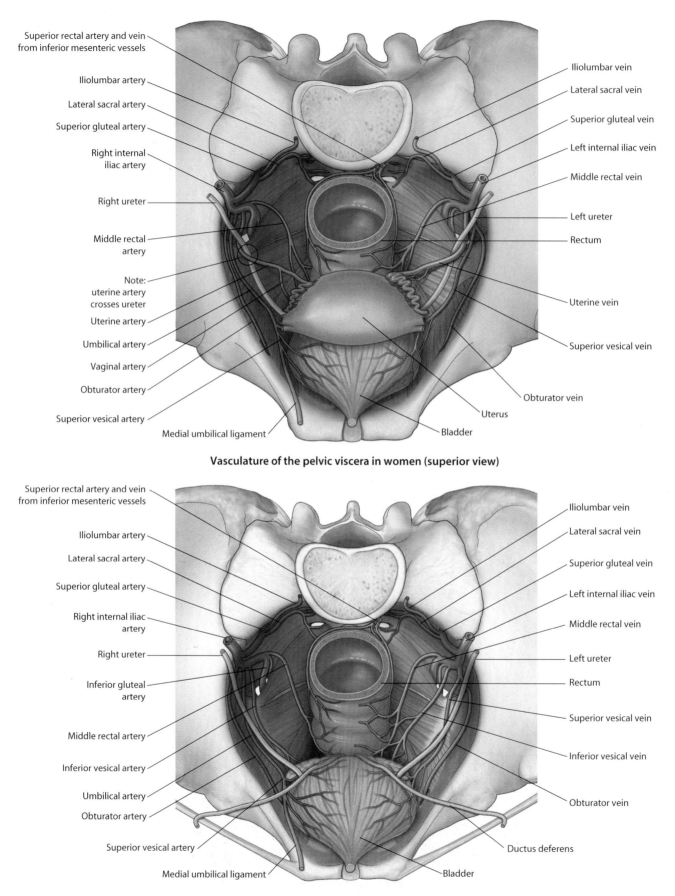

Superior rectal artery and vein
from inferior mesenteric vessels

Iliolumbar artery

Lateral sacral artery

Superior gluteal artery

Right internal
iliac artery

Right ureter

Middle rectal
artery

Note:
uterine artery
crosses ureter

Uterine artery

Umbilical artery

Vaginal artery

Obturator artery

Superior vesical artery

Medial umbilical ligament

Iliolumbar vein

Lateral sacral vein

Superior gluteal vein

Left internal iliac vein

Middle rectal vein

Left ureter

Rectum

Uterine vein

Superior vesical vein

Obturator vein

Uterus

Bladder

**Vasculature of the pelvic viscera in women (superior view)**

Superior rectal artery and vein
from inferior mesenteric vessels

Iliolumbar artery

Lateral sacral artery

Superior gluteal artery

Right internal iliac
artery

Right ureter

Inferior gluteal
artery

Middle rectal artery

Inferior vesical artery

Umbilical artery

Obturator artery

Superior vesical artery

Medial umbilical ligament

Iliolumbar vein

Lateral sacral vein

Superior gluteal vein

Left internal iliac vein

Middle rectal vein

Left ureter

Rectum

Superior vesical vein

Inferior vesical vein

Obturator vein

Ductus deferens

Bladder

**Vasculature of the pelvic viscera in men (superior view)**

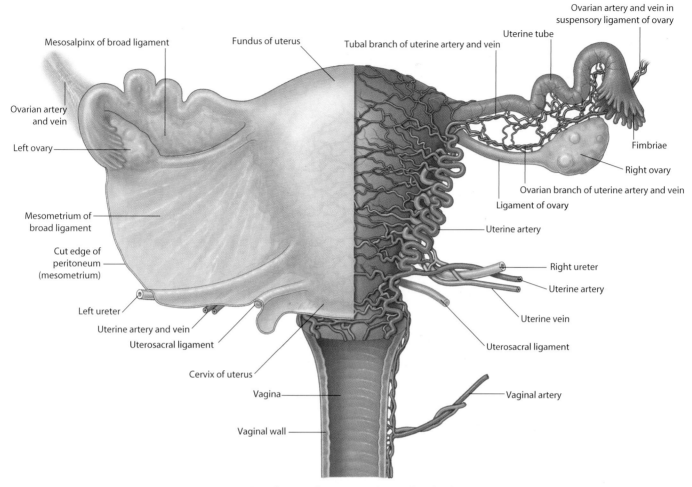

Mesosalpinx of broad ligament

Fundus of uterus

Tubal branch of uterine artery and vein

Uterine tube

Ovarian artery and vein in suspensory ligament of ovary

Ovarian artery and vein

Left ovary

Fimbriae

Right ovary

Ovarian branch of uterine artery and vein

Ligament of ovary

Mesometrium of broad ligament

Uterine artery

Cut edge of peritoneum (mesometrium)

Right ureter

Uterine artery

Left ureter

Uterine vein

Uterine artery and vein

Uterosacral ligament

Uterosacral ligament

Cervix of uterus

Vagina

Vaginal artery

Vaginal wall

**Vascular supply to uterus (posterior view)**

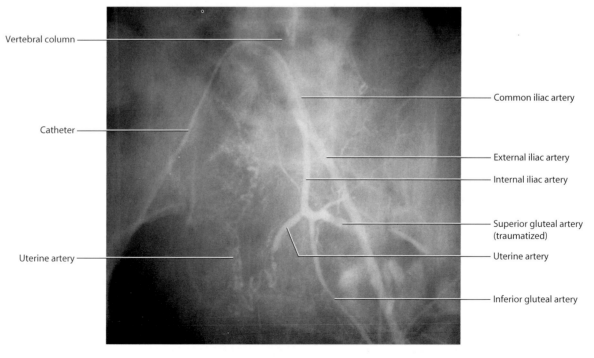

Vertebral column

Common iliac artery

Catheter

External iliac artery

Internal iliac artery

Superior gluteal artery (traumatized)

Uterine artery

Uterine artery

Inferior gluteal artery

**Vascular supply to uterus.**
Angiogram

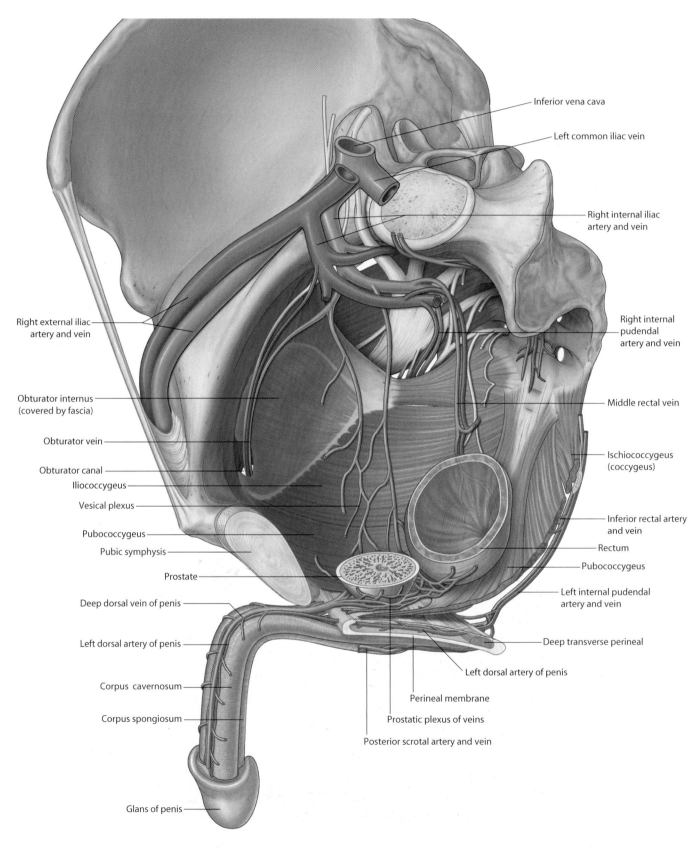

Inferior vena cava

Left common iliac vein

Right internal iliac artery and vein

Right internal pudendal artery and vein

Right external iliac artery and vein

Obturator internus (covered by fascia)

Obturator vein

Obturator canal

Iliococcygeus

Vesical plexus

Pubococcygeus

Pubic symphysis

Prostate

Deep dorsal vein of penis

Left dorsal artery of penis

Corpus cavernosum

Corpus spongiosum

Glans of penis

Middle rectal vein

Ischiococcygeus (coccygeus)

Inferior rectal artery and vein

Rectum

Pubococcygeus

Left internal pudendal artery and vein

Deep transverse perineal

Left dorsal artery of penis

Perineal membrane

Prostatic plexus of veins

Posterior scrotal artery and vein

**Venous drainage of pelvic viscera in men
(oblique sagittal view)**

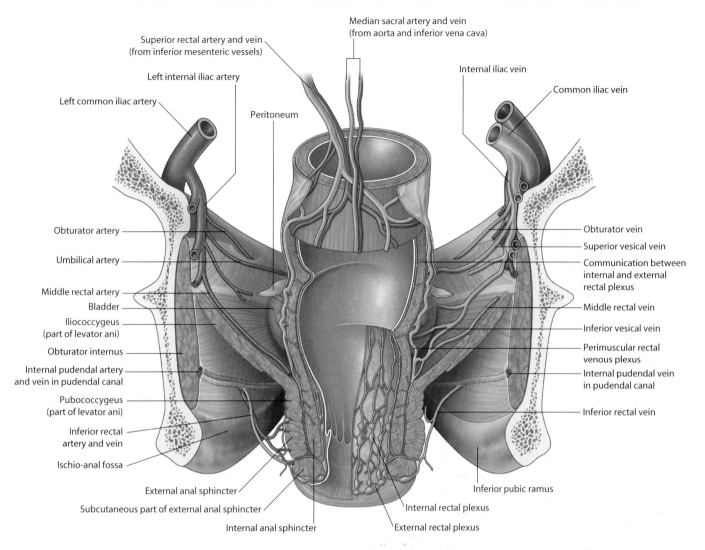

Median sacral artery and vein
(from aorta and inferior vena cava)

Superior rectal artery and vein
(from inferior mesenteric vessels)

Left internal iliac artery

Left common iliac artery

Peritoneum

Internal iliac vein

Common iliac vein

Obturator artery

Umbilical artery

Middle rectal artery

Bladder

Iliococcygeus
(part of levator ani)

Obturator internus

Internal pudendal artery
and vein in pudendal canal

Pubococcygeus
(part of levator ani)

Inferior rectal
artery and vein

Ischio-anal fossa

Obturator vein

Superior vesical vein

Communication between
internal and external
rectal plexus

Middle rectal vein

Inferior vesical vein

Perimuscular rectal
venous plexus

Internal pudendal vein
in pudendal canal

Inferior rectal vein

External anal sphincter

Subcutaneous part of external anal sphincter

Internal anal sphincter

Internal rectal plexus

External rectal plexus

Inferior pubic ramus

**Vasculature of the rectum (posterior view)**

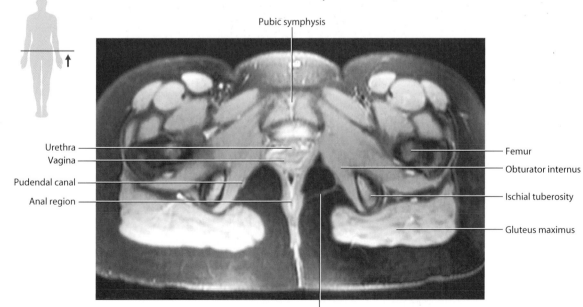

Pubic symphysis

Urethra

Vagina

Pudendal canal

Anal region

Femur

Obturator internus

Ischial tuberosity

Gluteus maximus

Inferior rectal branch to anal region

**Inferior rectal neurovascular bundle crossing the ischio-anal fossa.**
T2-weighted MR image in axial plane

**237**

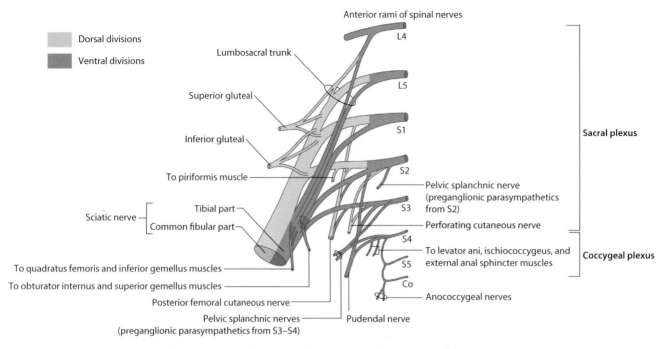

Dorsal divisions

Ventral divisions

Anterior rami of spinal nerves

L4

Lumbosacral trunk

L5

Superior gluteal

S1

Inferior gluteal

S2

To piriformis muscle

Pelvic splanchnic nerve
(preganglionic parasympathetics
from S2)

S3

Sciatic nerve

Tibial part

Common fibular part

Perforating cutaneous nerve

S4

To quadratus femoris and inferior gemellus muscles

S5

To levator ani, ischiococcygeus, and
external anal sphincter muscles

To obturator internus and superior gemellus muscles

Co

Posterior femoral cutaneous nerve

Anococcygeal nerves

Pelvic splanchnic nerves
(preganglionic parasympathetics from S3–S4)

Pudendal nerve

Sacral plexus

Coccygeal plexus

**Components and branches of the sacral and coccygeal nerve plexuses**

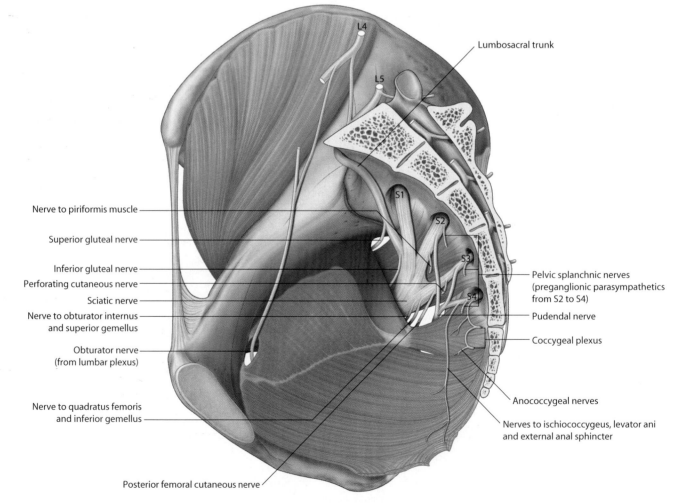

L4

Lumbosacral trunk

L5

Nerve to piriformis muscle

S1

Superior gluteal nerve

S2

Inferior gluteal nerve

Perforating cutaneous nerve

S3

Pelvic splanchnic nerves
(preganglionic parasympathetics
from S2 to S4)

Sciatic nerve

S4

Nerve to obturator internus
and superior gemellus

Pudendal nerve

Obturator nerve
(from lumbar plexus)

Coccygeal plexus

Nerve to quadratus femoris
and inferior gemellus

Anococcygeal nerves

Nerves to ischiococcygeus, levator ani
and external anal sphincter

Posterior femoral cutaneous nerve

**Sacral and coccygeal nerve plexuses within the pelvic cavity (sagittal view)**

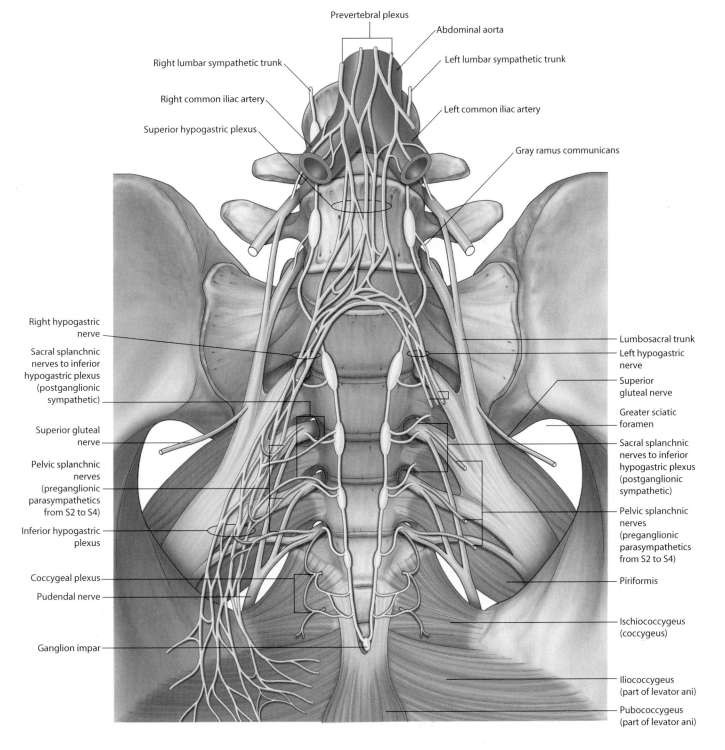

Prevertebral plexus

Abdominal aorta

Right lumbar sympathetic trunk

Left lumbar sympathetic trunk

Right common iliac artery

Left common iliac artery

Superior hypogastric plexus

Gray ramus communicans

Right hypogastric nerve

Lumbosacral trunk

Sacral splanchnic nerves to inferior hypogastric plexus (postganglionic sympathetic)

Left hypogastric nerve

Superior gluteal nerve

Greater sciatic foramen

Superior gluteal nerve

Sacral splanchnic nerves to inferior hypogastric plexus (postganglionic sympathetic)

Pelvic splanchnic nerves (preganglionic parasympathetics from S2 to S4)

Pelvic splanchnic nerves (preganglionic parasympathetics from S2 to S4)

Inferior hypogastric plexus

Coccygeal plexus

Piriformis

Pudendal nerve

Ischiococcygeus (coccygeus)

Ganglion impar

Iliococcygeus (part of levator ani)

Pubococcygeus (part of levator ani)

**Pelvic extensions of the prevertebral nerve plexus (anterior view)**

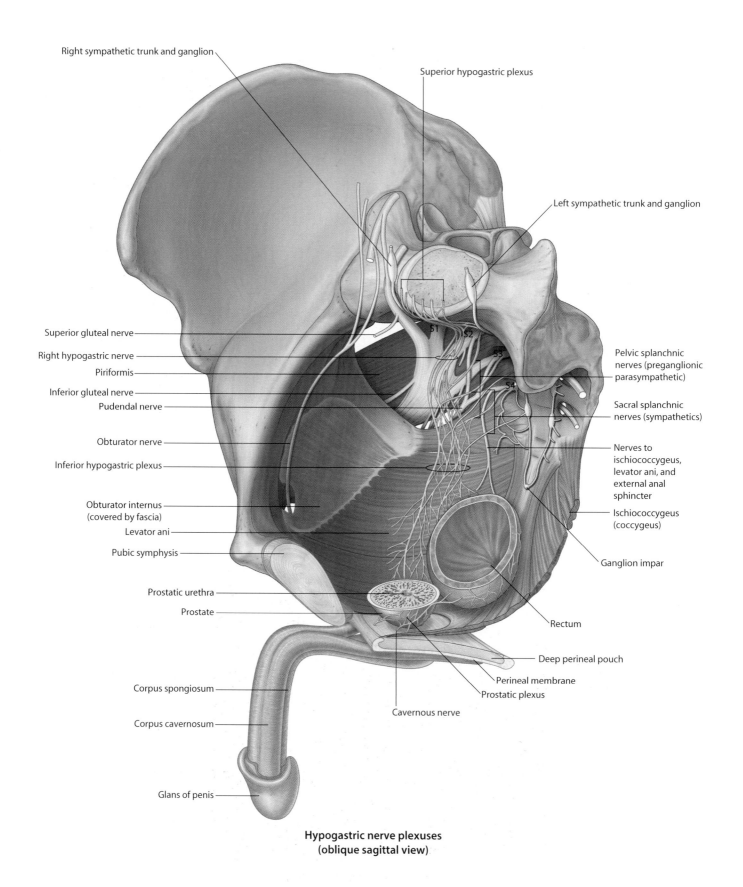

Right sympathetic trunk and ganglion

Superior hypogastric plexus

Left sympathetic trunk and ganglion

S1

S2

S3

S4

Superior gluteal nerve

Right hypogastric nerve

Piriformis

Inferior gluteal nerve

Pudendal nerve

Obturator nerve

Inferior hypogastric plexus

Obturator internus
(covered by fascia)

Levator ani

Pubic symphysis

Prostatic urethra

Prostate

Corpus spongiosum

Corpus cavernosum

Glans of penis

Pelvic splanchnic
nerves (preganglionic
parasympathetic)

Sacral splanchnic
nerves (sympathetics)

Nerves to
ischiococcygeus,
levator ani, and
external anal
sphincter

Ischiococcygeus
(coccygeus)

Ganglion impar

Rectum

Deep perineal pouch

Perineal membrane

Prostatic plexus

Cavernous nerve

**Hypogastric nerve plexuses
(oblique sagittal view)**

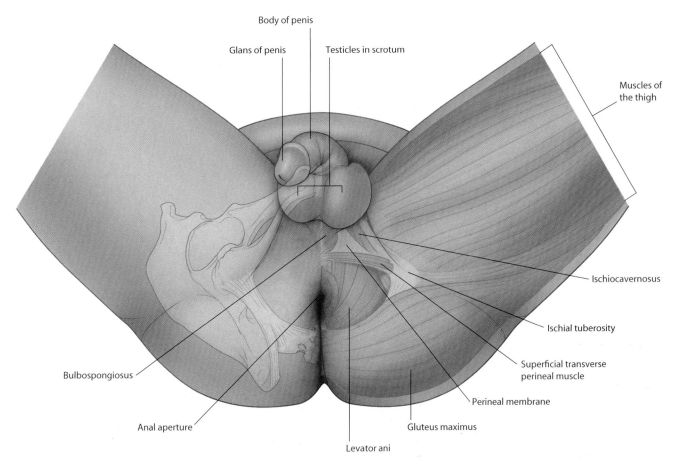

Body of penis

Glans of penis

Testicles in scrotum

Muscles of the thigh

Ischiocavernosus

Ischial tuberosity

Superficial transverse perineal muscle

Perineal membrane

Gluteus maximus

Levator ani

Anal aperture

Bulbospongiosus

**Structures of the perineum in men**

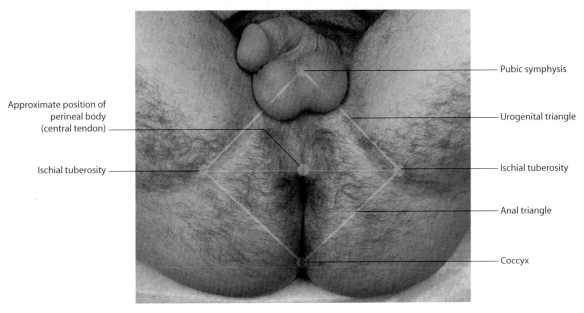

Pubic symphysis

Urogenital triangle

Approximate position of perineal body (central tendon)

Ischial tuberosity

Ischial tuberosity

Anal triangle

Coccyx

**Surface anatomy of the perineum in men**

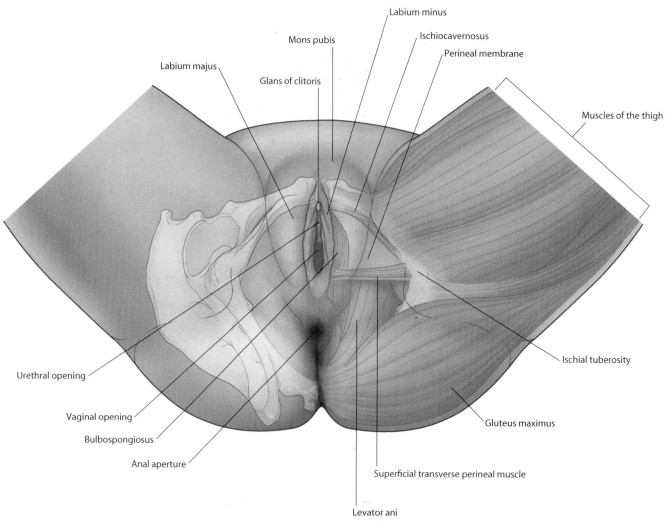

Labium minus

Mons pubis

Ischiocavernosus

Perineal membrane

Labium majus

Glans of clitoris

Muscles of the thigh

Urethral opening

Vaginal opening

Bulbospongiosus

Anal aperture

Ischial tuberosity

Gluteus maximus

Superficial transverse perineal muscle

Levator ani

**Structures of the perineum in women**

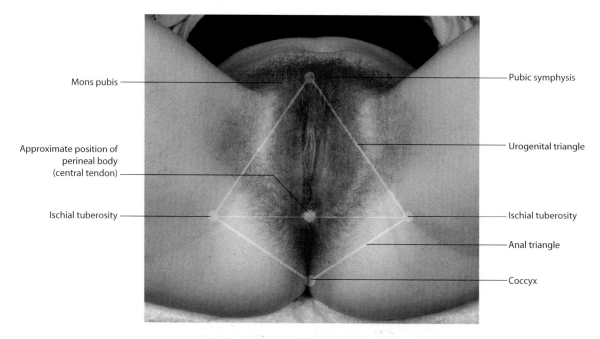

Mons pubis

Pubic symphysis

Approximate position of perineal body (central tendon)

Urogenital triangle

Ischial tuberosity

Ischial tuberosity

Anal triangle

Coccyx

**Surface anatomy of the perineum in women**

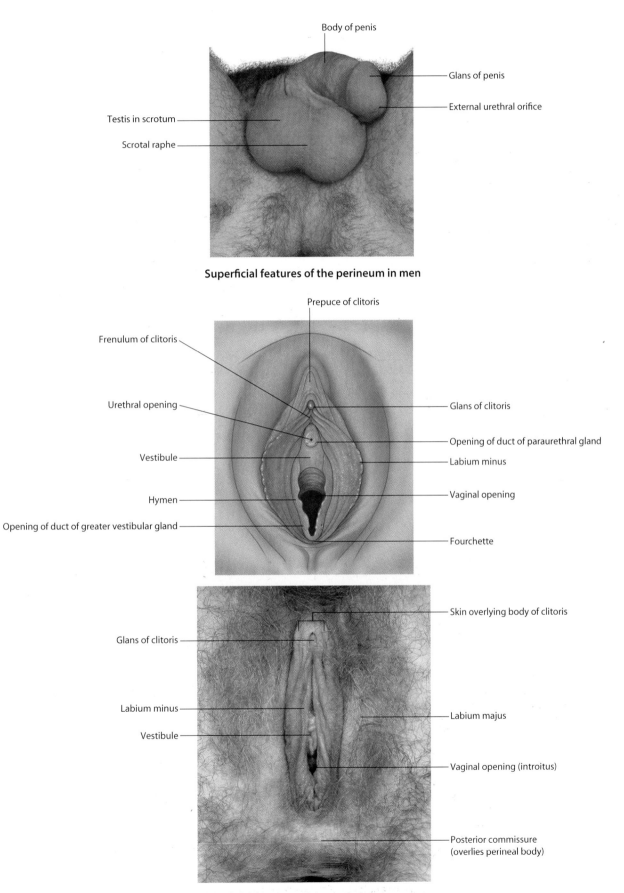

Body of penis

Glans of penis

External urethral orifice

Testis in scrotum

Scrotal raphe

**Superficial features of the perineum in men**

Prepuce of clitoris

Frenulum of clitoris

Glans of clitoris

Urethral opening

Opening of duct of paraurethral gland

Vestibule

Labium minus

Hymen

Vaginal opening

Opening of duct of greater vestibular gland

Fourchette

Skin overlying body of clitoris

Glans of clitoris

Labium minus

Labium majus

Vestibule

Vaginal opening (introitus)

Posterior commissure
(overlies perineal body)

**Superficial features of the perineum in women**

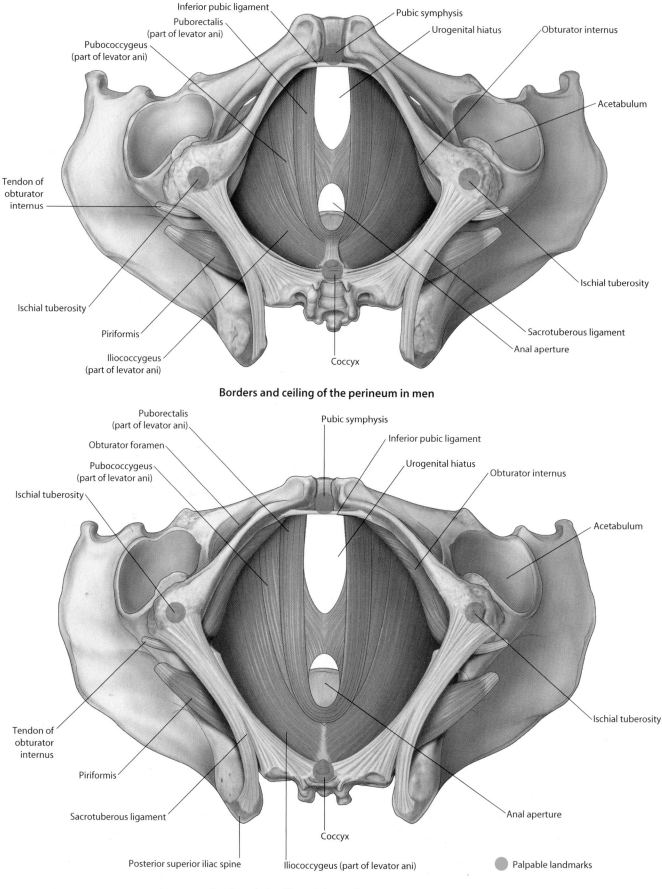

Inferior pubic ligament

Puborectalis
(part of levator ani)

Pubococcygeus
(part of levator ani)

Pubic symphysis

Urogenital hiatus

Obturator internus

Acetabulum

Tendon of
obturator
internus

Ischial tuberosity

Ischial tuberosity

Sacrotuberous ligament

Piriformis

Anal aperture

Iliococcygeus
(part of levator ani)

Coccyx

**Borders and ceiling of the perineum in men**

Puborectalis
(part of levator ani)

Obturator foramen

Pubococcygeus
(part of levator ani)

Ischial tuberosity

Pubic symphysis

Inferior pubic ligament

Urogenital hiatus

Obturator internus

Acetabulum

Ischial tuberosity

Tendon of
obturator
internus

Piriformis

Anal aperture

Sacrotuberous ligament

Coccyx

Posterior superior iliac spine

Iliococcygeus (part of levator ani)

Palpable landmarks

**Borders and ceiling of the perineum in women**

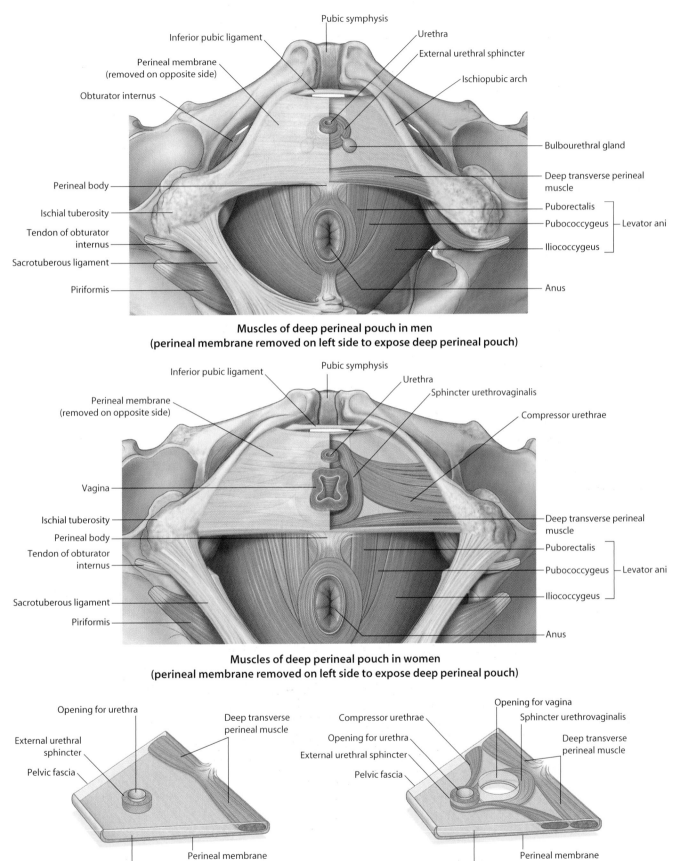

**Muscles of deep perineal pouch in men**
**(perineal membrane removed on left side to expose deep perineal pouch)**

**Muscles of deep perineal pouch in women**
**(perineal membrane removed on left side to expose deep perineal pouch)**

**Muscles of deep perineal pouch in men**

**Muscles of deep perineal pouch in women**

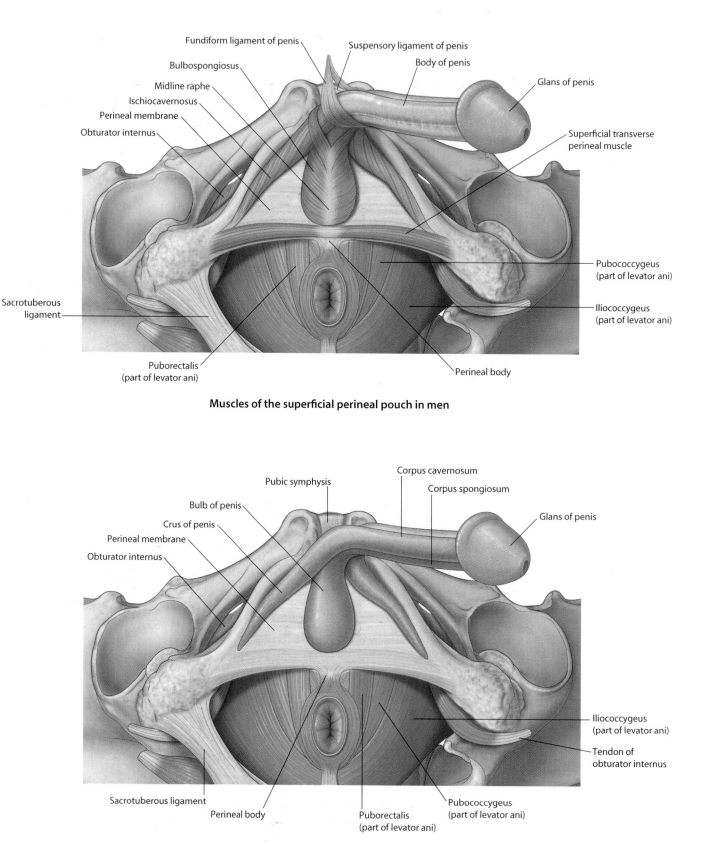

**Muscles of the superficial perineal pouch in men**

**Erectile tissues of the superficial perineal pouch in men**

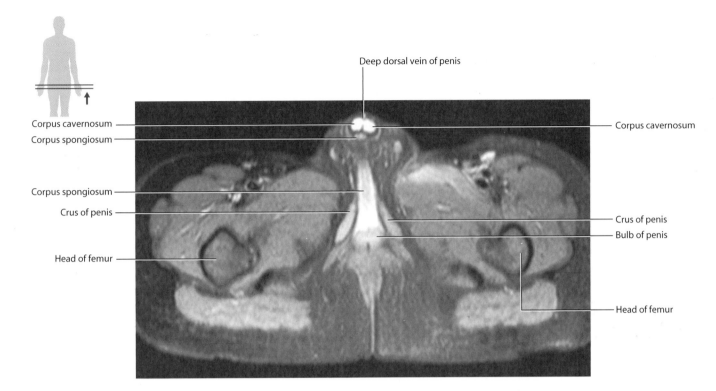

Deep dorsal vein of penis

Corpus cavernosum

Corpus spongiosum

Corpus spongiosum

Crus of penis

Head of femur

Corpus cavernosum

Crus of penis

Bulb of penis

Head of femur

**Erectile tissues in relation to other structures in the male perineum.**
T2-weighted MR image in axial plane

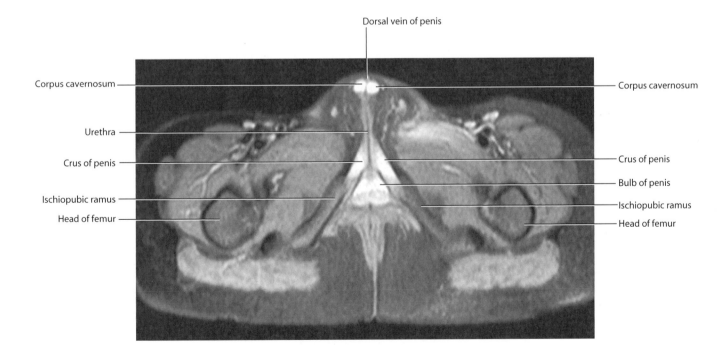

Dorsal vein of penis

Corpus cavernosum

Urethra

Crus of penis

Ischiopubic ramus

Head of femur

Corpus cavernosum

Crus of penis

Bulb of penis

Ischiopubic ramus

Head of femur

**Erectile tissues in relation to other structures in the male perineum.**
T2-weighted MR image in axial plane

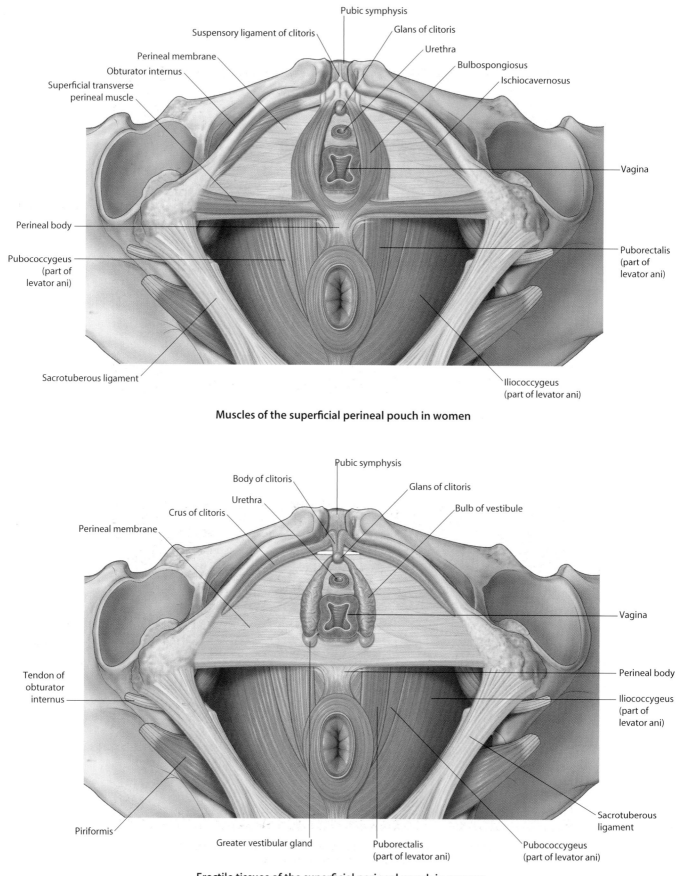

Pubic symphysis

Suspensory ligament of clitoris

Glans of clitoris

Perineal membrane

Urethra

Obturator internus

Bulbospongiosus

Superficial transverse perineal muscle

Ischiocavernosus

Vagina

Perineal body

Puborectalis (part of levator ani)

Pubococcygeus (part of levator ani)

Sacrotuberous ligament

Iliococcygeus (part of levator ani)

**Muscles of the superficial perineal pouch in women**

Pubic symphysis

Body of clitoris

Glans of clitoris

Urethra

Crus of clitoris

Bulb of vestibule

Perineal membrane

Vagina

Tendon of obturator internus

Perineal body

Iliococcygeus (part of levator ani)

Sacrotuberous ligament

Piriformis

Greater vestibular gland

Puborectalis (part of levator ani)

Pubococcygeus (part of levator ani)

**Erectile tissues of the superficial perineal pouch in women**

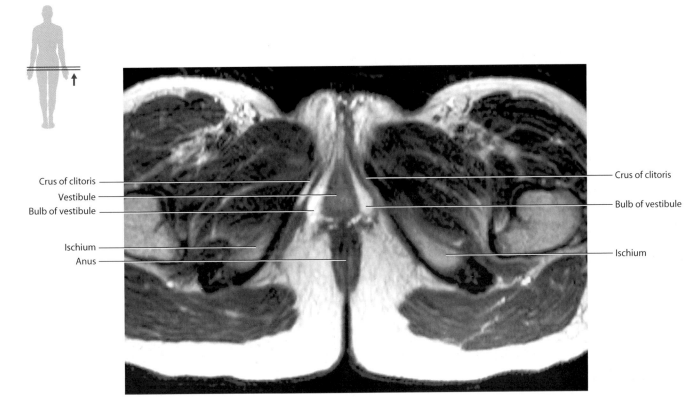

Crus of clitoris
Vestibule
Bulb of vestibule

Ischium
Anus

Crus of clitoris

Bulb of vestibule

Ischium

**Erectile tissues in relation to other structures in the female perineum.**
T2-weighted MR image in axial plane

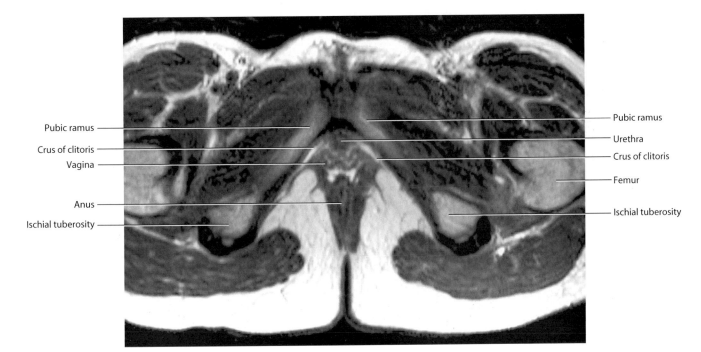

Pubic ramus

Crus of clitoris

Vagina

Anus

Ischial tuberosity

Pubic ramus

Urethra

Crus of clitoris

Femur

Ischial tuberosity

**Erectile tissues in relation to other structures in the female perineum.**
T2-weighted MR image in axial plane

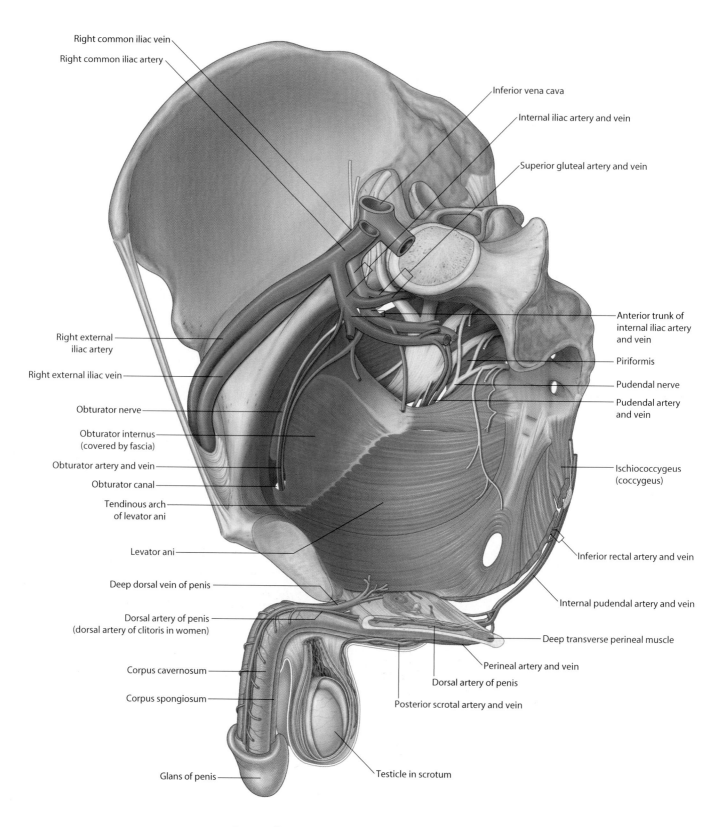

Right common iliac vein

Right common iliac artery

Inferior vena cava

Internal iliac artery and vein

Superior gluteal artery and vein

Right external iliac artery

Right external iliac vein

Obturator nerve

Obturator internus (covered by fascia)

Obturator artery and vein

Obturator canal

Tendinous arch of levator ani

Levator ani

Deep dorsal vein of penis

Dorsal artery of penis (dorsal artery of clitoris in women)

Corpus cavernosum

Corpus spongiosum

Glans of penis

Anterior trunk of internal iliac artery and vein

Piriformis

Pudendal nerve

Pudendal artery and vein

Ischiococcygeus (coccygeus)

Inferior rectal artery and vein

Internal pudendal artery and vein

Deep transverse perineal muscle

Perineal artery and vein

Dorsal artery of penis

Posterior scrotal artery and vein

Testicle in scrotum

**Course of internal pudendal artery and vein in men
(oblique sagittal view)**

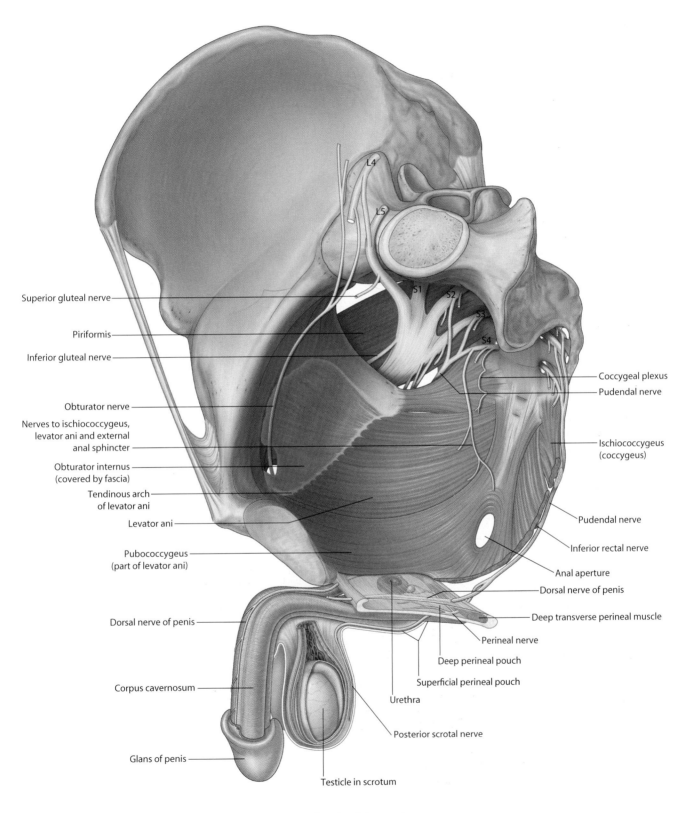

Superior gluteal nerve

Piriformis

Inferior gluteal nerve

Obturator nerve

Nerves to ischiococcygeus, levator ani and external anal sphincter

Obturator internus (covered by fascia)

Tendinous arch of levator ani

Levator ani

Pubococcygeus (part of levator ani)

Dorsal nerve of penis

Corpus cavernosum

Glans of penis

L4

L5

S1

S2

S3

S4

Coccygeal plexus

Pudendal nerve

Ischiococcygeus (coccygeus)

Pudendal nerve

Inferior rectal nerve

Anal aperture

Dorsal nerve of penis

Deep transverse perineal muscle

Perineal nerve

Deep perineal pouch

Superficial perineal pouch

Urethra

Posterior scrotal nerve

Testicle in scrotum

**Course of pudendal nerve in men
(oblique sagittal view)**

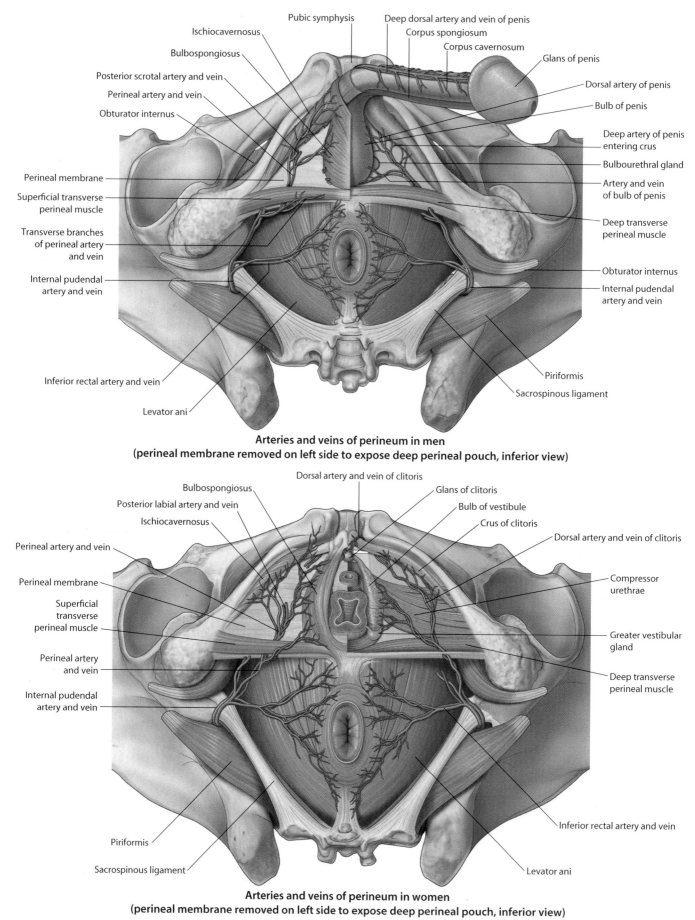

Pubic symphysis

Ischiocavernosus

Bulbospongiosus

Posterior scrotal artery and vein

Perineal artery and vein

Obturator internus

Perineal membrane

Superficial transverse perineal muscle

Transverse branches of perineal artery and vein

Internal pudendal artery and vein

Inferior rectal artery and vein

Levator ani

Deep dorsal artery and vein of penis

Corpus spongiosum

Corpus cavernosum

Glans of penis

Dorsal artery of penis

Bulb of penis

Deep artery of penis entering crus

Bulbourethral gland

Artery and vein of bulb of penis

Deep transverse perineal muscle

Obturator internus

Internal pudendal artery and vein

Piriformis

Sacrospinous ligament

**Arteries and veins of perineum in men**
**(perineal membrane removed on left side to expose deep perineal pouch, inferior view)**

Bulbospongiosus

Posterior labial artery and vein

Ischiocavernosus

Perineal artery and vein

Perineal membrane

Superficial transverse perineal muscle

Perineal artery and vein

Internal pudendal artery and vein

Piriformis

Sacrospinous ligament

Dorsal artery and vein of clitoris

Glans of clitoris

Bulb of vestibule

Crus of clitoris

Dorsal artery and vein of clitoris

Compressor urethrae

Greater vestibular gland

Deep transverse perineal muscle

Inferior rectal artery and vein

Levator ani

**Arteries and veins of perineum in women**
**(perineal membrane removed on left side to expose deep perineal pouch, inferior view)**

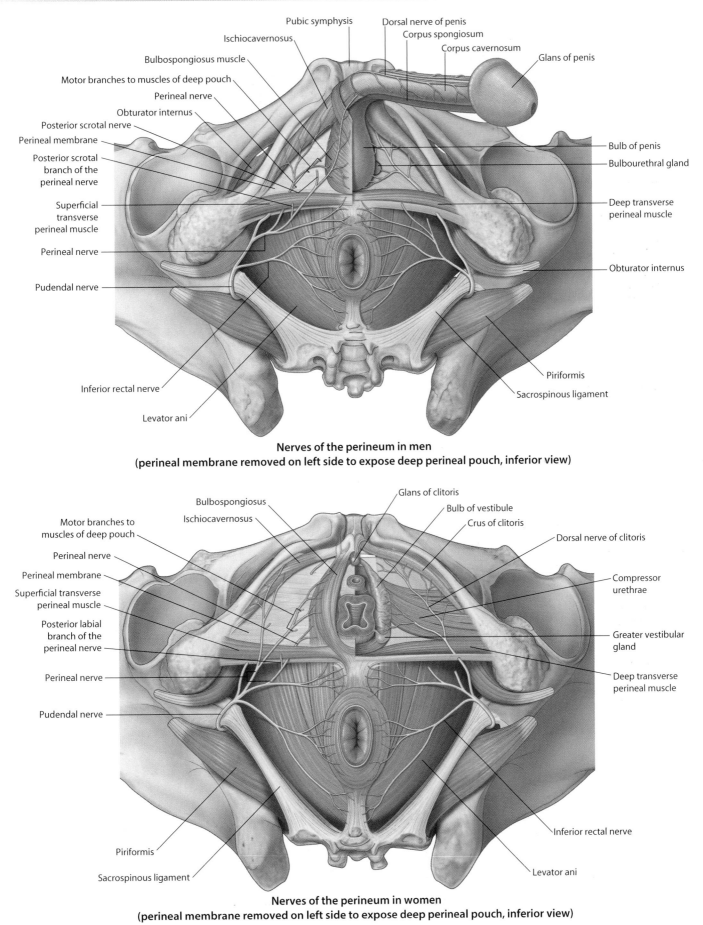

Pubic symphysis
Ischiocavernosus
Bulbospongiosus muscle
Motor branches to muscles of deep pouch
Perineal nerve
Obturator internus
Posterior scrotal nerve
Perineal membrane
Posterior scrotal branch of the perineal nerve
Superficial transverse perineal muscle
Perineal nerve
Pudendal nerve
Inferior rectal nerve
Levator ani

Dorsal nerve of penis
Corpus spongiosum
Corpus cavernosum
Glans of penis
Bulb of penis
Bulbourethral gland
Deep transverse perineal muscle
Obturator internus
Piriformis
Sacrospinous ligament

**Nerves of the perineum in men**
**(perineal membrane removed on left side to expose deep perineal pouch, inferior view)**

Motor branches to muscles of deep pouch
Perineal nerve
Perineal membrane
Superficial transverse perineal muscle
Posterior labial branch of the perineal nerve
Perineal nerve
Pudendal nerve
Piriformis
Sacrospinous ligament

Bulbospongiosus
Ischiocavernosus
Glans of clitoris
Bulb of vestibule
Crus of clitoris
Dorsal nerve of clitoris
Compressor urethrae
Greater vestibular gland
Deep transverse perineal muscle
Inferior rectal nerve
Levator ani

**Nerves of the perineum in women**
**(perineal membrane removed on left side to expose deep perineal pouch, inferior view)**

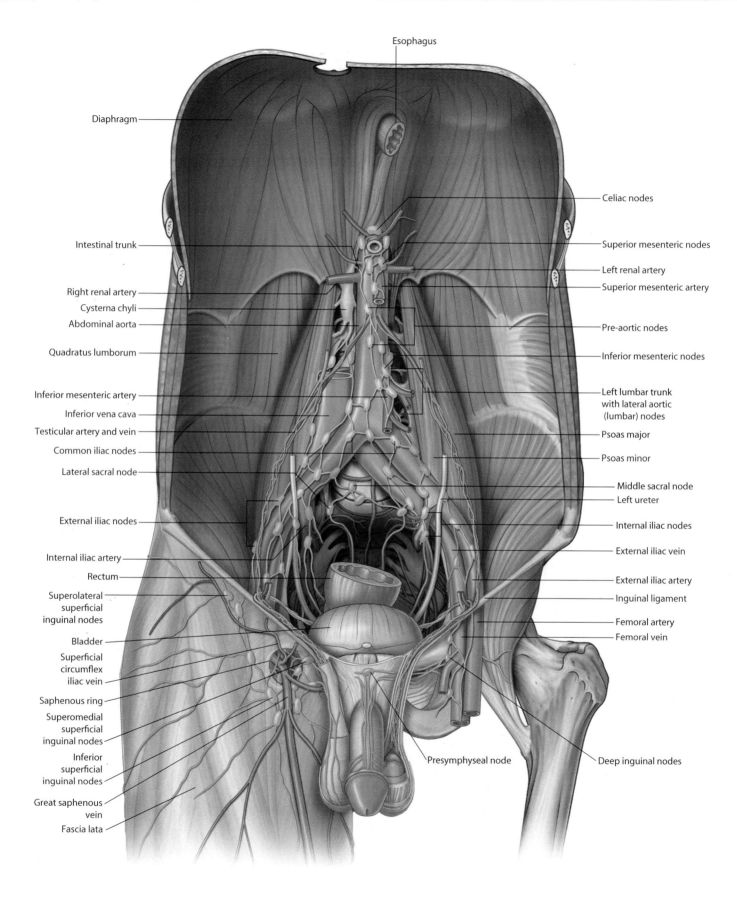

Esophagus

Diaphragm

Celiac nodes

Intestinal trunk

Superior mesenteric nodes

Left renal artery

Superior mesenteric artery

Right renal artery

Cysterna chyli

Abdominal aorta

Pre-aortic nodes

Quadratus lumborum

Inferior mesenteric nodes

Inferior mesenteric artery

Left lumbar trunk with lateral aortic (lumbar) nodes

Inferior vena cava

Psoas major

Testicular artery and vein

Psoas minor

Common iliac nodes

Lateral sacral node

Middle sacral node

Left ureter

External iliac nodes

Internal iliac nodes

External iliac vein

Internal iliac artery

Rectum

External iliac artery

Superolateral superficial inguinal nodes

Inguinal ligament

Femoral artery

Bladder

Femoral vein

Superficial circumflex iliac vein

Saphenous ring

Superomedial superficial inguinal nodes

Inferior superficial inguinal nodes

Great saphenous vein

Fascia lata

Presymphyseal node

Deep inguinal nodes

Lymphatics of pelvis and perineum in men

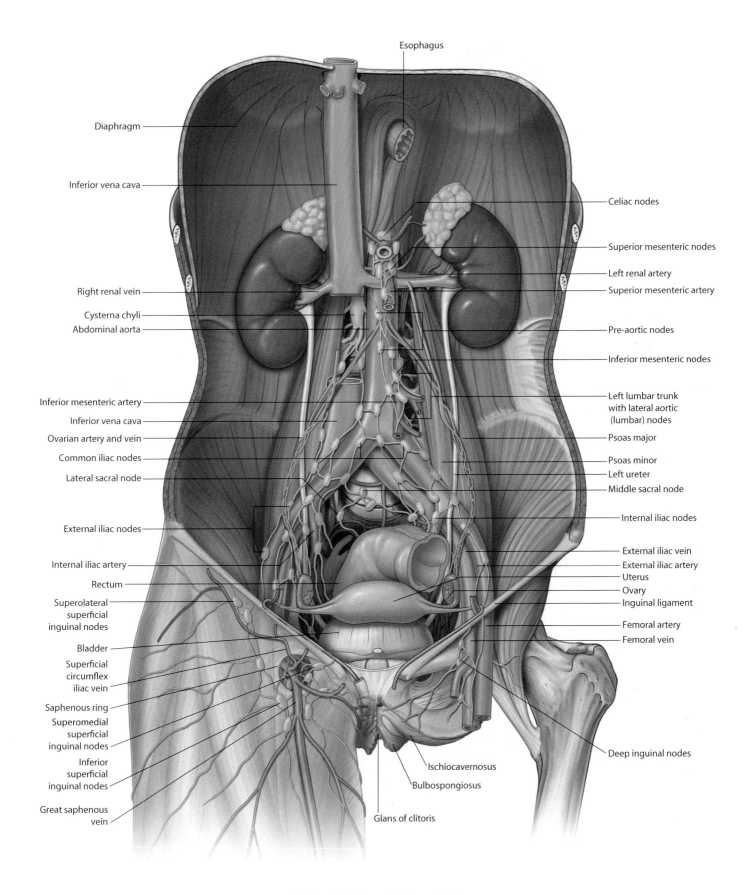

Esophagus

Diaphragm

Inferior vena cava

Celiac nodes

Superior mesenteric nodes

Left renal artery

Right renal vein

Superior mesenteric artery

Cysterna chyli

Abdominal aorta

Pre-aortic nodes

Inferior mesenteric nodes

Inferior mesenteric artery

Inferior vena cava

Ovarian artery and vein

Common iliac nodes

Lateral sacral node

Left lumbar trunk with lateral aortic (lumbar) nodes

Psoas major

Psoas minor

Left ureter

Middle sacral node

Internal iliac nodes

External iliac nodes

Internal iliac artery

External iliac vein

External iliac artery

Uterus

Rectum

Ovary

Superolateral superficial inguinal nodes

Inguinal ligament

Femoral artery

Femoral vein

Bladder

Superficial circumflex iliac vein

Saphenous ring

Superomedial superficial inguinal nodes

Inferior superficial inguinal nodes

Deep inguinal nodes

Ischiocavernosus

Bulbospongiosus

Great saphenous vein

Glans of clitoris

**Lymphatics of pelvis and perineum in women**

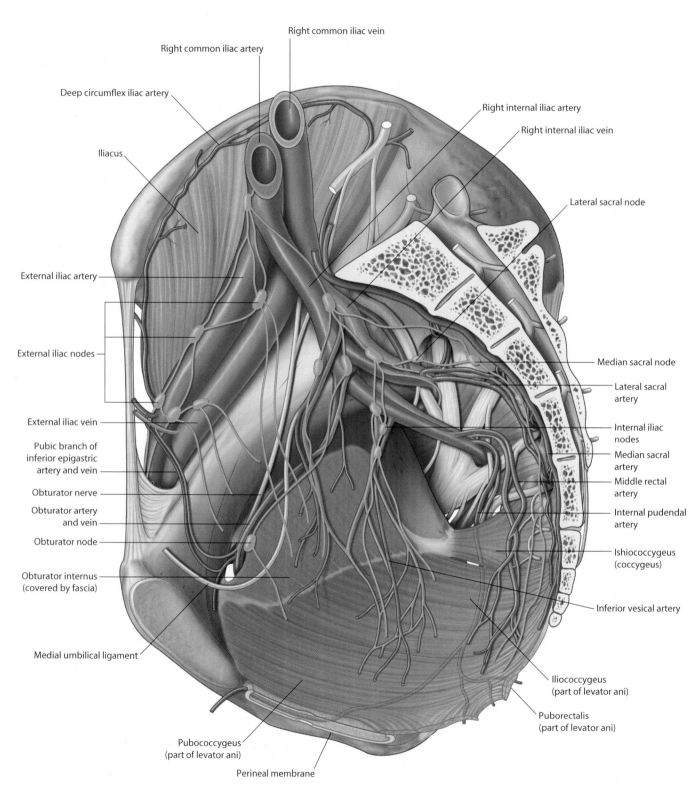

Right common iliac vein

Right common iliac artery

Deep circumflex iliac artery

Iliacus

External iliac artery

External iliac nodes

External iliac vein

Pubic branch of inferior epigastric artery and vein

Obturator nerve

Obturator artery and vein

Obturator node

Obturator internus (covered by fascia)

Medial umbilical ligament

Pubococcygeus (part of levator ani)

Perineal membrane

Right internal iliac artery

Right internal iliac vein

Lateral sacral node

Median sacral node

Lateral sacral artery

Internal iliac nodes

Median sacral artery

Middle rectal artery

Internal pudendal artery

Ischiococcygeus (coccygeus)

Inferior vesical artery

Iliococcygeus (part of levator ani)

Puborectalis (part of levator ani)

**Lymphatics of pelvic cavity (sagittal view)**

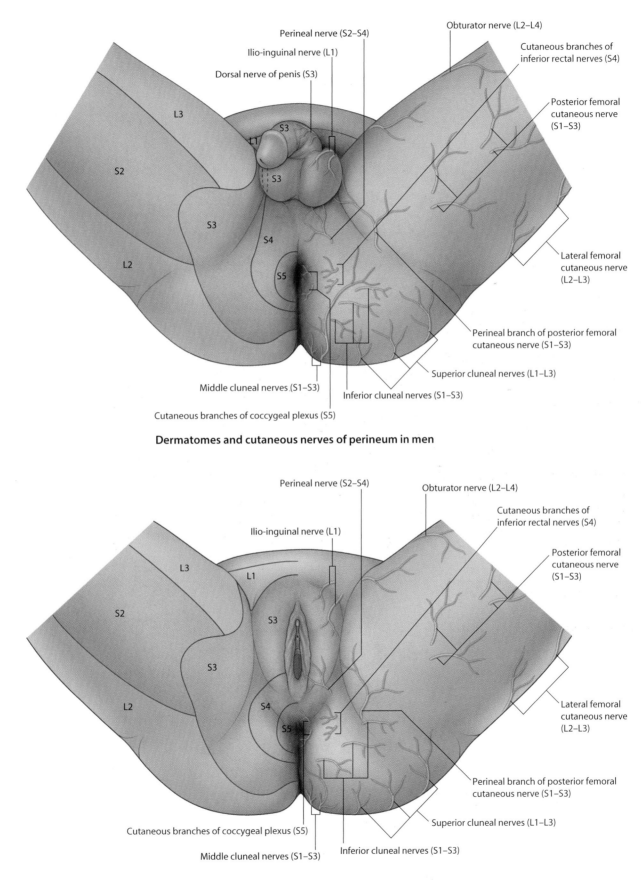

Perineal nerve (S2–S4)

Ilio-inguinal nerve (L1)

Dorsal nerve of penis (S3)

Obturator nerve (L2–L4)

Cutaneous branches of inferior rectal nerves (S4)

Posterior femoral cutaneous nerve (S1–S3)

L3

S3

L1

S2

S3

S4

L2

S5

Lateral femoral cutaneous nerve (L2–L3)

Perineal branch of posterior femoral cutaneous nerve (S1–S3)

Superior cluneal nerves (L1–L3)

Middle cluneal nerves (S1–S3)

Inferior cluneal nerves (S1–S3)

Cutaneous branches of coccygeal plexus (S5)

**Dermatomes and cutaneous nerves of perineum in men**

Perineal nerve (S2–S4)

Ilio-inguinal nerve (L1)

Obturator nerve (L2–L4)

Cutaneous branches of inferior rectal nerves (S4)

Posterior femoral cutaneous nerve (S1–S3)

L3

L1

S2

S3

S3

L2

S4

S5

Lateral femoral cutaneous nerve (L2–L3)

Perineal branch of posterior femoral cutaneous nerve (S1–S3)

Superior cluneal nerves (L1–L3)

Cutaneous branches of coccygeal plexus (S5)

Middle cluneal nerves (S1–S3)

Inferior cluneal nerves (S1–S3)

**Dermatomes and cutaneous nerves of perineum in women**

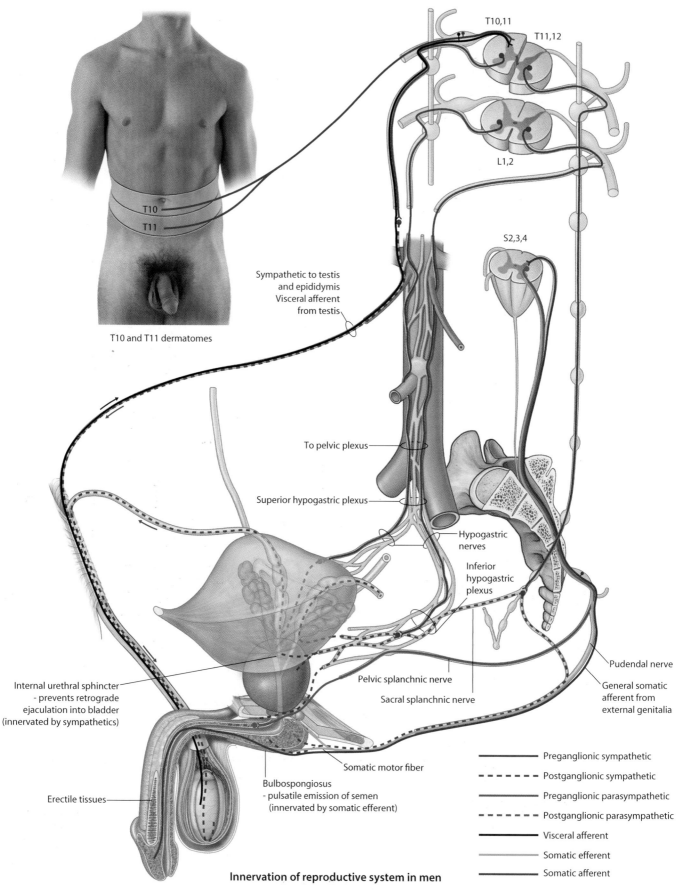

T10,11

T11,12

L1,2

S2,3,4

T10

T11

Sympathetic to testis
and epididymis
Visceral afferent
from testis

T10 and T11 dermatomes

To pelvic plexus

Superior hypogastric plexus

Hypogastric
nerves

Inferior
hypogastric
plexus

Pudendal nerve

General somatic
afferent from
external genitalia

Internal urethral sphincter
- prevents retrograde
ejaculation into bladder
(innervated by sympathetics)

Pelvic splanchnic nerve

Sacral splanchnic nerve

Somatic motor fiber

Bulbospongiosus
- pulsatile emission of semen
(innervated by somatic efferent)

Erectile tissues

Preganglionic sympathetic

Postganglionic sympathetic

Preganglionic parasympathetic

Postganglionic parasympathetic

Visceral afferent

Somatic efferent

Somatic afferent

**Innervation of reproductive system in men**

258

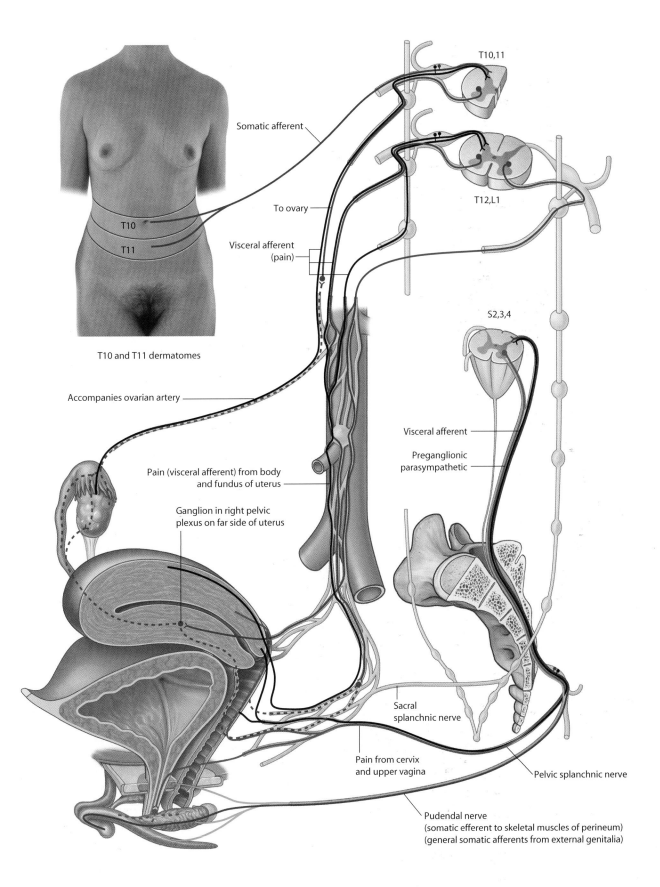

Somatic afferent

T10,11

To ovary

Visceral afferent
(pain)

T12,L1

T10

T11

S2,3,4

T10 and T11 dermatomes

Accompanies ovarian artery

Visceral afferent

Preganglionic
parasympathetic

Pain (visceral afferent) from body
and fundus of uterus

Ganglion in right pelvic
plexus on far side of uterus

Sacral
splanchnic nerve

Pain from cervix
and upper vagina

Pelvic splanchnic nerve

Pudendal nerve
(somatic efferent to skeletal muscles of perineum)
(general somatic afferents from external genitalia)

**Innervation of reproductive system in women**

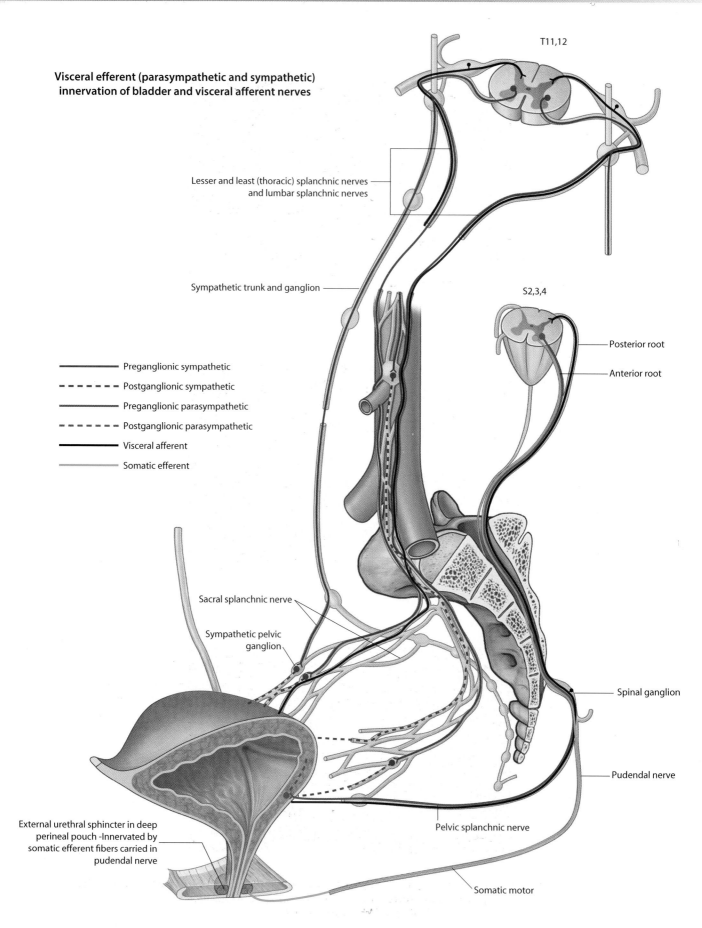

T11,12

**Visceral efferent (parasympathetic and sympathetic) innervation of bladder and visceral afferent nerves**

Lesser and least (thoracic) splanchnic nerves and lumbar splanchnic nerves

Sympathetic trunk and ganglion

S2,3,4

Posterior root

Anterior root

——————— Preganglionic sympathetic

- - - - - - Postganglionic sympathetic

——————— Preganglionic parasympathetic

- - - - - - Postganglionic parasympathetic

——————— Visceral afferent

——————— Somatic efferent

Sacral splanchnic nerve

Sympathetic pelvic ganglion

Spinal ganglion

Pudendal nerve

External urethral sphincter in deep perineal pouch -Innervated by somatic efferent fibers carried in pudendal nerve

Pelvic splanchnic nerve

Somatic motor

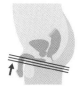

**A**

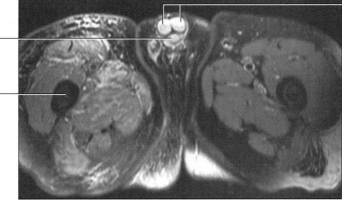

Corpora cavernosa

Corpus spongiosum

Femur

**B**

Corpora cavernosa

Corpus spongiosum

Femur

**C**

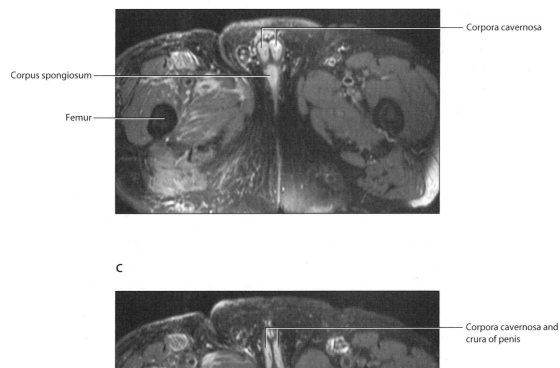

Corpora cavernosa and crura of penis

Corpus spongiosum and bulb of penis

Femur

Anus

**A through C – Series of axial images that pass through the pelvic cavity and perineum from inferior to superior showing the various structures and their relationships with each other.**
T2-weighted MR images in axial plane

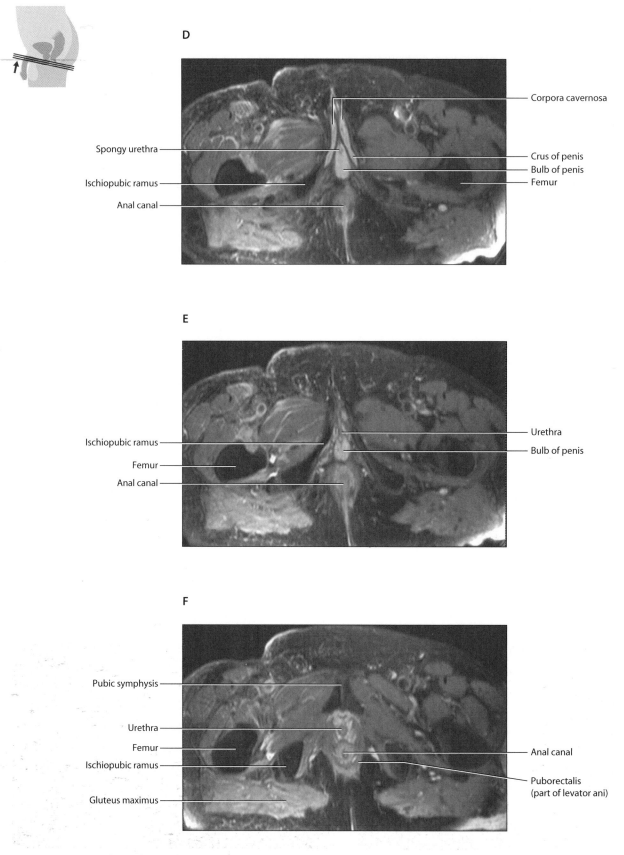

**D**

Corpora cavernosa

Spongy urethra

Crus of penis
Bulb of penis
Femur

Ischiopubic ramus

Anal canal

**E**

Ischiopubic ramus

Urethra
Bulb of penis

Femur

Anal canal

**F**

Pubic symphysis

Urethra

Femur

Ischiopubic ramus

Anal canal

Puborectalis
(part of levator ani)

Gluteus maximus

**D through J – Series of axial images that pass through the pelvic cavity and perineum from inferior to superior showing the various structures and their relationships with each other.**
T2-weighted MR images in axial plane

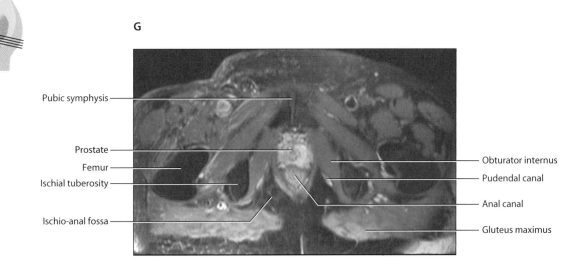

**G**

Pubic symphysis

Prostate

Femur

Ischial tuberosity

Ischio-anal fossa

Obturator internus

Pudendal canal

Anal canal

Gluteus maximus

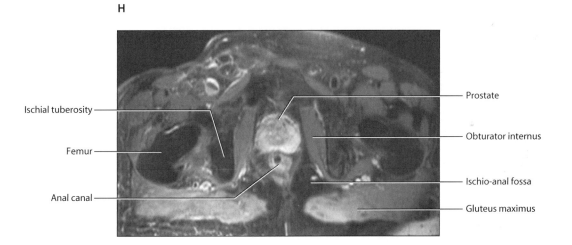

**H**

Ischial tuberosity

Femur

Anal canal

Prostate

Obturator internus

Ischio-anal fossa

Gluteus maximus

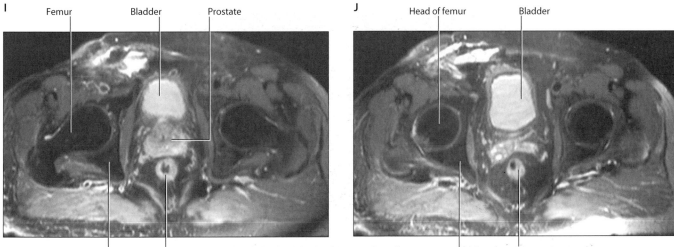

**I**   Femur      Bladder      Prostate

Ischium      Rectum

**J**   Head of femur      Bladder

Ischium      Rectum

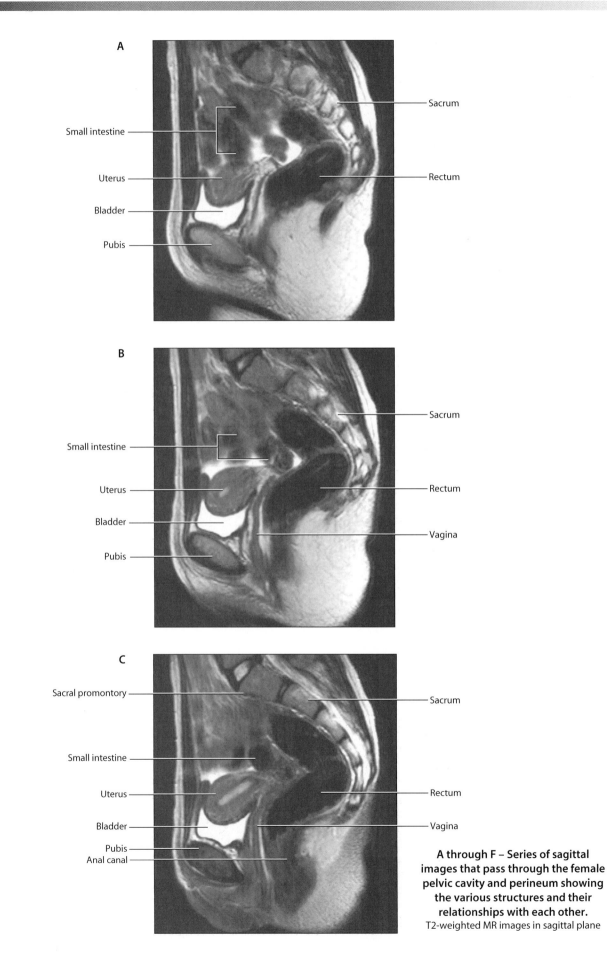

**A**

Small intestine

Uterus

Bladder

Pubis

Sacrum

Rectum

**B**

Small intestine

Uterus

Bladder

Pubis

Sacrum

Rectum

Vagina

**C**

Sacral promontory

Small intestine

Uterus

Bladder

Pubis

Anal canal

Sacrum

Rectum

Vagina

**A through F – Series of sagittal images that pass through the female pelvic cavity and perineum showing the various structures and their relationships with each other.**
T2-weighted MR images in sagittal plane

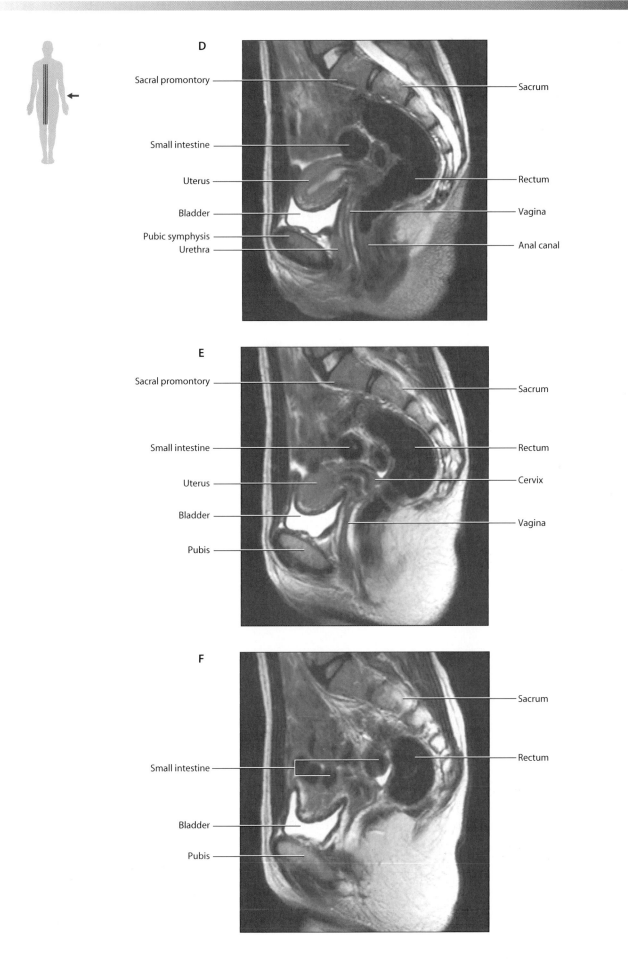

**D**

Sacral promontory

Small intestine

Uterus

Bladder

Pubic symphysis

Urethra

Sacrum

Rectum

Vagina

Anal canal

**E**

Sacral promontory

Small intestine

Uterus

Bladder

Pubis

Sacrum

Rectum

Cervix

Vagina

**F**

Small intestine

Bladder

Pubis

Sacrum

Rectum

**A**

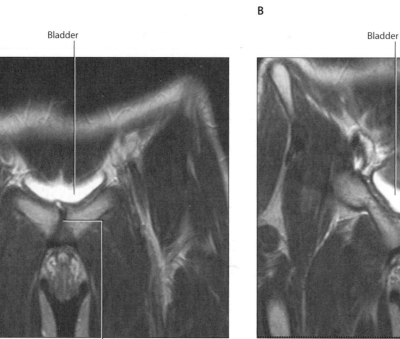

Bladder

Pubic symphysis

**B**

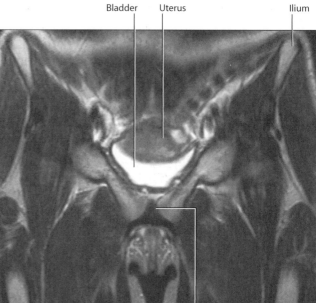

Bladder   Uterus

Ilium

Pubic symphysis

**C**

Uterus   Small intestine   Iliacus   Ilium

Bladder   Head of femur   Neck of femur

**D**

Acetabulum   Small intestine   Uterus   Ilium

Bladder   Head of femur   Neck of femur

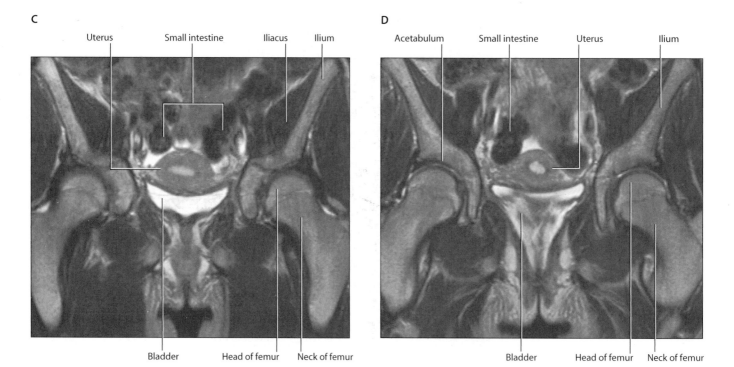

**A through G – Series of coronal images that pass through the pelvic cavity and perineum from anterior to posterior showing the various structures and their relationships with each other.**
T2-weighted MR images in coronal plane

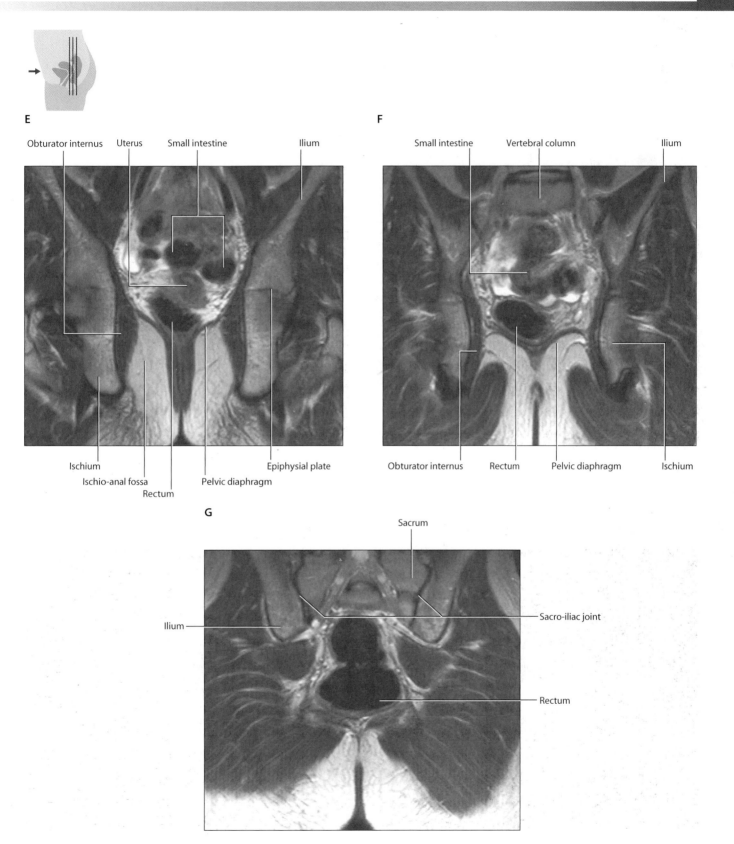

**E**

Obturator internus  Uterus  Small intestine  Ilium

Ischium

Ischio-anal fossa  Pelvic diaphragm

Rectum

Epiphysial plate

**F**

Small intestine  Vertebral column  Ilium

Obturator internus  Rectum  Pelvic diaphragm  Ischium

**G**

Sacrum

Ilium

Sacro-iliac joint

Rectum

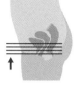

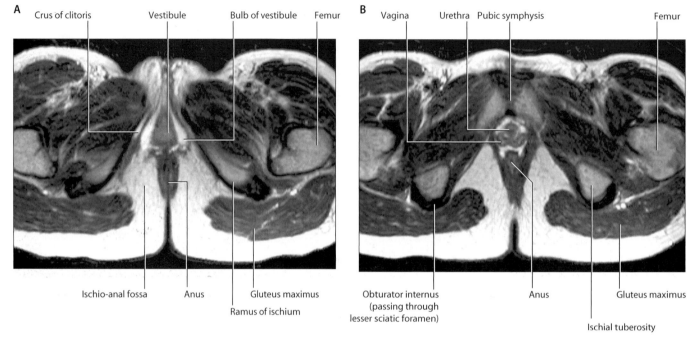

**A** — Crus of clitoris — Vestibule — Bulb of vestibule — Femur

Ischio-anal fossa — Anus — Gluteus maximus — Ramus of ischium

**B** — Vagina — Urethra — Pubic symphysis — Femur

Obturator internus (passing through lesser sciatic foramen) — Anus — Gluteus maximus — Ischial tuberosity

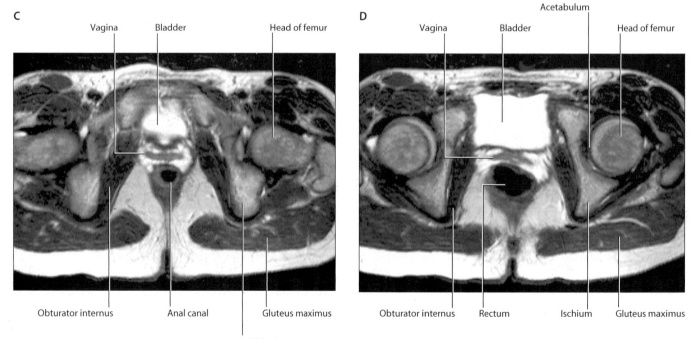

**C** — Vagina — Bladder — Head of femur

Obturator internus — Anal canal — Gluteus maximus — Ischial tuberosity

**D** — Acetabulum — Vagina — Bladder — Head of femur

Obturator internus — Rectum — Ischium — Gluteus maximus

**A through H – Series of axial images that pass through the pelvic cavity and perineum from inferior to superior showing the various structures and their relationships with each other.**
T2-weighted MR images in axial plane

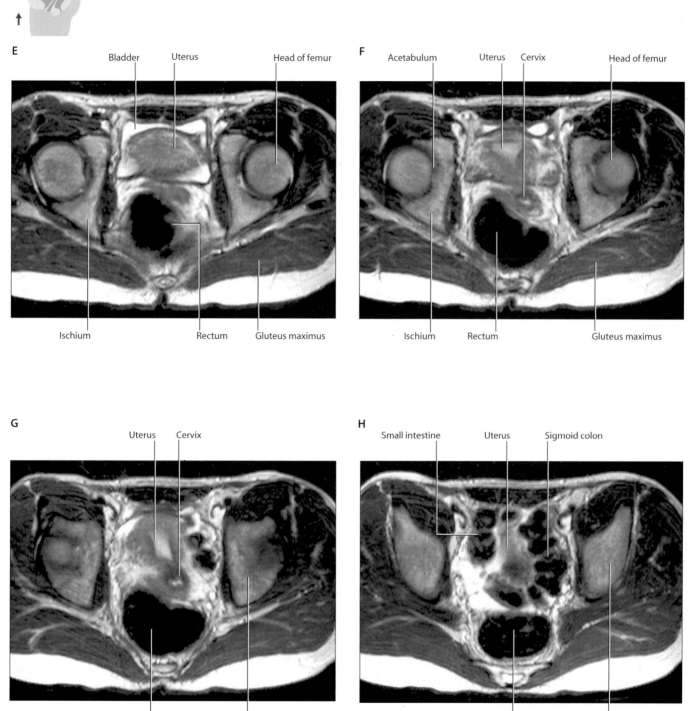

**E**

Bladder  Uterus  Head of femur

Ischium  Rectum  Gluteus maximus

**F**

Acetabulum  Uterus  Cervix  Head of femur

Ischium  Rectum  Gluteus maximus

**G**

Uterus  Cervix

Rectum  Ilium

**H**

Small intestine  Uterus  Sigmoid colon

Rectum  Ilium

# 6 *LOWER LIMB*

## CONTENTS

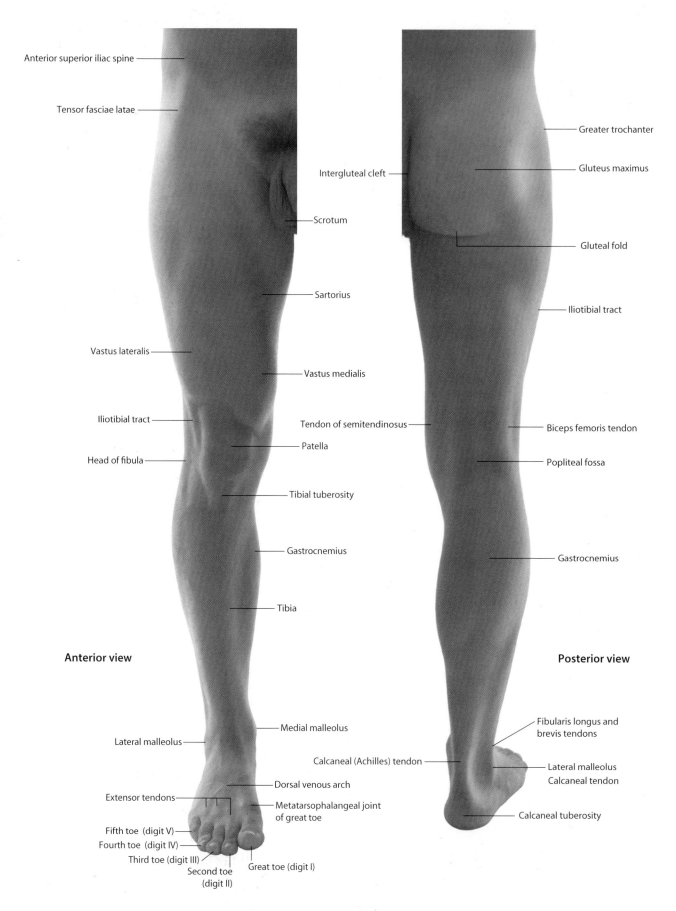

Anterior superior iliac spine

Tensor fasciae latae

Greater trochanter

Intergluteal cleft

Gluteus maximus

Scrotum

Gluteal fold

Sartorius

Iliotibial tract

Vastus lateralis

Vastus medialis

Iliotibial tract

Tendon of semitendinosus

Biceps femoris tendon

Patella

Popliteal fossa

Head of fibula

Tibial tuberosity

Gastrocnemius

Gastrocnemius

Tibia

**Anterior view**

**Posterior view**

Medial malleolus

Fibularis longus and brevis tendons

Lateral malleolus

Calcaneal (Achilles) tendon

Lateral malleolus
Calcaneal tendon

Dorsal venous arch

Extensor tendons

Metatarsophalangeal joint of great toe

Calcaneal tuberosity

Fifth toe (digit V)

Fourth toe (digit IV)

Third toe (digit III)

Great toe (digit I)

Second toe (digit II)

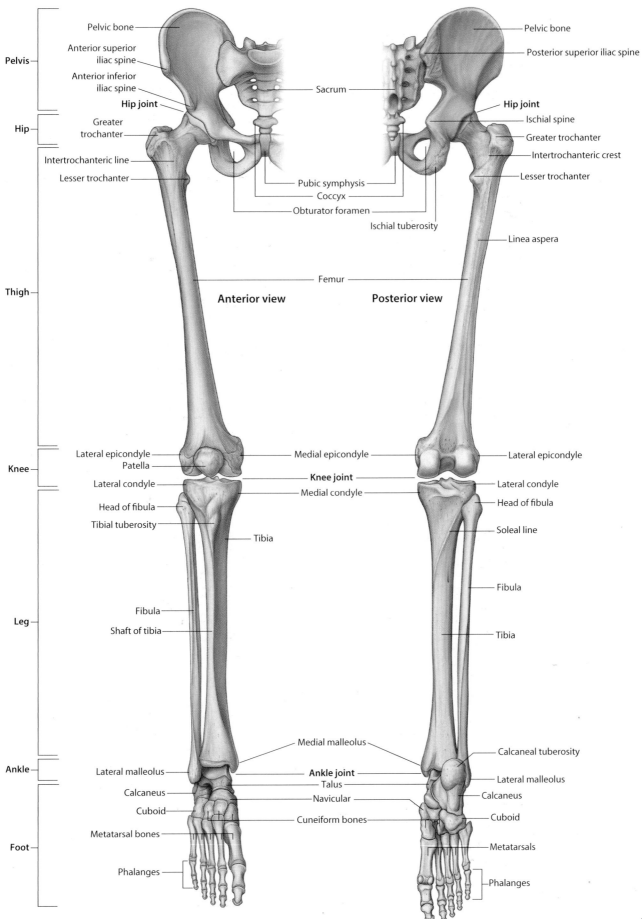

Pelvis
- Pelvic bone
- Anterior superior iliac spine
- Anterior inferior iliac spine
- **Hip joint**

Hip
- Greater trochanter
- Intertrochanteric line
- Lesser trochanter

Thigh

Sacrum

Pubic symphysis
Coccyx
Obturator foramen

Femur

**Anterior view**

- Pelvic bone
- Posterior superior iliac spine
- **Hip joint**
- Ischial spine
- Greater trochanter
- Intertrochanteric crest
- Lesser trochanter

Ischial tuberosity

Linea aspera

**Posterior view**

Knee
- Lateral epicondyle
- Patella
- Lateral condyle
- Head of fibula
- Tibial tuberosity

- Medial epicondyle
- **Knee joint**
- Medial condyle

- Tibia

- Lateral epicondyle
- Lateral condyle
- Head of fibula
- Soleal line

Leg
- Fibula
- Shaft of tibia

- Fibula
- Tibia

Ankle
- Lateral malleolus

- Medial malleolus
- **Ankle joint**
- Talus

- Calcaneal tuberosity
- Lateral malleolus

Foot
- Calcaneus
- Cuboid
- Metatarsal bones
- Phalanges

- Navicular
- Cuneiform bones

- Metatarsals

- Calcaneus
- Cuboid

- Phalanges

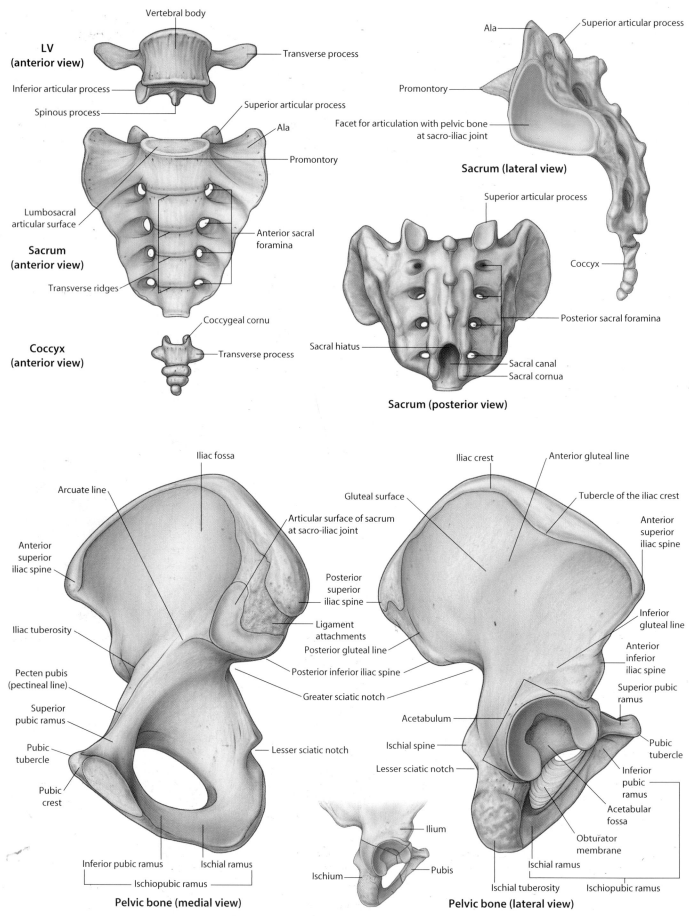

LV
(anterior view)

Vertebral body

Transverse process

Inferior articular process

Spinous process

Superior articular process

Ala

Promontory

Sacrum
(anterior view)

Lumbosacral
articular surface

Anterior sacral
foramina

Transverse ridges

Coccygeal cornu

Coccyx
(anterior view)

Transverse process

Ala

Superior articular process

Promontory

Facet for articulation with pelvic bone
at sacro-iliac joint

**Sacrum (lateral view)**

Superior articular process

Coccyx

Sacrum (posterior view)

Posterior sacral foramina

Sacral hiatus

Sacral canal

Sacral cornua

Iliac fossa

Arcuate line

Anterior
superior
iliac spine

Iliac tuberosity

Pecten pubis
(pectineal line)

Superior
pubic ramus

Pubic
tubercle

Pubic
crest

Inferior pubic ramus

Ischial ramus

Ischiopubic ramus

**Pelvic bone (medial view)**

Gluteal surface

Articular surface of sacrum
at sacro-iliac joint

Posterior
superior
iliac spine

Ligament
attachments

Posterior gluteal line

Posterior inferior iliac spine

Greater sciatic notch

Lesser sciatic notch

Iliac crest

Anterior gluteal line

Tubercle of the iliac crest

Anterior
superior
iliac spine

Inferior
gluteal line

Anterior
inferior
iliac spine

Superior pubic
ramus

Pubic
tubercle

Inferior
pubic
ramus

Acetabular
fossa

Obturator
membrane

Ischial ramus

Ischiopubic ramus

Acetabulum

Ischial spine

Lesser sciatic notch

Ilium

Pubis

Ischium

Ischial tuberosity

**Pelvic bone (lateral view)**

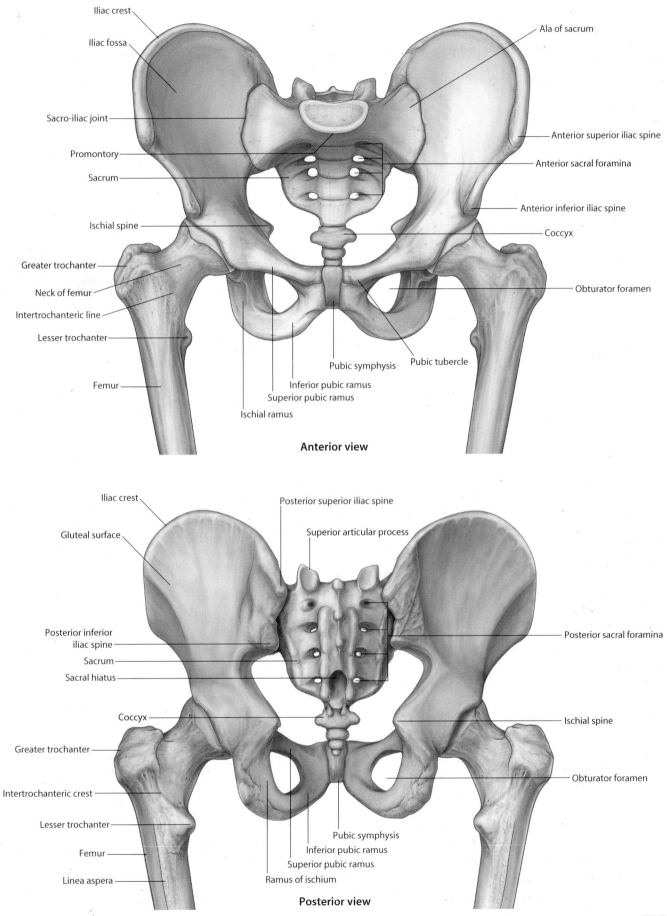

**Anterior view**

Iliac crest

Iliac fossa

Sacro-iliac joint

Promontory

Sacrum

Ischial spine

Greater trochanter

Neck of femur

Intertrochanteric line

Lesser trochanter

Femur

Ischial ramus

Superior pubic ramus

Inferior pubic ramus

Pubic symphysis

Pubic tubercle

Ala of sacrum

Anterior superior iliac spine

Anterior sacral foramina

Anterior inferior iliac spine

Coccyx

Obturator foramen

**Posterior view**

Iliac crest

Gluteal surface

Posterior inferior iliac spine

Sacrum

Sacral hiatus

Coccyx

Greater trochanter

Intertrochanteric crest

Lesser trochanter

Femur

Linea aspera

Ramus of ischium

Superior pubic ramus

Inferior pubic ramus

Pubic symphysis

Posterior superior iliac spine

Superior articular process

Posterior sacral foramina

Ischial spine

Obturator foramen

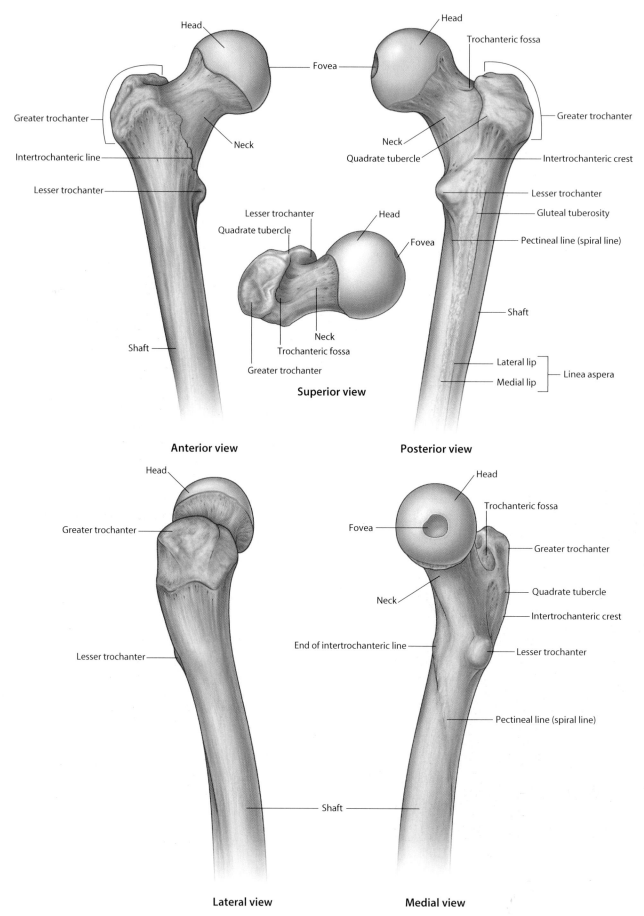

**Anterior view**

Head

Greater trochanter

Intertrochanteric line

Lesser trochanter

Shaft

Fovea

Neck

**Superior view**

Lesser trochanter

Quadrate tubercle

Head

Fovea

Greater trochanter

Neck

Trochanteric fossa

**Posterior view**

Head

Trochanteric fossa

Greater trochanter

Neck

Quadrate tubercle

Intertrochanteric crest

Lesser trochanter

Gluteal tuberosity

Pectineal line (spiral line)

Shaft

Lateral lip

Medial lip

Linea aspera

**Lateral view**

Head

Greater trochanter

Lesser trochanter

Shaft

**Medial view**

Head

Trochanteric fossa

Fovea

Greater trochanter

Quadrate tubercle

Intertrochanteric crest

Neck

Lesser trochanter

End of intertrochanteric line

Pectineal line (spiral line)

Shaft

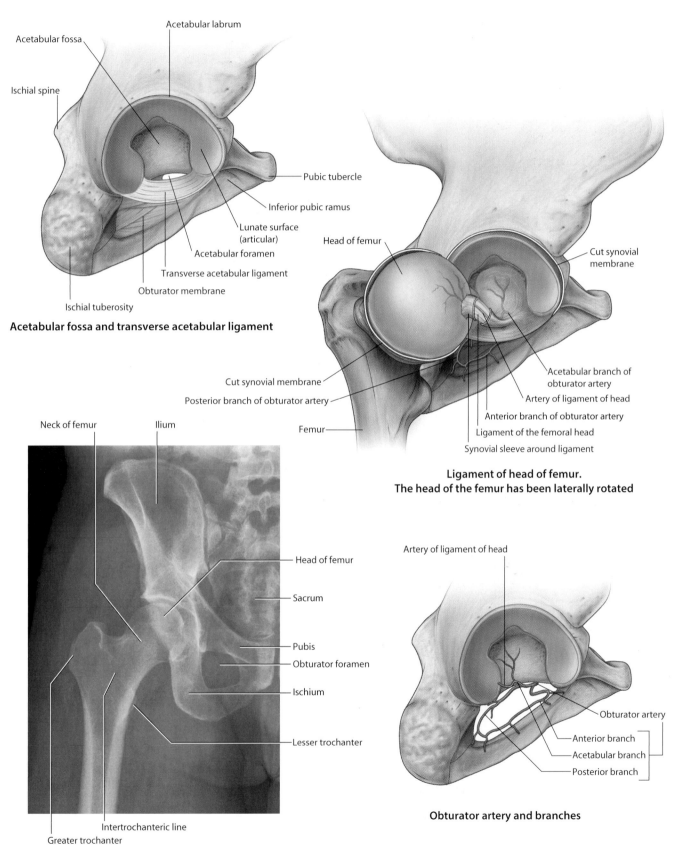

**Acetabular fossa and transverse acetabular ligament**

Acetabular fossa

Acetabular labrum

Ischial spine

Pubic tubercle

Inferior pubic ramus

Lunate surface (articular)

Acetabular foramen

Transverse acetabular ligament

Obturator membrane

Ischial tuberosity

Head of femur

Cut synovial membrane

Cut synovial membrane

Posterior branch of obturator artery

Acetabular branch of obturator artery

Artery of ligament of head

Anterior branch of obturator artery

Ligament of the femoral head

Synovial sleeve around ligament

Femur

**Ligament of head of femur.
The head of the femur has been laterally rotated**

Neck of femur

Ilium

Head of femur

Sacrum

Pubis

Obturator foramen

Ischium

Lesser trochanter

Intertrochanteric line

Greater trochanter

**Normal hip joint.**
Radiograph, AP view

Artery of ligament of head

Obturator artery

Anterior branch

Acetabular branch

Posterior branch

**Obturator artery and branches**

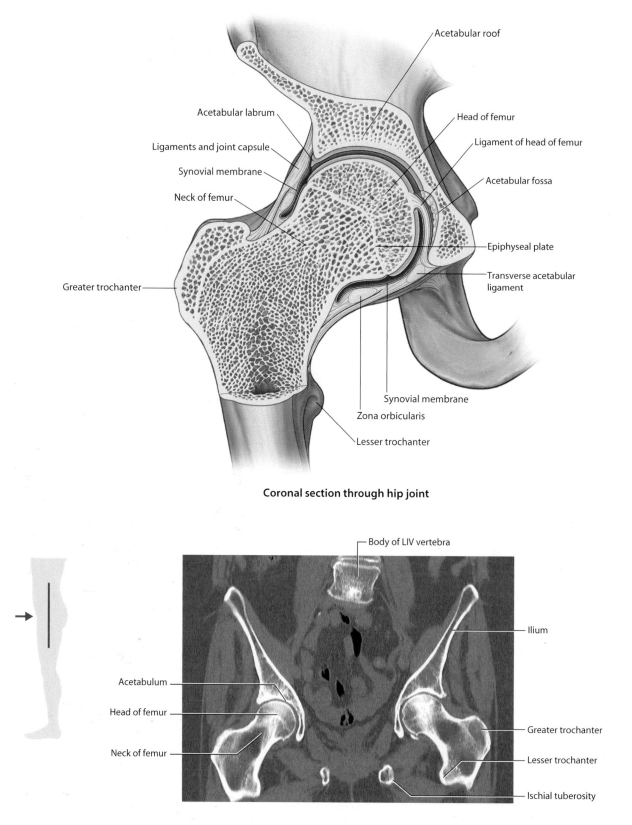

Acetabular roof

Acetabular labrum

Ligaments and joint capsule

Synovial membrane

Neck of femur

Greater trochanter

Head of femur

Ligament of head of femur

Acetabular fossa

Epiphyseal plate

Transverse acetabular ligament

Synovial membrane

Zona orbicularis

Lesser trochanter

**Coronal section through hip joint**

Body of LIV vertebra

Acetabulum

Head of femur

Neck of femur

Ilium

Greater trochanter

Lesser trochanter

Ischial tuberosity

**Hip joints.**
CT image in coronal plane

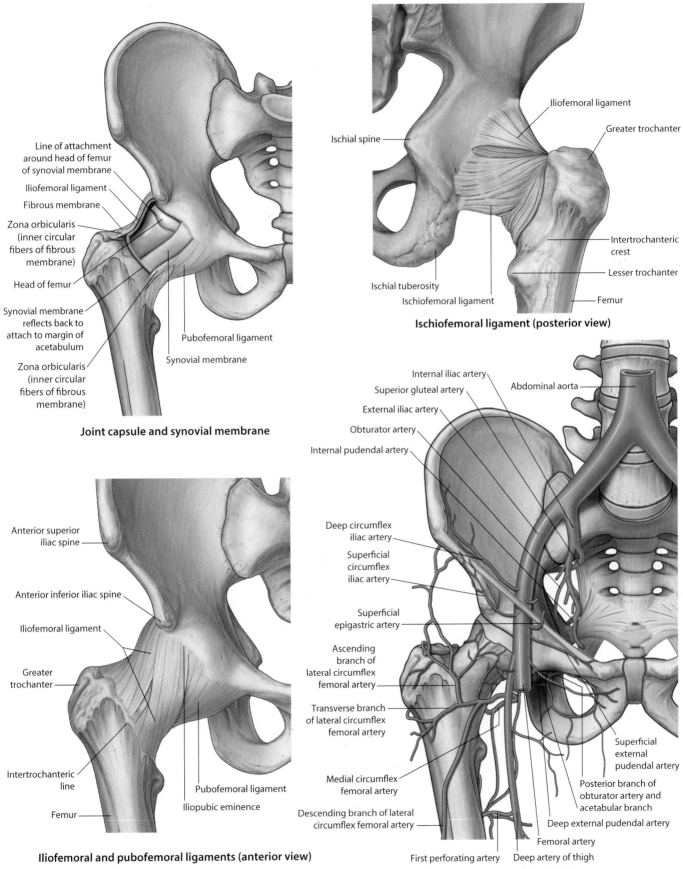

Line of attachment around head of femur of synovial membrane
Iliofemoral ligament
Fibrous membrane
Zona orbicularis (inner circular fibers of fibrous membrane)
Head of femur
Synovial membrane reflects back to attach to margin of acetabulum
Zona orbicularis (inner circular fibers of fibrous membrane)
Pubofemoral ligament
Synovial membrane

**Joint capsule and synovial membrane**

Ischial spine
Iliofemoral ligament
Greater trochanter
Intertrochanteric crest
Lesser trochanter
Femur
Ischial tuberosity
Ischiofemoral ligament

**Ischiofemoral ligament (posterior view)**

Anterior superior iliac spine
Anterior inferior iliac spine
Iliofemoral ligament
Greater trochanter
Intertrochanteric line
Femur
Pubofemoral ligament
Iliopubic eminence

**Iliofemoral and pubofemoral ligaments (anterior view)**

Internal iliac artery
Superior gluteal artery
External iliac artery
Obturator artery
Internal pudendal artery
Abdominal aorta
Deep circumflex iliac artery
Superficial circumflex iliac artery
Superficial epigastric artery
Ascending branch of lateral circumflex femoral artery
Transverse branch of lateral circumflex femoral artery
Medial circumflex femoral artery
Descending branch of lateral circumflex femoral artery
Superficial external pudendal artery
Posterior branch of obturator artery and acetabular branch
Deep external pudendal artery
Femoral artery
Deep artery of thigh
First perforating artery

**Arterial supply of the hip joint**

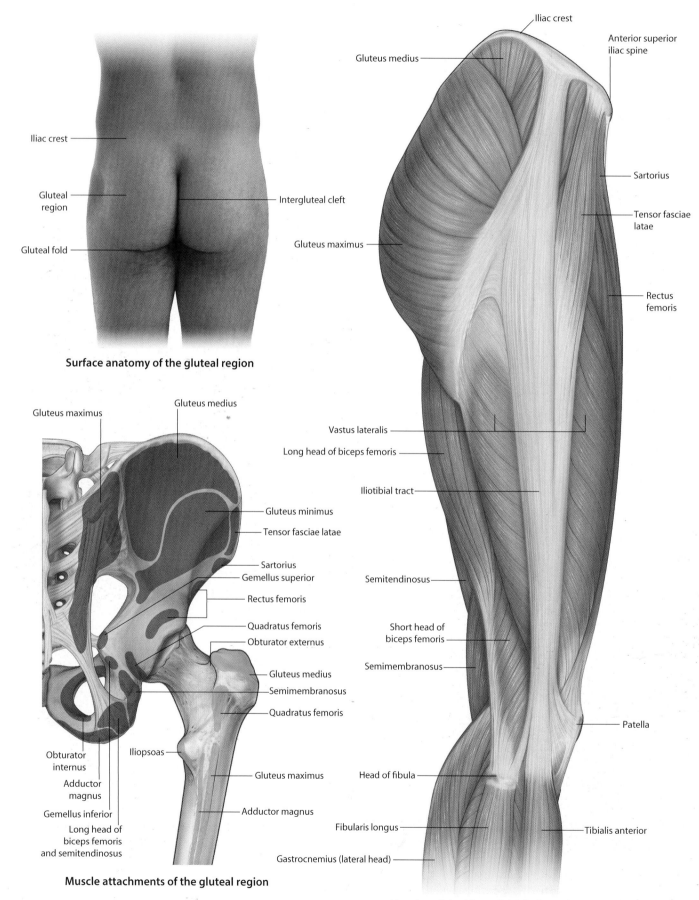

**Surface anatomy of the gluteal region**

Iliac crest

Gluteal region

Gluteal fold

Intergluteal cleft

Iliac crest

Gluteus medius

Anterior superior iliac spine

Sartorius

Tensor fasciae latae

Gluteus maximus

Rectus femoris

Vastus lateralis

Long head of biceps femoris

Iliotibial tract

Semitendinosus

Short head of biceps femoris

Semimembranosus

Patella

Head of fibula

Fibularis longus

Tibialis anterior

Gastrocnemius (lateral head)

**Muscles of the hip and thigh (lateral view)**

Gluteus maximus

Gluteus medius

Gluteus minimus

Tensor fasciae latae

Sartorius

Gemellus superior

Rectus femoris

Quadratus femoris

Obturator externus

Gluteus medius

Semimembranosus

Quadratus femoris

Obturator internus

Iliopsoas

Gluteus maximus

Adductor magnus

Gemellus inferior

Adductor magnus

Long head of biceps femoris and semitendinosus

**Muscle attachments of the gluteal region**

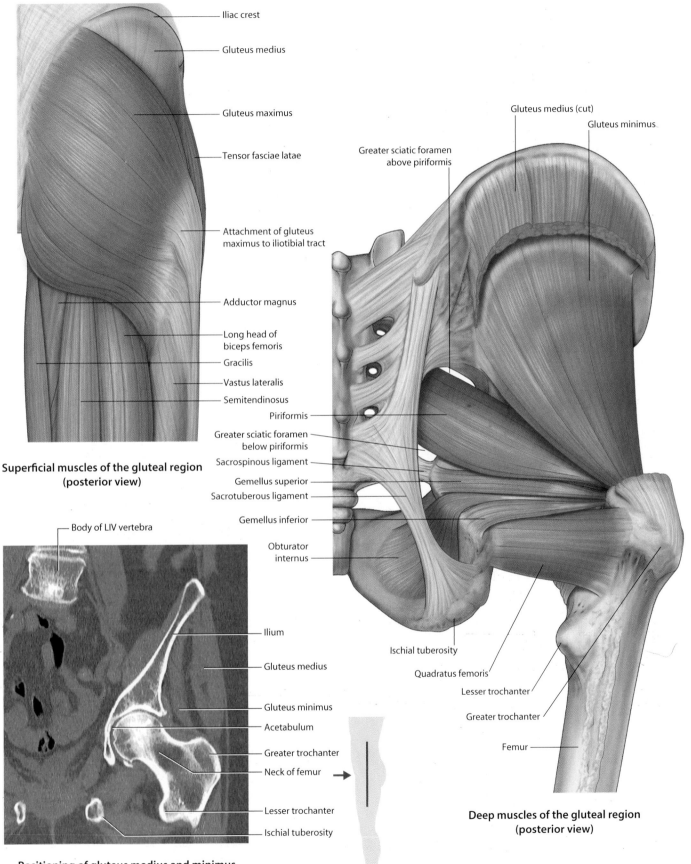

Iliac crest

Gluteus medius

Gluteus maximus

Tensor fasciae latae

Attachment of gluteus maximus to iliotibial tract

Adductor magnus

Long head of biceps femoris

Gracilis

Vastus lateralis

Semitendinosus

**Superficial muscles of the gluteal region (posterior view)**

Gluteus medius (cut)

Gluteus minimus

Greater sciatic foramen above piriformis

Piriformis

Greater sciatic foramen below piriformis

Sacrospinous ligament

Gemellus superior

Sacrotuberous ligament

Gemellus inferior

Obturator internus

Ischial tuberosity

Quadratus femoris

Lesser trochanter

Greater trochanter

Femur

**Deep muscles of the gluteal region (posterior view)**

Body of LIV vertebra

Ilium

Gluteus medius

Gluteus minimus

Acetabulum

Greater trochanter

Neck of femur

Lesser trochanter

Ischial tuberosity

**Positioning of gluteus medius and minimus muscles in relation to the hip joint.**
CT image in coronal plane

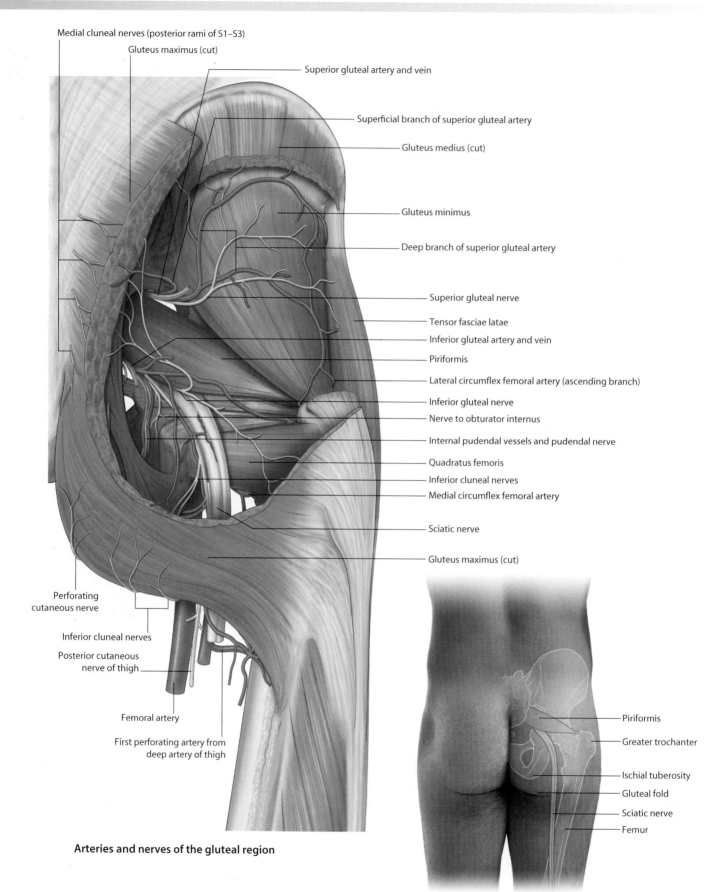

Medial cluneal nerves (posterior rami of S1–S3)

Gluteus maximus (cut)

Superior gluteal artery and vein

Superficial branch of superior gluteal artery

Gluteus medius (cut)

Gluteus minimus

Deep branch of superior gluteal artery

Superior gluteal nerve

Tensor fasciae latae

Inferior gluteal artery and vein

Piriformis

Lateral circumflex femoral artery (ascending branch)

Inferior gluteal nerve

Nerve to obturator internus

Internal pudendal vessels and pudendal nerve

Quadratus femoris

Inferior cluneal nerves

Medial circumflex femoral artery

Sciatic nerve

Gluteus maximus (cut)

Perforating cutaneous nerve

Inferior cluneal nerves

Posterior cutaneous nerve of thigh

Femoral artery

First perforating artery from deep artery of thigh

**Arteries and nerves of the gluteal region**

Piriformis

Greater trochanter

Ischial tuberosity

Gluteal fold

Sciatic nerve

Femur

**Sciatic nerve in the gluteal region as it relates to the surface (posterior view)**

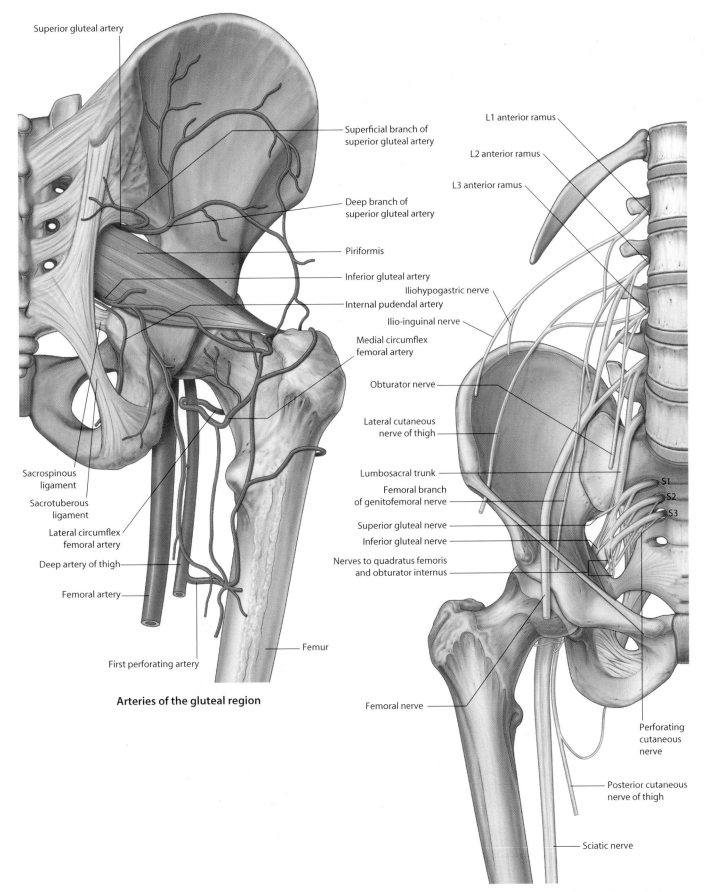

**Arteries of the gluteal region**

Superior gluteal artery

Superficial branch of superior gluteal artery

Deep branch of superior gluteal artery

Piriformis

Inferior gluteal artery

Internal pudendal artery

Medial circumflex femoral artery

Sacrospinous ligament

Sacrotuberous ligament

Lateral circumflex femoral artery

Deep artery of thigh

Femoral artery

First perforating artery

Femur

**Branches of the lumbosacral plexus related to lower limb**

L1 anterior ramus

L2 anterior ramus

L3 anterior ramus

Iliohypogastric nerve

Ilio-inguinal nerve

Obturator nerve

Lateral cutaneous nerve of thigh

Lumbosacral trunk

Femoral branch of genitofemoral nerve

Superior gluteal nerve

Inferior gluteal nerve

Nerves to quadratus femoris and obturator internus

Femoral nerve

S1

S2

S3

Perforating cutaneous nerve

Posterior cutaneous nerve of thigh

Sciatic nerve

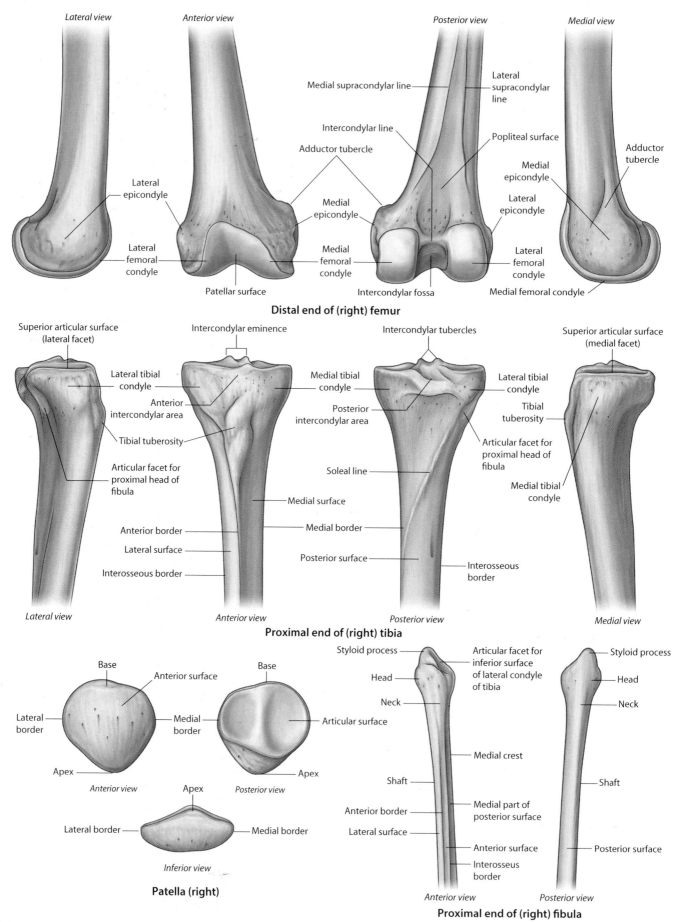

*Lateral view*   *Anterior view*   *Posterior view*   *Medial view*

Lateral epicondyle

Lateral femoral condyle

Medial supracondylar line

Intercondylar line

Adductor tubercle

Medial epicondyle

Medial femoral condyle

Patellar surface

Lateral supracondylar line

Popliteal surface

Medial epicondyle

Lateral epicondyle

Intercondylar fossa

Lateral femoral condyle

Medial femoral condyle

Adductor tubercle

**Distal end of (right) femur**

Superior articular surface (lateral facet)

Lateral tibial condyle

Anterior intercondylar area

Tibial tuberosity

Articular facet for proximal head of fibula

Anterior border

Lateral surface

Interosseous border

*Lateral view*

Intercondylar eminence

Intercondylar tubercles

Medial tibial condyle

Posterior intercondylar area

Soleal line

Medial surface

Medial border

Posterior surface

*Anterior view*

Lateral tibial condyle

Tibial tuberosity

Articular facet for proximal head of fibula

Medial tibial condyle

Interosseous border

*Posterior view*

Superior articular surface (medial facet)

*Medial view*

**Proximal end of (right) tibia**

Base

Anterior surface

Base

Lateral border

Medial border

Medial border

Apex

Apex

Apex

*Anterior view*

*Posterior view*

Articular surface

Lateral border

Medial border

*Inferior view*

**Patella (right)**

Styloid process

Head

Neck

Shaft

Anterior border

Lateral surface

Articular facet for inferior surface of lateral condyle of tibia

Medial crest

Medial part of posterior surface

Anterior surface

Interosseus border

*Anterior view*

Styloid process

Head

Neck

Shaft

Posterior surface

*Posterior view*

**Proximal end of (right) fibula**

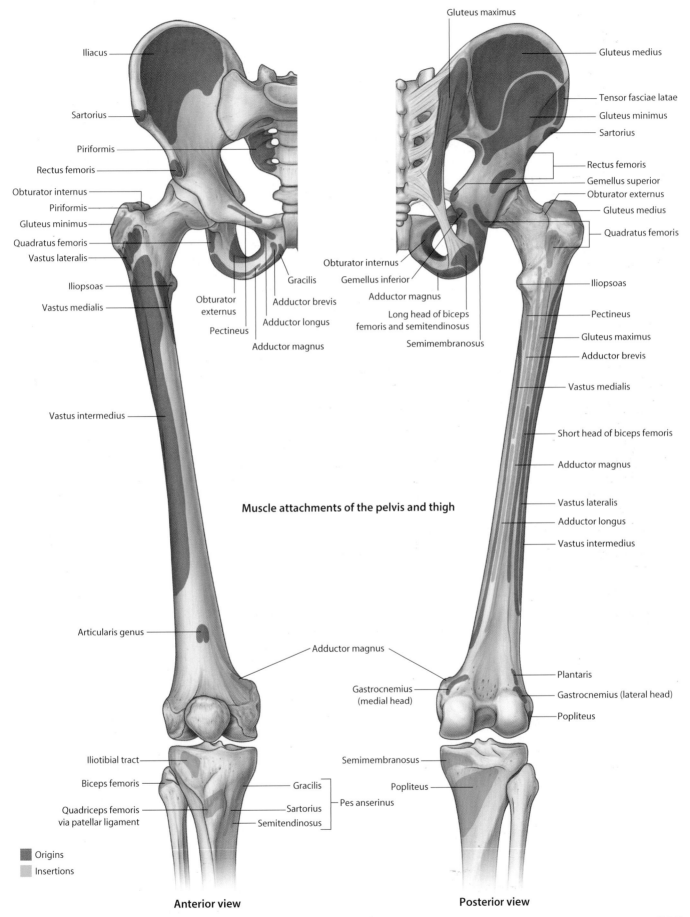

**Muscle attachments of the pelvis and thigh**

Iliacus

Sartorius

Piriformis

Rectus femoris

Obturator internus

Piriformis

Gluteus minimus

Quadratus femoris

Vastus lateralis

Iliopsoas

Vastus medialis

Obturator externus

Pectineus

Gracilis

Adductor brevis

Adductor longus

Adductor magnus

Vastus intermedius

Articularis genus

Adductor magnus

Iliotibial tract

Biceps femoris

Quadriceps femoris via patellar ligament

Gracilis

Sartorius

Semitendinosus

Pes anserinus

Gluteus maximus

Gluteus medius

Tensor fasciae latae

Gluteus minimus

Sartorius

Rectus femoris

Gemellus superior

Obturator externus

Gluteus medius

Quadratus femoris

Obturator internus

Gemellus inferior

Adductor magnus

Long head of biceps femoris and semitendinosus

Semimembranosus

Iliopsoas

Pectineus

Gluteus maximus

Adductor brevis

Vastus medialis

Short head of biceps femoris

Adductor magnus

Vastus lateralis

Adductor longus

Vastus intermedius

Gastrocnemius (medial head)

Plantaris

Gastrocnemius (lateral head)

Popliteus

Semimembranosus

Popliteus

■ Origins

■ Insertions

**Anterior view**

**Posterior view**

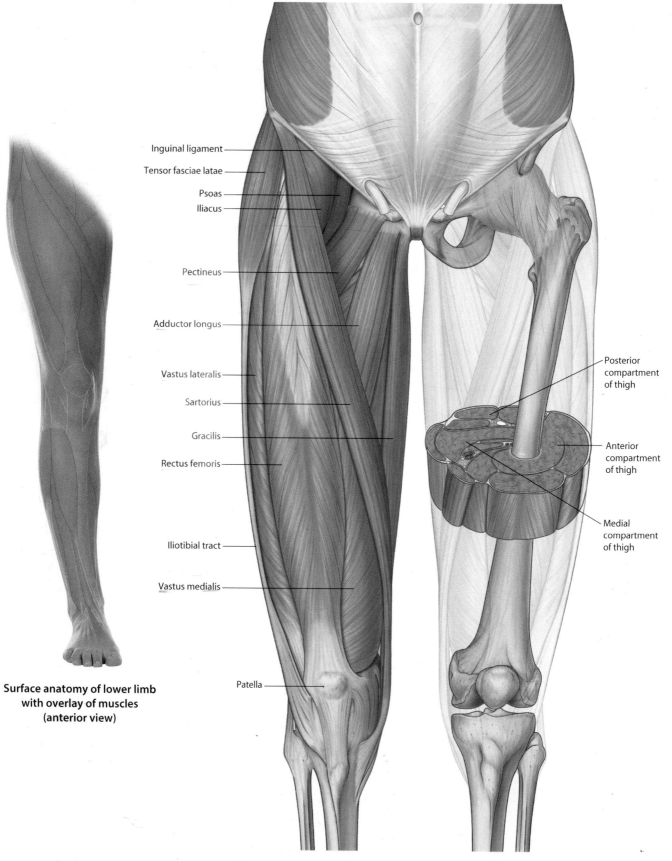

Inguinal ligament

Tensor fasciae latae

Psoas

Iliacus

Pectineus

Adductor longus

Vastus lateralis

Sartorius

Gracilis

Rectus femoris

Iliotibial tract

Vastus medialis

Patella

Posterior
compartment
of thigh

Anterior
compartment
of thigh

Medial
compartment
of thigh

**Surface anatomy of lower limb
with overlay of muscles
(anterior view)**

**Superficial muscles of the thigh (anterior view)**

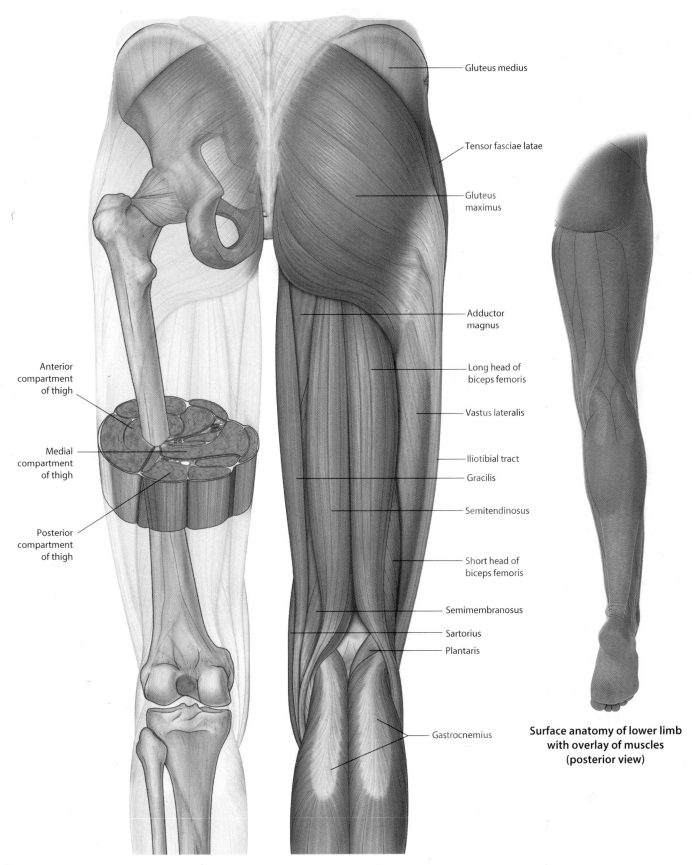

Gluteus medius

Tensor fasciae latae

Gluteus maximus

Adductor magnus

Long head of biceps femoris

Vastus lateralis

Iliotibial tract

Gracilis

Semitendinosus

Short head of biceps femoris

Semimembranosus

Sartorius

Plantaris

Gastrocnemius

Anterior compartment of thigh

Medial compartment of thigh

Posterior compartment of thigh

**Surface anatomy of lower limb with overlay of muscles (posterior view)**

**Superficial muscles of the thigh (posterior view)**

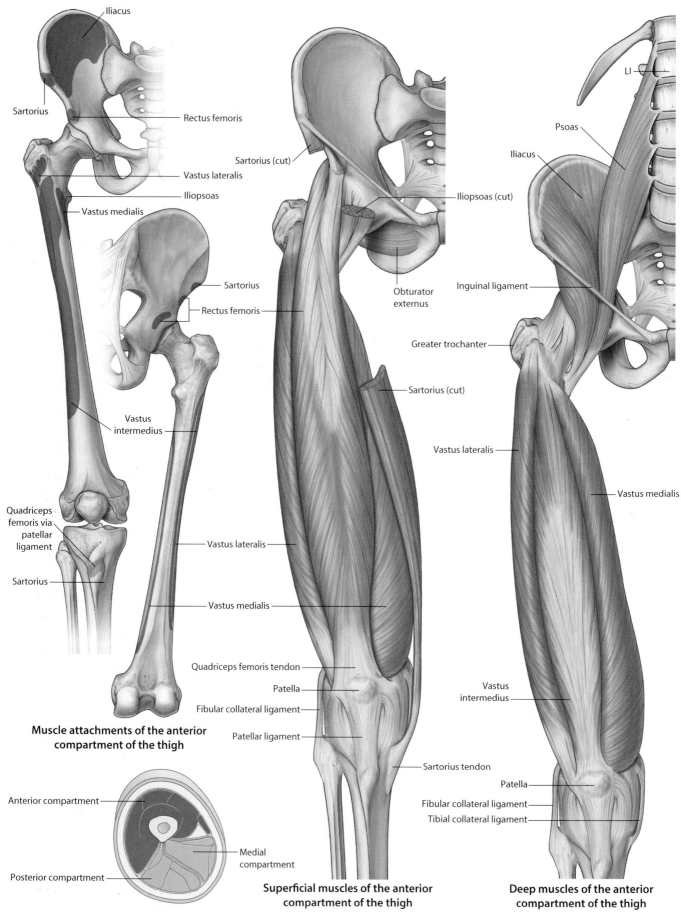

Iliacus

Sartorius

Rectus femoris

Vastus lateralis

Iliopsoas

Vastus medialis

Sartorius

Rectus femoris

Vastus intermedius

Quadriceps femoris via patellar ligament

Sartorius

**Muscle attachments of the anterior compartment of the thigh**

Anterior compartment

Posterior compartment

Medial compartment

Sartorius (cut)

Iliopsoas (cut)

Obturator externus

Vastus lateralis

Vastus medialis

Quadriceps femoris tendon

Patella

Fibular collateral ligament

Patellar ligament

Sartorius tendon

**Superficial muscles of the anterior compartment of the thigh**

L1

Psoas

Iliacus

Inguinal ligament

Greater trochanter

Sartorius (cut)

Vastus lateralis

Vastus medialis

Vastus intermedius

Patella

Fibular collateral ligament

Tibial collateral ligament

**Deep muscles of the anterior compartment of the thigh**

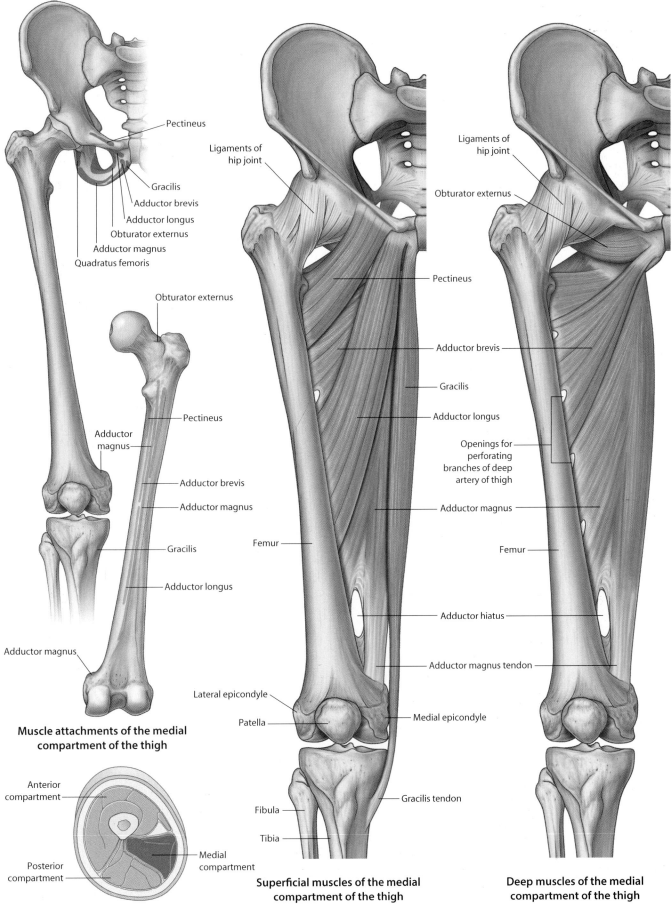

Pectineus

Gracilis

Adductor brevis

Adductor longus

Obturator externus

Adductor magnus

Quadratus femoris

Obturator externus

Pectineus

Adductor
magnus

Adductor brevis

Adductor magnus

Gracilis

Adductor longus

Adductor magnus

**Muscle attachments of the medial
compartment of the thigh**

Anterior
compartment

Posterior
compartment

Medial
compartment

Ligaments of
hip joint

Pectineus

Adductor brevis

Gracilis

Adductor longus

Femur

Lateral epicondyle

Patella

Medial epicondyle

Fibula

Tibia

Gracilis tendon

**Superficial muscles of the medial
compartment of the thigh**

Ligaments of
hip joint

Obturator externus

Pectineus

Adductor brevis

Gracilis

Adductor longus

Openings for
perforating
branches of deep
artery of thigh

Adductor magnus

Femur

Adductor hiatus

Adductor magnus tendon

**Deep muscles of the medial
compartment of the thigh**

**289**

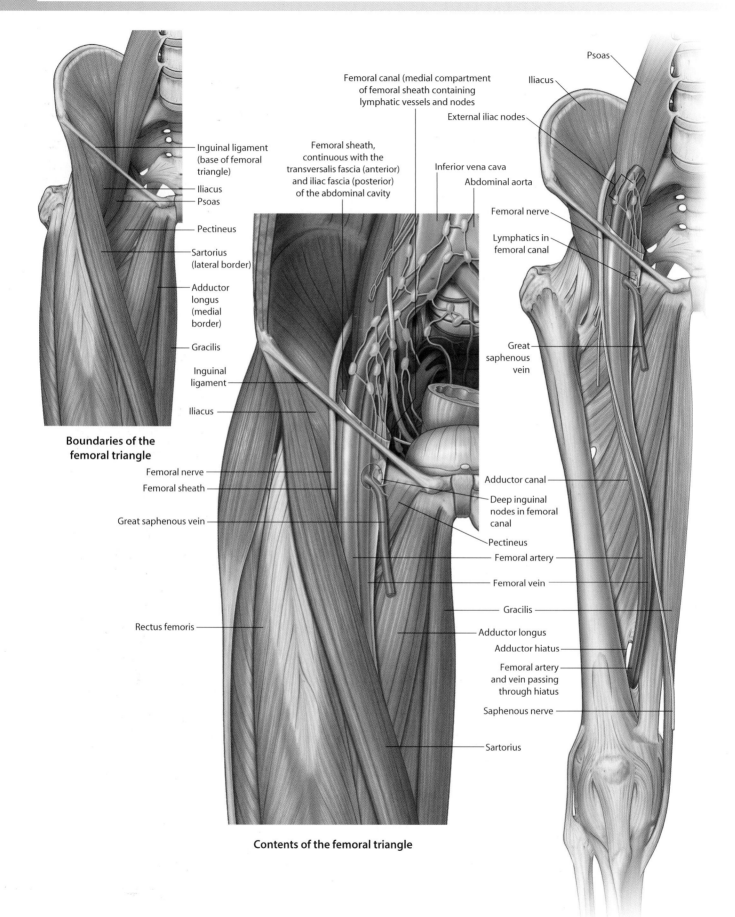

Inguinal ligament (base of femoral triangle)

Iliacus

Psoas

Pectineus

Sartorius (lateral border)

Adductor longus (medial border)

Gracilis

Inguinal ligament

Iliacus

**Boundaries of the femoral triangle**

Femoral nerve

Femoral sheath

Great saphenous vein

Rectus femoris

Femoral sheath, continuous with the transversalis fascia (anterior) and iliac fascia (posterior) of the abdominal cavity

Femoral canal (medial compartment of femoral sheath containing lymphatic vessels and nodes

Inferior vena cava

Abdominal aorta

Deep inguinal nodes in femoral canal

Pectineus

Femoral artery

Femoral vein

Gracilis

Adductor longus

Sartorius

**Contents of the femoral triangle**

Psoas

Iliacus

External iliac nodes

Femoral nerve

Lymphatics in femoral canal

Great saphenous vein

Adductor canal

Femoral artery

Adductor hiatus

Femoral artery and vein passing through hiatus

Saphenous nerve

**Adductor canal**

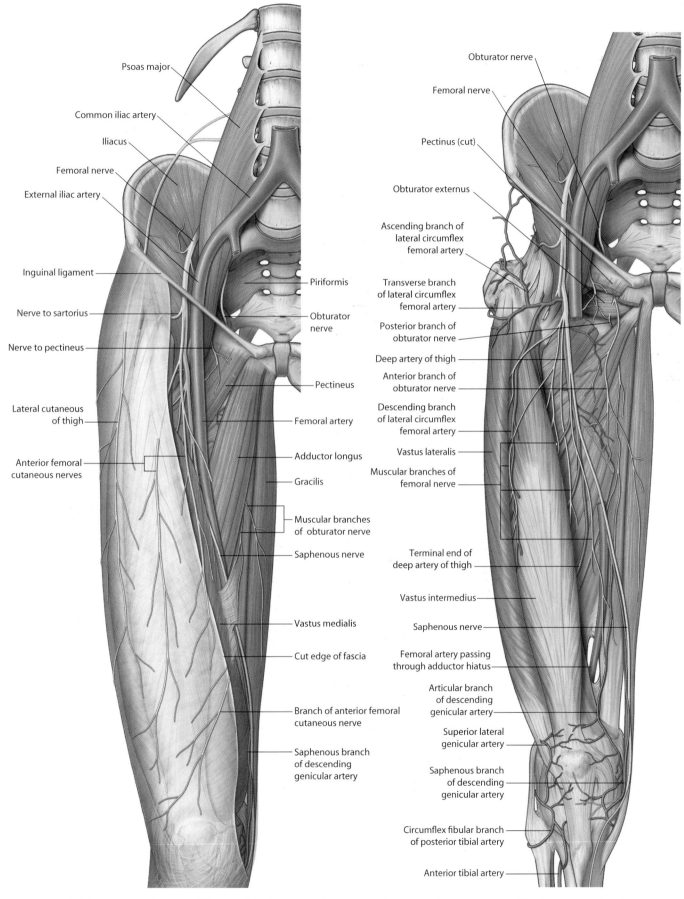

Psoas major

Common iliac artery

Iliacus

Femoral nerve

External iliac artery

Inguinal ligament

Nerve to sartorius

Nerve to pectineus

Lateral cutaneous of thigh

Anterior femoral cutaneous nerves

Piriformis

Obturator nerve

Pectineus

Femoral artery

Adductor longus

Gracilis

Muscular branches of obturator nerve

Saphenous nerve

Vastus medialis

Cut edge of fascia

Branch of anterior femoral cutaneous nerve

Saphenous branch of descending genicular artery

Obturator nerve

Femoral nerve

Pectinus (cut)

Obturator externus

Ascending branch of lateral circumflex femoral artery

Transverse branch of lateral circumflex femoral artery

Posterior branch of obturator nerve

Deep artery of thigh

Anterior branch of obturator nerve

Descending branch of lateral circumflex femoral artery

Vastus lateralis

Muscular branches of femoral nerve

Terminal end of deep artery of thigh

Vastus intermedius

Saphenous nerve

Femoral artery passing through adductor hiatus

Articular branch of descending genicular artery

Superior lateral genicular artery

Saphenous branch of descending genicular artery

Circumflex fibular branch of posterior tibial artery

Anterior tibial artery

**Superficial arteries and nerves of the thigh (anterior view)**    **Deep arteries and nerves of the thigh (anterior view)**

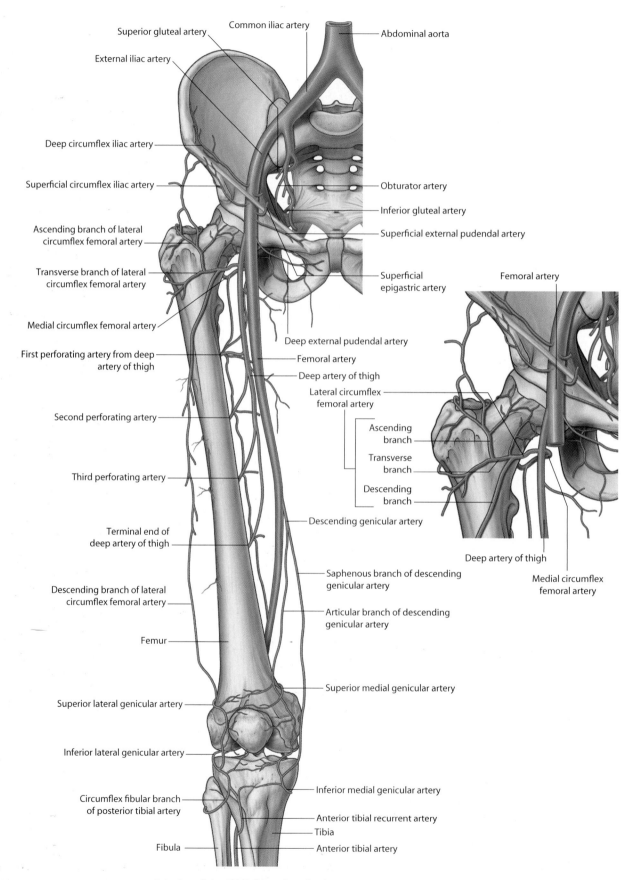

Superior gluteal artery

Common iliac artery

Abdominal aorta

External iliac artery

Deep circumflex iliac artery

Superficial circumflex iliac artery

Ascending branch of lateral circumflex femoral artery

Transverse branch of lateral circumflex femoral artery

Medial circumflex femoral artery

First perforating artery from deep artery of thigh

Second perforating artery

Third perforating artery

Terminal end of deep artery of thigh

Descending branch of lateral circumflex femoral artery

Femur

Superior lateral genicular artery

Inferior lateral genicular artery

Circumflex fibular branch of posterior tibial artery

Fibula

Obturator artery

Inferior gluteal artery

Superficial external pudendal artery

Superficial epigastric artery

Deep external pudendal artery

Femoral artery

Deep artery of thigh

Descending genicular artery

Saphenous branch of descending genicular artery

Articular branch of descending genicular artery

Superior medial genicular artery

Inferior medial genicular artery

Anterior tibial recurrent artery

Tibia

Anterior tibial artery

Femoral artery

Lateral circumflex femoral artery

Ascending branch

Transverse branch

Descending branch

Deep artery of thigh

Medial circumflex femoral artery

**Arteries of the thigh (anterior view)**

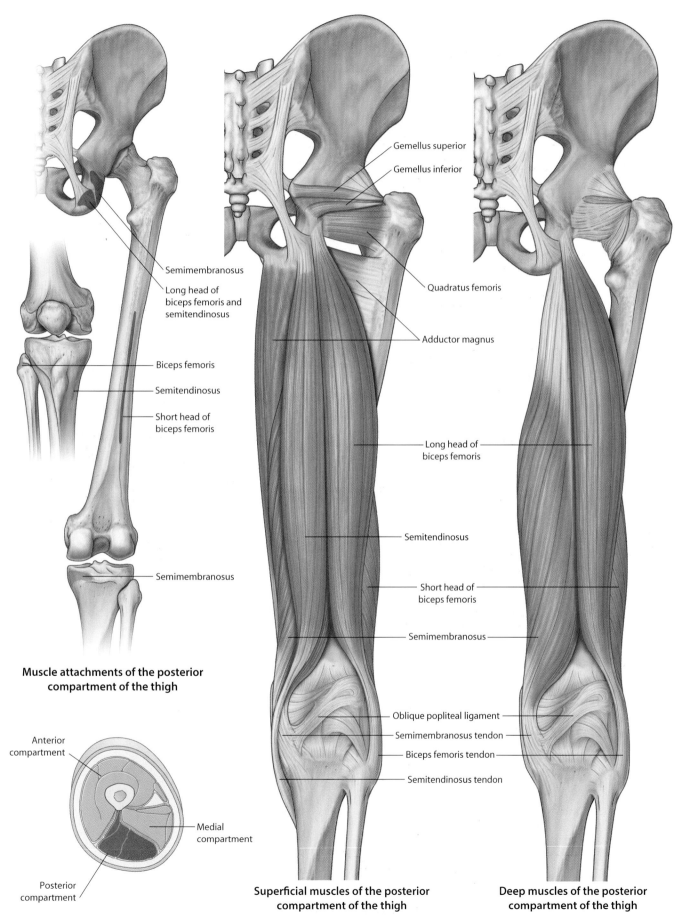

Semimembranosus

Long head of
biceps femoris and
semitendinosus

Biceps femoris

Semitendinosus

Short head of
biceps femoris

Semimembranosus

**Muscle attachments of the posterior
compartment of the thigh**

Anterior
compartment

Medial
compartment

Posterior
compartment

Gemellus superior

Gemellus inferior

Quadratus femoris

Adductor magnus

Long head of
biceps femoris

Semitendinosus

Short head of
biceps femoris

Semimembranosus

Oblique popliteal ligament

Semimembranosus tendon

Biceps femoris tendon

Semitendinosus tendon

**Superficial muscles of the posterior
compartment of the thigh**

**Deep muscles of the posterior
compartment of the thigh**

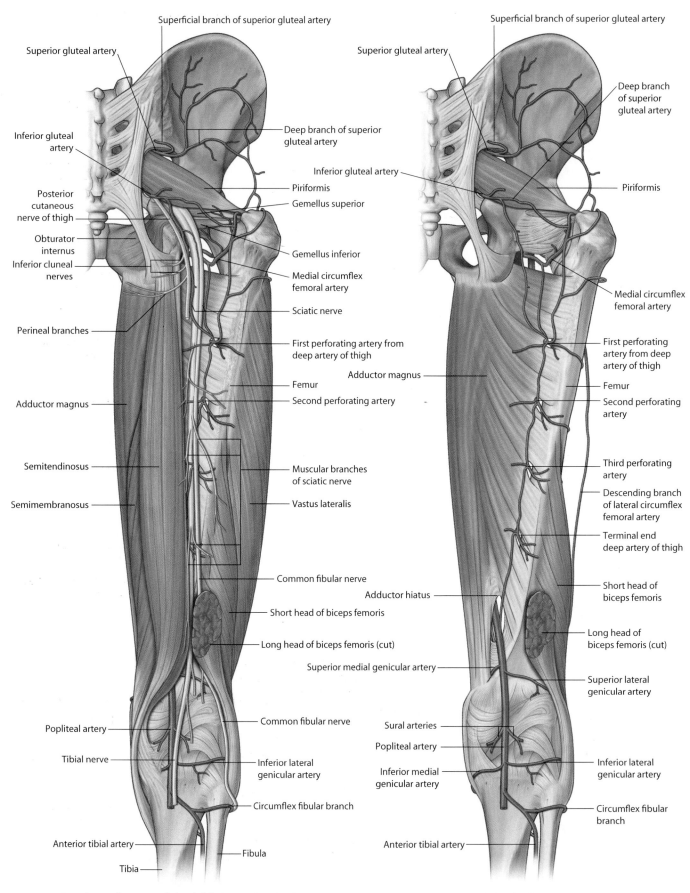

Superficial branch of superior gluteal artery

Superior gluteal artery

Inferior gluteal artery

Posterior cutaneous nerve of thigh

Obturator internus

Inferior cluneal nerves

Perineal branches

Adductor magnus

Semitendinosus

Semimembranosus

Popliteal artery

Tibial nerve

Anterior tibial artery

Tibia

Deep branch of superior gluteal artery

Piriformis

Gemellus superior

Gemellus inferior

Medial circumflex femoral artery

Sciatic nerve

First perforating artery from deep artery of thigh

Femur

Second perforating artery

Muscular branches of sciatic nerve

Vastus lateralis

Common fibular nerve

Short head of biceps femoris

Long head of biceps femoris (cut)

Common fibular nerve

Inferior lateral genicular artery

Circumflex fibular branch

Fibula

**Arteries and nerves of the thigh (posterior view)**

Superficial branch of superior gluteal artery

Superior gluteal artery

Inferior gluteal artery

Deep branch of superior gluteal artery

Piriformis

Medial circumflex femoral artery

First perforating artery from deep artery of thigh

Femur

Second perforating artery

Third perforating artery

Descending branch of lateral circumflex femoral artery

Terminal end deep artery of thigh

Short head of biceps femoris

Adductor magnus

Adductor hiatus

Long head of biceps femoris (cut)

Superior medial genicular artery

Superior lateral genicular artery

Sural arteries

Popliteal artery

Inferior medial genicular artery

Inferior lateral genicular artery

Circumflex fibular branch

Anterior tibial artery

**Deep arteries of the thigh (posterior view)**

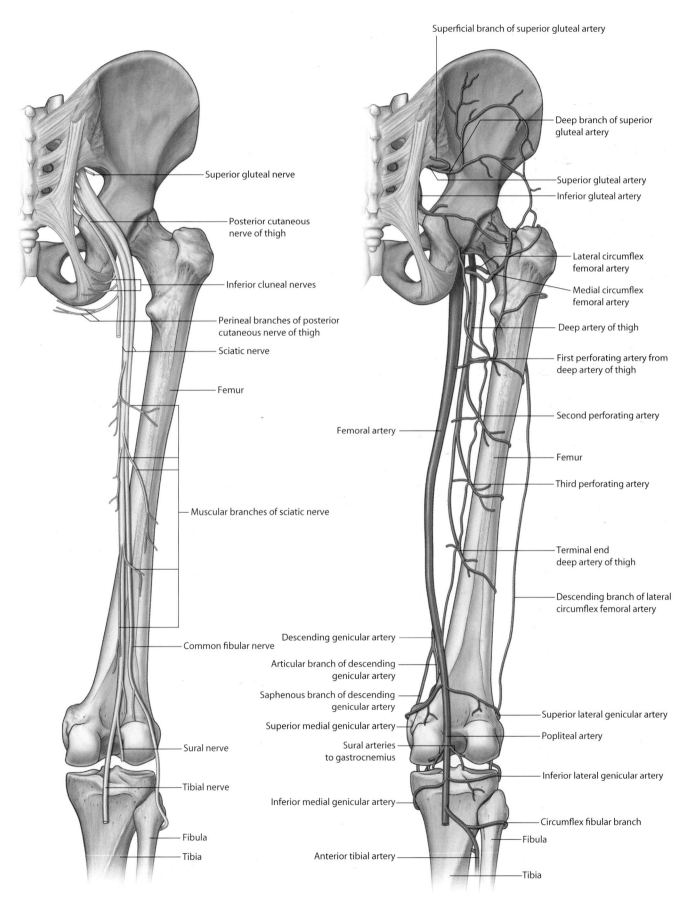

Superficial branch of superior gluteal artery

Superior gluteal nerve

Posterior cutaneous
nerve of thigh

Inferior cluneal nerves

Perineal branches of posterior
cutaneous nerve of thigh

Sciatic nerve

Femur

Muscular branches of sciatic nerve

Common fibular nerve

Sural nerve

Tibial nerve

Fibula

Tibia

Deep branch of superior
gluteal artery

Superior gluteal artery

Inferior gluteal artery

Lateral circumflex
femoral artery

Medial circumflex
femoral artery

Deep artery of thigh

First perforating artery from
deep artery of thigh

Second perforating artery

Femoral artery

Femur

Third perforating artery

Terminal end
deep artery of thigh

Descending branch of lateral
circumflex femoral artery

Descending genicular artery

Articular branch of descending
genicular artery

Saphenous branch of descending
genicular artery

Superior medial genicular artery

Sural arteries
to gastrocnemius

Inferior medial genicular artery

Anterior tibial artery

Superior lateral genicular artery

Popliteal artery

Inferior lateral genicular artery

Circumflex fibular branch

Fibula

Tibia

**Nerves of the thigh (posterior view)**

**Arteries of the thigh (posterior view)**

**295**

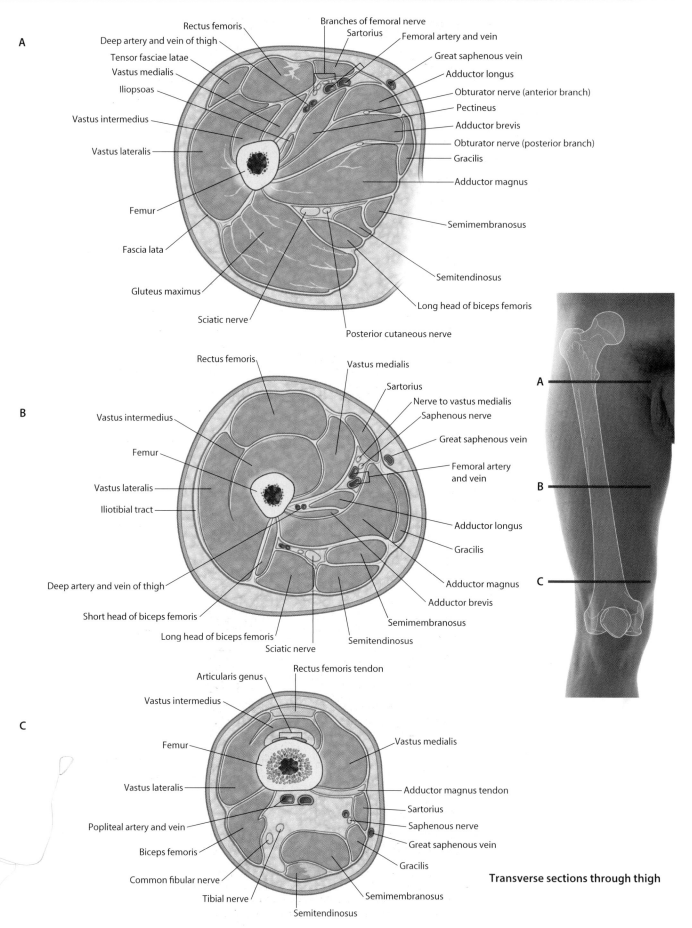

A

Rectus femoris
Deep artery and vein of thigh
Tensor fasciae latae
Vastus medialis
Iliopsoas
Vastus intermedius
Vastus lateralis
Femur
Fascia lata
Gluteus maximus
Sciatic nerve

Branches of femoral nerve
Sartorius
Femoral artery and vein
Great saphenous vein
Adductor longus
Obturator nerve (anterior branch)
Pectineus
Adductor brevis
Obturator nerve (posterior branch)
Gracilis
Adductor magnus
Semimembranosus
Semitendinosus
Long head of biceps femoris
Posterior cutaneous nerve

B

Rectus femoris
Vastus intermedius
Femur
Vastus lateralis
Iliotibial tract
Deep artery and vein of thigh
Short head of biceps femoris
Long head of biceps femoris
Sciatic nerve

Vastus medialis
Sartorius
Nerve to vastus medialis
Saphenous nerve
Great saphenous vein
Femoral artery and vein
Adductor longus
Gracilis
Adductor magnus
Adductor brevis
Semimembranosus
Semitendinosus

C

Articularis genus
Vastus intermedius
Femur
Vastus lateralis
Popliteal artery and vein
Biceps femoris
Common fibular nerve
Tibial nerve
Semitendinosus

Rectus femoris tendon
Vastus medialis
Adductor magnus tendon
Sartorius
Saphenous nerve
Great saphenous vein
Gracilis
Semimembranosus

A

B

C

**Transverse sections through thigh**

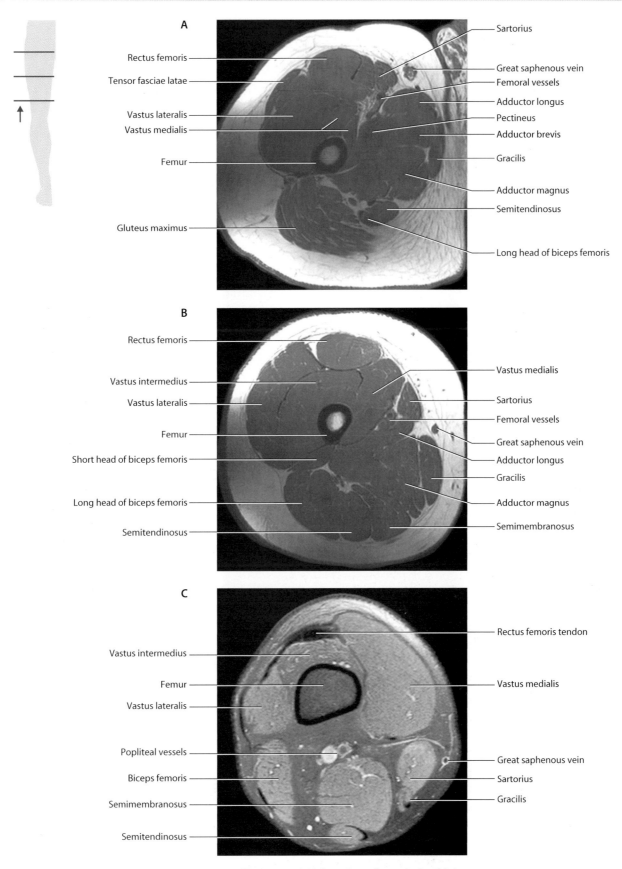

**A**

Rectus femoris
Tensor fasciae latae
Vastus lateralis
Vastus medialis
Femur
Gluteus maximus

Sartorius
Great saphenous vein
Femoral vessels
Adductor longus
Pectineus
Adductor brevis
Gracilis
Adductor magnus
Semitendinosus
Long head of biceps femoris

**B**

Rectus femoris
Vastus intermedius
Vastus lateralis
Femur
Short head of biceps femoris
Long head of biceps femoris
Semitendinosus

Vastus medialis
Sartorius
Femoral vessels
Great saphenous vein
Adductor longus
Gracilis
Adductor magnus
Semimembranosus

**C**

Vastus intermedius
Femur
Vastus lateralis
Popliteal vessels
Biceps femoris
Semimembranosus
Semitendinosus

Rectus femoris tendon
Vastus medialis
Great saphenous vein
Sartorius
Gracilis

**Transverse/axial sections through the thigh.**
A. Proximal/upper thigh. T1-weighted MR image in axial plane
B. Middle thigh. T1-weighted MR image in axial plane
C. Distal/lower thigh. T2-weighted MR image in axial plane

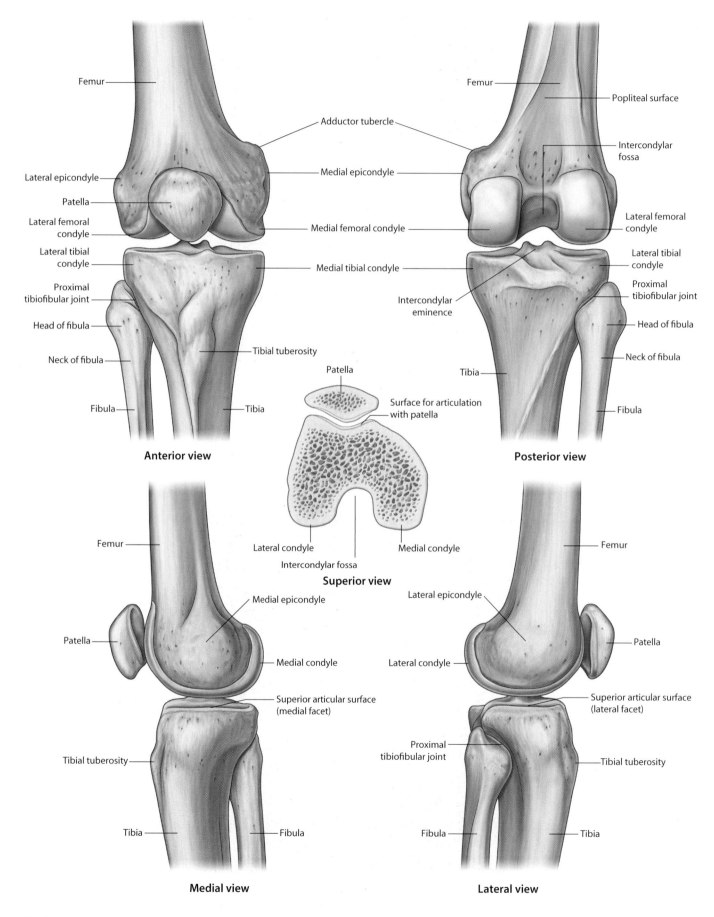

Femur

Adductor tubercle

Lateral epicondyle

Patella

Lateral femoral condyle

Lateral tibial condyle

Proximal tibiofibular joint

Head of fibula

Neck of fibula

Fibula

Medial epicondyle

Medial femoral condyle

Medial tibial condyle

Tibial tuberosity

Tibia

**Anterior view**

Femur

Popliteal surface

Intercondylar fossa

Lateral femoral condyle

Lateral tibial condyle

Proximal tibiofibular joint

Head of fibula

Neck of fibula

Fibula

Intercondylar eminence

Tibia

**Posterior view**

Patella

Surface for articulation with patella

Lateral condyle

Medial condyle

Intercondylar fossa

**Superior view**

Femur

Patella

Medial epicondyle

Medial condyle

Superior articular surface (medial facet)

Tibial tuberosity

Tibia

Fibula

**Medial view**

Femur

Lateral epicondyle

Patella

Lateral condyle

Superior articular surface (lateral facet)

Proximal tibiofibular joint

Tibial tuberosity

Fibula

Tibia

**Lateral view**

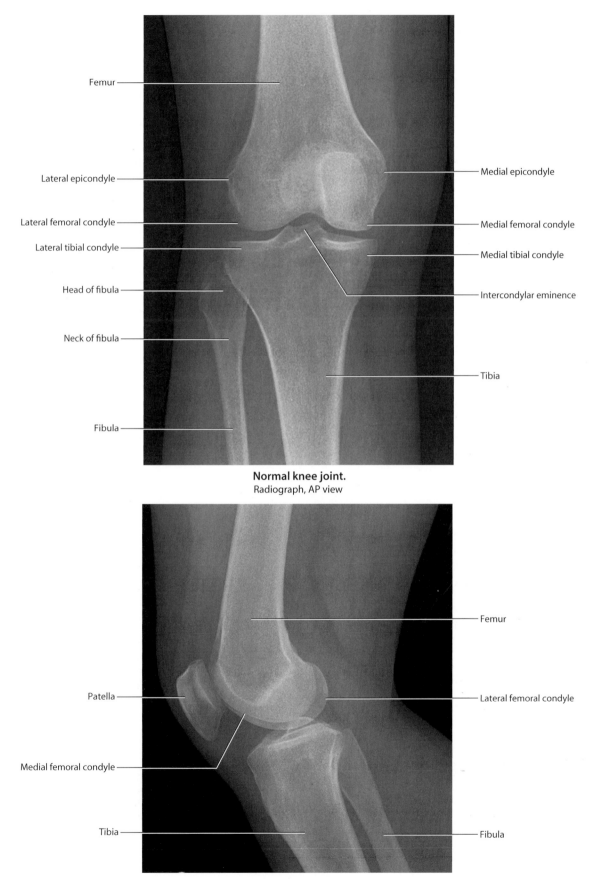

**Normal knee joint.**
Radiograph, AP view

**Normal knee joint.**
Radiograph, lateral view

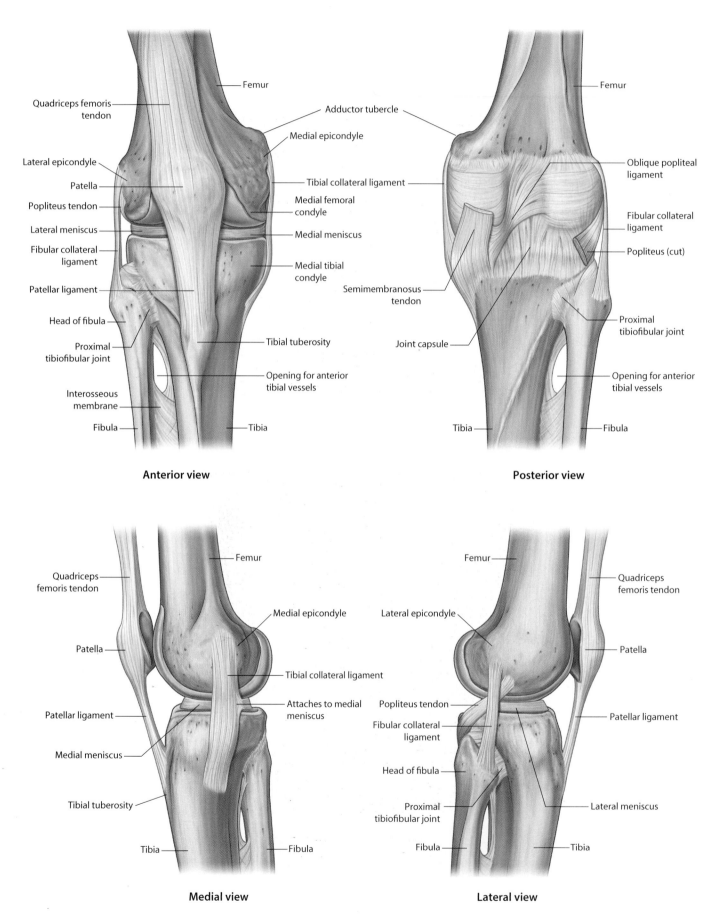

Quadriceps femoris tendon

Femur

Adductor tubercle

Medial epicondyle

Lateral epicondyle

Patella

Tibial collateral ligament

Popliteus tendon

Medial femoral condyle

Lateral meniscus

Medial meniscus

Fibular collateral ligament

Medial tibial condyle

Patellar ligament

Head of fibula

Tibial tuberosity

Proximal tibiofibular joint

Opening for anterior tibial vessels

Interosseous membrane

Fibula

Tibia

**Anterior view**

Femur

Adductor tubercle

Oblique popliteal ligament

Fibular collateral ligament

Popliteus (cut)

Semimembranosus tendon

Joint capsule

Proximal tibiofibular joint

Opening for anterior tibial vessels

Tibia

Fibula

**Posterior view**

Quadriceps femoris tendon

Femur

Medial epicondyle

Patella

Tibial collateral ligament

Patellar ligament

Attaches to medial meniscus

Medial meniscus

Tibial tuberosity

Tibia

Fibula

**Medial view**

Femur

Quadriceps femoris tendon

Lateral epicondyle

Patella

Popliteus tendon

Patellar ligament

Fibular collateral ligament

Head of fibula

Proximal tibiofibular joint

Lateral meniscus

Fibula

Tibia

**Lateral view**

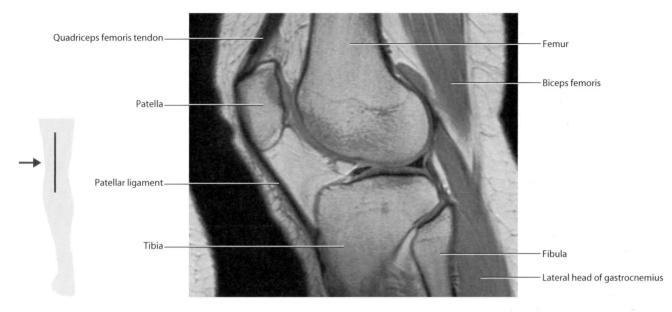

Quadriceps femoris tendon — — Femur

— Biceps femoris

Patella —

Patellar ligament —

Tibia —

— Fibula

— Lateral head of gastrocnemius

**Normal knee joint.**
T2-weighted MR image in sagittal plane

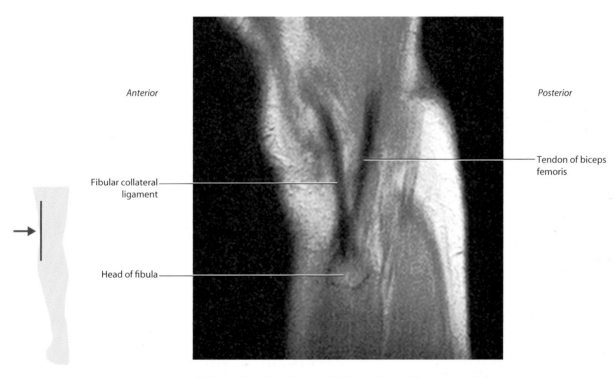

*Anterior*

*Posterior*

— Tendon of biceps femoris

Fibular collateral ligament —

Head of fibula —

**Unique view showing the fibular collateral ligament and the tendon of the biceps femoris muscle attaching to the head of the fibula.**
T2-weighted MR image in sagittal plane

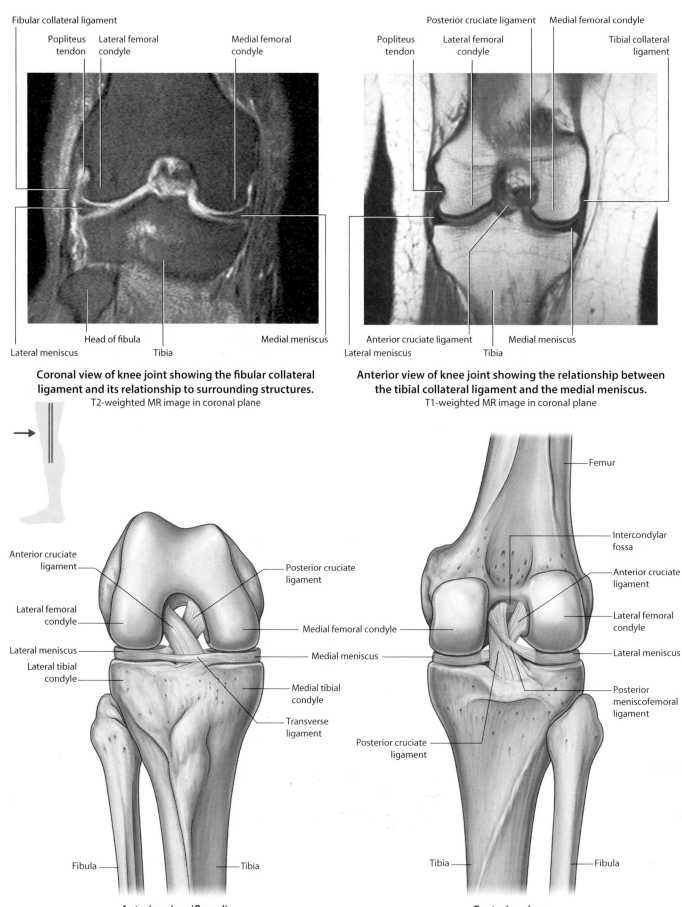

Fibular collateral ligament

Popliteus tendon

Lateral femoral condyle

Medial femoral condyle

Lateral meniscus

Head of fibula

Tibia

Medial meniscus

**Coronal view of knee joint showing the fibular collateral ligament and its relationship to surrounding structures.**
T2-weighted MR image in coronal plane

Posterior cruciate ligament

Medial femoral condyle

Popliteus tendon

Lateral femoral condyle

Tibial collateral ligament

Lateral meniscus

Anterior cruciate ligament

Medial meniscus

Tibia

**Anterior view of knee joint showing the relationship between the tibial collateral ligament and the medial meniscus.**
T1-weighted MR image in coronal plane

Anterior cruciate ligament

Lateral femoral condyle

Lateral meniscus

Lateral tibial condyle

Posterior cruciate ligament

Medial femoral condyle

Medial meniscus

Medial tibial condyle

Transverse ligament

Fibula

Tibia

**Anterior view (flexed)**

Femur

Intercondylar fossa

Anterior cruciate ligament

Lateral femoral condyle

Lateral meniscus

Posterior meniscofemoral ligament

Medial femoral condyle

Posterior cruciate ligament

Tibia

Fibula

**Posterior view**

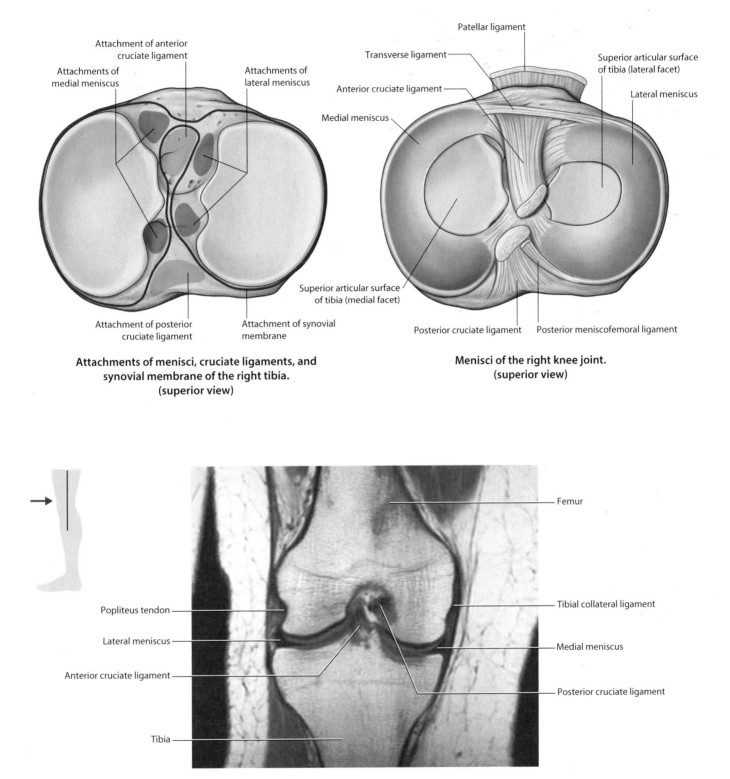

Attachment of anterior
cruciate ligament

Attachments of
medial meniscus

Attachments of
lateral meniscus

Attachment of posterior
cruciate ligament

Attachment of synovial
membrane

**Attachments of menisci, cruciate ligaments, and
synovial membrane of the right tibia.
(superior view)**

Patellar ligament

Transverse ligament

Anterior cruciate ligament

Medial meniscus

Superior articular surface
of tibia (lateral facet)

Lateral meniscus

Superior articular surface
of tibia (medial facet)

Posterior cruciate ligament

Posterior meniscofemoral ligament

**Menisci of the right knee joint.
(superior view)**

Femur

Popliteus tendon

Lateral meniscus

Anterior cruciate ligament

Tibia

Tibial collateral ligament

Medial meniscus

Posterior cruciate ligament

**Anterior view of knee joint showing the anterior and posterior cruciate ligaments.**
T2-weighted MR image in coronal plane

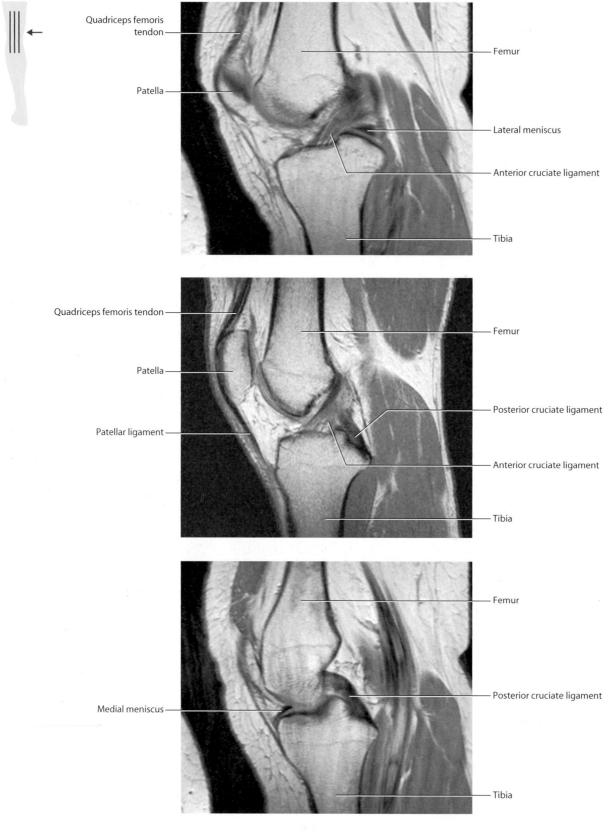

Quadriceps femoris tendon

Patella

Femur

Lateral meniscus

Anterior cruciate ligament

Tibia

Quadriceps femoris tendon

Patella

Patellar ligament

Femur

Posterior cruciate ligament

Anterior cruciate ligament

Tibia

Femur

Posterior cruciate ligament

Medial meniscus

Tibia

**A series of images moving from lateral to medial showing the relationship between anterior and posterior cruciate ligaments.**
T2-weighted MR images in sagittal plane

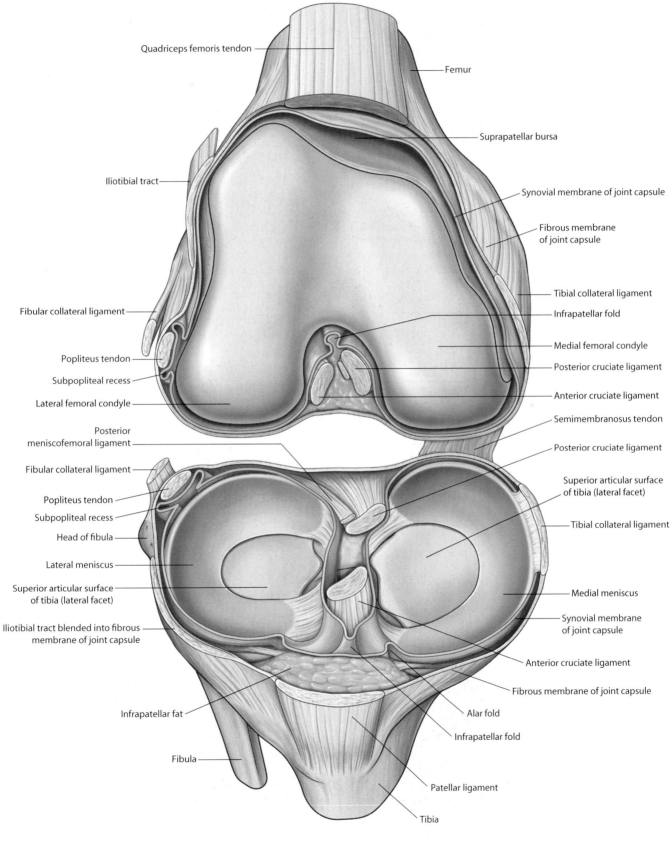

Quadriceps femoris tendon

Femur

Suprapatellar bursa

Iliotibial tract

Synovial membrane of joint capsule

Fibrous membrane of joint capsule

Tibial collateral ligament

Fibular collateral ligament

Infrapatellar fold

Medial femoral condyle

Popliteus tendon

Posterior cruciate ligament

Subpopliteal recess

Anterior cruciate ligament

Lateral femoral condyle

Semimembranosus tendon

Posterior meniscofemoral ligament

Posterior cruciate ligament

Fibular collateral ligament

Superior articular surface of tibia (lateral facet)

Popliteus tendon

Subpopliteal recess

Head of fibula

Tibial collateral ligament

Lateral meniscus

Superior articular surface of tibia (lateral facet)

Medial meniscus

Iliotibial tract blended into fibrous membrane of joint capsule

Synovial membrane of joint capsule

Anterior cruciate ligament

Fibrous membrane of joint capsule

Infrapatellar fat

Alar fold

Infrapatellar fold

Fibula

Patellar ligament

Tibia

**Knee joint (anterosuperior view)**

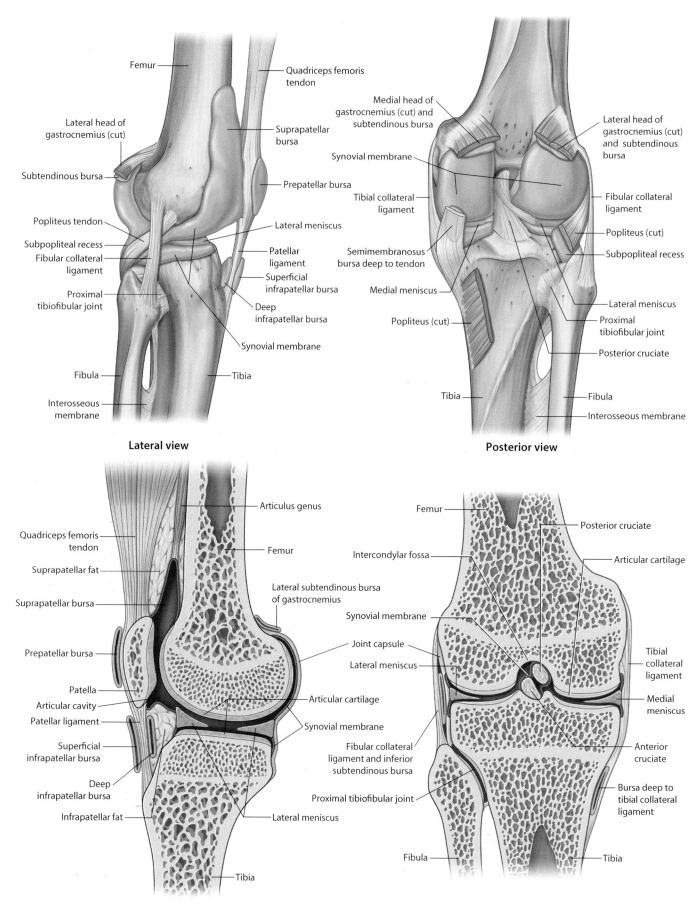

Femur

Quadriceps femoris tendon

Lateral head of gastrocnemius (cut)

Suprapatellar bursa

Subtendinous bursa

Prepatellar bursa

Popliteus tendon

Lateral meniscus

Subpopliteal recess

Patellar ligament

Fibular collateral ligament

Superficial infrapatellar bursa

Proximal tibiofibular joint

Deep infrapatellar bursa

Synovial membrane

Fibula

Tibia

Interosseous membrane

**Lateral view**

Medial head of gastrocnemius (cut) and subtendinous bursa

Lateral head of gastrocnemius (cut) and subtendinous bursa

Synovial membrane

Tibial collateral ligament

Fibular collateral ligament

Popliteus (cut)

Semimembranosus bursa deep to tendon

Subpopliteal recess

Medial meniscus

Lateral meniscus

Popliteus (cut)

Proximal tibiofibular joint

Posterior cruciate

Tibia

Fibula

Interosseous membrane

**Posterior view**

Articulus genus

Quadriceps femoris tendon

Femur

Suprapatellar fat

Lateral subtendinous bursa of gastrocnemius

Suprapatellar bursa

Prepatellar bursa

Patella

Articular cartilage

Articular cavity

Synovial membrane

Patellar ligament

Superficial infrapatellar bursa

Fibular collateral ligament and inferior subtendinous bursa

Deep infrapatellar bursa

Proximal tibiofibular joint

Infrapatellar fat

Lateral meniscus

Tibia

**Paramedian section through knee joint**

Femur

Posterior cruciate

Intercondylar fossa

Articular cartilage

Synovial membrane

Joint capsule

Tibial collateral ligament

Lateral meniscus

Medial meniscus

Articular cartilage

Synovial membrane

Anterior cruciate

Fibular collateral ligament

Bursa deep to tibial collateral ligament

Fibula

Tibia

**Coronal section through knee joint (anterior view)**

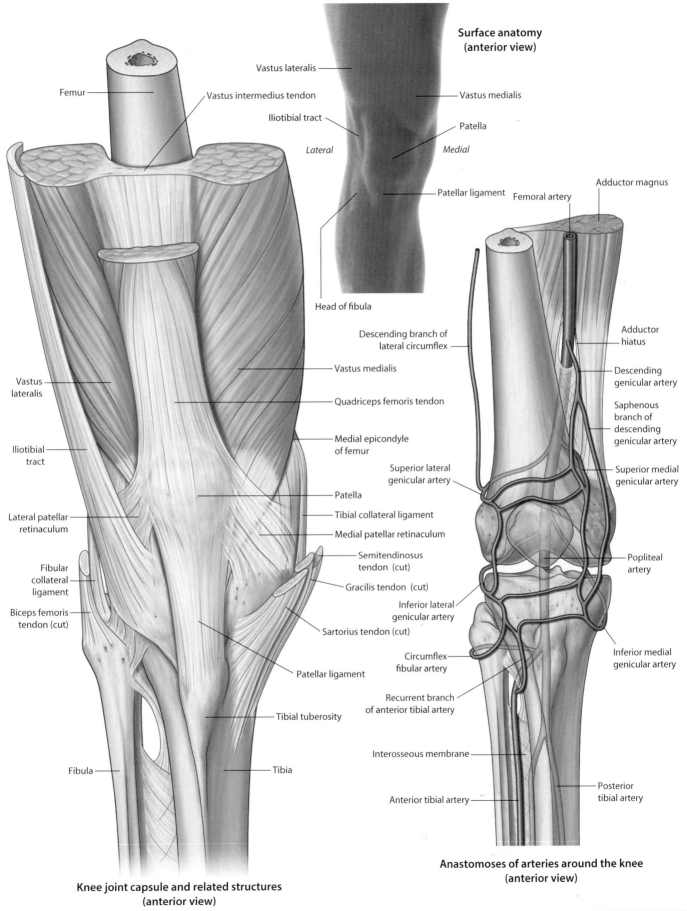

Surface anatomy
(anterior view)

Vastus lateralis

Vastus medialis

Iliotibial tract

Patella

*Lateral*

*Medial*

Patellar ligament

Head of fibula

Femur

Vastus intermedius tendon

Adductor magnus

Femoral artery

Adductor hiatus

Descending branch of lateral circumflex

Descending genicular artery

Vastus medialis

Saphenous branch of descending genicular artery

Quadriceps femoris tendon

Superior medial genicular artery

Medial epicondyle of femur

Superior lateral genicular artery

Vastus lateralis

Patella

Iliotibial tract

Tibial collateral ligament

Popliteal artery

Lateral patellar retinaculum

Medial patellar retinaculum

Semitendinosus tendon (cut)

Inferior lateral genicular artery

Fibular collateral ligament

Gracilis tendon (cut)

Biceps femoris tendon (cut)

Sartorius tendon (cut)

Inferior medial genicular artery

Circumflex fibular artery

Patellar ligament

Recurrent branch of anterior tibial artery

Tibial tuberosity

Interosseous membrane

Fibula

Tibia

Posterior tibial artery

Anterior tibial artery

**Knee joint capsule and related structures
(anterior view)**

**Anastomoses of arteries around the knee
(anterior view)**

**307**

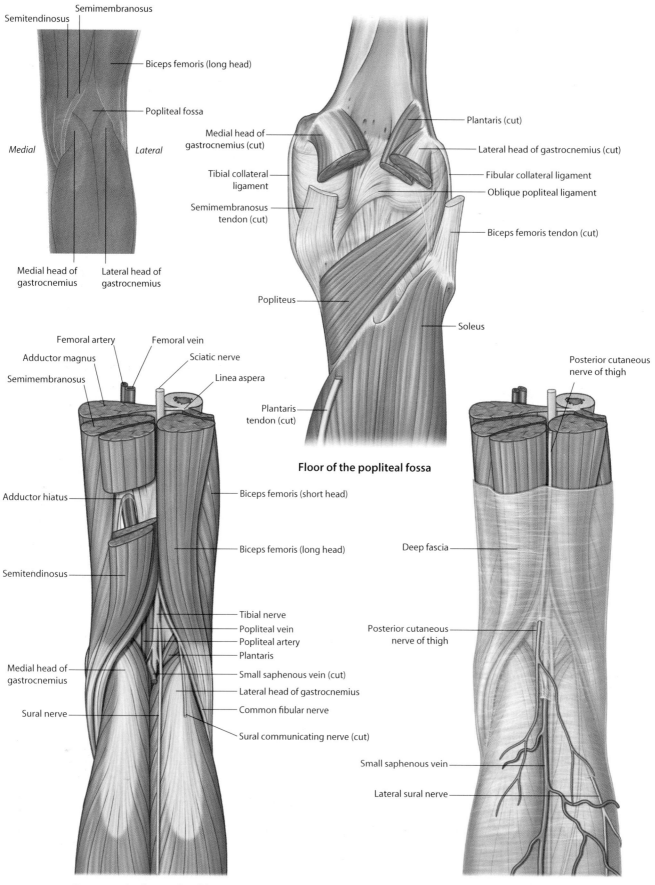

Semitendinosus

Semimembranosus

Biceps femoris (long head)

Popliteal fossa

*Medial*

*Lateral*

Medial head of gastrocnemius

Lateral head of gastrocnemius

Medial head of gastrocnemius (cut)

Tibial collateral ligament

Semimembranosus tendon (cut)

Popliteus

Plantaris (cut)

Lateral head of gastrocnemius (cut)

Fibular collateral ligament

Oblique popliteal ligament

Biceps femoris tendon (cut)

Soleus

Plantaris tendon (cut)

**Floor of the popliteal fossa**

Femoral artery

Adductor magnus

Semimembranosus

Femoral vein

Sciatic nerve

Linea aspera

Adductor hiatus

Semitendinosus

Medial head of gastrocnemius

Sural nerve

Biceps femoris (short head)

Biceps femoris (long head)

Tibial nerve

Popliteal vein

Popliteal artery

Plantaris

Small saphenous vein (cut)

Lateral head of gastrocnemius

Common fibular nerve

Sural communicating nerve (cut)

**Structures in the popliteal fossa**

Posterior cutaneous nerve of thigh

Deep fascia

Posterior cutaneous nerve of thigh

Small saphenous vein

Lateral sural nerve

**Superficial structures**

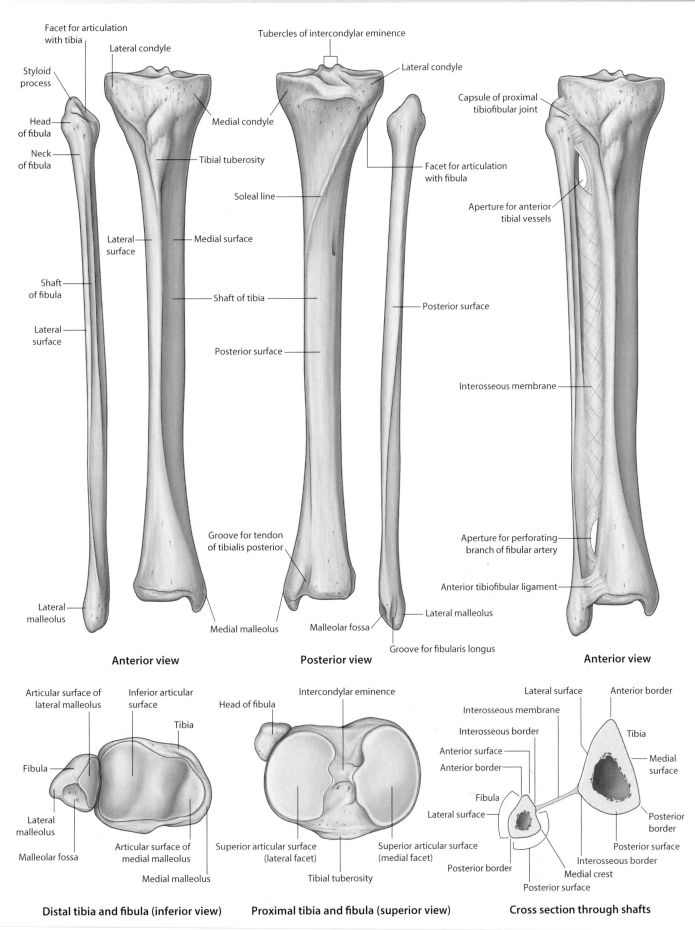

Facet for articulation with tibia

Styloid process

Head of fibula

Neck of fibula

Lateral condyle

Medial condyle

Tibial tuberosity

Lateral surface

Medial surface

Shaft of fibula

Lateral surface

Shaft of tibia

Posterior surface

Lateral malleolus

Groove for tendon of tibialis posterior

Medial malleolus

**Anterior view**

Tubercles of intercondylar eminence

Lateral condyle

Facet for articulation with fibula

Soleal line

Posterior surface

Malleolar fossa

Lateral malleolus

Groove for fibularis longus

**Posterior view**

Capsule of proximal tibiofibular joint

Aperture for anterior tibial vessels

Interosseous membrane

Aperture for perforating branch of fibular artery

Anterior tibiofibular ligament

**Anterior view**

Articular surface of lateral malleolus

Inferior articular surface

Tibia

Fibula

Lateral malleolus

Malleolar fossa

Articular surface of medial malleolus

Medial malleolus

**Distal tibia and fibula (inferior view)**

Head of fibula

Intercondylar eminence

Superior articular surface (lateral facet)

Tibial tuberosity

Superior articular surface (medial facet)

**Proximal tibia and fibula (superior view)**

Lateral surface

Anterior border

Interosseous membrane

Interosseous border

Anterior surface

Anterior border

Fibula

Lateral surface

Tibia

Medial surface

Posterior border

Posterior surface

Interosseous border

Medial crest

Posterior border

Posterior surface

**Cross section through shafts**

**309**

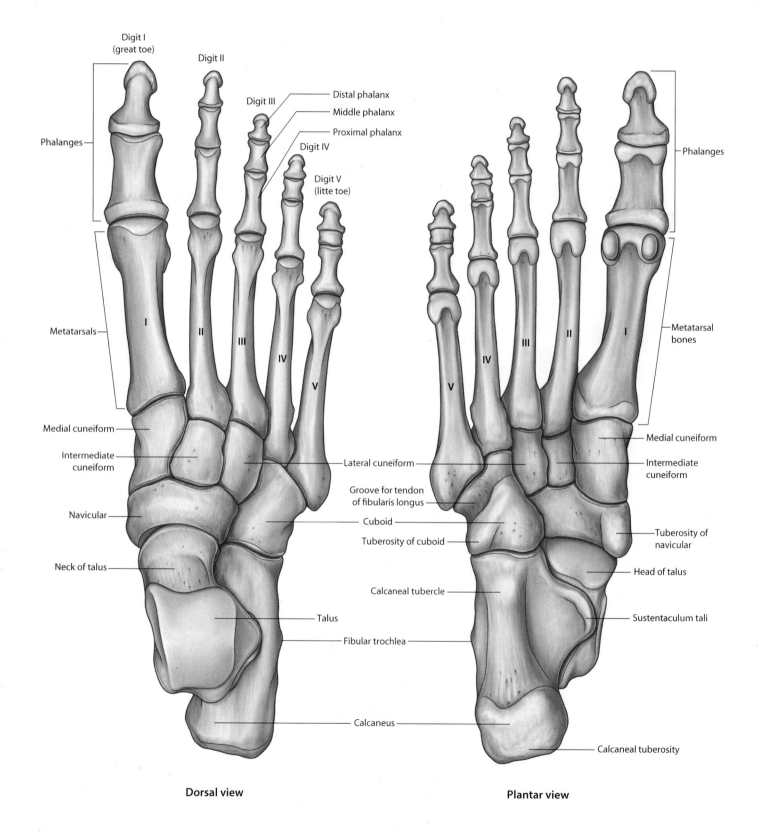

Digit I
(great toe)

Digit II

Digit III

Distal phalanx

Middle phalanx

Proximal phalanx

Digit IV

Digit V
(litte toe)

Phalanges

Phalanges

Metatarsals

Metatarsal
bones

Medial cuneiform

Intermediate
cuneiform

Lateral cuneiform

Navicular

Groove for tendon
of fibularis longus

Cuboid

Tuberosity of cuboid

Neck of talus

Medial cuneiform

Intermediate
cuneiform

Tuberosity of
navicular

Head of talus

Sustentaculum tali

Talus

Fibular trochlea

Calcaneal tubercle

Calcaneus

Calcaneal tuberosity

**Dorsal view**

**Plantar view**

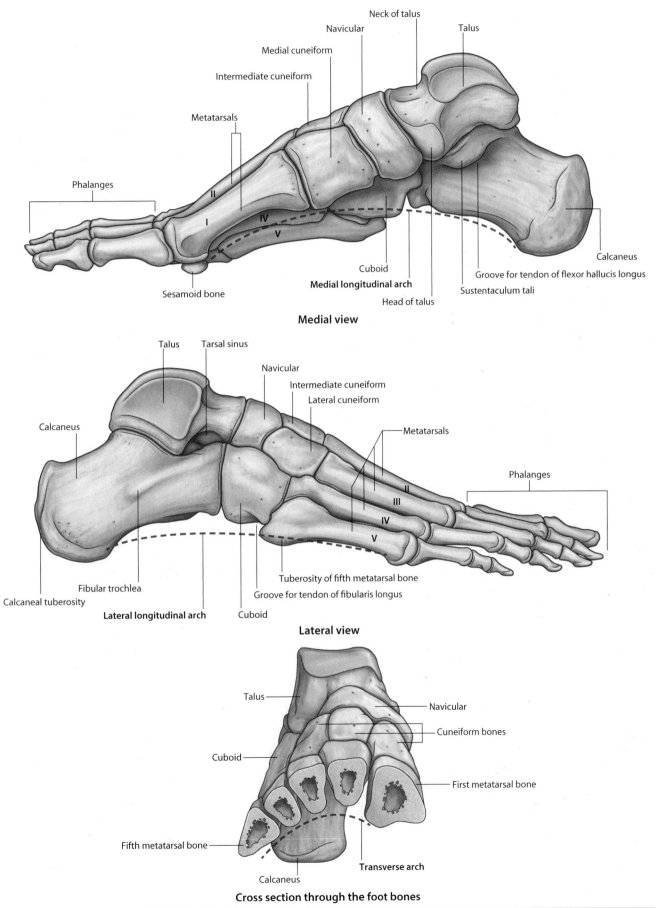

Neck of talus

Navicular

Talus

Medial cuneiform

Intermediate cuneiform

Metatarsals

Phalanges

II

I

IV

V

Sesamoid bone

Cuboid

**Medial longitudinal arch**

Head of talus

Groove for tendon of flexor hallucis longus

Sustentaculum tali

Calcaneus

**Medial view**

Talus    Tarsal sinus

Navicular

Intermediate cuneiform

Lateral cuneiform

Metatarsals

Calcaneus

Phalanges

II

III

IV

V

Tuberosity of fifth metatarsal bone

Groove for tendon of fibularis longus

Fibular trochlea

Calcaneal tuberosity

**Lateral longitudinal arch**    Cuboid

**Lateral view**

Talus

Navicular

Cuneiform bones

Cuboid

First metatarsal bone

Fifth metatarsal bone

Calcaneus

**Transverse arch**

**Cross section through the foot bones**

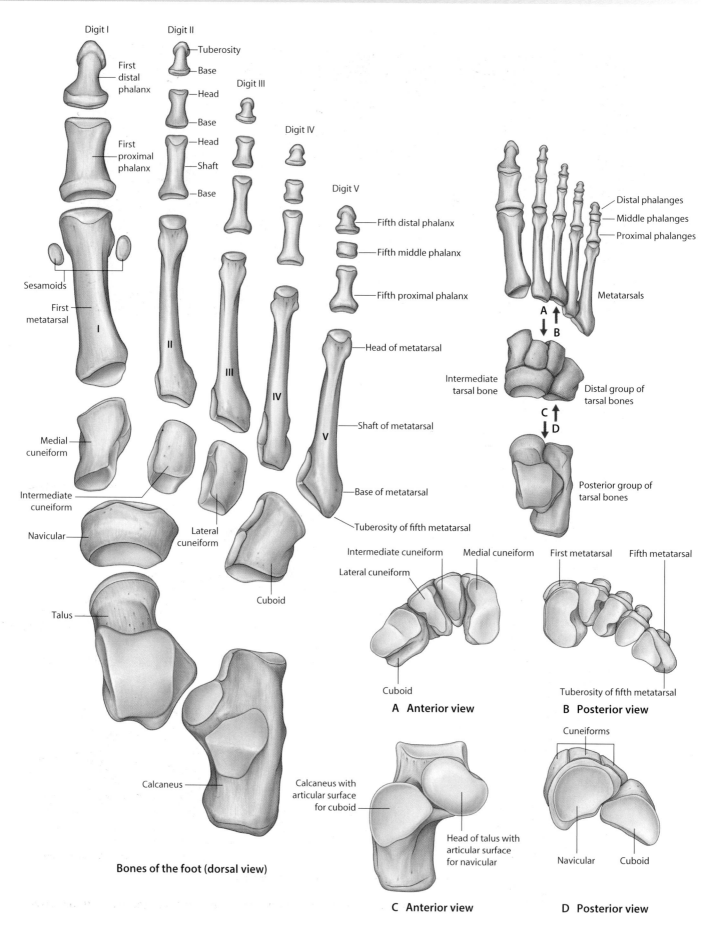

Digit I

First
distal
phalanx

First
proximal
phalanx

Sesamoids

First
metatarsal

I

Medial
cuneiform

Intermediate
cuneiform

Navicular

Talus

Calcaneus

Digit II

Tuberosity

Base

Head

Base

Digit III

Head

Shaft

Base

II

Digit IV

III

IV

Lateral
cuneiform

Cuboid

Digit V

Fifth distal phalanx

Fifth middle phalanx

Fifth proximal phalanx

Head of metatarsal

V

Shaft of metatarsal

Base of metatarsal

Tuberosity of fifth metatarsal

**Bones of the foot (dorsal view)**

Distal phalanges

Middle phalanges

Proximal phalanges

Metatarsals

A        B

Intermediate
tarsal bone

Distal group of
tarsal bones

C        D

Posterior group of
tarsal bones

Intermediate cuneiform      Medial cuneiform

Lateral cuneiform

First metatarsal      Fifth metatarsal

Cuboid

**A   Anterior view**

Tuberosity of fifth metatarsal

**B   Posterior view**

Calcaneus with
articular surface
for cuboid

Head of talus with
articular surface
for navicular

**C   Anterior view**

Cuneiforms

Navicular      Cuboid

**D   Posterior view**

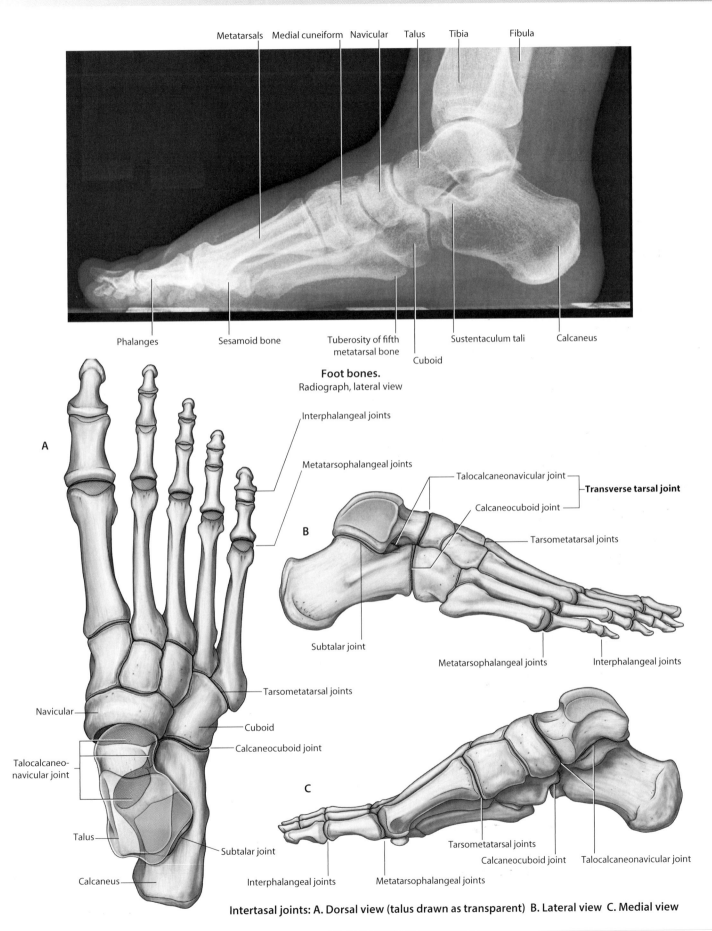

Metatarsals  Medial cuneiform  Navicular  Talus  Tibia  Fibula

Phalanges  Sesamoid bone  Tuberosity of fifth metatarsal bone  Cuboid  Sustentaculum tali  Calcaneus

**Foot bones.**
Radiograph, lateral view

A

Interphalangeal joints

Metatarsophalangeal joints

Navicular

Tarsometatarsal joints

Cuboid

Talocalcaneo-navicular joint

Calcaneocuboid joint

Talus

Subtalar joint

Calcaneus

B

Talocalcaneonavicular joint
Calcaneocuboid joint — **Transverse tarsal joint**

Tarsometatarsal joints

Subtalar joint

Metatarsophalangeal joints  Interphalangeal joints

C

Tarsometatarsal joints
Calcaneocuboid joint  Talocalcaneonavicular joint

Interphalangeal joints  Metatarsophalangeal joints

**Intertasal joints: A. Dorsal view (talus drawn as transparent)  B. Lateral view  C. Medial view**

**313**

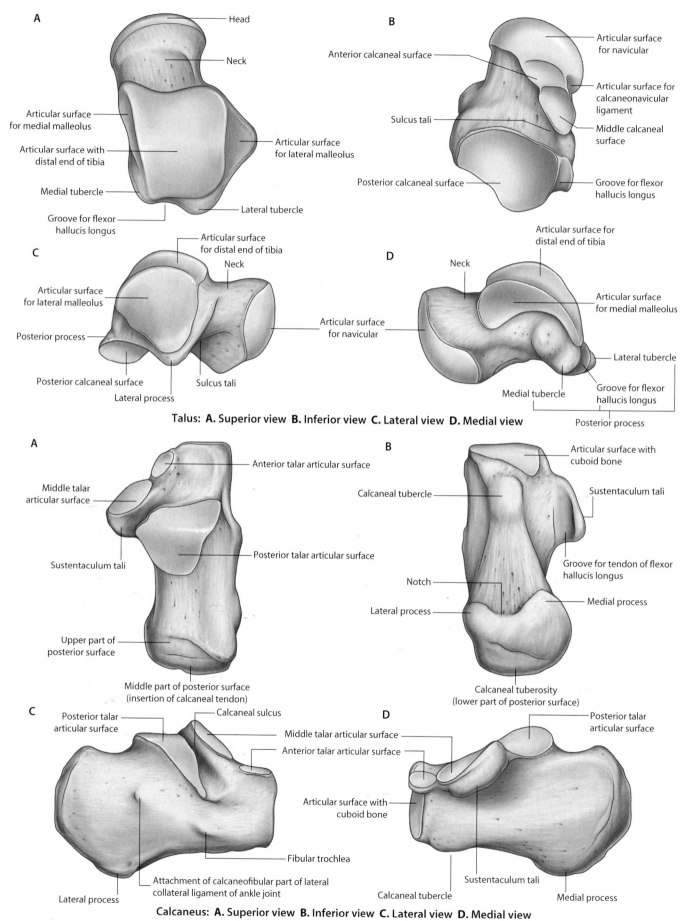

A

Head

Neck

Articular surface
for medial malleolus

Articular surface with
distal end of tibia

Medial tubercle

Groove for flexor
hallucis longus

Lateral tubercle

Articular surface
for lateral malleolus

B

Articular surface
for navicular

Anterior calcaneal surface

Articular surface for
calcaneonavicular
ligament

Sulcus tali

Middle calcaneal
surface

Posterior calcaneal surface

Groove for flexor
hallucis longus

C

Articular surface
for distal end of tibia

Neck

Articular surface
for lateral malleolus

Posterior process

Articular surface
for navicular

Posterior calcaneal surface

Lateral process

Sulcus tali

D

Articular surface for
distal end of tibia

Neck

Articular surface
for medial malleolus

Lateral tubercle

Medial tubercle

Groove for flexor
hallucis longus

Posterior process

Talus: **A. Superior view B. Inferior view C. Lateral view D. Medial view**

A

Anterior talar articular surface

Middle talar
articular surface

Posterior talar articular surface

Sustentaculum tali

Upper part of
posterior surface

Middle part of posterior surface
(insertion of calcaneal tendon)

B

Articular surface with
cuboid bone

Calcaneal tubercle

Sustentaculum tali

Groove for tendon of flexor
hallucis longus

Notch

Medial process

Lateral process

Calcaneal tuberosity
(lower part of posterior surface)

C

Posterior talar
articular surface

Calcaneal sulcus

Middle talar articular surface

Anterior talar articular surface

Fibular trochlea

Attachment of calcaneofibular part of lateral
collateral ligament of ankle joint

Lateral process

D

Posterior talar
articular surface

Articular surface with
cuboid bone

Sustentaculum tali

Calcaneal tubercle

Medial process

Calcaneus: **A. Superior view B. Inferior view C. Lateral view D. Medial view**

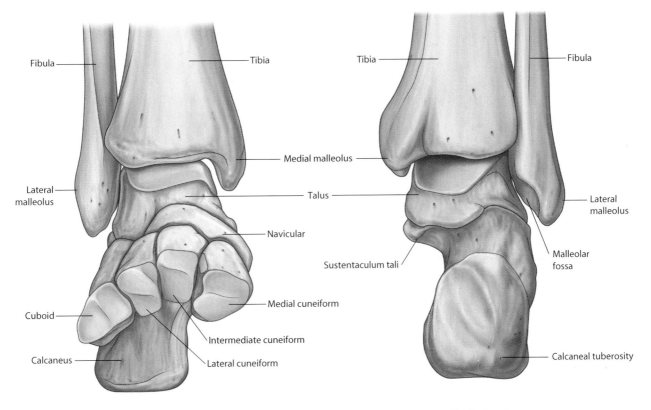

**Anterior view
(metatarsals and phalanges removed)**

**Posterior view**

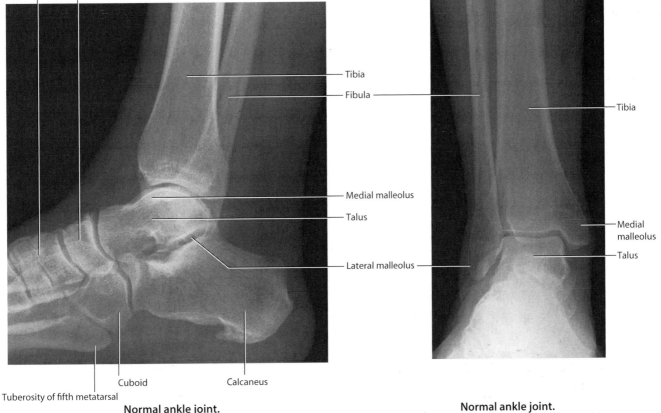

**Normal ankle joint.**
Radiograph, lateral view

**Normal ankle joint.**
Radiograph, AP view

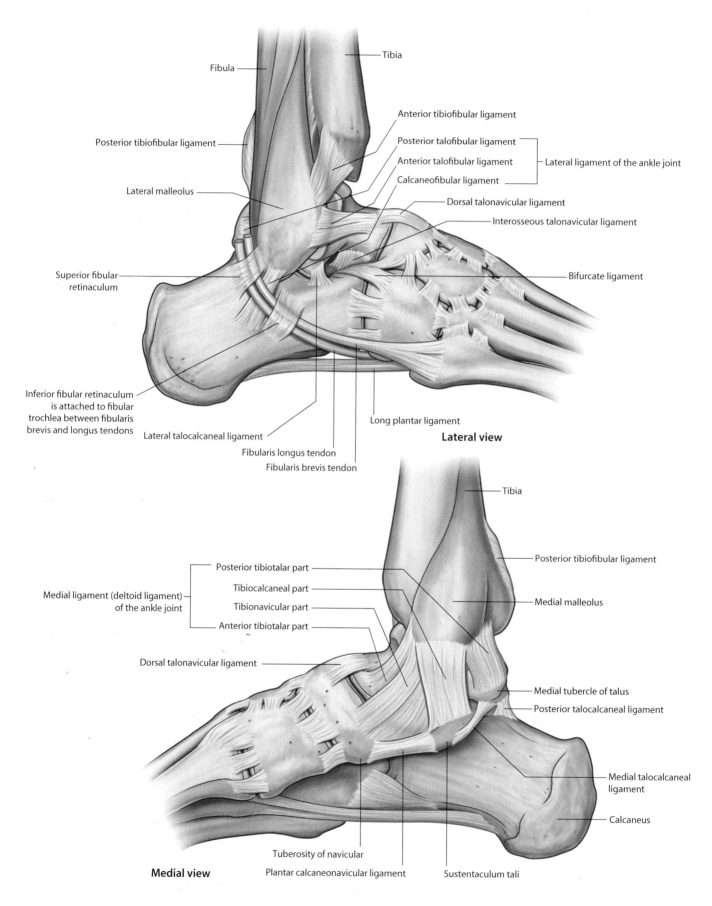

Fibula

Tibia

Anterior tibiofibular ligament

Posterior tibiofibular ligament

Posterior talofibular ligament

Anterior talofibular ligament

Calcaneofibular ligament

Lateral ligament of the ankle joint

Lateral malleolus

Dorsal talonavicular ligament

Interosseous talonavicular ligament

Superior fibular retinaculum

Bifurcate ligament

Inferior fibular retinaculum is attached to fibular trochlea between fibularis brevis and longus tendons

Lateral talocalcaneal ligament

Fibularis longus tendon

Fibularis brevis tendon

Long plantar ligament

**Lateral view**

Tibia

Posterior tibiofibular ligament

Posterior tibiotalar part

Tibiocalcaneal part

Medial ligament (deltoid ligament) of the ankle joint

Tibionavicular part

Anterior tibiotalar part

Medial malleolus

Dorsal talonavicular ligament

Medial tubercle of talus

Posterior talocalcaneal ligament

Medial talocalcaneal ligament

Calcaneus

Tuberosity of navicular

**Medial view**

Plantar calcaneonavicular ligament

Sustentaculum tali

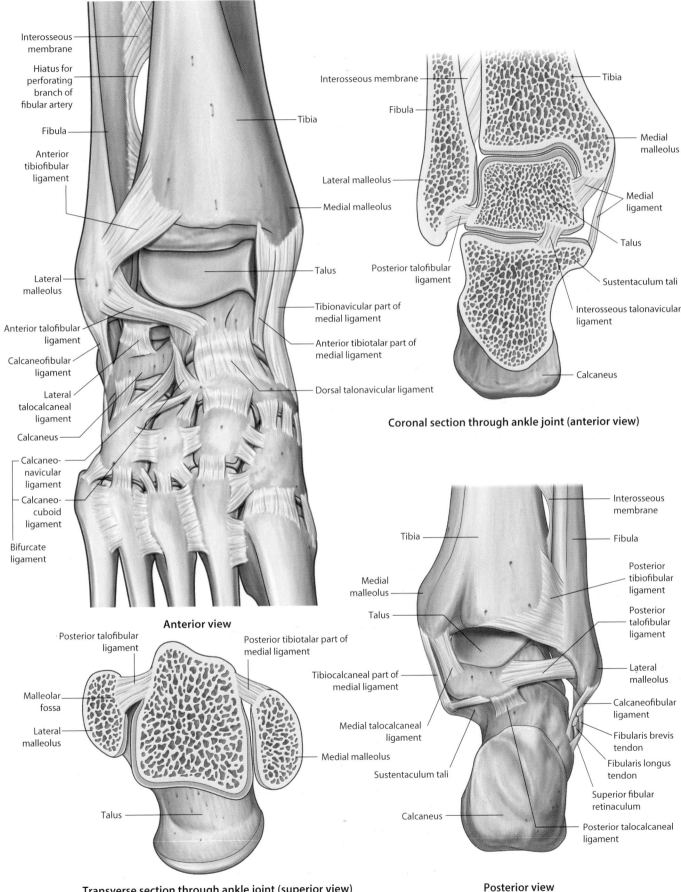

Interosseous membrane

Hiatus for perforating branch of fibular artery

Fibula

Anterior tibiofibular ligament

Lateral malleolus

Anterior talofibular ligament

Calcaneofibular ligament

Lateral talocalcaneal ligament

Calcaneus

Calcaneo-navicular ligament

Calcaneo-cuboid ligament

Bifurcate ligament

Tibia

Medial malleolus

Talus

Tibionavicular part of medial ligament

Anterior tibiotalar part of medial ligament

Dorsal talonavicular ligament

**Anterior view**

Interosseous membrane

Fibula

Lateral malleolus

Posterior talofibular ligament

Tibia

Medial malleolus

Medial ligament

Talus

Sustentaculum tali

Interosseous talonavicular ligament

Calcaneus

**Coronal section through ankle joint (anterior view)**

Posterior talofibular ligament

Malleolar fossa

Lateral malleolus

Posterior tibiotalar part of medial ligament

Medial malleolus

Talus

**Transverse section through ankle joint (superior view)**

Tibia

Medial malleolus

Talus

Tibiocalcaneal part of medial ligament

Medial talocalcaneal ligament

Sustentaculum tali

Calcaneus

Interosseous membrane

Fibula

Posterior tibiofibular ligament

Posterior talofibular ligament

Lateral malleolus

Calcaneofibular ligament

Fibularis brevis tendon

Fibularis longus tendon

Superior fibular retinaculum

Posterior talocalcaneal ligament

**Posterior view**

**317**

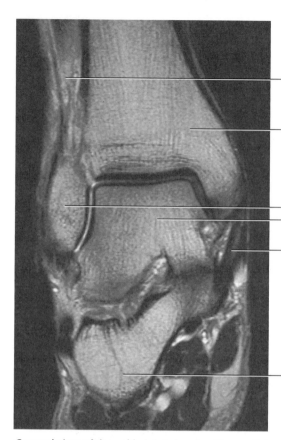

Fibula

Tibia

Lateral malleolus

Talus

Medial ligament of
ankle joint
(deltoid ligament)

Calcaneus

**Coronal view of the ankle joint showing the medial
ligament of the ankle joint (deltoid ligament).**
T2-weighted MR image in coronal plane

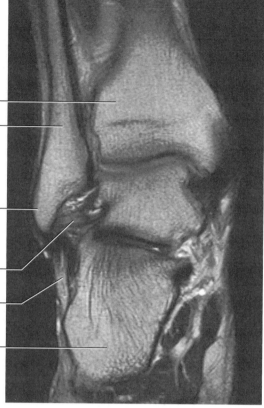

Tibia

Fibula

Lateral malleolus

Posterior talofibular ligament

Calcaneofibular ligament

Calcaneus

**Coronal view of the ankle joint showing the
posterior talofibular and calcaneofibular ligaments.**
T2-weighted MR image in coronal plane

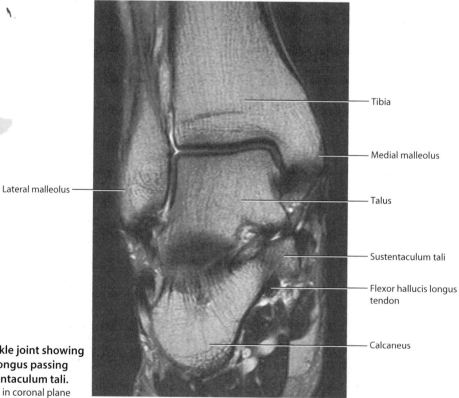

Lateral malleolus

Tibia

Medial malleolus

Talus

Sustentaculum tali

Flexor hallucis longus
tendon

Calcaneus

**Coronal view of the ankle joint showing
the flexor hallucis longus passing
inferior to the sustentaculum tali.**
T2-weighted MR image in coronal plane

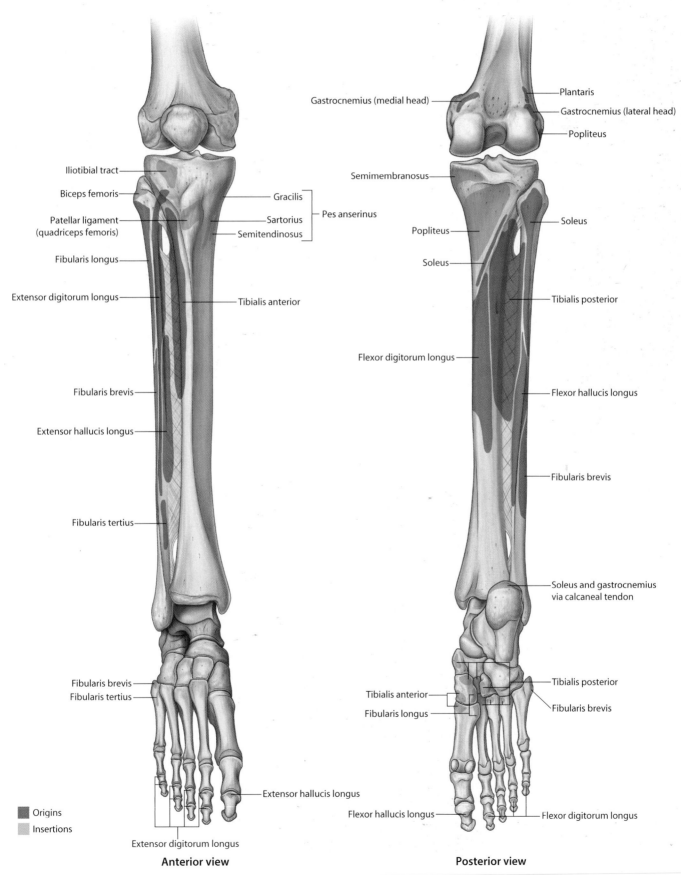

Gastrocnemius (medial head)

Plantaris

Gastrocnemius (lateral head)

Popliteus

Iliotibial tract

Biceps femoris

Patellar ligament
(quadriceps femoris)

Gracilis

Sartorius — Pes anserinus

Semitendinosus

Semimembranosus

Soleus

Fibularis longus

Popliteus

Soleus

Extensor digitorum longus

Tibialis anterior

Tibialis posterior

Flexor digitorum longus

Fibularis brevis

Flexor hallucis longus

Extensor hallucis longus

Fibularis brevis

Fibularis tertius

Soleus and gastrocnemius
via calcaneal tendon

Fibularis brevis

Fibularis tertius

Tibialis posterior

Tibialis anterior

Fibularis brevis

Fibularis longus

Extensor hallucis longus

Origins

Insertions

Flexor hallucis longus

Flexor digitorum longus

Extensor digitorum longus

**Anterior view**

**Posterior view**

**319**

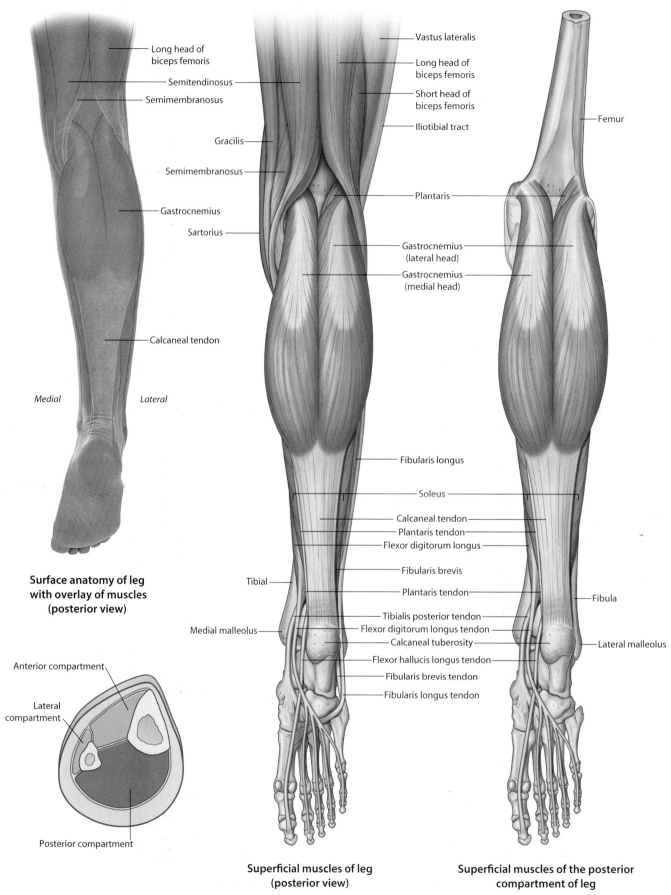

Long head of
biceps femoris

Semitendinosus

Semimembranosus

Gracilis

Semimembranosus

Gastrocnemius

Sartorius

Calcaneal tendon

*Medial*

*Lateral*

**Surface anatomy of leg
with overlay of muscles
(posterior view)**

Anterior compartment

Lateral
compartment

Posterior compartment

Vastus lateralis

Long head of
biceps femoris

Short head of
biceps femoris

Iliotibial tract

Femur

Plantaris

Gastrocnemius
(lateral head)

Gastrocnemius
(medial head)

Fibularis longus

Soleus

Calcaneal tendon

Plantaris tendon

Flexor digitorum longus

Fibularis brevis

Plantaris tendon

Tibial

Tibialis posterior tendon

Flexor digitorum longus tendon

Calcaneal tuberosity

Flexor hallucis longus tendon

Fibularis brevis tendon

Fibularis longus tendon

Medial malleolus

Fibula

Lateral malleolus

**Superficial muscles of leg
(posterior view)**

**Superficial muscles of the posterior
compartment of leg**

**320**

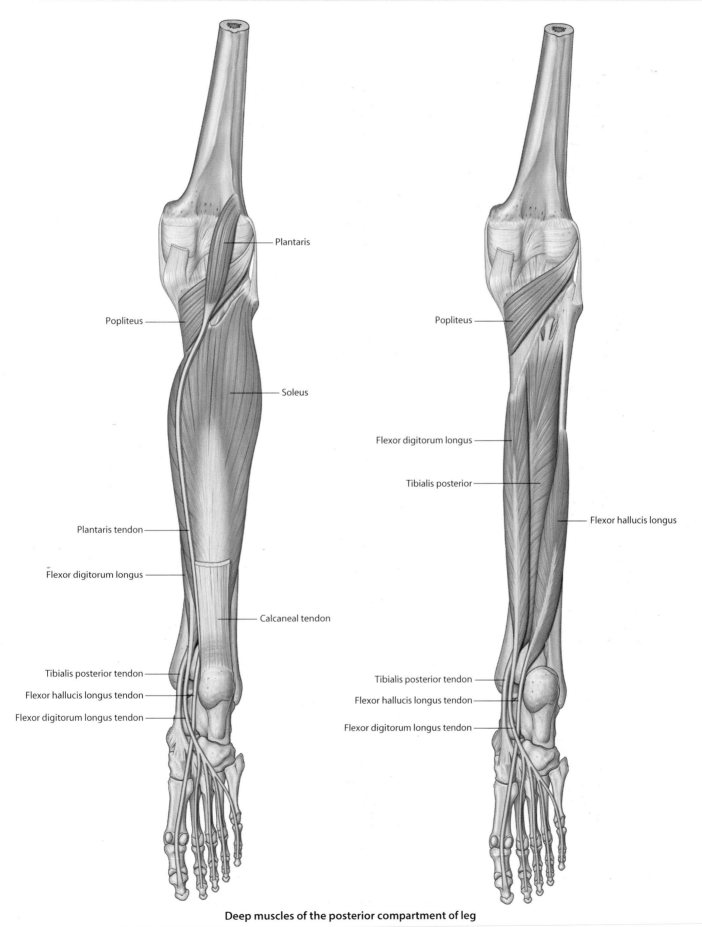

Plantaris

Popliteus

Soleus

Plantaris tendon

Flexor digitorum longus

Calcaneal tendon

Tibialis posterior tendon

Flexor hallucis longus tendon

Flexor digitorum longus tendon

Popliteus

Flexor digitorum longus

Tibialis posterior

Flexor hallucis longus

Tibialis posterior tendon

Flexor hallucis longus tendon

Flexor digitorum longus tendon

**Deep muscles of the posterior compartment of leg**

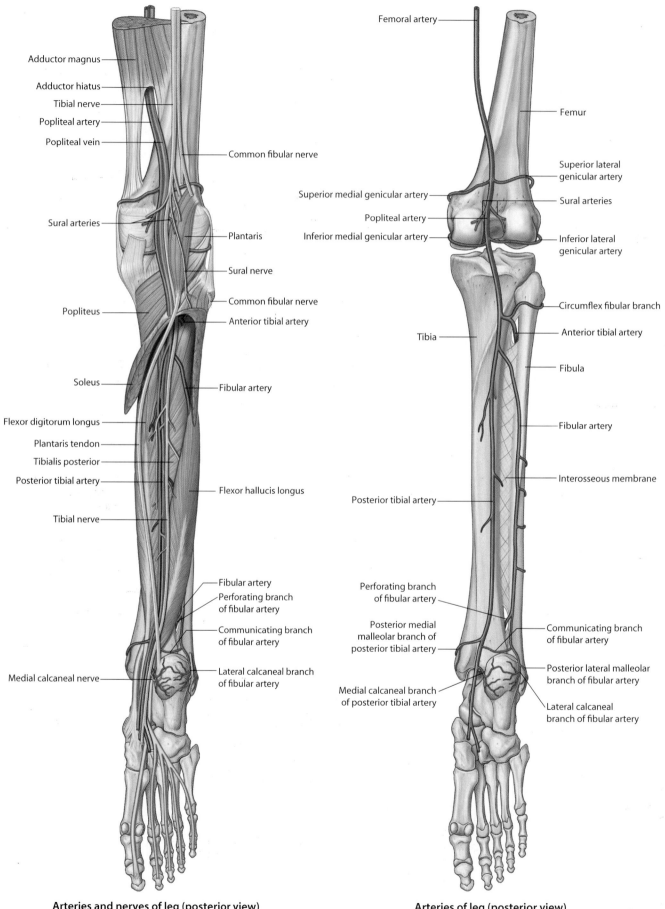

Adductor magnus

Adductor hiatus

Tibial nerve

Popliteal artery

Popliteal vein

Common fibular nerve

Sural arteries

Plantaris

Sural nerve

Common fibular nerve

Popliteus

Anterior tibial artery

Soleus

Fibular artery

Flexor digitorum longus

Plantaris tendon

Tibialis posterior

Posterior tibial artery

Flexor hallucis longus

Tibial nerve

Fibular artery

Perforating branch of fibular artery

Communicating branch of fibular artery

Medial calcaneal nerve

Lateral calcaneal branch of fibular artery

Femoral artery

Femur

Superior lateral genicular artery

Superior medial genicular artery

Sural arteries

Popliteal artery

Inferior medial genicular artery

Inferior lateral genicular artery

Circumflex fibular branch

Anterior tibial artery

Tibia

Fibula

Fibular artery

Interosseous membrane

Posterior tibial artery

Perforating branch of fibular artery

Posterior medial malleolar branch of posterior tibial artery

Communicating branch of fibular artery

Medial calcaneal branch of posterior tibial artery

Posterior lateral malleolar branch of fibular artery

Lateral calcaneal branch of fibular artery

**Arteries and nerves of leg (posterior view)**

**Arteries of leg (posterior view)**

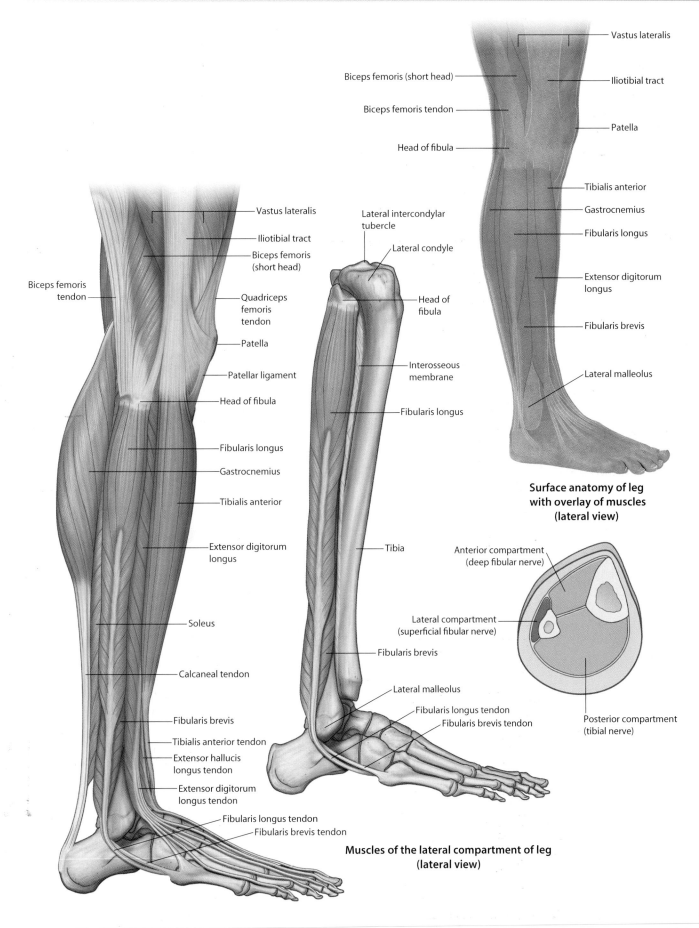

Vastus lateralis

Biceps femoris (short head)

Iliotibial tract

Biceps femoris tendon

Patella

Head of fibula

Tibialis anterior

Gastrocnemius

Fibularis longus

Extensor digitorum longus

Fibularis brevis

Lateral malleolus

**Surface anatomy of leg with overlay of muscles (lateral view)**

Vastus lateralis

Iliotibial tract

Biceps femoris (short head)

Quadriceps femoris tendon

Biceps femoris tendon

Patella

Patellar ligament

Head of fibula

Fibularis longus

Gastrocnemius

Tibialis anterior

Extensor digitorum longus

Soleus

Calcaneal tendon

Fibularis brevis

Tibialis anterior tendon

Extensor hallucis longus tendon

Extensor digitorum longus tendon

Fibularis longus tendon

Fibularis brevis tendon

Lateral intercondylar tubercle

Lateral condyle

Head of fibula

Interosseous membrane

Fibularis longus

Tibia

Fibularis brevis

Lateral malleolus

Fibularis longus tendon

Fibularis brevis tendon

**Muscles of the lateral compartment of leg (lateral view)**

Anterior compartment (deep fibular nerve)

Lateral compartment (superficial fibular nerve)

Posterior compartment (tibial nerve)

**323**

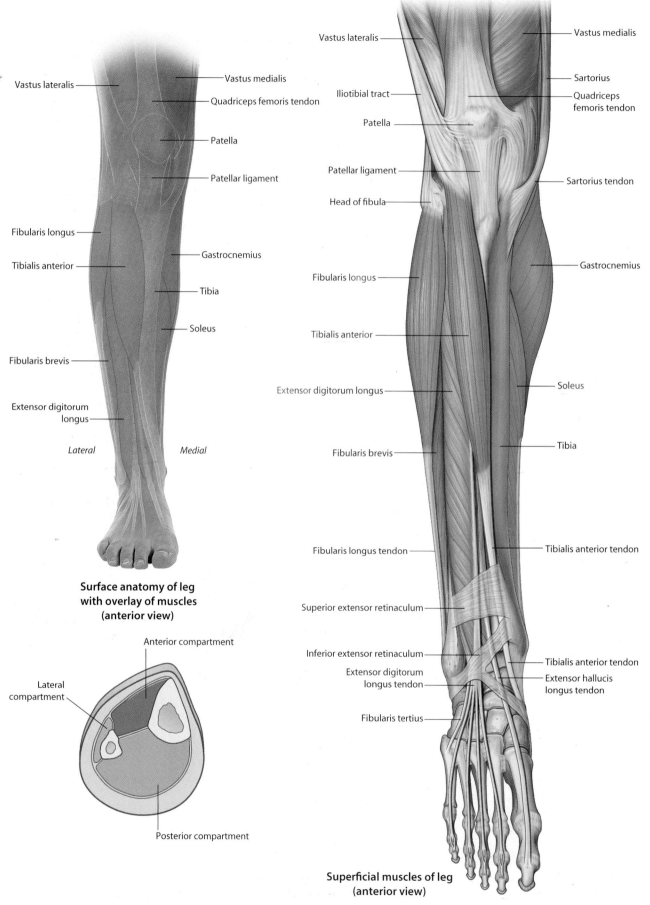

Vastus lateralis

Vastus medialis

Quadriceps femoris tendon

Patella

Patellar ligament

Fibularis longus

Tibialis anterior

Gastrocnemius

Tibia

Soleus

Fibularis brevis

Extensor digitorum longus

*Lateral*

*Medial*

**Surface anatomy of leg
with overlay of muscles
(anterior view)**

Anterior compartment

Lateral
compartment

Posterior compartment

Vastus lateralis

Iliotibial tract

Patella

Patellar ligament

Head of fibula

Fibularis longus

Tibialis anterior

Extensor digitorum longus

Fibularis brevis

Fibularis longus tendon

Superior extensor retinaculum

Inferior extensor retinaculum

Extensor digitorum
longus tendon

Fibularis tertius

Vastus medialis

Sartorius

Quadriceps
femoris tendon

Sartorius tendon

Gastrocnemius

Soleus

Tibia

Tibialis anterior tendon

Tibialis anterior tendon

Extensor hallucis
longus tendon

**Superficial muscles of leg
(anterior view)**

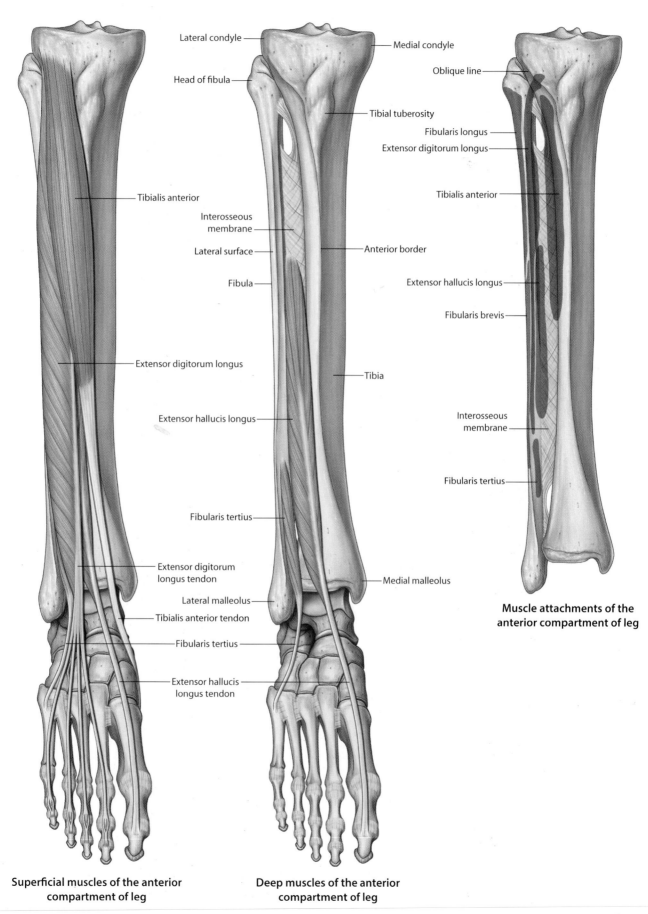

Lateral condyle

Medial condyle

Head of fibula

Oblique line

Tibial tuberosity

Fibularis longus

Extensor digitorum longus

Tibialis anterior

Tibialis anterior

Interosseous membrane

Lateral surface

Anterior border

Fibula

Extensor hallucis longus

Extensor digitorum longus

Fibularis brevis

Tibia

Extensor hallucis longus

Interosseous membrane

Fibularis tertius

Fibularis tertius

Extensor digitorum longus tendon

Lateral malleolus

Medial malleolus

Tibialis anterior tendon

Fibularis tertius

Extensor hallucis longus tendon

**Muscle attachments of the anterior compartment of leg**

**Superficial muscles of the anterior compartment of leg**

**Deep muscles of the anterior compartment of leg**

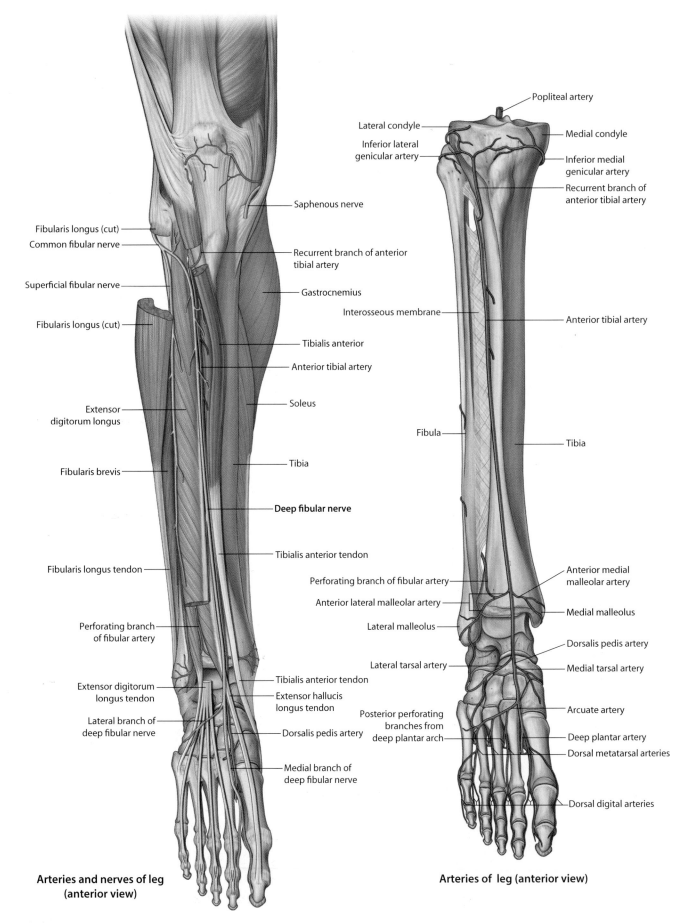

Popliteal artery

Lateral condyle

Medial condyle

Inferior lateral genicular artery

Inferior medial genicular artery

Recurrent branch of anterior tibial artery

Saphenous nerve

Fibularis longus (cut)

Common fibular nerve

Recurrent branch of anterior tibial artery

Superficial fibular nerve

Gastrocnemius

Interosseous membrane

Anterior tibial artery

Fibularis longus (cut)

Tibialis anterior

Anterior tibial artery

Extensor digitorum longus

Soleus

Fibula

Tibia

Fibularis brevis

Tibia

Deep fibular nerve

Tibialis anterior tendon

Fibularis longus tendon

Anterior medial malleolar artery

Perforating branch of fibular artery

Medial malleolus

Anterior lateral malleolar artery

Lateral malleolus

Dorsalis pedis artery

Perforating branch of fibular artery

Lateral tarsal artery

Medial tarsal artery

Extensor digitorum longus tendon

Tibialis anterior tendon

Extensor hallucis longus tendon

Arcuate artery

Lateral branch of deep fibular nerve

Posterior perforating branches from deep plantar arch

Deep plantar artery

Dorsalis pedis artery

Dorsal metatarsal arteries

Medial branch of deep fibular nerve

Dorsal digital arteries

**Arteries and nerves of leg (anterior view)**

**Arteries of leg (anterior view)**

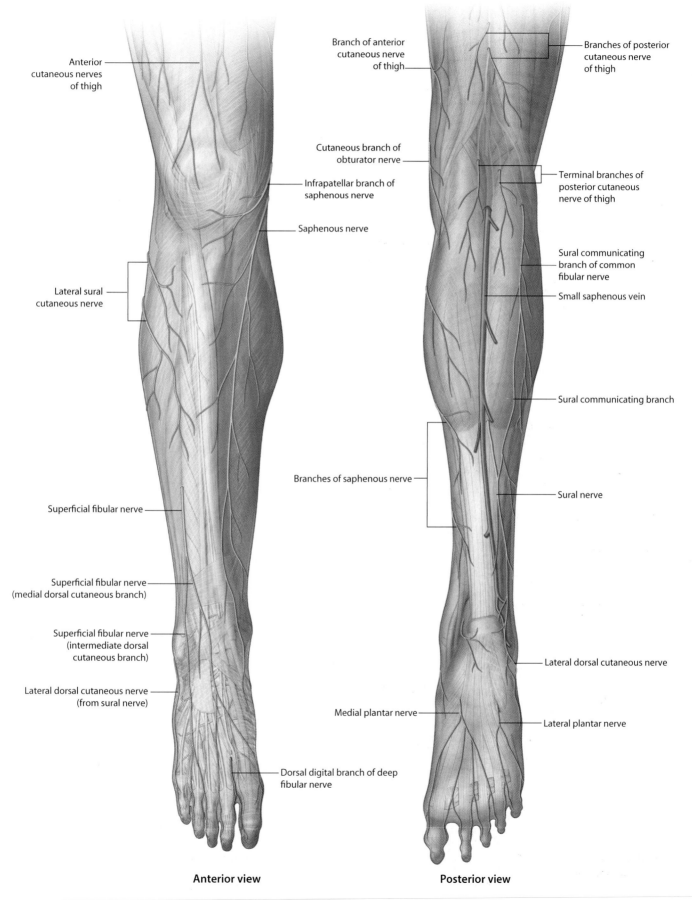

Anterior cutaneous nerves of thigh

Branch of anterior cutaneous nerve of thigh

Branches of posterior cutaneous nerve of thigh

Cutaneous branch of obturator nerve

Infrapatellar branch of saphenous nerve

Saphenous nerve

Terminal branches of posterior cutaneous nerve of thigh

Sural communicating branch of common fibular nerve

Small saphenous vein

Lateral sural cutaneous nerve

Superficial fibular nerve

Branches of saphenous nerve

Sural communicating branch

Sural nerve

Superficial fibular nerve (medial dorsal cutaneous branch)

Superficial fibular nerve (intermediate dorsal cutaneous branch)

Lateral dorsal cutaneous nerve (from sural nerve)

Lateral dorsal cutaneous nerve

Medial plantar nerve

Lateral plantar nerve

Dorsal digital branch of deep fibular nerve

**Anterior view**

**Posterior view**

A

Patellar ligament — Bursa of tibial tuberosity

Tibialis anterior —

Tibia

Extensor digitorum longus —

Sartorius tendon

Interosseous membrane —

Semimembranosus tendon

Fibularis longus —

Great saphenous vein

Fibula —

Gracilis tendon

Popliteal vessels —

Semitendinosus tendon

Common fibular nerve —

Anserine bursa

Soleus —

Popliteus

Gastrocnemius (lateral head) —

Gastrocnemius (medial head)

Plantaris

Tibial nerve

B

Tibialis anterior — Deep fibular nerve

Extensor hallucis longus —

Anterior tibial vessels

Interosseous membrane —

Extensor digitorum longus —

Tibia

Superficial fibular nerve —

Fibularis longus —

Great saphenous vein

Fibularis brevis —

Fibula —

Tibialis posterior

Flexor hallucis longus —

Flexor digitorum longus

Soleus —

Posterior tibial vessels

Fibular vessels —

Tibial nerve

Gastrocnemius (lateral head) —

Plantaris tendon

Sural nerve — Small saphenous vein

Gastrocnemius (medial head)

C

Extensor hallucis longus — Tibialis anterior

Extensor digitorum longus —

Tibia

Fibula —

Tibialis posterior

Flexor digitorum longus

Posterior tibial vessels

Fibularis longus —

Fibularis brevis —

Tibial nerve

Flexor hallucis longus —

Calcaneal tendon

**Transverse sections through leg**

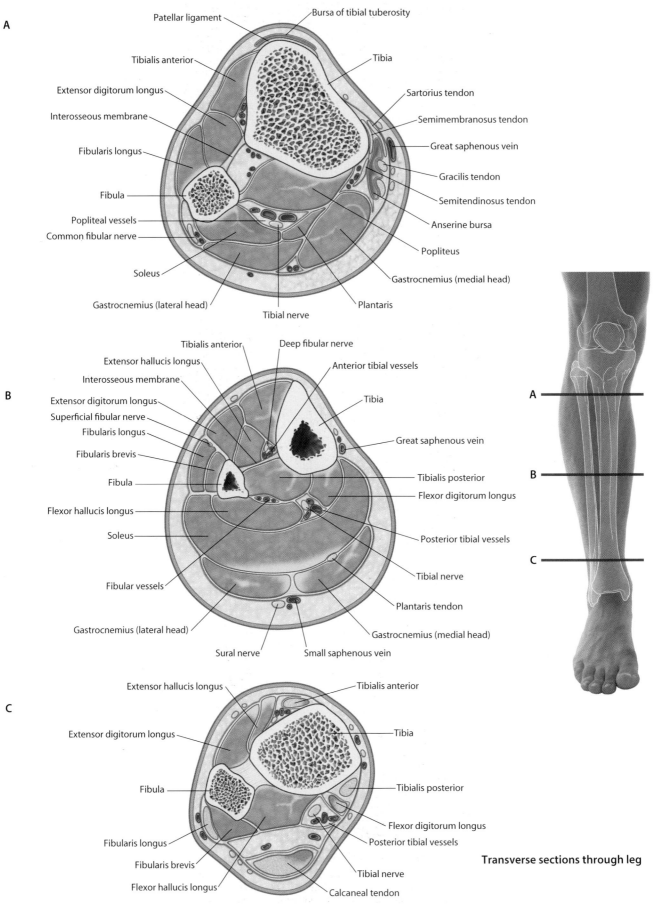

A

B

C

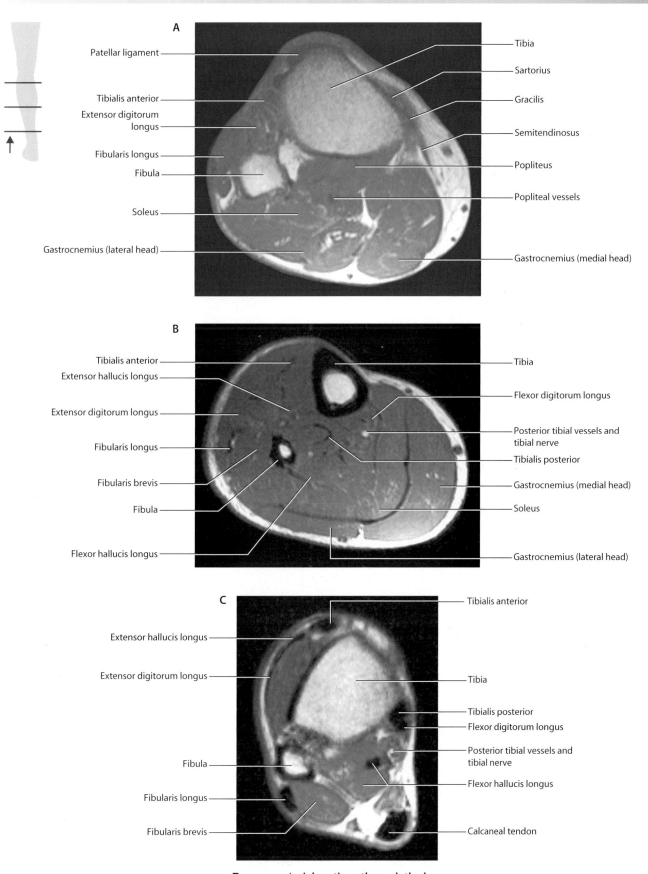

**A**

Patellar ligament

Tibialis anterior

Extensor digitorum longus

Fibularis longus

Fibula

Soleus

Gastrocnemius (lateral head)

Tibia

Sartorius

Gracilis

Semitendinosus

Popliteus

Popliteal vessels

Gastrocnemius (medial head)

**B**

Tibialis anterior

Extensor hallucis longus

Extensor digitorum longus

Fibularis longus

Fibularis brevis

Fibula

Flexor hallucis longus

Tibia

Flexor digitorum longus

Posterior tibial vessels and tibial nerve

Tibialis posterior

Gastrocnemius (medial head)

Soleus

Gastrocnemius (lateral head)

**C**

Extensor hallucis longus

Extensor digitorum longus

Fibula

Fibularis longus

Fibularis brevis

Tibialis anterior

Tibia

Tibialis posterior

Flexor digitorum longus

Posterior tibial vessels and tibial nerve

Flexor hallucis longus

Calcaneal tendon

**Transverse/axial sections through the leg.**

A. Proximal/upper leg. T1-weighted MR image in axial plane
B. Middle leg. T1-weighted MR image in axial plane
C. Distal/lower leg. T1-weighted MR image in axial plane

## Muscle attachments of the foot

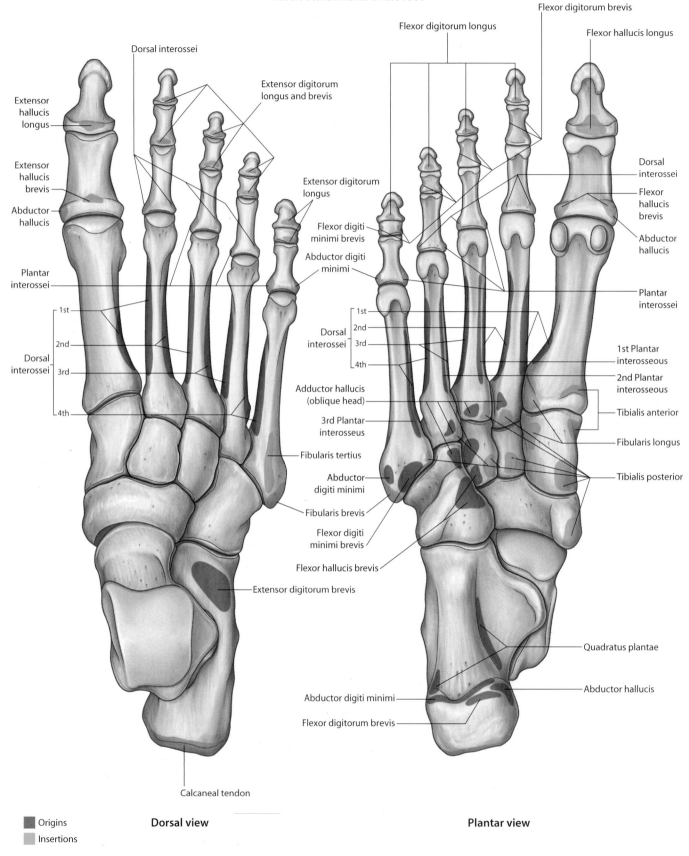

Extensor hallucis longus

Dorsal interossei

Extensor digitorum longus and brevis

Flexor digitorum longus

Flexor digitorum brevis

Flexor hallucis longus

Extensor hallucis longus

Extensor hallucis brevis

Abductor hallucis

Extensor digitorum longus

Dorsal interossei

Flexor hallucis brevis

Abductor hallucis

Flexor digiti minimi brevis

Abductor digiti minimi

Plantar interossei

Plantar interossei

Dorsal interossei
— 1st
— 2nd
— 3rd
— 4th

Dorsal interossei
— 1st
— 2nd
— 3rd
— 4th

1st Plantar interosseous

2nd Plantar interosseous

Tibialis anterior

Adductor hallucis (oblique head)

3rd Plantar interosseus

Fibularis longus

Tibialis posterior

Fibularis tertius

Abductor digiti minimi

Fibularis brevis

Flexor digiti minimi brevis

Flexor hallucis brevis

Flexor digitorum brevis

Extensor digitorum brevis

Quadratus plantae

Abductor hallucis

Abductor digiti minimi

Flexor digitorum brevis

Calcaneal tendon

■ Origins
■ Insertions

**Dorsal view**

**Plantar view**

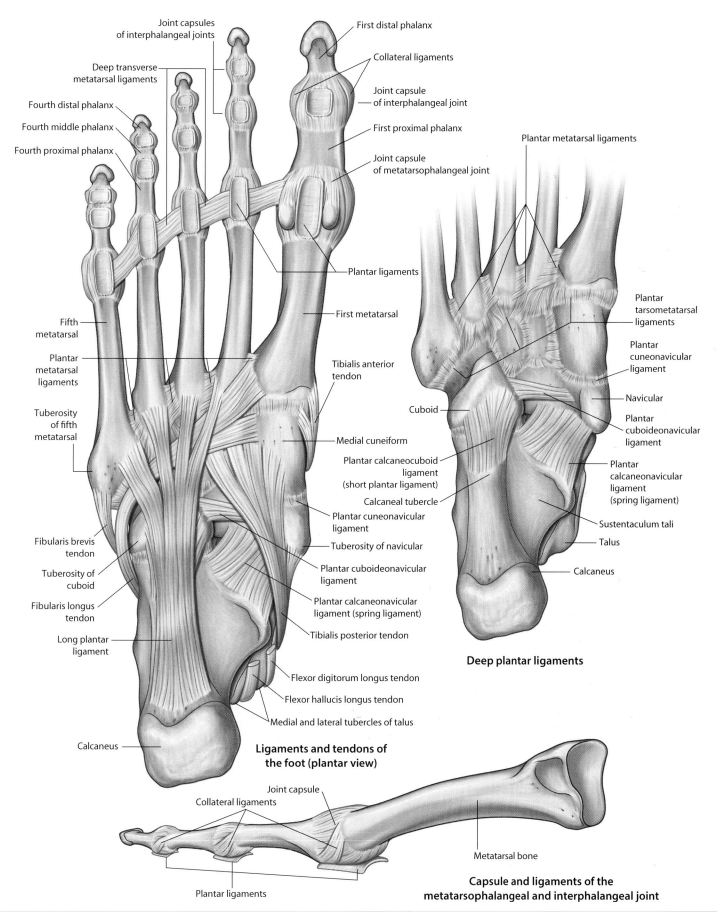

Joint capsules of interphalangeal joints

First distal phalanx

Deep transverse metatarsal ligaments

Collateral ligaments

Fourth distal phalanx

Joint capsule of interphalangeal joint

Fourth middle phalanx

First proximal phalanx

Fourth proximal phalanx

Joint capsule of metatarsophalangeal joint

Plantar metatarsal ligaments

Fifth metatarsal

Plantar metatarsal ligaments

Plantar ligaments

First metatarsal

Plantar tarsometatarsal ligaments

Tibialis anterior tendon

Plantar cuneonavicular ligament

Tuberosity of fifth metatarsal

Navicular

Medial cuneiform

Cuboid

Plantar cuboideonavicular ligament

Plantar calcaneocuboid ligament (short plantar ligament)

Calcaneal tubercle

Plantar calcaneonavicular ligament (spring ligament)

Plantar cuneonavicular ligament

Sustentaculum tali

Fibularis brevis tendon

Tuberosity of navicular

Talus

Tuberosity of cuboid

Plantar cuboideonavicular ligament

Calcaneus

Fibularis longus tendon

Plantar calcaneonavicular ligament (spring ligament)

Long plantar ligament

Tibialis posterior tendon

**Deep plantar ligaments**

Flexor digitorum longus tendon

Flexor hallucis longus tendon

Calcaneus

Medial and lateral tubercles of talus

**Ligaments and tendons of the foot (plantar view)**

Joint capsule

Collateral ligaments

Metatarsal bone

Plantar ligaments

**Capsule and ligaments of the metatarsophalangeal and interphalangeal joint**

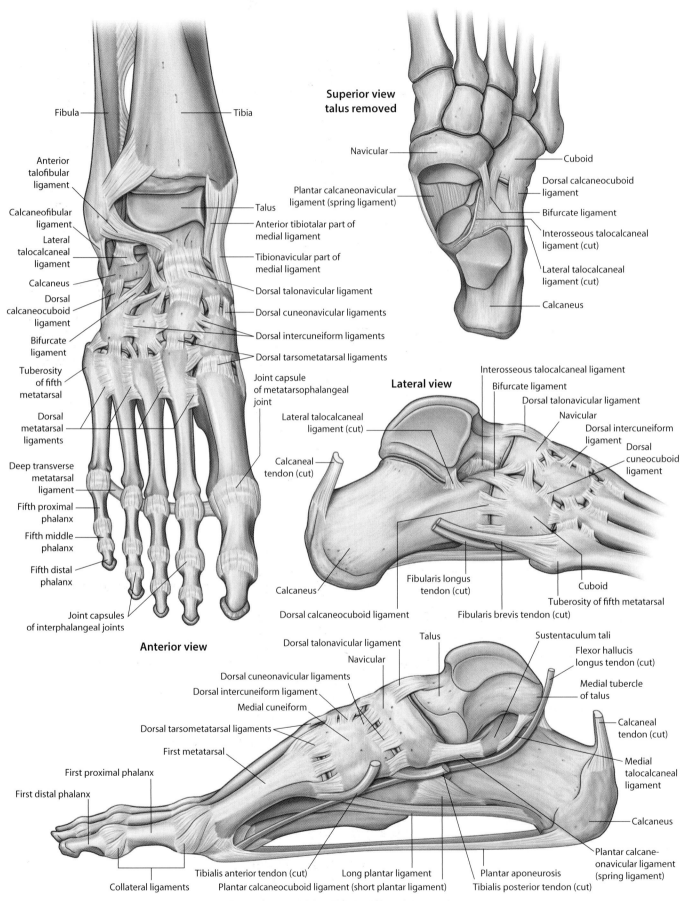

**Superior view talus removed**

Navicular

Cuboid

Plantar calcaneonavicular ligament (spring ligament)

Dorsal calcaneocuboid ligament

Bifurcate ligament

Interosseous talocalcaneal ligament (cut)

Lateral talocalcaneal ligament (cut)

Calcaneus

Fibula

Tibia

Anterior talofibular ligament

Calcaneofibular ligament

Lateral talocalcaneal ligament

Calcaneus

Dorsal calcaneocuboid ligament

Bifurcate ligament

Tuberosity of fifth metatarsal

Dorsal metatarsal ligaments

Deep transverse metatarsal ligament

Fifth proximal phalanx

Fifth middle phalanx

Fifth distal phalanx

Talus

Anterior tibiotalar part of medial ligament

Tibionavicular part of medial ligament

Dorsal talonavicular ligament

Dorsal cuneonavicular ligaments

Dorsal intercuneiform ligaments

Dorsal tarsometatarsal ligaments

Joint capsule of metatarsophalangeal joint

Joint capsules of interphalangeal joints

**Anterior view**

**Lateral view**

Lateral talocalcaneal ligament (cut)

Calcaneal tendon (cut)

Interosseous talocalcaneal ligament

Bifurcate ligament

Dorsal talonavicular ligament

Navicular

Dorsal intercuneiform ligament

Dorsal cuneocuboid ligament

Calcaneus

Dorsal calcaneocuboid ligament

Fibularis longus tendon (cut)

Fibularis brevis tendon (cut)

Cuboid

Tuberosity of fifth metatarsal

Dorsal talonavicular ligament

Navicular

Dorsal cuneonavicular ligaments

Dorsal intercuneiform ligament

Medial cuneiform

Dorsal tarsometatarsal ligaments

First metatarsal

First proximal phalanx

First distal phalanx

Collateral ligaments

Tibialis anterior tendon (cut)

Plantar calcaneocuboid ligament (short plantar ligament)

Long plantar ligament

Talus

Sustentaculum tali

Flexor hallucis longus tendon (cut)

Medial tubercle of talus

Calcaneal tendon (cut)

Medial talocalcaneal ligament

Calcaneus

Plantar calcaneonavicular ligament (spring ligament)

Plantar aponeurosis

Tibialis posterior tendon (cut)

**Medial view**

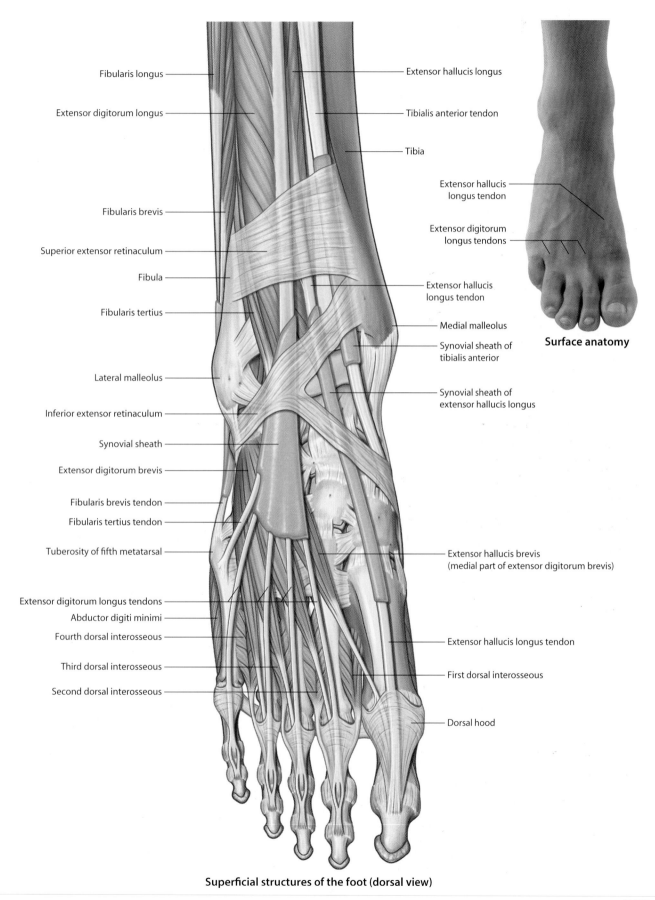

Fibularis longus

Extensor digitorum longus

Fibularis brevis

Superior extensor retinaculum

Fibula

Fibularis tertius

Lateral malleolus

Inferior extensor retinaculum

Synovial sheath

Extensor digitorum brevis

Fibularis brevis tendon

Fibularis tertius tendon

Tuberosity of fifth metatarsal

Extensor digitorum longus tendons

Abductor digiti minimi

Fourth dorsal interosseous

Third dorsal interosseous

Second dorsal interosseous

Extensor hallucis longus

Tibialis anterior tendon

Tibia

Extensor hallucis longus tendon

Extensor digitorum longus tendons

Extensor hallucis longus tendon

Medial malleolus

Synovial sheath of tibialis anterior

Synovial sheath of extensor hallucis longus

Extensor hallucis brevis (medial part of extensor digitorum brevis)

Extensor hallucis longus tendon

First dorsal interosseous

Dorsal hood

**Surface anatomy**

**Superficial structures of the foot (dorsal view)**

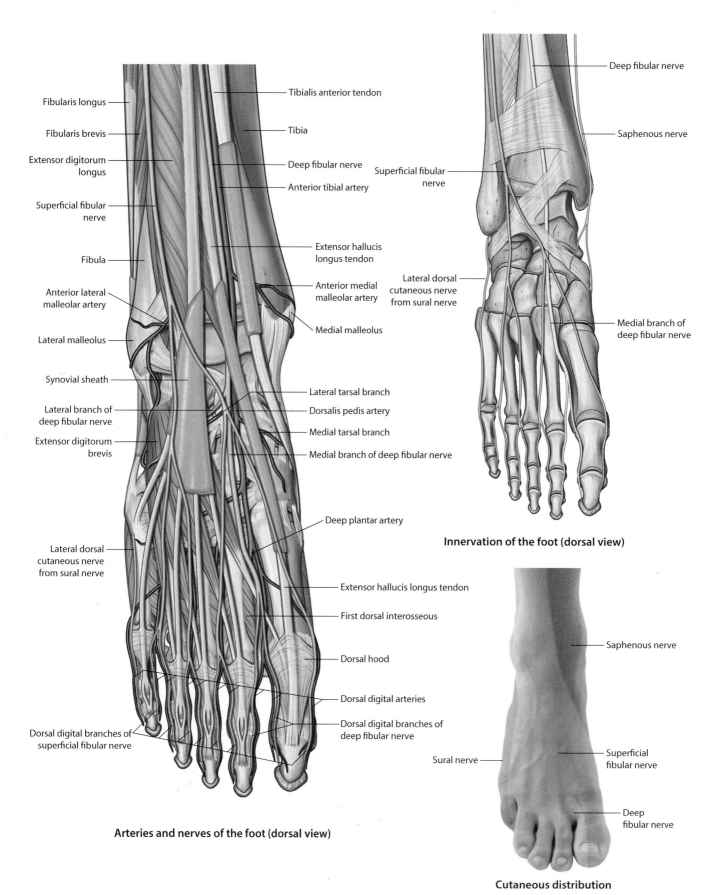

Fibularis longus

Fibularis brevis

Extensor digitorum longus

Superficial fibular nerve

Fibula

Anterior lateral malleolar artery

Lateral malleolus

Synovial sheath

Lateral branch of deep fibular nerve

Extensor digitorum brevis

Lateral dorsal cutaneous nerve from sural nerve

Dorsal digital branches of superficial fibular nerve

Tibialis anterior tendon

Tibia

Deep fibular nerve

Anterior tibial artery

Extensor hallucis longus tendon

Anterior medial malleolar artery

Medial malleolus

Lateral tarsal branch

Dorsalis pedis artery

Medial tarsal branch

Medial branch of deep fibular nerve

Deep plantar artery

Extensor hallucis longus tendon

First dorsal interosseous

Dorsal hood

Dorsal digital arteries

Dorsal digital branches of deep fibular nerve

**Arteries and nerves of the foot (dorsal view)**

Deep fibular nerve

Saphenous nerve

Superficial fibular nerve

Lateral dorsal cutaneous nerve from sural nerve

Medial branch of deep fibular nerve

**Innervation of the foot (dorsal view)**

Saphenous nerve

Superficial fibular nerve

Sural nerve

Deep fibular nerve

**Cutaneous distribution**

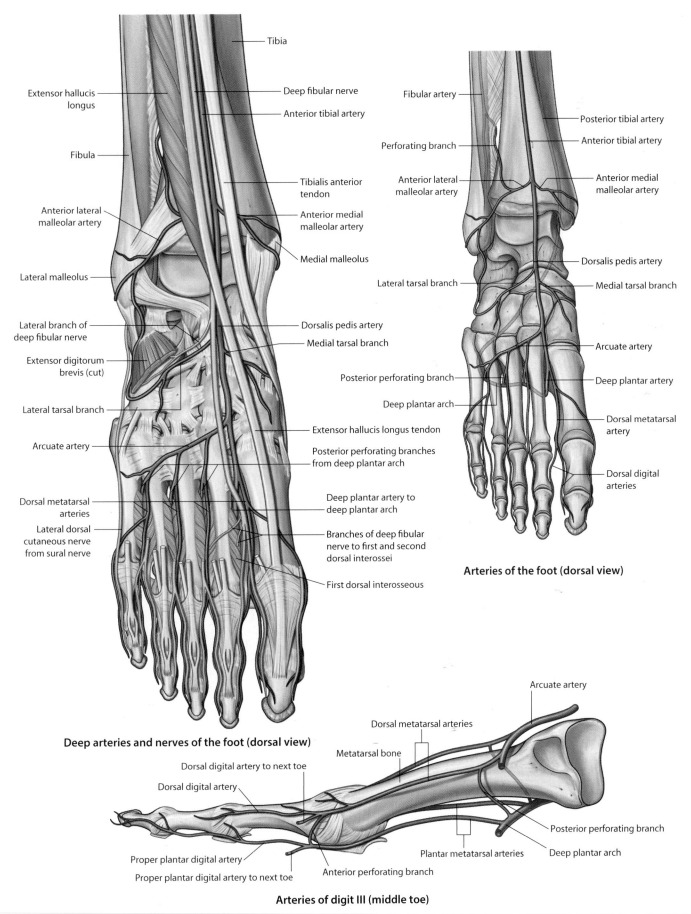

Tibia

Extensor hallucis longus

Deep fibular nerve

Anterior tibial artery

Fibula

Tibialis anterior tendon

Anterior lateral malleolar artery

Anterior medial malleolar artery

Medial malleolus

Lateral malleolus

Lateral branch of deep fibular nerve

Dorsalis pedis artery

Medial tarsal branch

Extensor digitorum brevis (cut)

Lateral tarsal branch

Arcuate artery

Extensor hallucis longus tendon

Posterior perforating branches from deep plantar arch

Dorsal metatarsal arteries

Deep plantar artery to deep plantar arch

Lateral dorsal cutaneous nerve from sural nerve

Branches of deep fibular nerve to first and second dorsal interossei

First dorsal interosseous

**Deep arteries and nerves of the foot (dorsal view)**

Fibular artery

Posterior tibial artery

Perforating branch

Anterior tibial artery

Anterior lateral malleolar artery

Anterior medial malleolar artery

Dorsalis pedis artery

Lateral tarsal branch

Medial tarsal branch

Arcuate artery

Posterior perforating branch

Deep plantar artery

Deep plantar arch

Dorsal metatarsal artery

Dorsal digital arteries

**Arteries of the foot (dorsal view)**

Arcuate artery

Dorsal metatarsal arteries

Metatarsal bone

Dorsal digital artery to next toe

Dorsal digital artery

Posterior perforating branch

Plantar metatarsal arteries

Deep plantar arch

Proper plantar digital artery

Proper plantar digital artery to next toe

Anterior perforating branch

**Arteries of digit III (middle toe)**

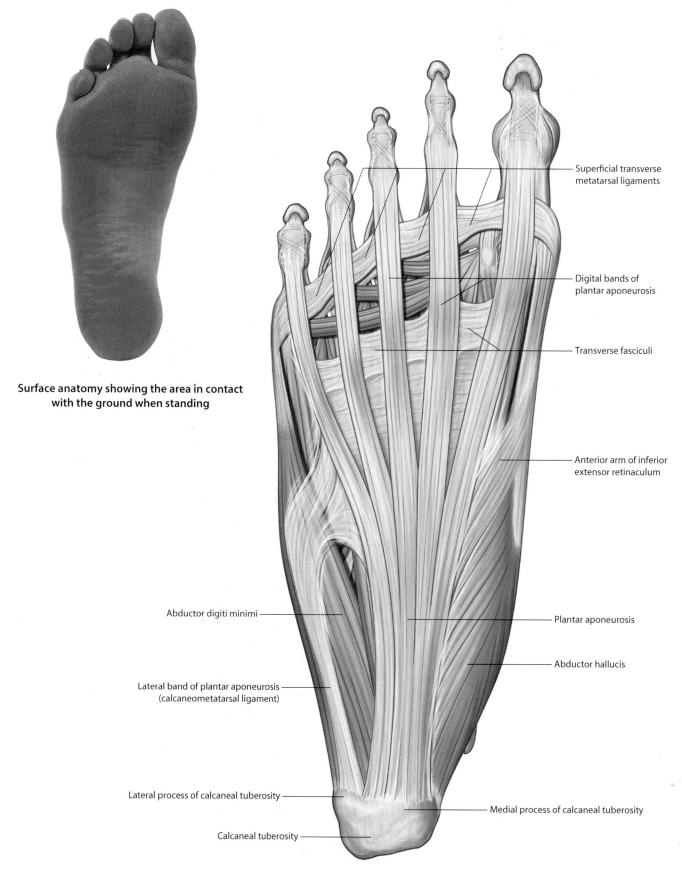

**Surface anatomy showing the area in contact with the ground when standing**

Superficial transverse metatarsal ligaments

Digital bands of plantar aponeurosis

Transverse fasciculi

Anterior arm of inferior extensor retinaculum

Abductor digiti minimi

Plantar aponeurosis

Abductor hallucis

Lateral band of plantar aponeurosis (calcaneometatarsal ligament)

Lateral process of calcaneal tuberosity

Medial process of calcaneal tuberosity

Calcaneal tuberosity

**Superficial structures of the foot (plantar view)**

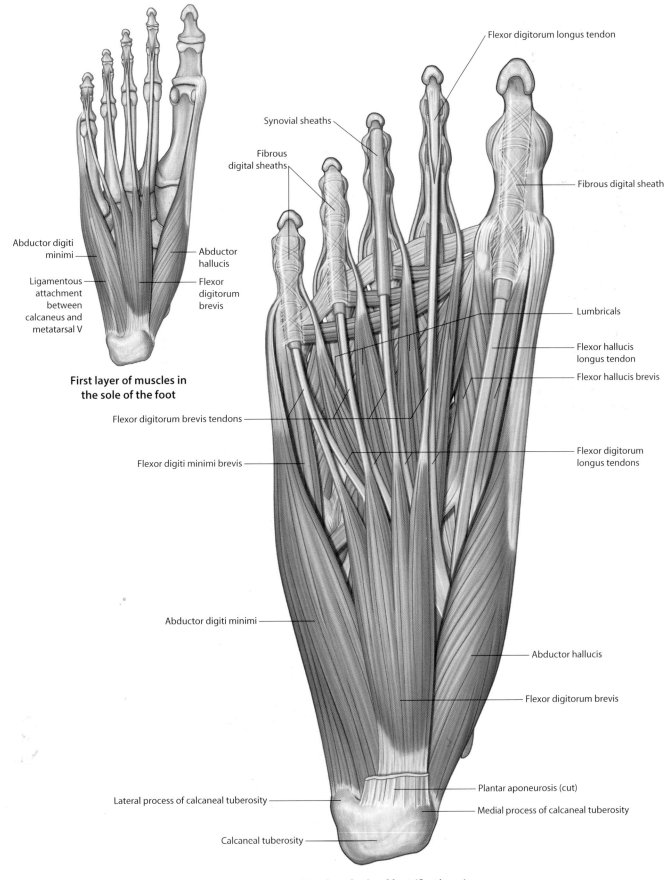

Flexor digitorum longus tendon

Synovial sheaths

Fibrous digital sheaths

Fibrous digital sheath

Abductor digiti minimi

Abductor hallucis

Ligamentous attachment between calcaneus and metatarsal V

Flexor digitorum brevis

Lumbricals

Flexor hallucis longus tendon

Flexor hallucis brevis

**First layer of muscles in the sole of the foot**

Flexor digitorum brevis tendons

Flexor digiti minimi brevis

Flexor digitorum longus tendons

Abductor digiti minimi

Abductor hallucis

Flexor digitorum brevis

Plantar aponeurosis (cut)

Lateral process of calcaneal tuberosity

Medial process of calcaneal tuberosity

Calcaneal tuberosity

**Muscles of sole of foot (first layer)**

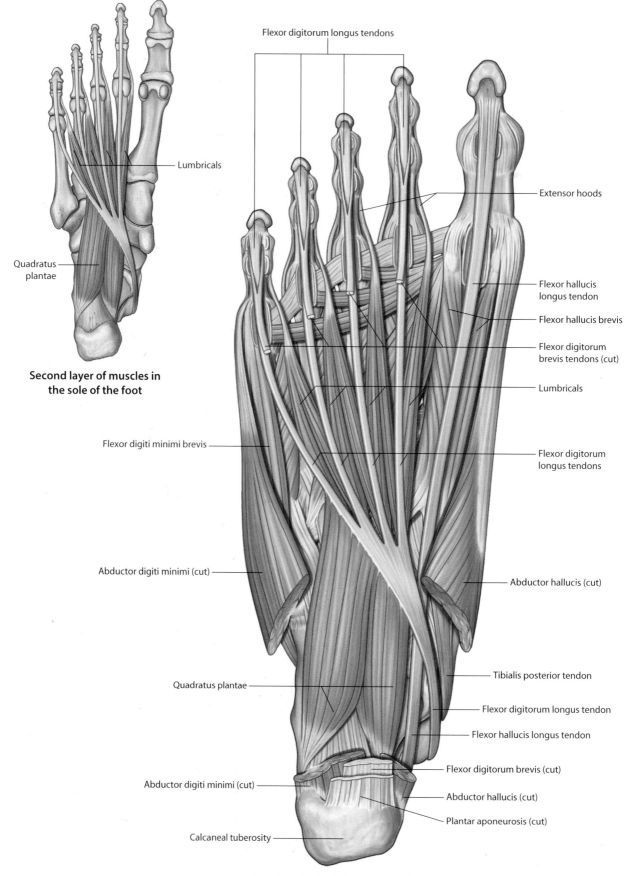

Flexor digitorum longus tendons

Lumbricals

Quadratus plantae

**Second layer of muscles in the sole of the foot**

Extensor hoods

Flexor hallucis longus tendon

Flexor hallucis brevis

Flexor digitorum brevis tendons (cut)

Lumbricals

Flexor digiti minimi brevis

Flexor digitorum longus tendons

Abductor digiti minimi (cut)

Abductor hallucis (cut)

Quadratus plantae

Tibialis posterior tendon

Flexor digitorum longus tendon

Flexor hallucis longus tendon

Flexor digitorum brevis (cut)

Abductor digiti minimi (cut)

Abductor hallucis (cut)

Plantar aponeurosis (cut)

Calcaneal tuberosity

**Muscles of sole of foot (second layer)**

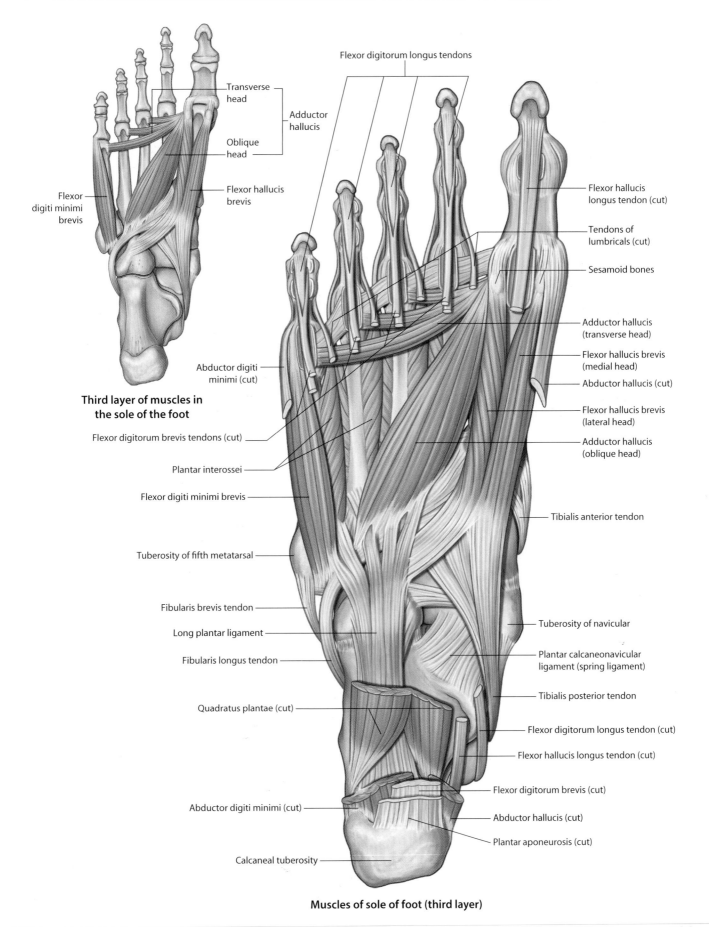

Flexor digitorum longus tendons

Transverse head

Adductor hallucis

Oblique head

Flexor hallucis brevis

Flexor digiti minimi brevis

Flexor hallucis longus tendon (cut)

Tendons of lumbricals (cut)

Sesamoid bones

Adductor hallucis (transverse head)

Flexor hallucis brevis (medial head)

Abductor hallucis (cut)

Flexor hallucis brevis (lateral head)

Adductor hallucis (oblique head)

Abductor digiti minimi (cut)

**Third layer of muscles in the sole of the foot**

Flexor digitorum brevis tendons (cut)

Plantar interossei

Flexor digiti minimi brevis

Tuberosity of fifth metatarsal

Fibularis brevis tendon

Long plantar ligament

Fibularis longus tendon

Quadratus plantae (cut)

Abductor digiti minimi (cut)

Calcaneal tuberosity

Tibialis anterior tendon

Tuberosity of navicular

Plantar calcaneonavicular ligament (spring ligament)

Tibialis posterior tendon

Flexor digitorum longus tendon (cut)

Flexor hallucis longus tendon (cut)

Flexor digitorum brevis (cut)

Abductor hallucis (cut)

Plantar aponeurosis (cut)

**Muscles of sole of foot (third layer)**

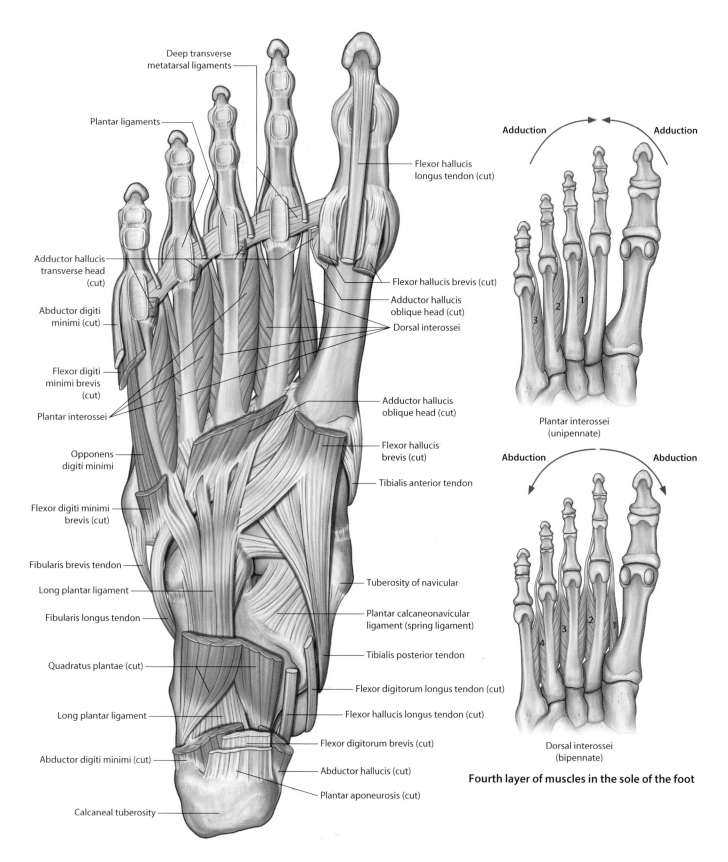

Deep transverse metatarsal ligaments

Plantar ligaments

Adductor hallucis transverse head (cut)

Abductor digiti minimi (cut)

Flexor digiti minimi brevis (cut)

Plantar interossei

Opponens digiti minimi

Flexor digiti minimi brevis (cut)

Fibularis brevis tendon

Long plantar ligament

Fibularis longus tendon

Quadratus plantae (cut)

Long plantar ligament

Abductor digiti minimi (cut)

Calcaneal tuberosity

Flexor hallucis longus tendon (cut)

Flexor hallucis brevis (cut)

Adductor hallucis oblique head (cut)

Dorsal interossei

Adductor hallucis oblique head (cut)

Flexor hallucis brevis (cut)

Tibialis anterior tendon

Tuberosity of navicular

Plantar calcaneonavicular ligament (spring ligament)

Tibialis posterior tendon

Flexor digitorum longus tendon (cut)

Flexor hallucis longus tendon (cut)

Flexor digitorum brevis (cut)

Abductor hallucis (cut)

Plantar aponeurosis (cut)

**Muscles of sole of foot (fourth layer)**

Adduction          Adduction

3   2   1

Plantar interossei (unipennate)

Abduction          Abduction

4   3   2   1

Dorsal interossei (bipennate)

**Fourth layer of muscles in the sole of the foot**

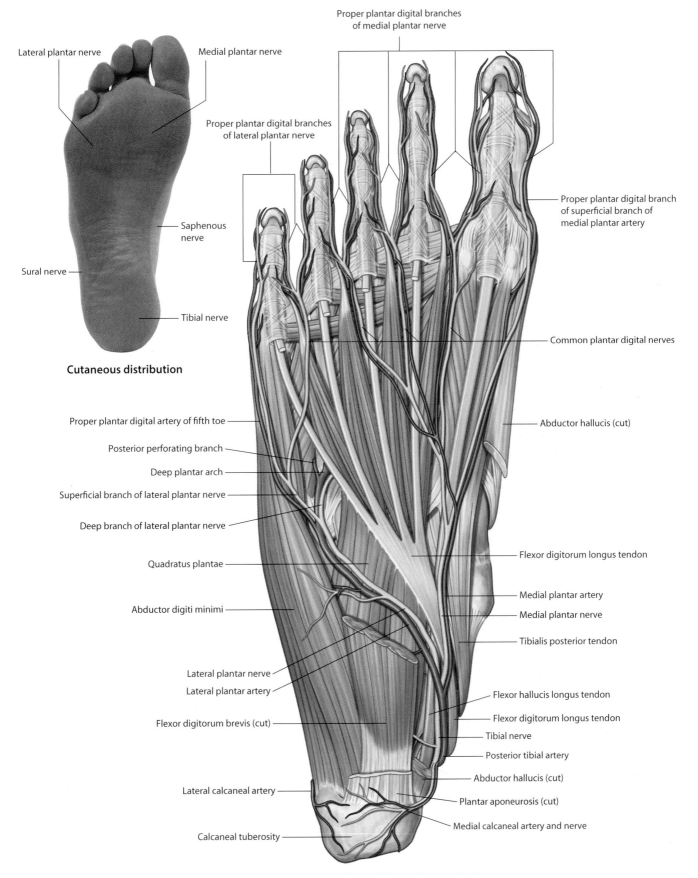

Lateral plantar nerve

Medial plantar nerve

Proper plantar digital branches
of medial plantar nerve

Proper plantar digital branches
of lateral plantar nerve

Proper plantar digital branch
of superficial branch of
medial plantar artery

Saphenous
nerve

Sural nerve

Tibial nerve

Common plantar digital nerves

**Cutaneous distribution**

Proper plantar digital artery of fifth toe

Abductor hallucis (cut)

Posterior perforating branch

Deep plantar arch

Superficial branch of lateral plantar nerve

Deep branch of lateral plantar nerve

Flexor digitorum longus tendon

Quadratus plantae

Medial plantar artery

Medial plantar nerve

Abductor digiti minimi

Tibialis posterior tendon

Lateral plantar nerve

Lateral plantar artery

Flexor hallucis longus tendon

Flexor digitorum longus tendon

Flexor digitorum brevis (cut)

Tibial nerve

Posterior tibial artery

Abductor hallucis (cut)

Lateral calcaneal artery

Plantar aponeurosis (cut)

Medial calcaneal artery and nerve

Calcaneal tuberosity

**Arteries and nerves of sole of foot (plantar view)**

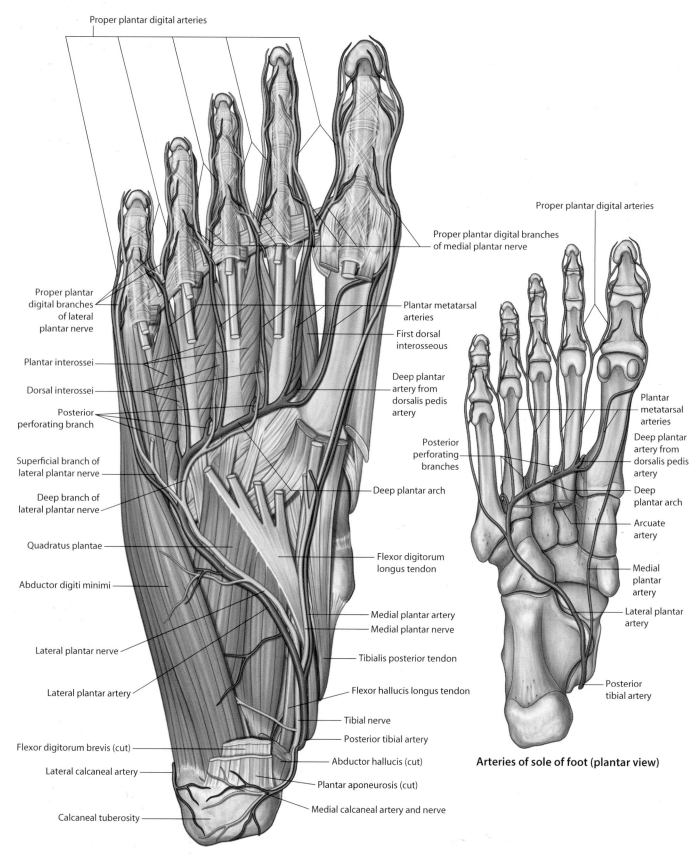

Proper plantar digital arteries

Proper plantar digital branches
of medial plantar nerve

Proper plantar
digital branches
of lateral
plantar nerve

Plantar metatarsal
arteries

First dorsal
interosseous

Plantar interossei

Dorsal interossei

Deep plantar
artery from
dorsalis pedis
artery

Posterior
perforating branch

Posterior
perforating
branches

Superficial branch of
lateral plantar nerve

Deep branch of
lateral plantar nerve

Deep plantar arch

Quadratus plantae

Flexor digitorum
longus tendon

Abductor digiti minimi

Medial plantar artery

Medial plantar nerve

Lateral plantar nerve

Tibialis posterior tendon

Lateral plantar artery

Flexor hallucis longus tendon

Tibial nerve

Posterior tibial artery

Flexor digitorum brevis (cut)

Abductor hallucis (cut)

Lateral calcaneal artery

Plantar aponeurosis (cut)

Medial calcaneal artery and nerve

Calcaneal tuberosity

**Arteries and nerves of sole of foot (plantar view)**

Proper plantar digital arteries

Plantar
metatarsal
arteries

Deep plantar
artery from
dorsalis pedis
artery

Deep
plantar arch

Arcuate
artery

Medial
plantar
artery

Lateral plantar
artery

Posterior
tibial artery

**Arteries of sole of foot (plantar view)**

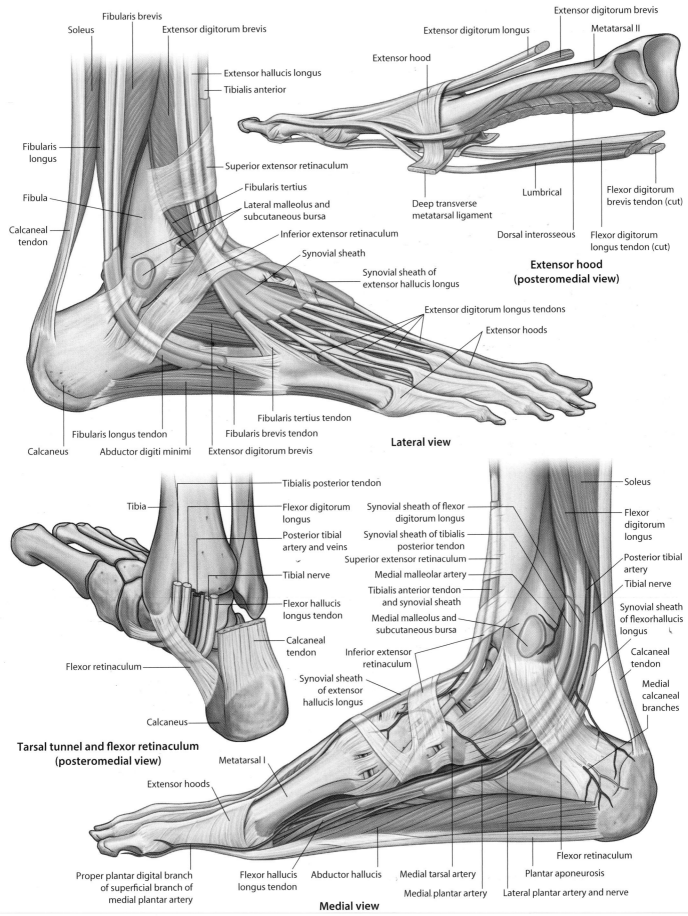

Soleus
Fibularis brevis
Extensor digitorum brevis
Extensor hallucis longus
Tibialis anterior
Fibularis longus
Fibula
Calcaneal tendon
Superior extensor retinaculum
Fibularis tertius
Lateral malleolus and subcutaneous bursa
Inferior extensor retinaculum
Synovial sheath
Synovial sheath of extensor hallucis longus
Fibularis longus tendon
Abductor digiti minimi
Calcaneus
Extensor digitorum brevis
Fibularis brevis tendon
Fibularis tertius tendon
Extensor digitorum longus tendons
Extensor hoods

**Lateral view**

Extensor digitorum longus
Extensor hood
Extensor digitorum brevis
Metatarsal II
Deep transverse metatarsal ligament
Lumbrical
Dorsal interosseous
Flexor digitorum brevis tendon (cut)
Flexor digitorum longus tendon (cut)

**Extensor hood (posteromedial view)**

Tibia
Tibialis posterior tendon
Flexor digitorum longus
Posterior tibial artery and veins
Tibial nerve
Flexor hallucis longus tendon
Calcaneal tendon
Flexor retinaculum
Calcaneus

**Tarsal tunnel and flexor retinaculum (posteromedial view)**

Extensor hoods
Metatarsal I
Proper plantar digital branch of superficial branch of medial plantar artery
Flexor hallucis longus tendon
Abductor hallucis
Medial plantar artery
Medial tarsal artery
Lateral plantar artery and nerve
Plantar aponeurosis
Flexor retinaculum

Soleus
Flexor digitorum longus
Posterior tibial artery
Tibial nerve
Synovial sheath of flexor hallucis longus
Calcaneal tendon
Medial calcaneal branches

Synovial sheath of flexor digitorum longus
Synovial sheath of tibialis posterior tendon
Superior extensor retinaculum
Medial malleolar artery
Tibialis anterior tendon and synovial sheath
Medial malleolus and subcutaneous bursa
Inferior extensor retinaculum
Synovial sheath of extensor hallucis longus

**Medial view**

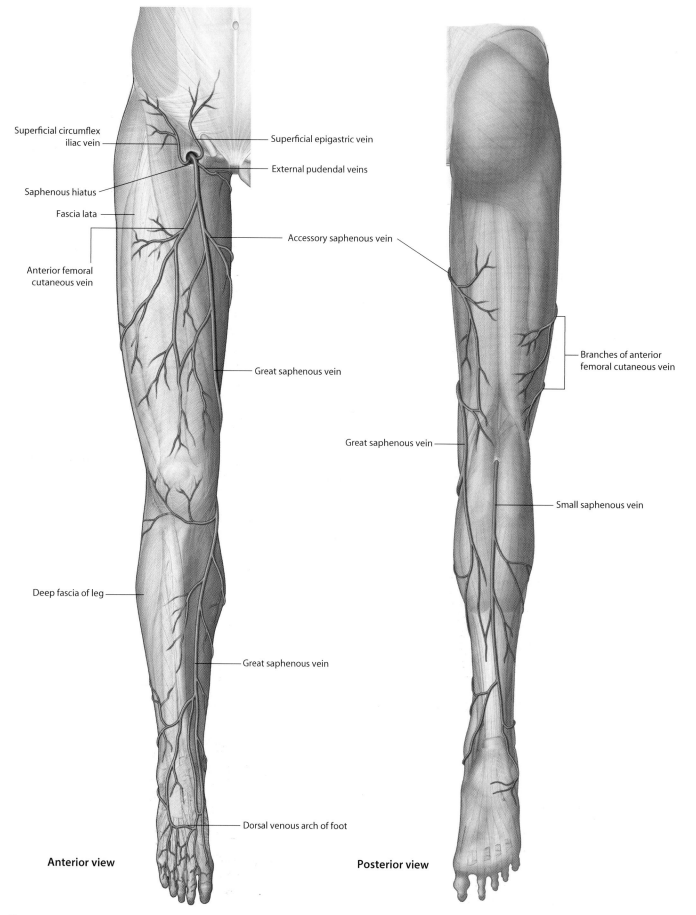

Superficial circumflex iliac vein

Saphenous hiatus

Fascia lata

Anterior femoral cutaneous vein

Deep fascia of leg

Superficial epigastric vein

External pudendal veins

Accessory saphenous vein

Great saphenous vein

Great saphenous vein

Dorsal venous arch of foot

Branches of anterior femoral cutaneous vein

Great saphenous vein

Small saphenous vein

**Anterior view**

**Posterior view**

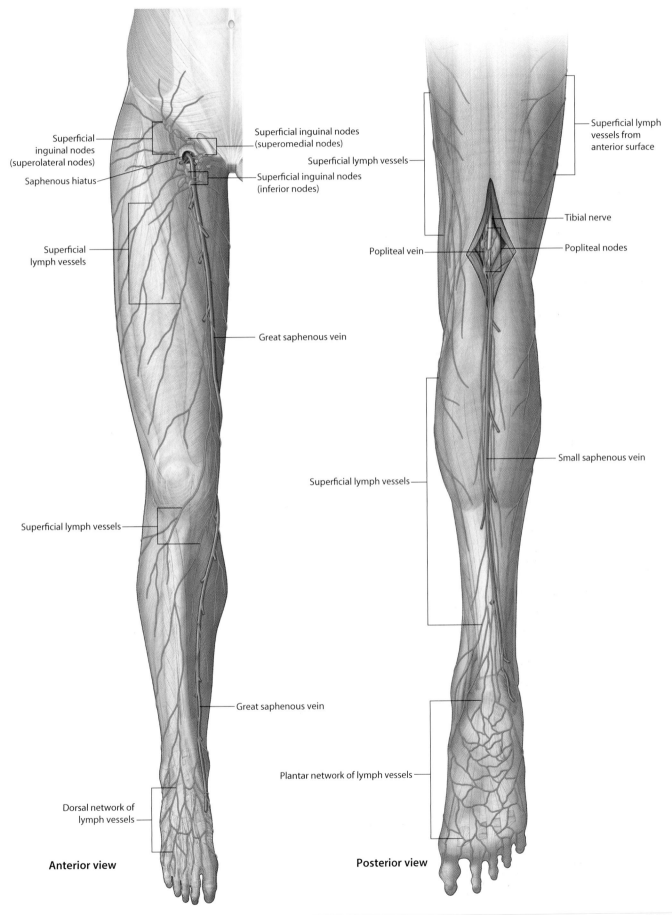

Superficial
inguinal nodes
(superolateral nodes)

Saphenous hiatus

Superficial
lymph vessels

Superficial lymph vessels

Great saphenous vein

Dorsal network of
lymph vessels

**Anterior view**

Superficial inguinal nodes
(superomedial nodes)

Superficial lymph vessels

Superficial inguinal nodes
(inferior nodes)

Great saphenous vein

Superficial lymph
vessels from
anterior surface

Tibial nerve

Popliteal vein

Popliteal nodes

Small saphenous vein

Superficial lymph vessels

Plantar network of lymph vessels

**Posterior view**

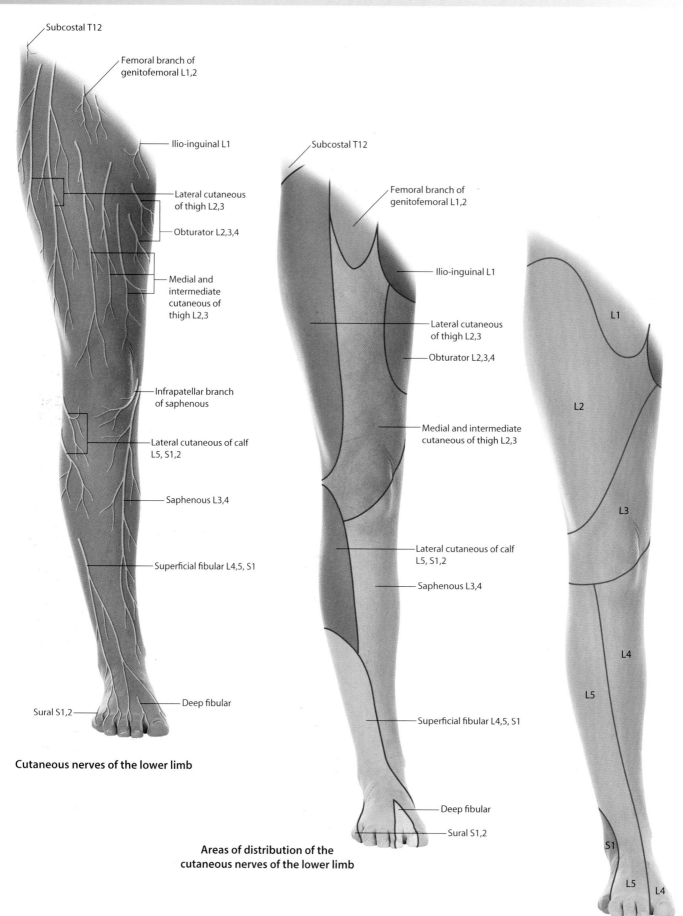

Subcostal T12

Femoral branch of
genitofemoral L1,2

Ilio-inguinal L1

Lateral cutaneous
of thigh L2,3

Obturator L2,3,4

Medial and
intermediate
cutaneous of
thigh L2,3

Infrapatellar branch
of saphenous

Lateral cutaneous of calf
L5, S1,2

Saphenous L3,4

Superficial fibular L4,5, S1

Sural S1,2

Deep fibular

**Cutaneous nerves of the lower limb**

Subcostal T12

Femoral branch of
genitofemoral L1,2

Ilio-inguinal L1

Lateral cutaneous
of thigh L2,3

Obturator L2,3,4

Medial and intermediate
cutaneous of thigh L2,3

Lateral cutaneous of calf
L5, S1,2

Saphenous L3,4

Superficial fibular L4,5, S1

Deep fibular

Sural S1,2

**Areas of distribution of the
cutaneous nerves of the lower limb**

L1

L2

L3

L4

L5

S1

L5

L4

**Dermatomes of the lower limb**

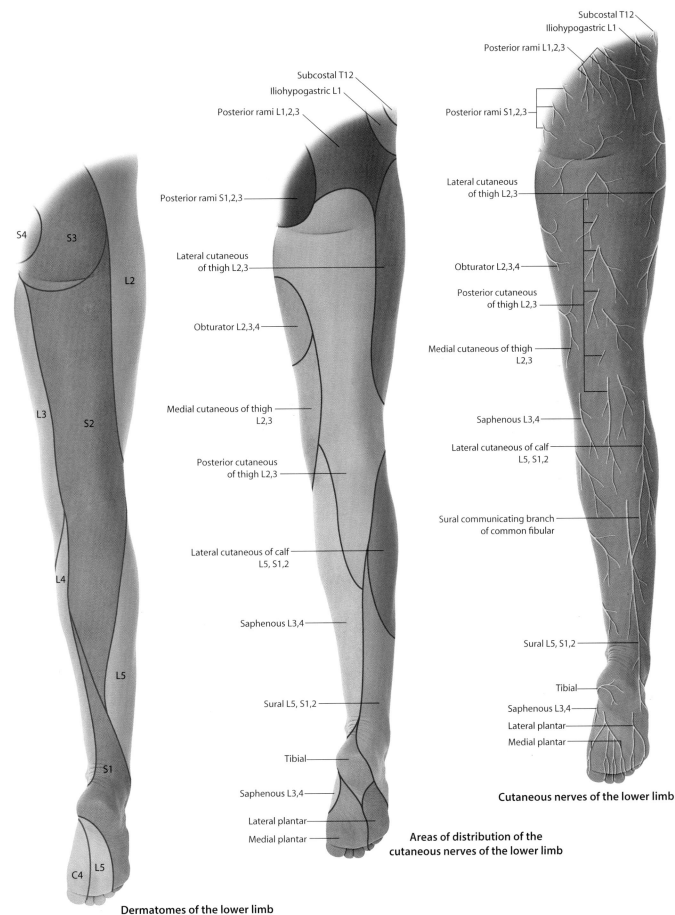

Subcostal T12
Iliohypogastric L1
Posterior rami L1,2,3

Posterior rami S1,2,3

Lateral cutaneous
of thigh L2,3

Obturator L2,3,4

Posterior cutaneous
of thigh L2,3

Medial cutaneous of thigh
L2,3

Saphenous L3,4

Lateral cutaneous of calf
L5, S1,2

Sural communicating branch
of common fibular

Sural L5, S1,2

Tibial

Saphenous L3,4

Lateral plantar

Medial plantar

**Cutaneous nerves of the lower limb**

Subcostal T12
Iliohypogastric L1
Posterior rami L1,2,3

Posterior rami S1,2,3

Lateral cutaneous
of thigh L2,3

Obturator L2,3,4

Medial cutaneous of thigh
L2,3

Posterior cutaneous
of thigh L2,3

Lateral cutaneous of calf
L5, S1,2

Saphenous L3,4

Sural L5, S1,2

Tibial

Saphenous L3,4

Lateral plantar

Medial plantar

**Areas of distribution of the
cutaneous nerves of the lower limb**

S4    S3

L2

L3    S2

L4

L5

S1

C4    L5

**Dermatomes of the lower limb**

**347**

# 7 UPPER LIMB

## CONTENTS

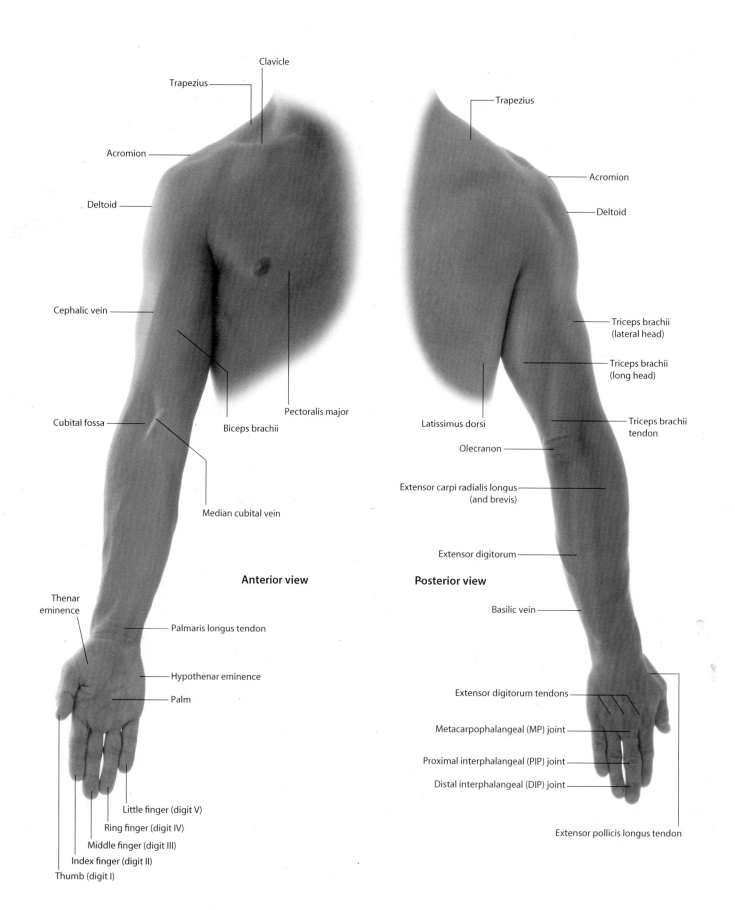

Clavicle

Trapezius

Acromion

Deltoid

Cephalic vein

Cubital fossa

Biceps brachii

Pectoralis major

Median cubital vein

**Anterior view**

Thenar eminence

Palmaris longus tendon

Hypothenar eminence

Palm

Little finger (digit V)

Ring finger (digit IV)

Middle finger (digit III)

Index finger (digit II)

Thumb (digit I)

Trapezius

Acromion

Deltoid

Triceps brachii (lateral head)

Triceps brachii (long head)

Triceps brachii tendon

Latissimus dorsi

Olecranon

Extensor carpi radialis longus (and brevis)

Extensor digitorum

**Posterior view**

Basilic vein

Extensor digitorum tendons

Metacarpophalangeal (MP) joint

Proximal interphalangeal (PIP) joint

Distal interphalangeal (DIP) joint

Extensor pollicis longus tendon

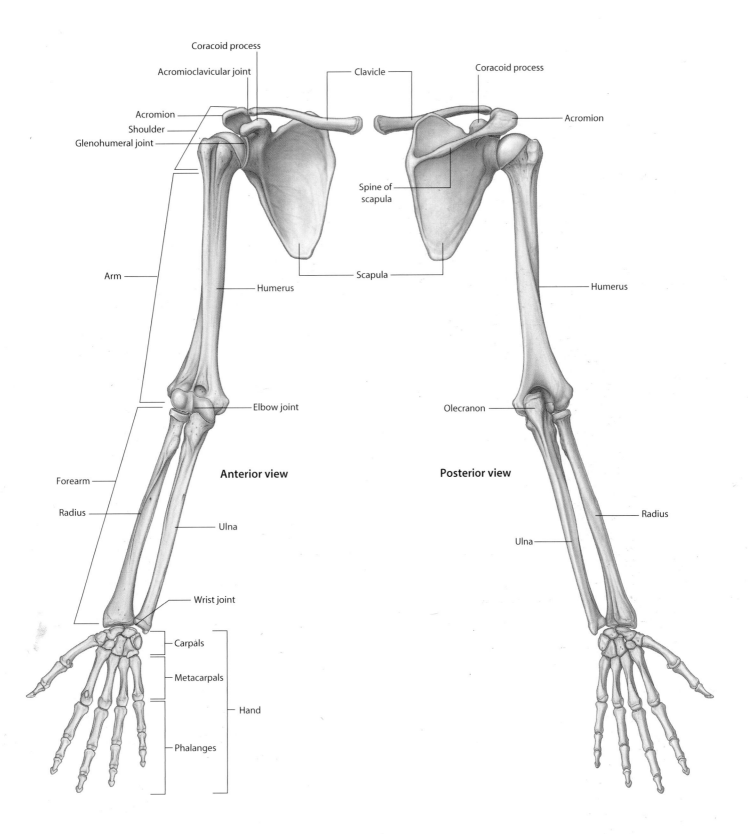

Coracoid process

Acromioclavicular joint

Clavicle

Coracoid process

Acromion

Acromion

Shoulder

Glenohumeral joint

Spine of
scapula

Arm

Humerus

Scapula

Humerus

Elbow joint

Olecranon

**Anterior view**

**Posterior view**

Forearm

Radius

Radius

Ulna

Ulna

Wrist joint

Carpals

Metacarpals

Hand

Phalanges

Cervical vertebrae CI-VII

Superior transverse scapular ligament

Rib I

Clavicle

Acromion

Coracoid process

Sterno-clavicular joint

Greater tubercle

Humerus

Manubrium of sternum

Supra-scapular notch

**Anterior view**

Rib I

Acromion

Clavicle

Supraspinous fossa

Greater tubercle

Spine of scapula

Humerus

Infraspinous fossa

Lesser tubercle

Sternal angle

Humerus

**Lateral view**

Scapula

Transverse process of TI

Supraspinous fossa

Rib I

Spine of scapula

Acromion

Head of humerus

Greater tubercle

Intertubercular sulcus

Lesser tubercle

Humerus

Lateral epicondyle

Coracoid process

**Bony framework of shoulder**

Medial epicondyle

Clavicle

Sternum

**Superior view**

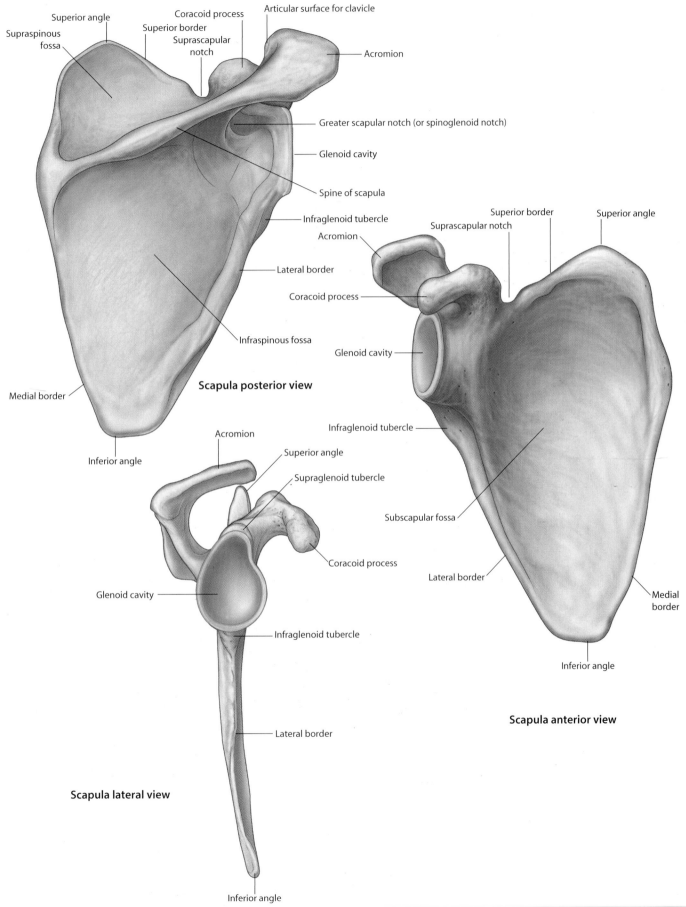

Superior angle

Supraspinous fossa

Superior border

Coracoid process

Suprascapular notch

Articular surface for clavicle

Acromion

Greater scapular notch (or spinoglenoid notch)

Glenoid cavity

Spine of scapula

Infraglenoid tubercle

Lateral border

Infraspinous fossa

Medial border

Inferior angle

**Scapula posterior view**

Acromion

Superior angle

Supraglenoid tubercle

Coracoid process

Glenoid cavity

Infraglenoid tubercle

Lateral border

Inferior angle

**Scapula lateral view**

Acromion

Suprascapular notch

Superior border

Superior angle

Coracoid process

Glenoid cavity

Infraglenoid tubercle

Subscapular fossa

Lateral border

Medial border

Inferior angle

**Scapula anterior view**

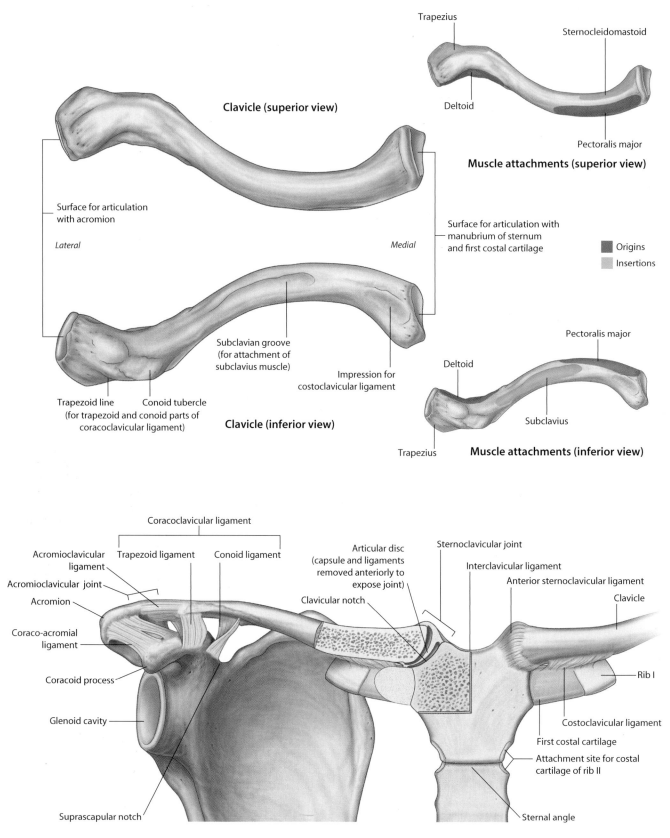

**Clavicle (superior view)**

Trapezius

Sternocleidomastoid

Deltoid

Pectoralis major

**Muscle attachments (superior view)**

Surface for articulation with acromion

*Lateral*

Surface for articulation with manubrium of sternum and first costal cartilage

*Medial*

Origins

Insertions

Subclavian groove (for attachment of subclavius muscle)

Impression for costoclavicular ligament

Trapezoid line       Conoid tubercle
(for trapezoid and conoid parts of coracoclavicular ligament)

**Clavicle (inferior view)**

Pectoralis major

Deltoid

Subclavius

Trapezius       **Muscle attachments (inferior view)**

Coracoclavicular ligament

Acromioclavicular ligament       Trapezoid ligament       Conoid ligament

Articular disc (capsule and ligaments removed anteriorly to expose joint)

Sternoclavicular joint

Interclavicular ligament

Anterior sternoclavicular ligament

Acromioclavicular joint

Acromion

Clavicular notch

Clavicle

Coraco-acromial ligament

Coracoid process

Rib I

Glenoid cavity

Costoclavicular ligament

First costal cartilage

Attachment site for costal cartilage of rib II

Suprascapular notch

Sternal angle

**Joints and ligaments of the clavicle (anterior view)**

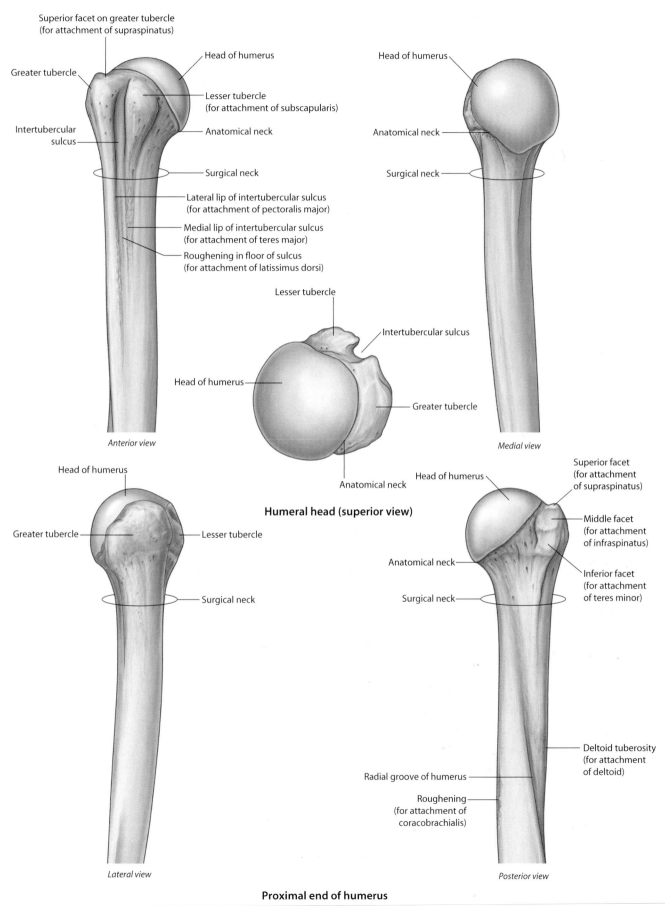

Superior facet on greater tubercle
(for attachment of supraspinatus)

Greater tubercle

Intertubercular
sulcus

Head of humerus

Lesser tubercle
(for attachment of subscapularis)

Anatomical neck

Surgical neck

Lateral lip of intertubercular sulcus
(for attachment of pectoralis major)

Medial lip of intertubercular sulcus
(for attachment of teres major)

Roughening in floor of sulcus
(for attachment of latissimus dorsi)

*Anterior view*

Lesser tubercle

Intertubercular sulcus

Head of humerus

Greater tubercle

Anatomical neck

**Humeral head (superior view)**

Head of humerus

Anatomical neck

Surgical neck

*Medial view*

Head of humerus

Greater tubercle

Lesser tubercle

Surgical neck

*Lateral view*

Head of humerus

Anatomical neck

Surgical neck

Superior facet
(for attachment
of supraspinatus)

Middle facet
(for attachment
of infraspinatus)

Inferior facet
(for attachment
of teres minor)

Deltoid tuberosity
(for attachment
of deltoid)

Radial groove of humerus

Roughening
(for attachment of
coracobrachialis)

*Posterior view*

**Proximal end of humerus**

**355**

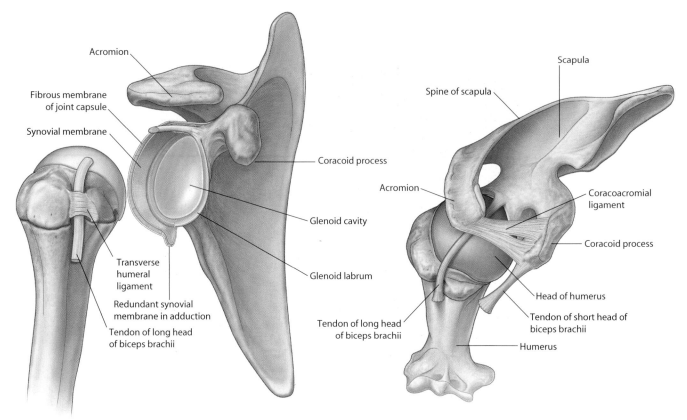

Acromion

Fibrous membrane
of joint capsule

Synovial membrane

Transverse
humeral
ligament

Redundant synovial
membrane in adduction

Tendon of long head
of biceps brachii

Coracoid process

Glenoid cavity

Glenoid labrum

Scapula

Spine of scapula

Acromion

Tendon of long head
of biceps brachii

Coracoacromial
ligament

Coracoid process

Head of humerus

Tendon of short head of
biceps brachii

Humerus

**Origins of biceps brachii tendons (superior view)**

**Articular surfaces of glenohumeral joint (anterolateral oblique view)**

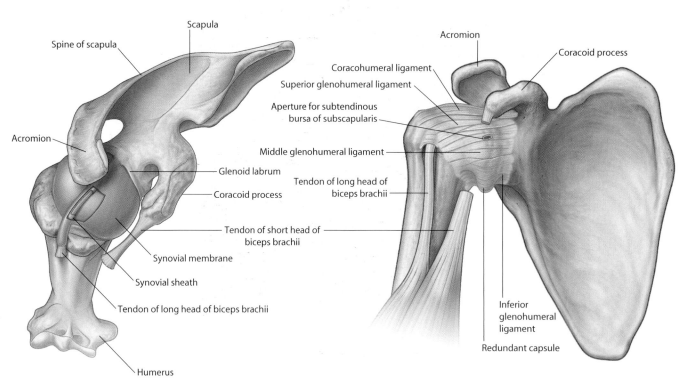

Spine of scapula

Scapula

Acromion

Glenoid labrum

Coracoid process

Synovial membrane

Synovial sheath

Tendon of long head of biceps brachii

Humerus

Tendon of short head of
biceps brachii

Acromion

Coracohumeral ligament

Superior glenohumeral ligament

Aperture for subtendinous
bursa of subscapularis

Middle glenohumeral ligament

Tendon of long head of
biceps brachii

Coracoid process

Scapula

Inferior
glenohumeral
ligament

Redundant capsule

**Synovial membrane (superior view)**

**Fibrous membrane of joint capsule (anterior view)**

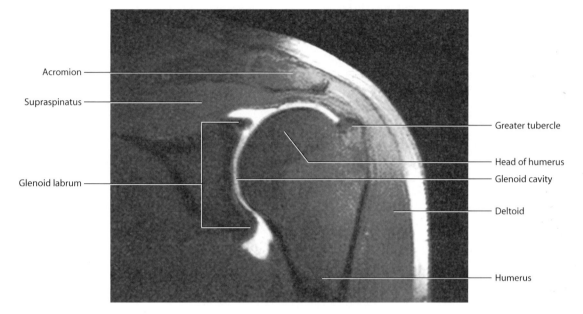

Acromion

Supraspinatus

Glenoid labrum

Greater tubercle

Head of humerus

Glenoid cavity

Deltoid

Humerus

**Anterior view of the glenohumeral joint.**
T1-weighted MR image in coronal plane

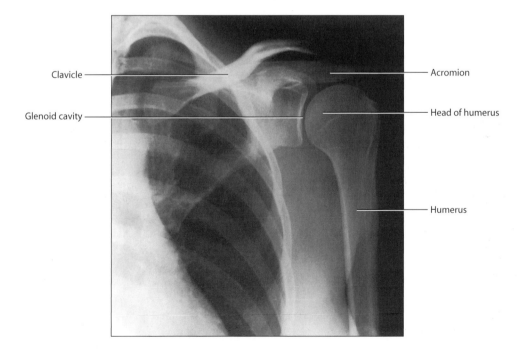

Clavicle

Glenoid cavity

Acromion

Head of humerus

Humerus

**Normal glenohumeral joint.**
Radiograph, AP view

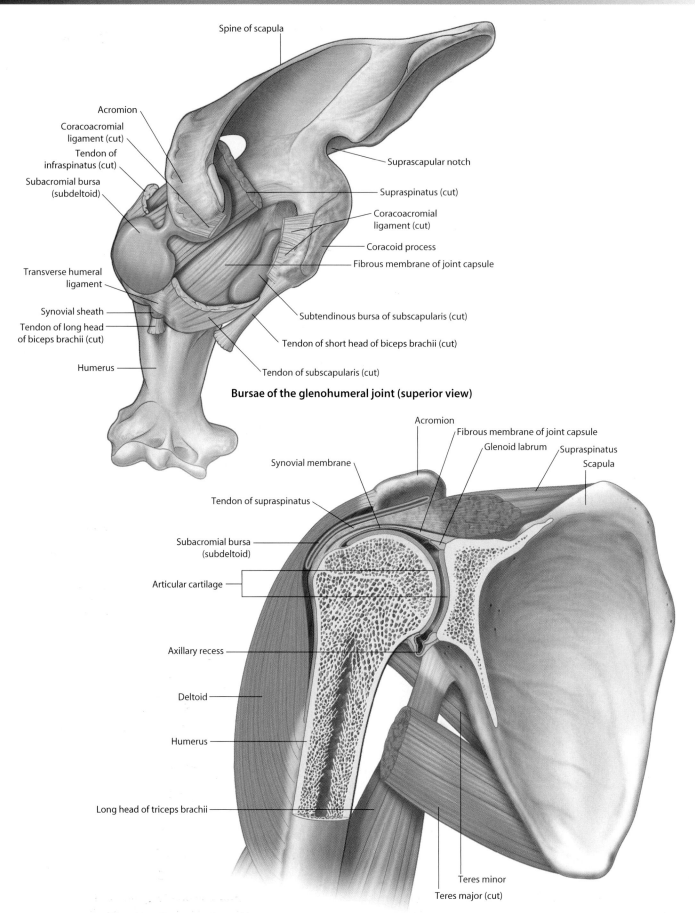

Spine of scapula

Acromion

Coracoacromial ligament (cut)

Tendon of infraspinatus (cut)

Subacromial bursa (subdeltoid)

Transverse humeral ligament

Synovial sheath

Tendon of long head of biceps brachii (cut)

Humerus

Suprascapular notch

Supraspinatus (cut)

Coracoacromial ligament (cut)

Coracoid process

Fibrous membrane of joint capsule

Subtendinous bursa of subscapularis (cut)

Tendon of short head of biceps brachii (cut)

Tendon of subscapularis (cut)

**Bursae of the glenohumeral joint (superior view)**

Acromion

Fibrous membrane of joint capsule

Glenoid labrum

Supraspinatus

Scapula

Synovial membrane

Tendon of supraspinatus

Subacromial bursa (subdeltoid)

Articular cartilage

Axillary recess

Deltoid

Humerus

Long head of triceps brachii

Teres minor

Teres major (cut)

**Glenohumeral joint (anterior view)**

**358**

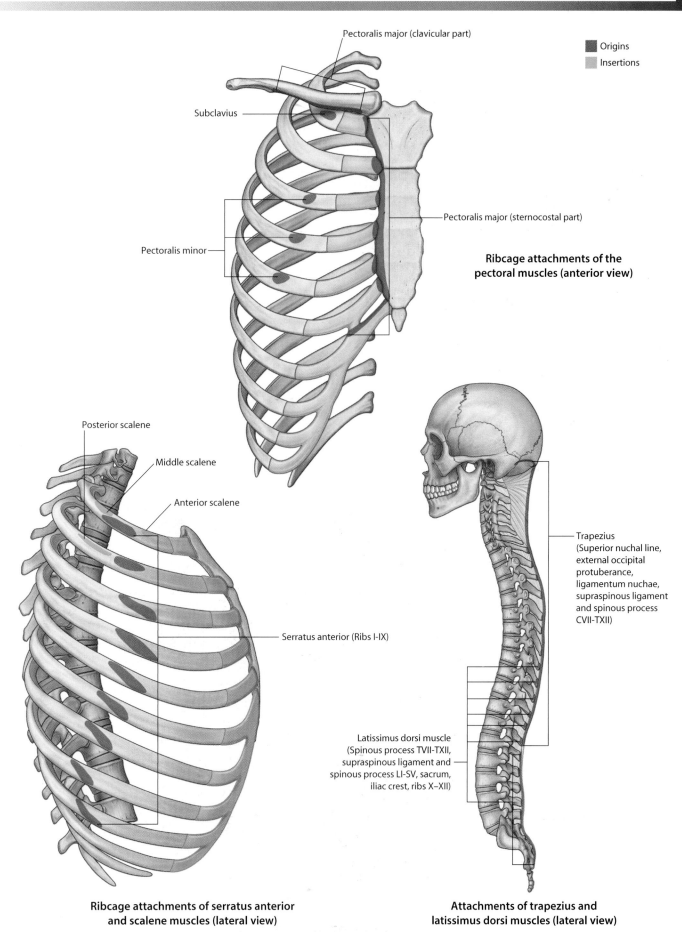

Pectoralis major (clavicular part)

Subclavius

Origins
Insertions

Pectoralis major (sternocostal part)

Pectoralis minor

**Ribcage attachments of the
pectoral muscles (anterior view)**

Posterior scalene

Middle scalene

Anterior scalene

Serratus anterior (Ribs I-IX)

Trapezius
(Superior nuchal line,
external occipital
protuberance,
ligamentum nuchae,
supraspinous ligament
and spinous process
CVII-TXII)

Latissimus dorsi muscle
(Spinous process TVII-TXII,
supraspinous ligament and
spinous process LI-SV, sacrum,
iliac crest, ribs X–XII)

**Ribcage attachments of serratus anterior
and scalene muscles (lateral view)**

**Attachments of trapezius and
latissimus dorsi muscles (lateral view)**

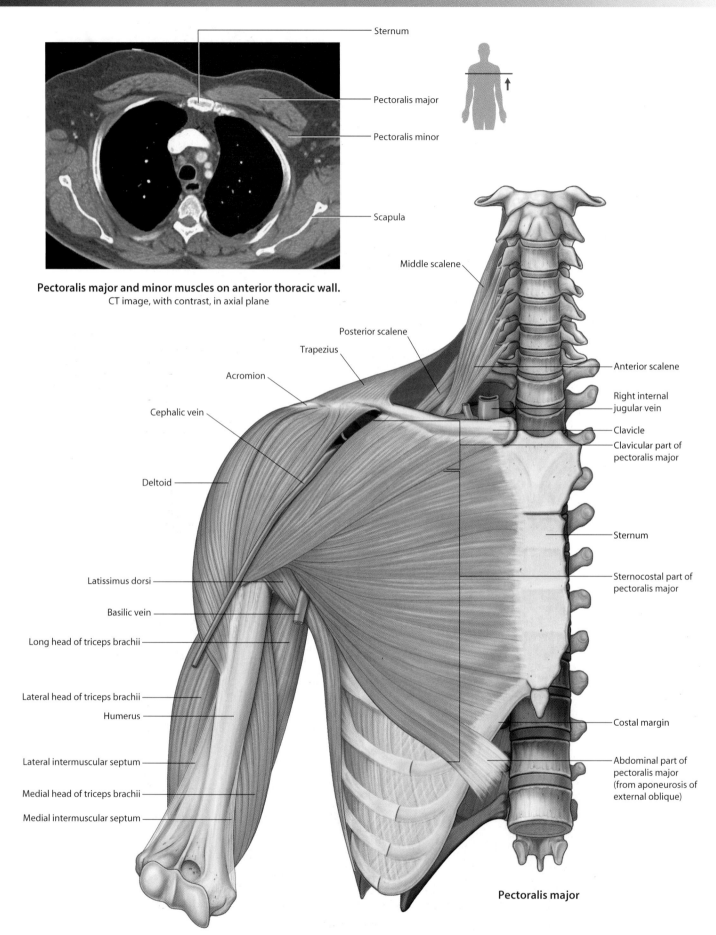

Sternum

Pectoralis major

Pectoralis minor

Scapula

**Pectoralis major and minor muscles on anterior thoracic wall.**
CT image, with contrast, in axial plane

Middle scalene

Posterior scalene

Trapezius

Acromion

Cephalic vein

Deltoid

Latissimus dorsi

Basilic vein

Long head of triceps brachii

Lateral head of triceps brachii

Humerus

Lateral intermuscular septum

Medial head of triceps brachii

Medial intermuscular septum

Anterior scalene

Right internal
jugular vein

Clavicle

Clavicular part of
pectoralis major

Sternum

Sternocostal part of
pectoralis major

Costal margin

Abdominal part of
pectoralis major
(from aponeurosis of
external oblique)

**Pectoralis major**

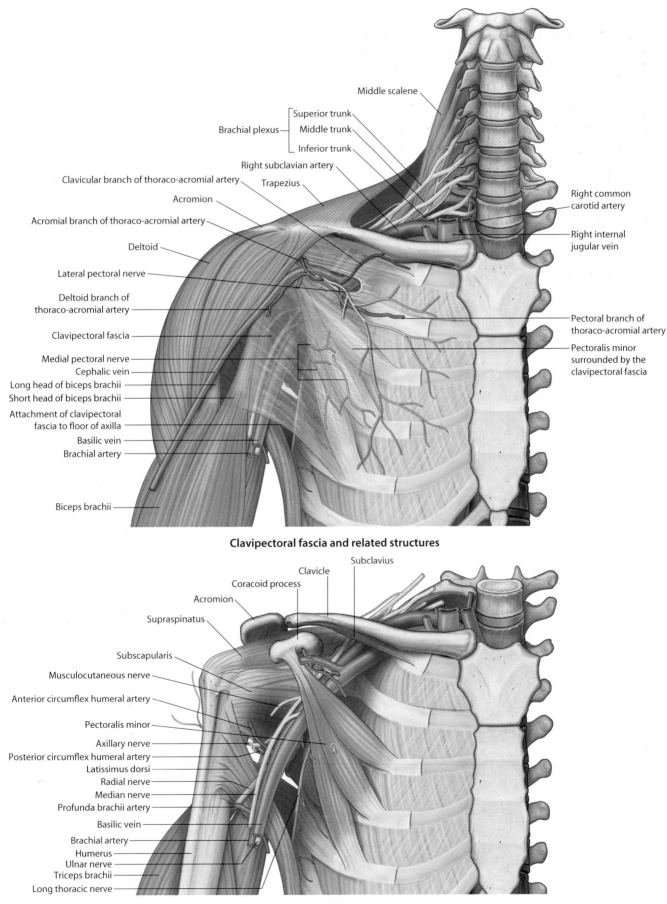

Middle scalene

Brachial plexus — Superior trunk
Middle trunk
Inferior trunk

Right subclavian artery

Clavicular branch of thoraco-acromial artery

Trapezius

Acromion

Acromial branch of thoraco-acromial artery

Deltoid

Lateral pectoral nerve

Deltoid branch of thoraco-acromial artery

Clavipectoral fascia

Medial pectoral nerve

Cephalic vein

Long head of biceps brachii

Short head of biceps brachii

Attachment of clavipectoral fascia to floor of axilla

Basilic vein

Brachial artery

Biceps brachii

Right common carotid artery

Right internal jugular vein

Pectoral branch of thoraco-acromial artery

Pectoralis minor surrounded by the clavipectoral fascia

**Clavipectoral fascia and related structures**

Subclavius

Clavicle

Coracoid process

Acromion

Supraspinatus

Subscapularis

Musculocutaneous nerve

Anterior circumflex humeral artery

Pectoralis minor

Axillary nerve

Posterior circumflex humeral artery

Latissimus dorsi

Radial nerve

Median nerve

Profunda brachii artery

Basilic vein

Brachial artery

Humerus

Ulnar nerve

Triceps brachii

Long thoracic nerve

**Pectoralis minor**

**361**

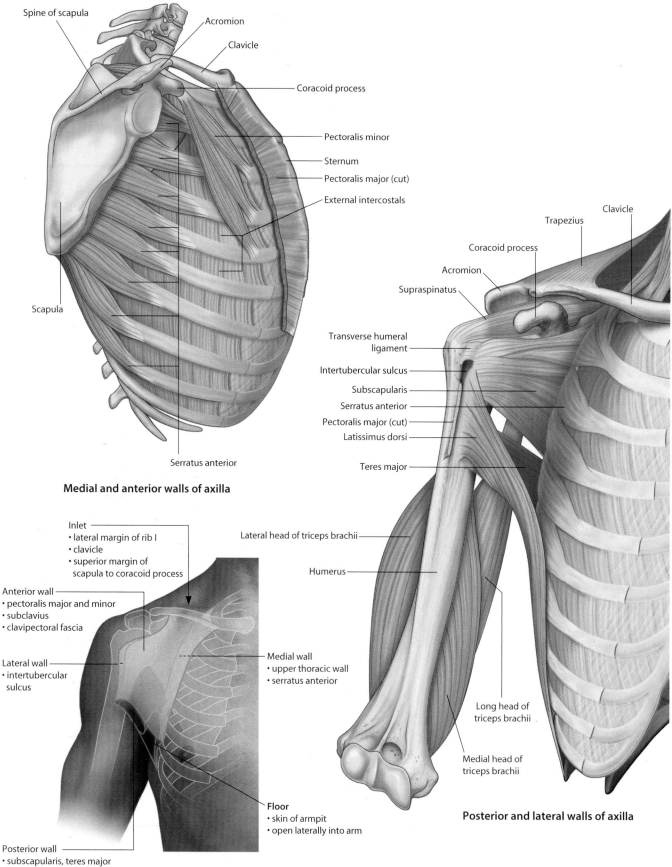

Spine of scapula

Acromion

Clavicle

Coracoid process

Pectoralis minor

Sternum

Pectoralis major (cut)

External intercostals

Scapula

Serratus anterior

**Medial and anterior walls of axilla**

Clavicle

Trapezius

Coracoid process

Acromion

Supraspinatus

Transverse humeral ligament

Intertubercular sulcus

Subscapularis

Serratus anterior

Pectoralis major (cut)

Latissimus dorsi

Teres major

Lateral head of triceps brachii

Humerus

Long head of triceps brachii

Medial head of triceps brachii

**Posterior and lateral walls of axilla**

Inlet
• lateral margin of rib I
• clavicle
• superior margin of scapula to coracoid process

Anterior wall
• pectoralis major and minor
• subclavius
• clavipectoral fascia

Lateral wall
• intertubercular sulcus

Medial wall
• upper thoracic wall
• serratus anterior

**Floor**
• skin of armpit
• open laterally into arm

Posterior wall
• subscapularis, teres major and latissimus dorsi, and long head of triceps brachii

**Boundaries of axilla**

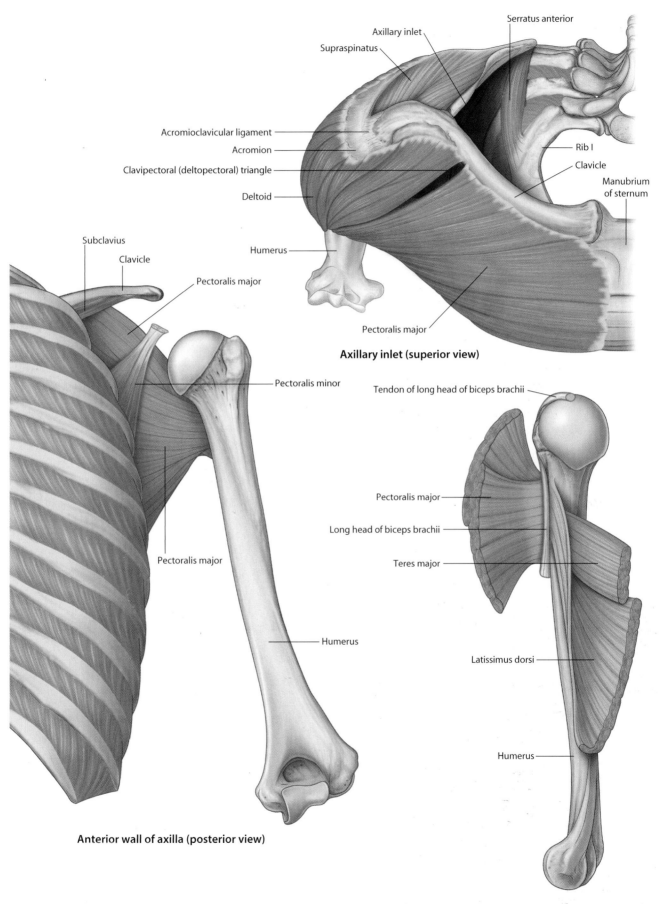

Axillary inlet (superior view)

Anterior wall of axilla (posterior view)

Lateral wall of axilla (medial view)

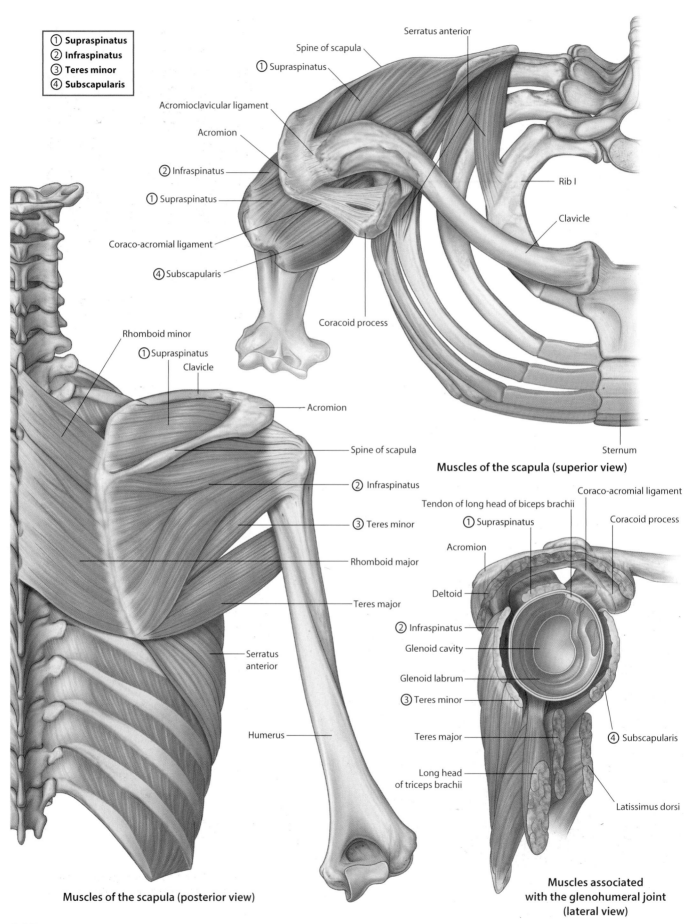

① **Supraspinatus**
② **Infraspinatus**
③ **Teres minor**
④ **Subscapularis**

Serratus anterior
Spine of scapula
① Supraspinatus
Acromioclavicular ligament
Acromion
② Infraspinatus
① Supraspinatus
Coraco-acromial ligament
④ Subscapularis
Coracoid process
Rib I
Clavicle
Sternum

**Muscles of the scapula (superior view)**

Rhomboid minor
① Supraspinatus
Clavicle
Acromion
Spine of scapula
② Infraspinatus
③ Teres minor
Rhomboid major
Teres major
Serratus anterior
Humerus

**Muscles of the scapula (posterior view)**

Coraco-acromial ligament
Tendon of long head of biceps brachii
Coracoid process
① Supraspinatus
Acromion
Deltoid
② Infraspinatus
Glenoid cavity
Glenoid labrum
③ Teres minor
Teres major
Long head of triceps brachii
④ Subscapularis
Latissimus dorsi

**Muscles associated with the glenohumeral joint (lateral view)**

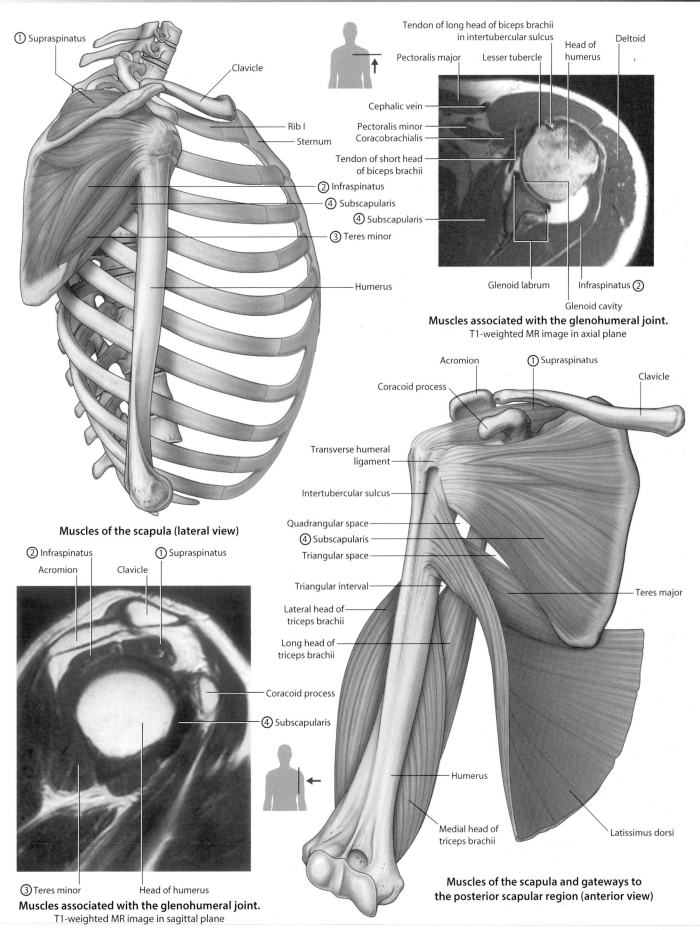

**Muscles of the scapula (lateral view)**

- ① Supraspinatus
- Clavicle
- Rib I
- Sternum
- ② Infraspinatus
- ④ Subscapularis
- ④ Subscapularis
- ③ Teres minor
- Humerus

Tendon of long head of biceps brachii in intertubercular sulcus
Pectoralis major — Lesser tubercle — Head of humerus — Deltoid
Cephalic vein
Pectoralis minor
Coracobrachialis
Tendon of short head of biceps brachii
Glenoid labrum — Infraspinatus ②
Glenoid cavity

**Muscles associated with the glenohumeral joint.**
T1-weighted MR image in axial plane

Acromion — ① Supraspinatus — Clavicle
Coracoid process
Transverse humeral ligament
Intertubercular sulcus
Quadrangular space
④ Subscapularis
Triangular space
Triangular interval
Lateral head of triceps brachii
Long head of triceps brachii
Teres major
Humerus
Medial head of triceps brachii
Latissimus dorsi

**Muscles of the scapula and gateways to the posterior scapular region (anterior view)**

② Infraspinatus — ① Supraspinatus
Acromion — Clavicle
Coracoid process
④ Subscapularis
③ Teres minor — Head of humerus

**Muscles associated with the glenohumeral joint.**
T1-weighted MR image in sagittal plane

**365**

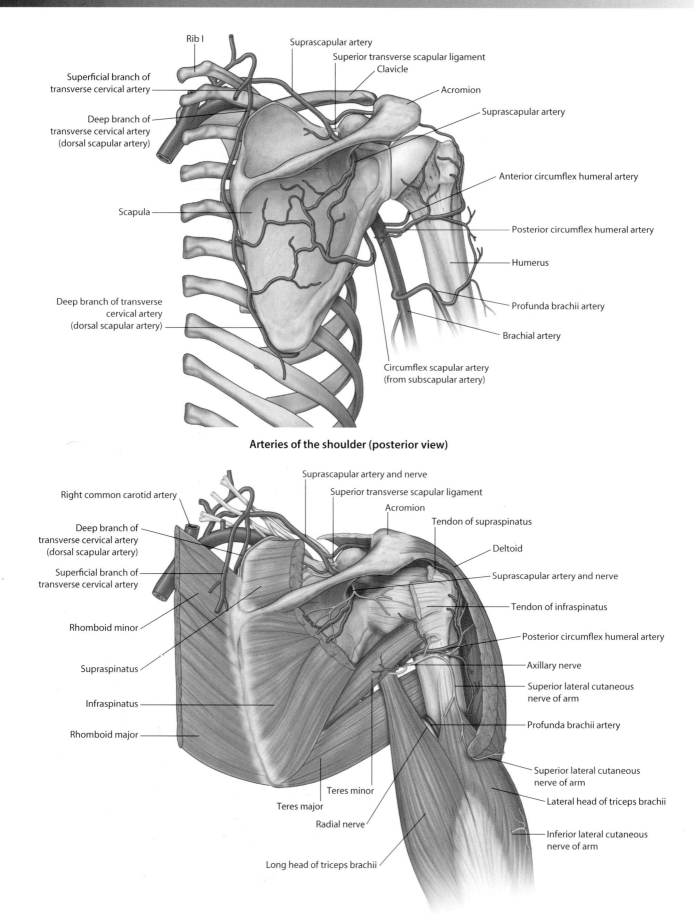

Rib I
Suprascapular artery
Superior transverse scapular ligament
Clavicle
Acromion
Suprascapular artery

Superficial branch of transverse cervical artery

Deep branch of transverse cervical artery (dorsal scapular artery)

Anterior circumflex humeral artery

Posterior circumflex humeral artery

Scapula

Humerus

Profunda brachii artery

Deep branch of transverse cervical artery (dorsal scapular artery)

Brachial artery

Circumflex scapular artery (from subscapular artery)

**Arteries of the shoulder (posterior view)**

Suprascapular artery and nerve
Superior transverse scapular ligament
Acromion
Tendon of supraspinatus

Right common carotid artery

Deltoid

Deep branch of transverse cervical artery (dorsal scapular artery)

Suprascapular artery and nerve

Superficial branch of transverse cervical artery

Tendon of infraspinatus

Rhomboid minor

Posterior circumflex humeral artery

Supraspinatus

Axillary nerve

Superior lateral cutaneous nerve of arm

Infraspinatus

Profunda brachii artery

Rhomboid major

Superior lateral cutaneous nerve of arm

Lateral head of triceps brachii

Teres minor

Teres major

Inferior lateral cutaneous nerve of arm

Radial nerve

Long head of triceps brachii

**Deep arteries and nerves of the shoulder (posterior view)**

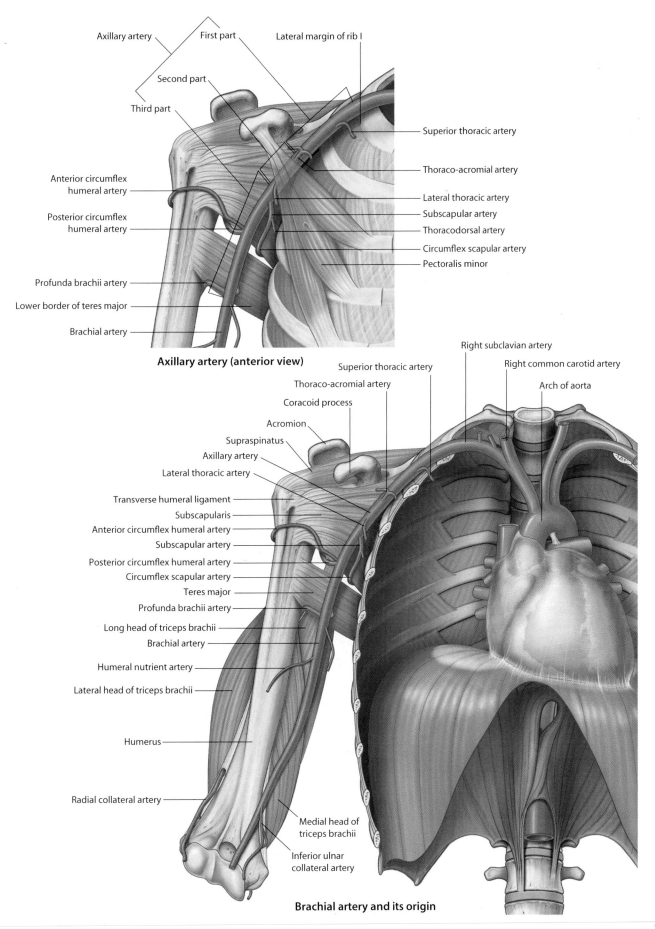

Axillary artery

First part

Lateral margin of rib I

Second part

Third part

Superior thoracic artery

Thoraco-acromial artery

Anterior circumflex
humeral artery

Lateral thoracic artery

Posterior circumflex
humeral artery

Subscapular artery

Thoracodorsal artery

Circumflex scapular artery

Pectoralis minor

Profunda brachii artery

Lower border of teres major

Brachial artery

**Axillary artery (anterior view)**

Superior thoracic artery

Right subclavian artery

Thoraco-acromial artery

Right common carotid artery

Coracoid process

Arch of aorta

Acromion

Supraspinatus

Axillary artery

Lateral thoracic artery

Transverse humeral ligament

Subscapularis

Anterior circumflex humeral artery

Subscapular artery

Posterior circumflex humeral artery

Circumflex scapular artery

Teres major

Profunda brachii artery

Long head of triceps brachii

Brachial artery

Humeral nutrient artery

Lateral head of triceps brachii

Humerus

Radial collateral artery

Medial head of
triceps brachii

Inferior ulnar
collateral artery

**Brachial artery and its origin**

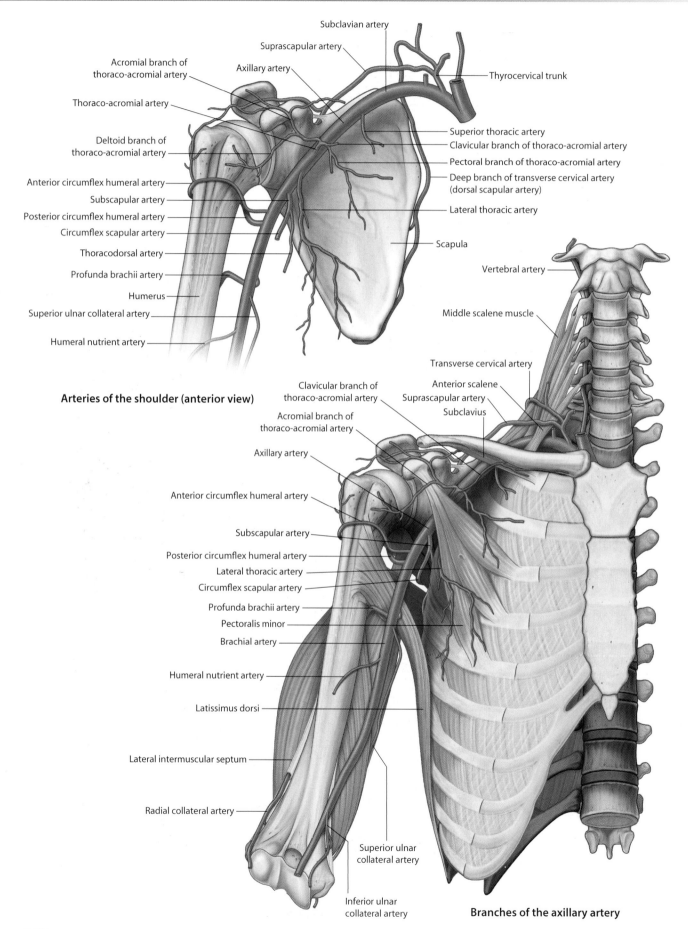

Acromial branch of
thoraco-acromial artery

Thoraco-acromial artery

Deltoid branch of
thoraco-acromial artery

Anterior circumflex humeral artery

Subscapular artery

Posterior circumflex humeral artery

Circumflex scapular artery

Thoracodorsal artery

Profunda brachii artery

Humerus

Superior ulnar collateral artery

Humeral nutrient artery

Subclavian artery

Suprascapular artery

Axillary artery

Thyrocervical trunk

Superior thoracic artery

Clavicular branch of thoraco-acromial artery

Pectoral branch of thoraco-acromial artery

Deep branch of transverse cervical artery
(dorsal scapular artery)

Lateral thoracic artery

Scapula

**Arteries of the shoulder (anterior view)**

Clavicular branch of
thoraco-acromial artery

Acromial branch of
thoraco-acromial artery

Axillary artery

Anterior circumflex humeral artery

Subscapular artery

Posterior circumflex humeral artery

Lateral thoracic artery

Circumflex scapular artery

Profunda brachii artery

Pectoralis minor

Brachial artery

Humeral nutrient artery

Latissimus dorsi

Lateral intermuscular septum

Radial collateral artery

Vertebral artery

Middle scalene muscle

Transverse cervical artery

Anterior scalene

Suprascapular artery

Subclavius

Superior ulnar
collateral artery

Inferior ulnar
collateral artery

**Branches of the axillary artery**

**368**

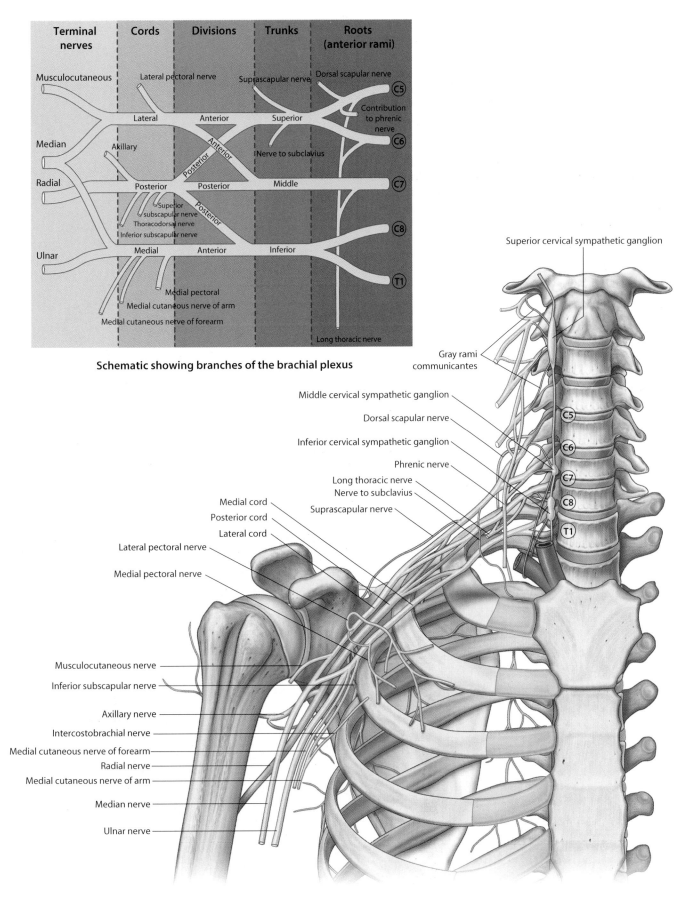

| Terminal nerves | Cords | Divisions | Trunks | Roots (anterior rami) |
|---|---|---|---|---|

Musculocutaneous

Lateral pectoral nerve

Suprascapular nerve

Dorsal scapular nerve

C5

Lateral

Anterior

Superior

Contribution to phrenic nerve

C6

Median

Axillary

Anterior

Nerve to subclavius

Radial

Posterior

Posterior

Middle

C7

Superior subscapular nerve
Thoracodorsal nerve
Inferior subscapular nerve

Posterior

C8

Ulnar

Medial

Anterior

Inferior

T1

Medial pectoral
Medial cutaneous nerve of arm
Medial cutaneous nerve of forearm

Long thoracic nerve

**Schematic showing branches of the brachial plexus**

Superior cervical sympathetic ganglion

Gray rami communicantes

Middle cervical sympathetic ganglion

Dorsal scapular nerve

Inferior cervical sympathetic ganglion

Phrenic nerve

Long thoracic nerve

Nerve to subclavius

Suprascapular nerve

Medial cord

Posterior cord

Lateral cord

Lateral pectoral nerve

Medial pectoral nerve

C5

C6

C7

C8

T1

Musculocutaneous nerve

Inferior subscapular nerve

Axillary nerve

Intercostobrachial nerve

Medial cutaneous nerve of forearm

Radial nerve

Medial cutaneous nerve of arm

Median nerve

Ulnar nerve

**Brachial plexus**

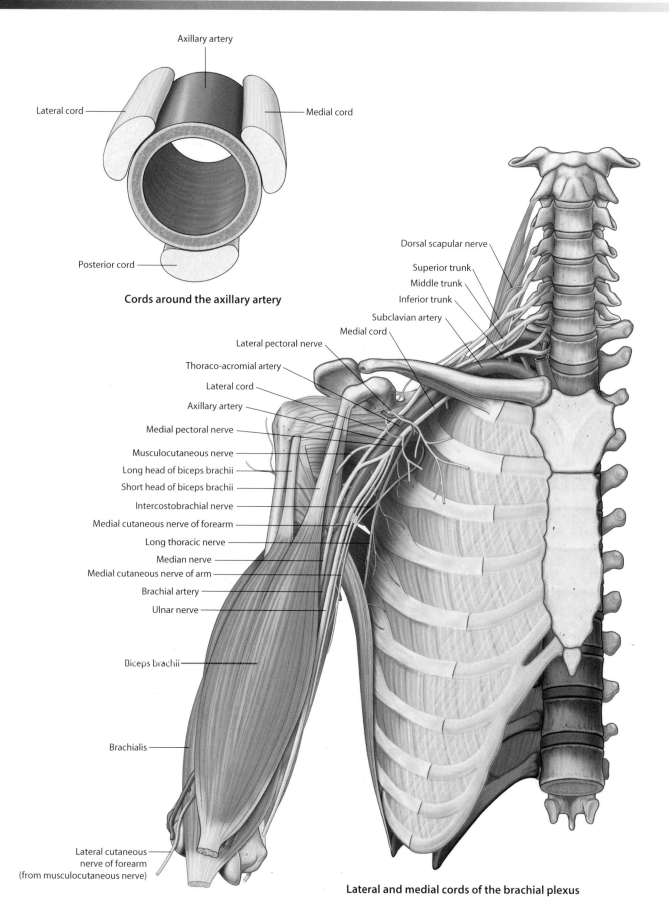

Axillary artery

Lateral cord

Medial cord

Posterior cord

**Cords around the axillary artery**

Dorsal scapular nerve

Superior trunk

Middle trunk

Inferior trunk

Subclavian artery

Medial cord

Lateral pectoral nerve

Thoraco-acromial artery

Lateral cord

Axillary artery

Medial pectoral nerve

Musculocutaneous nerve

Long head of biceps brachii

Short head of biceps brachii

Intercostobrachial nerve

Medial cutaneous nerve of forearm

Long thoracic nerve

Median nerve

Medial cutaneous nerve of arm

Brachial artery

Ulnar nerve

Biceps brachii

Brachialis

Lateral cutaneous
nerve of forearm
(from musculocutaneous nerve)

**Lateral and medial cords of the brachial plexus**

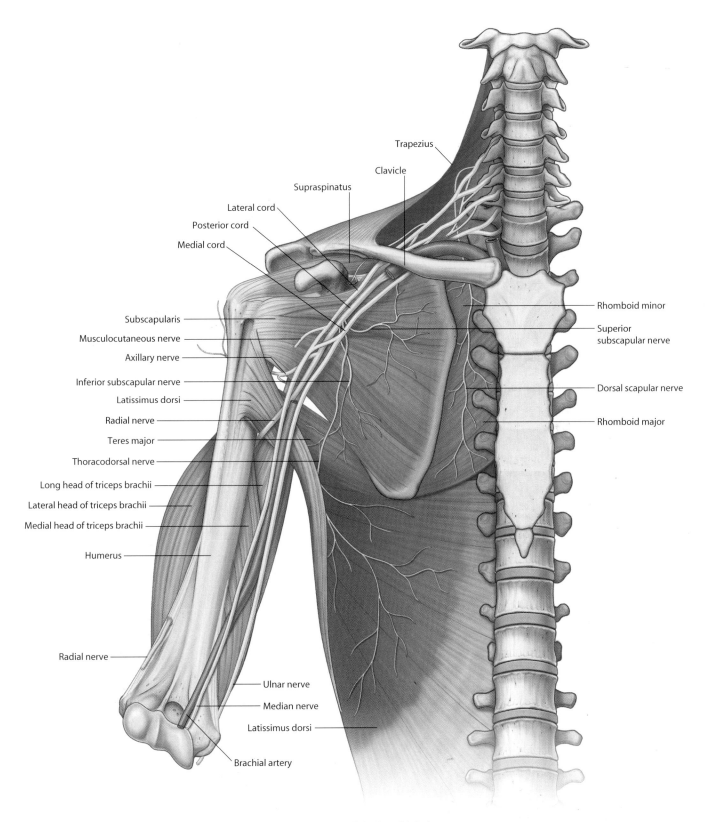

Trapezius

Clavicle

Supraspinatus

Lateral cord

Posterior cord

Medial cord

Subscapularis

Musculocutaneous nerve

Axillary nerve

Inferior subscapular nerve

Latissimus dorsi

Radial nerve

Teres major

Thoracodorsal nerve

Long head of triceps brachii

Lateral head of triceps brachii

Medial head of triceps brachii

Humerus

Radial nerve

Ulnar nerve

Median nerve

Latissimus dorsi

Brachial artery

Rhomboid minor

Superior subscapular nerve

Dorsal scapular nerve

Rhomboid major

**Posterior cord of the brachial plexus
(ribs and associated muscles removed)**

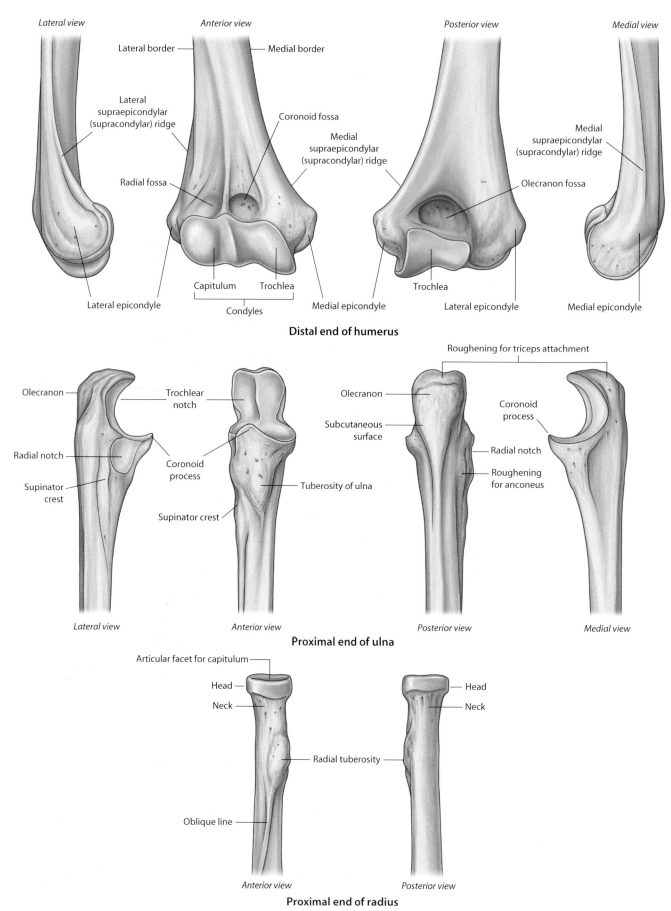

*Lateral view*　　*Anterior view*

Lateral border

Medial border

Lateral supraepicondylar (supracondylar) ridge

Coronoid fossa

Medial supraepicondylar (supracondylar) ridge

Radial fossa

Capitulum　　Trochlea

Condyles

Medial epicondyle

Lateral epicondyle

**Distal end of humerus**

*Posterior view*　　*Medial view*

Olecranon fossa

Medial supraepicondylar (supracondylar) ridge

Trochlea

Lateral epicondyle

Medial epicondyle

Roughening for triceps attachment

*Lateral view*　　*Anterior view*

Olecranon

Trochlear notch

Radial notch

Supinator crest

Coronoid process

Supinator crest

Tuberosity of ulna

*Posterior view*　　*Medial view*

Olecranon

Subcutaneous surface

Coronoid process

Radial notch

Roughening for anconeus

**Proximal end of ulna**

Articular facet for capitulum

Head

Neck

Radial tuberosity

Head

Neck

Oblique line

*Anterior view*　　*Posterior view*

**Proximal end of radius**

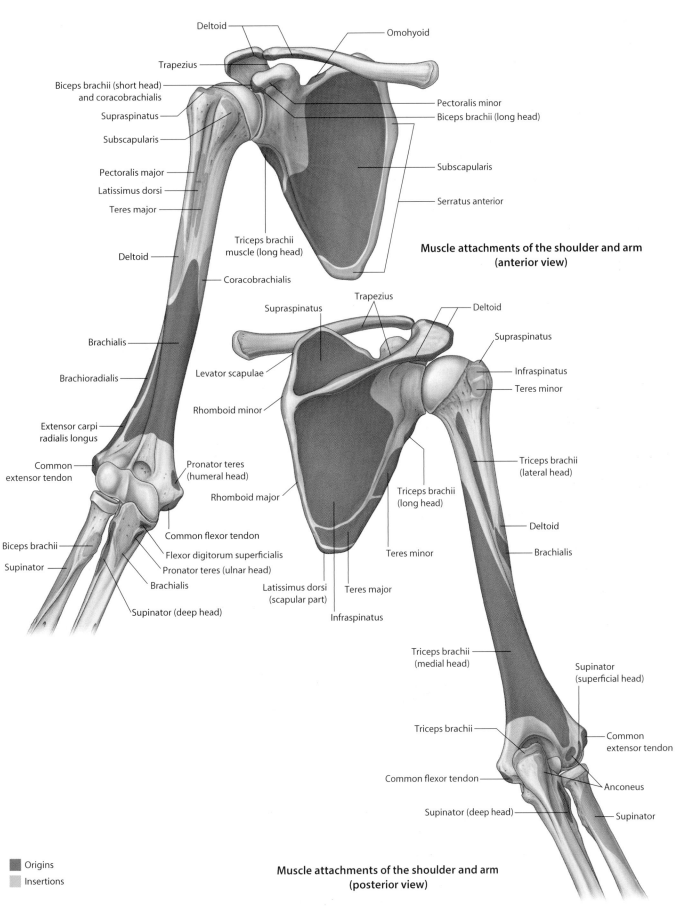

Muscle attachments of the shoulder and arm
(anterior view)

Muscle attachments of the shoulder and arm
(posterior view)

Deltoid
Omohyoid
Trapezius
Biceps brachii (short head)
and coracobrachialis
Supraspinatus
Subscapularis
Pectoralis major
Latissimus dorsi
Teres major
Deltoid
Triceps brachii
muscle (long head)
Coracobrachialis
Pectoralis minor
Biceps brachii (long head)
Subscapularis
Serratus anterior

Brachialis
Brachioradialis
Extensor carpi
radialis longus
Common
extensor tendon
Biceps brachii
Supinator

Supraspinatus
Levator scapulae
Rhomboid minor
Rhomboid major

Trapezius
Deltoid
Supraspinatus
Infraspinatus
Teres minor

Pronator teres
(humeral head)
Common flexor tendon
Flexor digitorum superficialis
Pronator teres (ulnar head)
Brachialis
Supinator (deep head)

Triceps brachii
(long head)
Teres minor
Latissimus dorsi
(scapular part)
Teres major
Infraspinatus

Triceps brachii
(lateral head)
Deltoid
Brachialis

Triceps brachii
(medial head)

Triceps brachii

Common flexor tendon

Supinator
(superficial head)

Common
extensor tendon
Anconeus
Supinator

Supinator (deep head)

Origins
Insertions

373

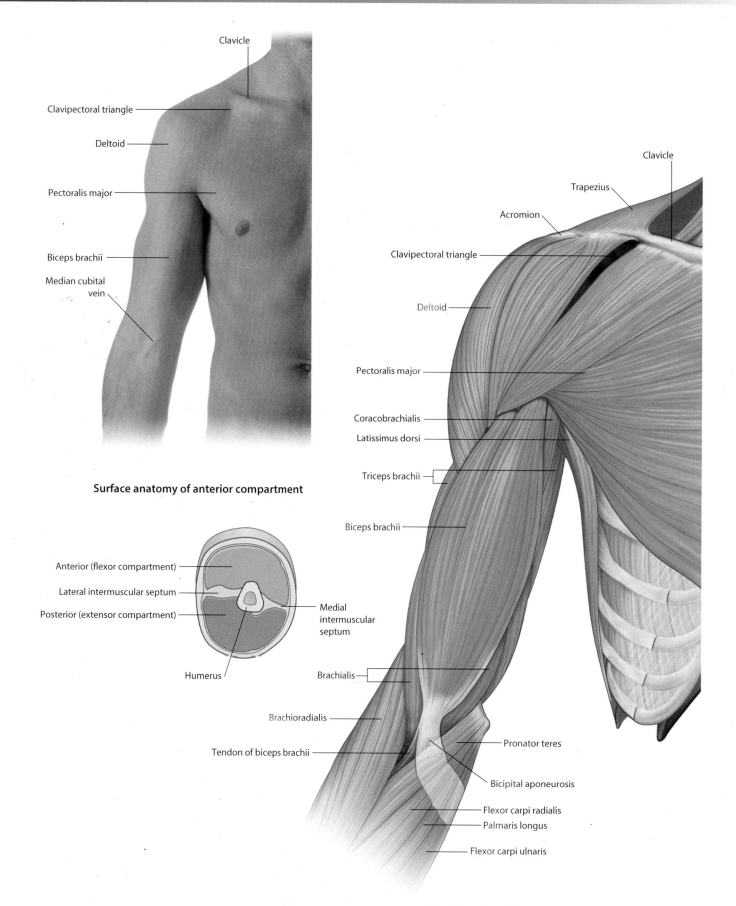

Clavicle

Clavipectoral triangle

Deltoid

Pectoralis major

Biceps brachii

Median cubital vein

**Surface anatomy of anterior compartment**

Anterior (flexor compartment)

Lateral intermuscular septum

Posterior (extensor compartment)

Medial intermuscular septum

Humerus

Clavicle

Trapezius

Acromion

Clavipectoral triangle

Deltoid

Pectoralis major

Coracobrachialis

Latissimus dorsi

Triceps brachii

Biceps brachii

Brachialis

Brachioradialis

Tendon of biceps brachii

Pronator teres

Bicipital aponeurosis

Flexor carpi radialis

Palmaris longus

Flexor carpi ulnaris

**Muscles of anterior compartment of arm**

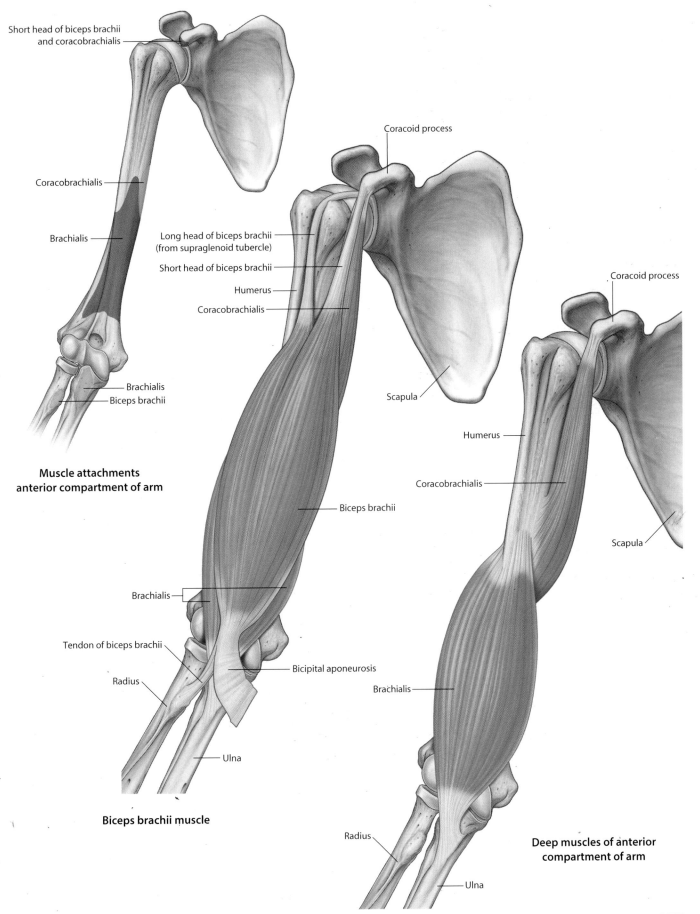

Short head of biceps brachii and coracobrachialis

Coracobrachialis

Brachialis

**Muscle attachments anterior compartment of arm**

Brachialis
Biceps brachii

Coracoid process

Long head of biceps brachii (from supraglenoid tubercle)

Short head of biceps brachii

Humerus

Coracobrachialis

Scapula

Biceps brachii

Brachialis

Tendon of biceps brachii

Radius

Bicipital aponeurosis

Ulna

**Biceps brachii muscle**

Coracoid process

Humerus

Coracobrachialis

Scapula

Brachialis

Radius

Ulna

**Deep muscles of anterior compartment of arm**

**375**

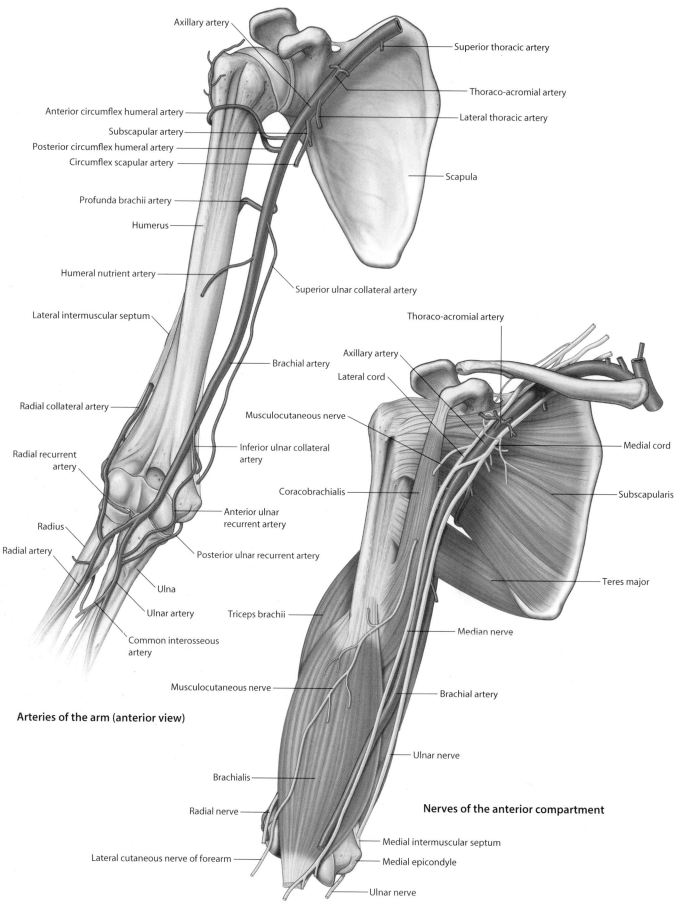

Axillary artery

Superior thoracic artery

Thoraco-acromial artery

Anterior circumflex humeral artery

Lateral thoracic artery

Subscapular artery

Posterior circumflex humeral artery

Circumflex scapular artery

Scapula

Profunda brachii artery

Humerus

Humeral nutrient artery

Superior ulnar collateral artery

Lateral intermuscular septum

Brachial artery

Thoraco-acromial artery

Axillary artery

Lateral cord

Radial collateral artery

Musculocutaneous nerve

Medial cord

Radial recurrent artery

Inferior ulnar collateral artery

Coracobrachialis

Subscapularis

Radius

Anterior ulnar recurrent artery

Radial artery

Posterior ulnar recurrent artery

Teres major

Ulna

Ulnar artery

Triceps brachii

Median nerve

Common interosseous artery

Musculocutaneous nerve

Brachial artery

**Arteries of the arm (anterior view)**

Ulnar nerve

Brachialis

Radial nerve

**Nerves of the anterior compartment**

Medial intermuscular septum

Medial epicondyle

Lateral cutaneous nerve of forearm

Ulnar nerve

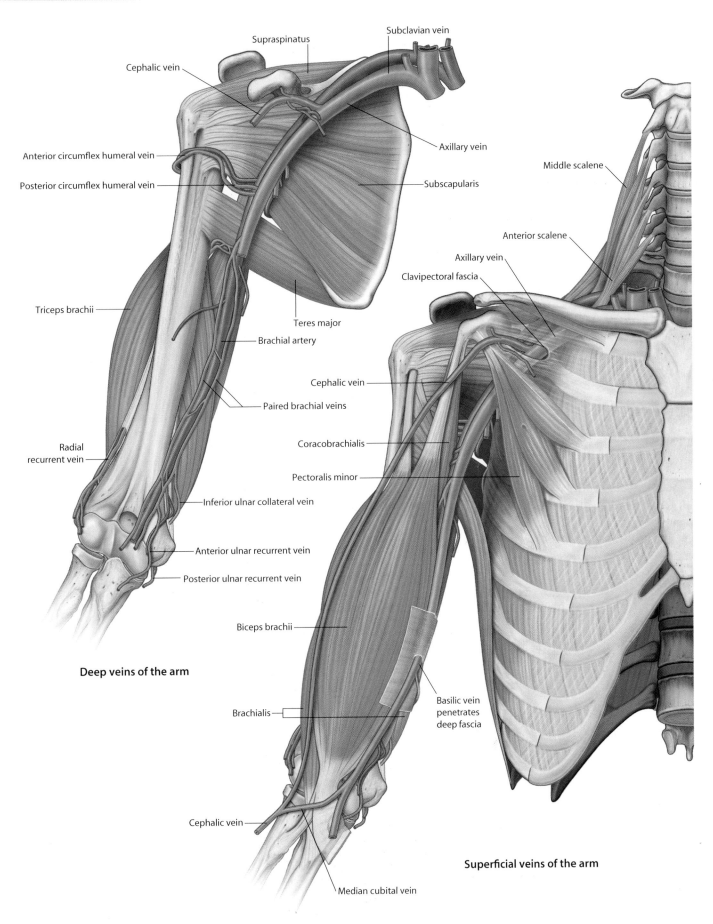

Supraspinatus

Subclavian vein

Cephalic vein

Anterior circumflex humeral vein

Posterior circumflex humeral vein

Axillary vein

Subscapularis

Middle scalene

Anterior scalene

Axillary vein

Clavipectoral fascia

Triceps brachii

Teres major

Brachial artery

Cephalic vein

Paired brachial veins

Coracobrachialis

Radial
recurrent vein

Pectoralis minor

Inferior ulnar collateral vein

Anterior ulnar recurrent vein

Posterior ulnar recurrent vein

Biceps brachii

**Deep veins of the arm**

Brachialis

Basilic vein
penetrates
deep fascia

Cephalic vein

**Superficial veins of the arm**

Median cubital vein

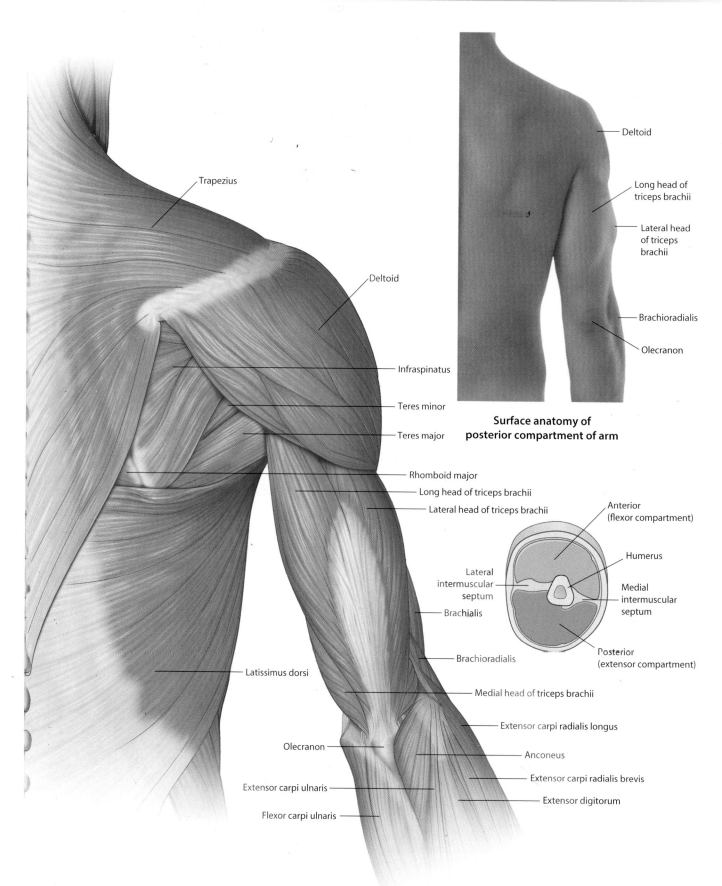

Trapezius

Deltoid

Infraspinatus

Teres minor

Teres major

Rhomboid major

Long head of triceps brachii

Lateral head of triceps brachii

Brachialis

Brachioradialis

Latissimus dorsi

Medial head of triceps brachii

Olecranon

Extensor carpi ulnaris

Flexor carpi ulnaris

Deltoid

Long head of triceps brachii

Lateral head of triceps brachii

Brachioradialis

Olecranon

**Surface anatomy of posterior compartment of arm**

Anterior (flexor compartment)

Humerus

Lateral intermuscular septum

Medial intermuscular septum

Brachialis

Posterior (extensor compartment)

Extensor carpi radialis longus

Anconeus

Extensor carpi radialis brevis

Extensor digitorum

**Muscles of posterior compartment of arm**

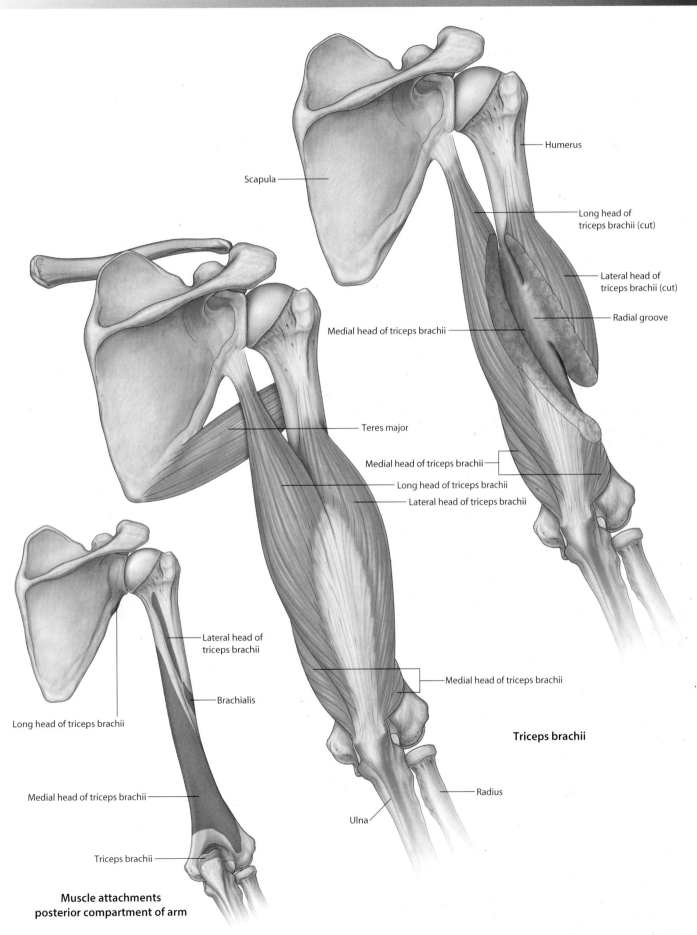

Humerus

Scapula

Long head of
triceps brachii (cut)

Lateral head of
triceps brachii (cut)

Radial groove

Medial head of triceps brachii

Medial head of triceps brachii

Long head of triceps brachii

Lateral head of triceps brachii

Teres major

**Triceps brachii**

Lateral head of
triceps brachii

Medial head of triceps brachii

Brachialis

Radius

Long head of triceps brachii

Medial head of triceps brachii

Ulna

Triceps brachii

**Muscle attachments
posterior compartment of arm**

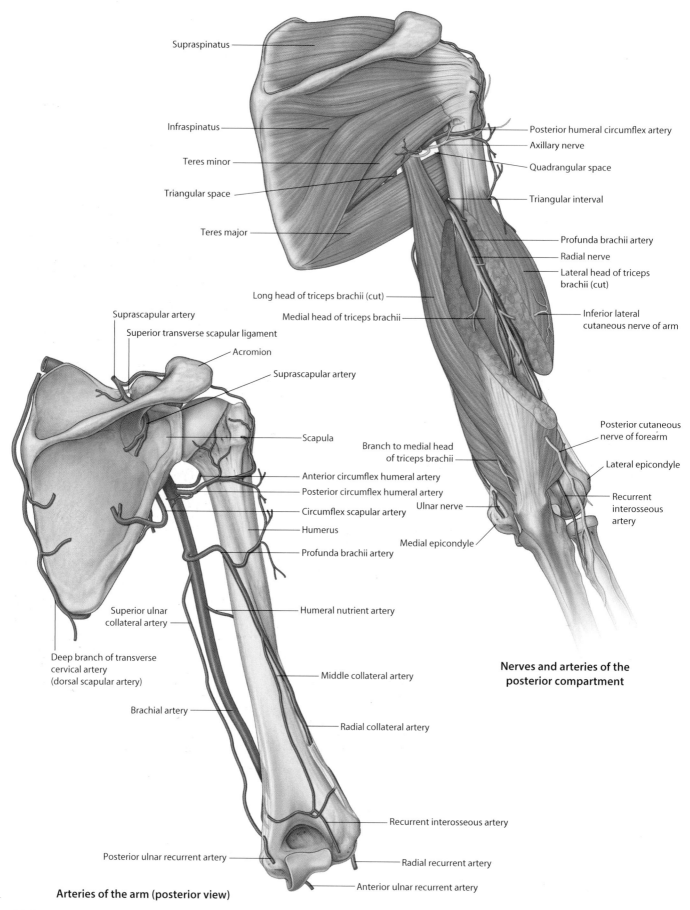

Supraspinatus

Infraspinatus

Teres minor

Triangular space

Teres major

Posterior humeral circumflex artery

Axillary nerve

Quadrangular space

Triangular interval

Profunda brachii artery

Radial nerve

Lateral head of triceps brachii (cut)

Long head of triceps brachii (cut)

Medial head of triceps brachii

Inferior lateral cutaneous nerve of arm

Suprascapular artery

Superior transverse scapular ligament

Acromion

Suprascapular artery

Scapula

Branch to medial head of triceps brachii

Anterior circumflex humeral artery

Posterior circumflex humeral artery

Circumflex scapular artery

Humerus

Profunda brachii artery

Humeral nutrient artery

Posterior cutaneous nerve of forearm

Lateral epicondyle

Ulnar nerve

Medial epicondyle

Recurrent interosseous artery

Superior ulnar collateral artery

Deep branch of transverse cervical artery (dorsal scapular artery)

Brachial artery

Middle collateral artery

Radial collateral artery

**Nerves and arteries of the posterior compartment**

Recurrent interosseous artery

Posterior ulnar recurrent artery

Radial recurrent artery

Anterior ulnar recurrent artery

**Arteries of the arm (posterior view)**

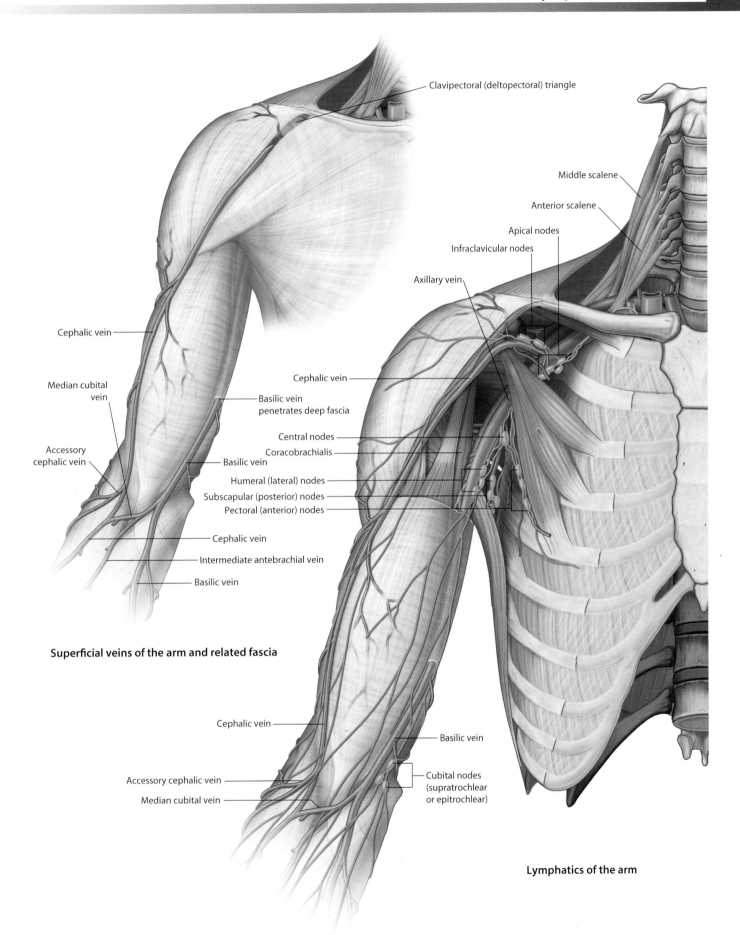

Clavipectoral (deltopectoral) triangle

Middle scalene

Anterior scalene

Apical nodes

Infraclavicular nodes

Axillary vein

Cephalic vein

Cephalic vein

Median cubital vein

Basilic vein penetrates deep fascia

Central nodes

Coracobrachialis

Accessory cephalic vein

Basilic vein

Humeral (lateral) nodes

Subscapular (posterior) nodes

Pectoral (anterior) nodes

Cephalic vein

Intermediate antebrachial vein

Basilic vein

**Superficial veins of the arm and related fascia**

Cephalic vein

Basilic vein

Accessory cephalic vein

Cubital nodes (supratrochlear or epitrochlear)

Median cubital vein

**Lymphatics of the arm**

**A**

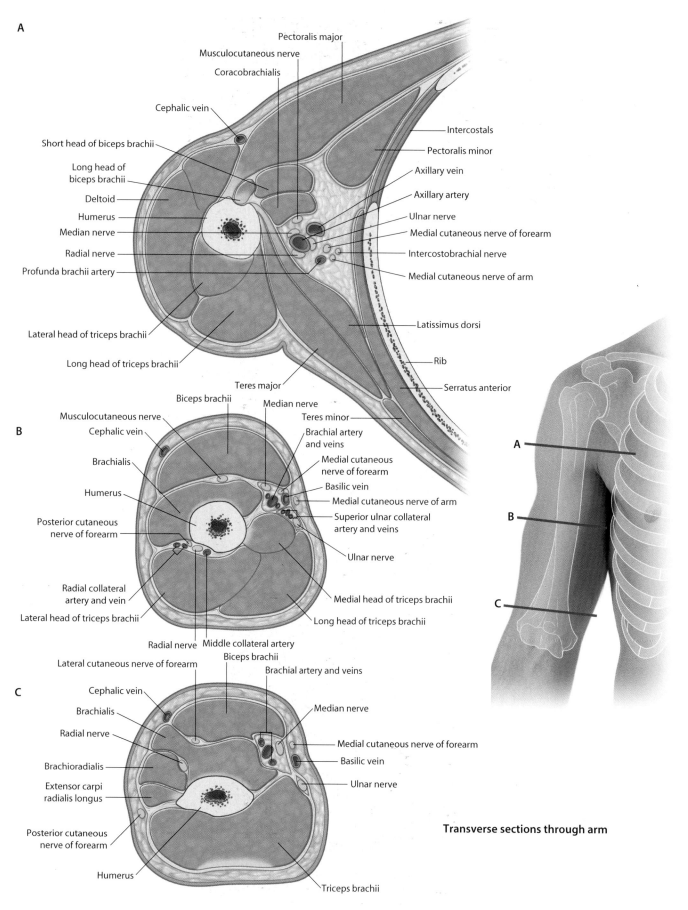

Pectoralis major

Musculocutaneous nerve

Coracobrachialis

Cephalic vein

Short head of biceps brachii

Long head of biceps brachii

Deltoid

Humerus

Median nerve

Radial nerve

Profunda brachii artery

Lateral head of triceps brachii

Long head of triceps brachii

Intercostals

Pectoralis minor

Axillary vein

Axillary artery

Ulnar nerve

Medial cutaneous nerve of forearm

Intercostobrachial nerve

Medial cutaneous nerve of arm

Latissimus dorsi

Rib

Serratus anterior

Teres major

**B**

Biceps brachii

Musculocutaneous nerve

Cephalic vein

Brachialis

Humerus

Posterior cutaneous nerve of forearm

Radial collateral artery and vein

Lateral head of triceps brachii

Radial nerve

Lateral cutaneous nerve of forearm

Median nerve

Teres minor

Brachial artery and veins

Medial cutaneous nerve of forearm

Basilic vein

Medial cutaneous nerve of arm

Superior ulnar collateral artery and veins

Ulnar nerve

Medial head of triceps brachii

Long head of triceps brachii

Middle collateral artery

Biceps brachii

**C**

Brachial artery and veins

Cephalic vein

Brachialis

Radial nerve

Brachioradialis

Extensor carpi radialis longus

Posterior cutaneous nerve of forearm

Humerus

Median nerve

Medial cutaneous nerve of forearm

Basilic vein

Ulnar nerve

Triceps brachii

**Transverse sections through arm**

**382**

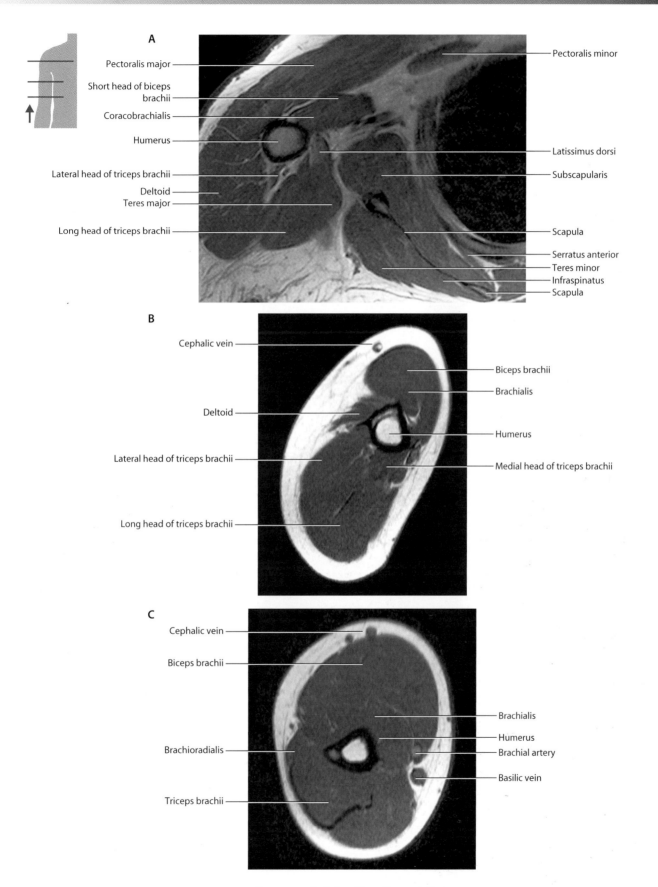

Pectoralis major

Short head of biceps brachii

Coracobrachialis

Humerus

Lateral head of triceps brachii

Deltoid

Teres major

Long head of triceps brachii

Pectoralis minor

Latissimus dorsi

Subscapularis

Scapula

Serratus anterior

Teres minor

Infraspinatus

Scapula

Cephalic vein

Deltoid

Lateral head of triceps brachii

Long head of triceps brachii

Biceps brachii

Brachialis

Humerus

Medial head of triceps brachii

Cephalic vein

Biceps brachii

Brachioradialis

Triceps brachii

Brachialis

Humerus

Brachial artery

Basilic vein

**Transverse/axial sections through the arm.**
**A. Proximal/upper arm.  B. Middle arm.  C. Distal/lower arm.**
T1-weighted MR image in axial plane

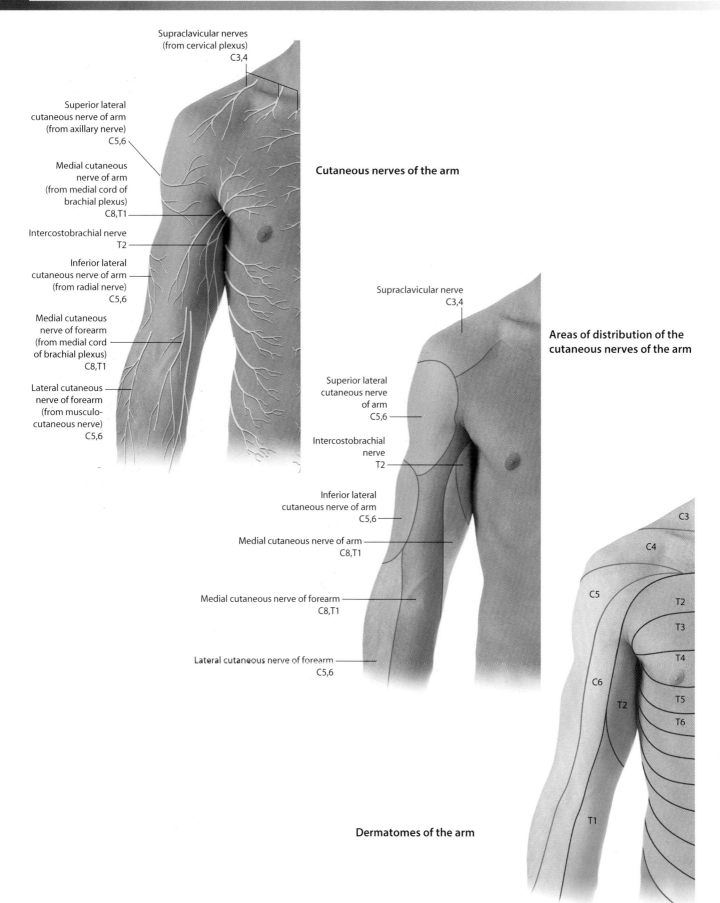

Supraclavicular nerves
(from cervical plexus)
C3,4

Superior lateral
cutaneous nerve of arm
(from axillary nerve)
C5,6

Medial cutaneous
nerve of arm
(from medial cord of
brachial plexus)
C8,T1

Intercostobrachial nerve
T2

Inferior lateral
cutaneous nerve of arm
(from radial nerve)
C5,6

Medial cutaneous
nerve of forearm
(from medial cord
of brachial plexus)
C8,T1

Lateral cutaneous
nerve of forearm
(from musculo-
cutaneous nerve)
C5,6

**Cutaneous nerves of the arm**

Supraclavicular nerve
C3,4

Superior lateral
cutaneous nerve
of arm
C5,6

Intercostobrachial
nerve
T2

Inferior lateral
cutaneous nerve of arm
C5,6

Medial cutaneous nerve of arm
C8,T1

Medial cutaneous nerve of forearm
C8,T1

Lateral cutaneous nerve of forearm
C5,6

**Areas of distribution of the
cutaneous nerves of the arm**

C3
C4
C5
T2
T3
T4
C6
T2
T5
T6
T1

**Dermatomes of the arm**

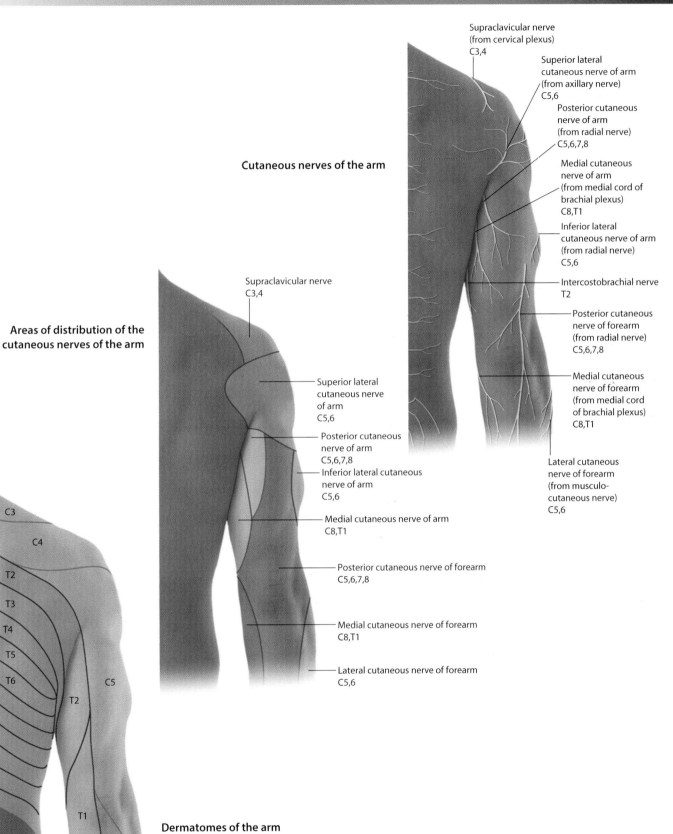

**Cutaneous nerves of the arm**

Supraclavicular nerve
(from cervical plexus)
C3,4

Superior lateral
cutaneous nerve of arm
(from axillary nerve)
C5,6

Posterior cutaneous
nerve of arm
(from radial nerve)
C5,6,7,8

Medial cutaneous
nerve of arm
(from medial cord of
brachial plexus)
C8,T1

Inferior lateral
cutaneous nerve of arm
(from radial nerve)
C5,6

Intercostobrachial nerve
T2

Posterior cutaneous
nerve of forearm
(from radial nerve)
C5,6,7,8

Medial cutaneous
nerve of forearm
(from medial cord
of brachial plexus)
C8,T1

Lateral cutaneous
nerve of forearm
(from musculo-
cutaneous nerve)
C5,6

**Areas of distribution of the
cutaneous nerves of the arm**

Supraclavicular nerve
C3,4

Superior lateral
cutaneous nerve
of arm
C5,6

Posterior cutaneous
nerve of arm
C5,6,7,8

Inferior lateral cutaneous
nerve of arm
C5,6

Medial cutaneous nerve of arm
C8,T1

Posterior cutaneous nerve of forearm
C5,6,7,8

Medial cutaneous nerve of forearm
C8,T1

Lateral cutaneous nerve of forearm
C5,6

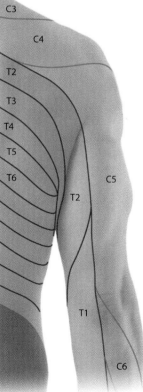

C3

C4

T2

T3

T4

T5

T6

C5

T2

T1

C6

**Dermatomes of the arm**

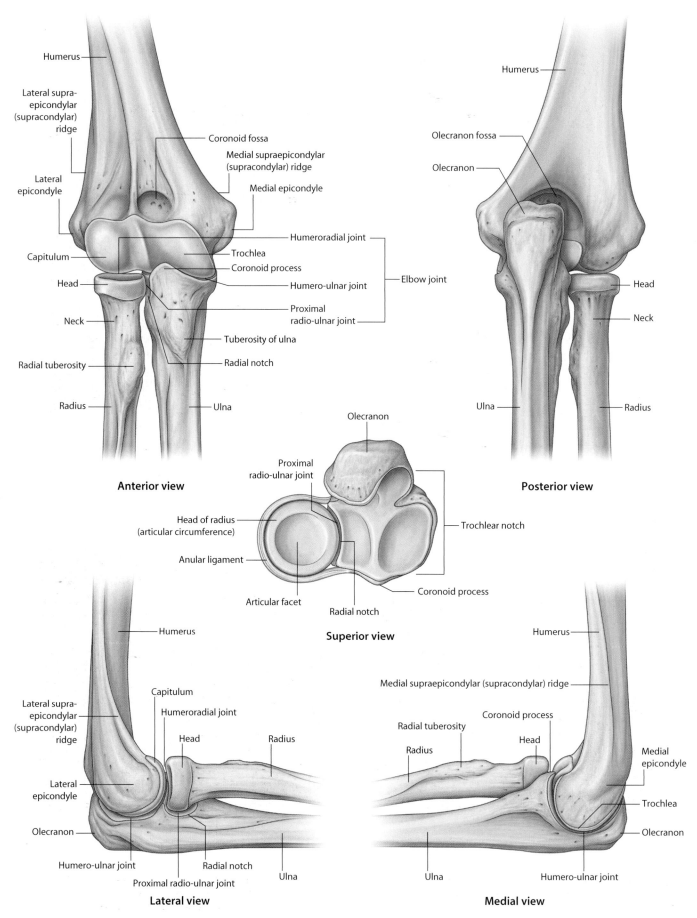

**Anterior view**

Humerus

Lateral supra-epicondylar (supracondylar) ridge

Lateral epicondyle

Capitulum

Head

Neck

Radial tuberosity

Radius

Coronoid fossa

Medial supraepicondylar (supracondylar) ridge

Medial epicondyle

Humeroradial joint

Trochlea

Coronoid process

Humero-ulnar joint

Proximal radio-ulnar joint

Tuberosity of ulna

Radial notch

Ulna

Elbow joint

**Posterior view**

Humerus

Olecranon fossa

Olecranon

Head

Neck

Ulna

Radius

**Superior view**

Olecranon

Proximal radio-ulnar joint

Head of radius (articular circumference)

Anular ligament

Articular facet

Radial notch

Trochlear notch

Coronoid process

**Lateral view**

Humerus

Lateral supra-epicondylar (supracondylar) ridge

Lateral epicondyle

Olecranon

Humero-ulnar joint

Proximal radio-ulnar joint

Capitulum

Humeroradial joint

Head

Radius

Radial notch

Ulna

**Medial view**

Humerus

Medial supraepicondylar (supracondylar) ridge

Radial tuberosity

Radius

Coronoid process

Head

Medial epicondyle

Trochlea

Olecranon

Ulna

Humero-ulnar joint

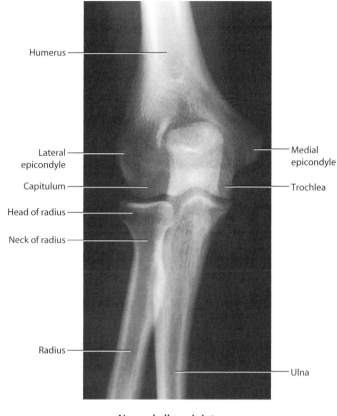

Normal elbow joint.
Radiograph, AP view

Humerus

Lateral epicondyle

Capitulum

Head of radius

Neck of radius

Radius

Medial epicondyle

Trochlea

Ulna

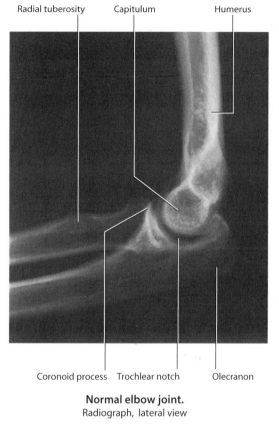

Normal elbow joint.
Radiograph, lateral view

Radial tuberosity  Capitulum  Humerus

Coronoid process  Trochlear notch  Olecranon

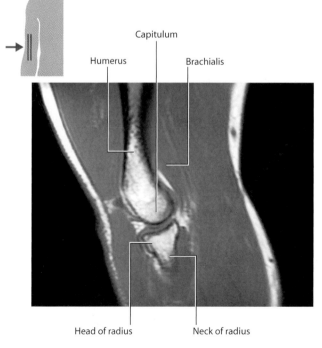

Capitulum

Humerus  Brachialis

Head of radius  Neck of radius

**Articulation of the capitulum of the humerus and the head of the radius at the elbow joint.**
T2-weighted MR image in sagittal plane

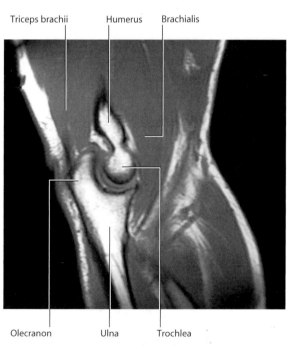

Triceps brachii  Humerus  Brachialis

Olecranon  Ulna  Trochlea

**Articulation of the trochlea of the humerus and the trochlear notch of the ulna.**
T2-weighted MR image in sagittal plane

**387**

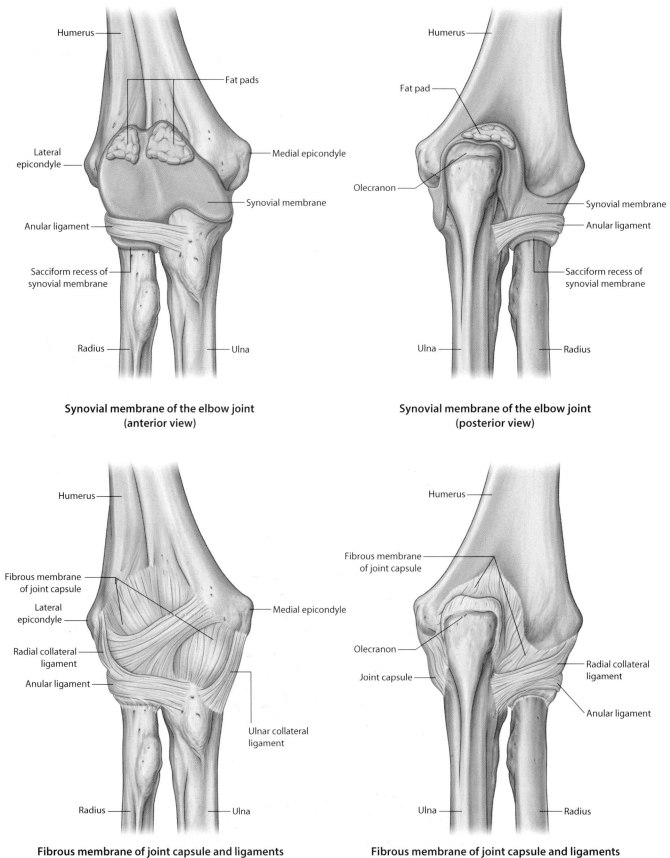

Humerus

Fat pads

Lateral epicondyle

Medial epicondyle

Synovial membrane

Anular ligament

Sacciform recess of synovial membrane

Radius

Ulna

**Synovial membrane of the elbow joint (anterior view)**

Humerus

Fat pad

Olecranon

Synovial membrane

Anular ligament

Sacciform recess of synovial membrane

Ulna

Radius

**Synovial membrane of the elbow joint (posterior view)**

Humerus

Fibrous membrane of joint capsule

Lateral epicondyle

Medial epicondyle

Radial collateral ligament

Anular ligament

Ulnar collateral ligament

Radius

Ulna

**Fibrous membrane of joint capsule and ligaments of the elbow joint (anterior view)**

Humerus

Fibrous membrane of joint capsule

Olecranon

Joint capsule

Radial collateral ligament

Anular ligament

Ulna

Radius

**Fibrous membrane of joint capsule and ligaments of the elbow joint (posterior view)**

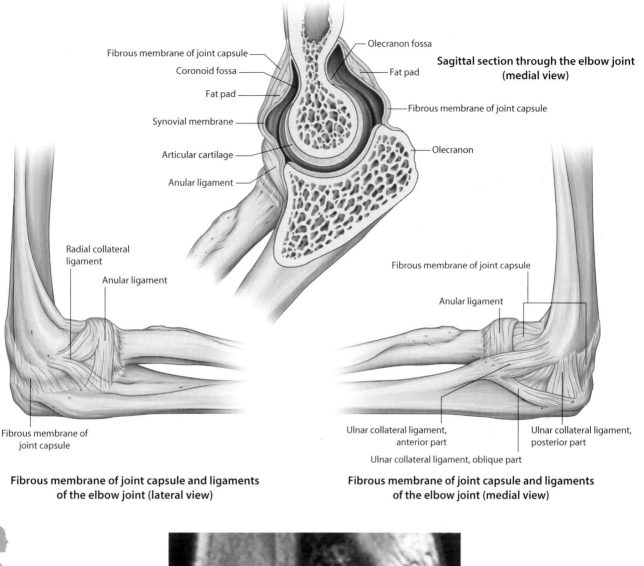

Fibrous membrane of joint capsule

Coronoid fossa

Fat pad

Synovial membrane

Articular cartilage

Anular ligament

Olecranon fossa

Fat pad

**Sagittal section through the elbow joint (medial view)**

Fibrous membrane of joint capsule

Olecranon

Radial collateral ligament

Anular ligament

Fibrous membrane of joint capsule

Fibrous membrane of joint capsule

Anular ligament

Ulnar collateral ligament, anterior part

Ulnar collateral ligament, oblique part

Ulnar collateral ligament, posterior part

**Fibrous membrane of joint capsule and ligaments of the elbow joint (lateral view)**

**Fibrous membrane of joint capsule and ligaments of the elbow joint (medial view)**

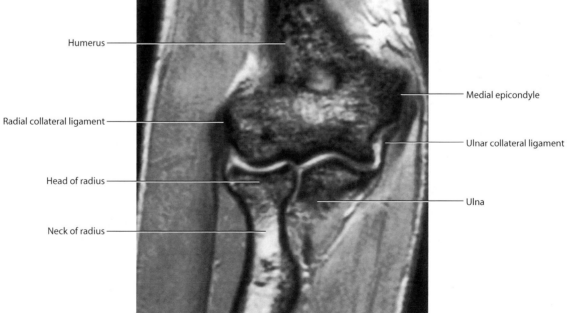

Humerus

Radial collateral ligament

Head of radius

Neck of radius

Medial epicondyle

Ulnar collateral ligament

Ulna

**Normal elbow joint.**
T2-weighted MR image in coronal plane

**389**

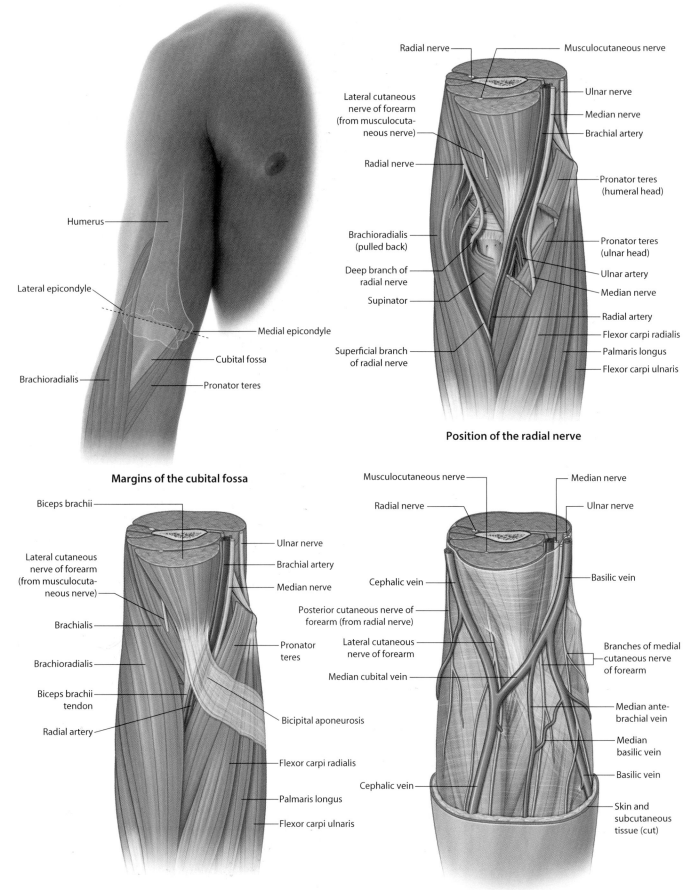

Radial nerve

Musculocutaneous nerve

Ulnar nerve

Median nerve

Brachial artery

Lateral cutaneous nerve of forearm (from musculocutaneous nerve)

Radial nerve

Pronator teres (humeral head)

Brachioradialis (pulled back)

Deep branch of radial nerve

Pronator teres (ulnar head)

Ulnar artery

Supinator

Median nerve

Radial artery

Flexor carpi radialis

Superficial branch of radial nerve

Palmaris longus

Flexor carpi ulnaris

**Position of the radial nerve**

Humerus

Lateral epicondyle

Medial epicondyle

Cubital fossa

Brachioradialis

Pronator teres

**Margins of the cubital fossa**

Biceps brachii

Ulnar nerve

Brachial artery

Median nerve

Lateral cutaneous nerve of forearm (from musculocutaneous nerve)

Brachialis

Brachioradialis

Pronator teres

Biceps brachii tendon

Radial artery

Bicipital aponeurosis

Flexor carpi radialis

Palmaris longus

Flexor carpi ulnaris

**Contents of the cubital fossa**

Musculocutaneous nerve

Median nerve

Radial nerve

Ulnar nerve

Cephalic vein

Basilic vein

Posterior cutaneous nerve of forearm (from radial nerve)

Lateral cutaneous nerve of forearm

Median cubital vein

Branches of medial cutaneous nerve of forearm

Median antebrachial vein

Median basilic vein

Basilic vein

Cephalic vein

Skin and subcutaneous tissue (cut)

**Superficial structures**

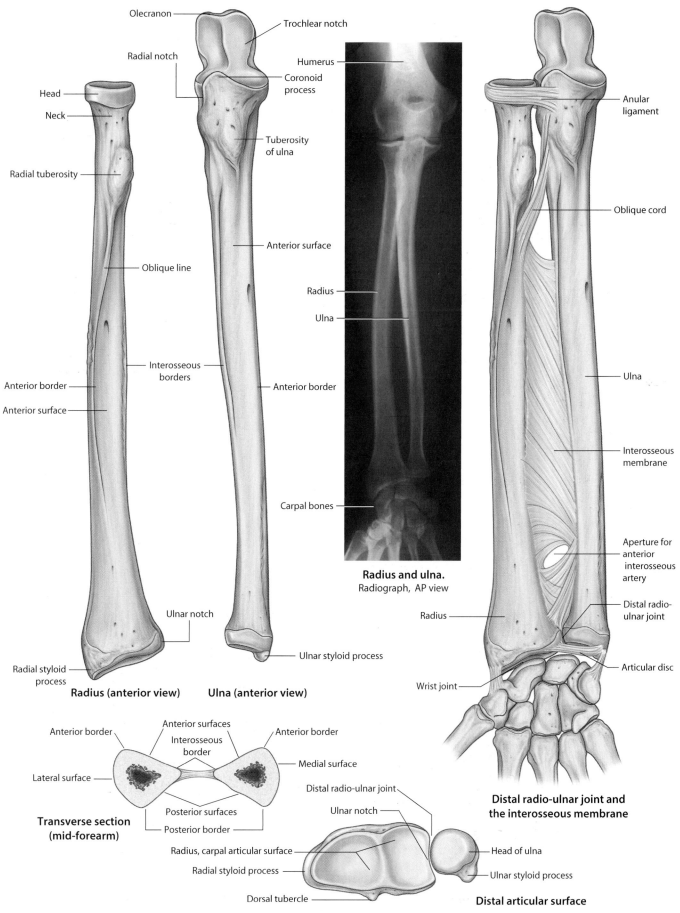

**Radius and ulna.**
Radiograph, AP view

**Radius (anterior view)**    **Ulna (anterior view)**

**Distal radio-ulnar joint and the interosseous membrane**

**Transverse section (mid-forearm)**

**Distal articular surface**

**391**

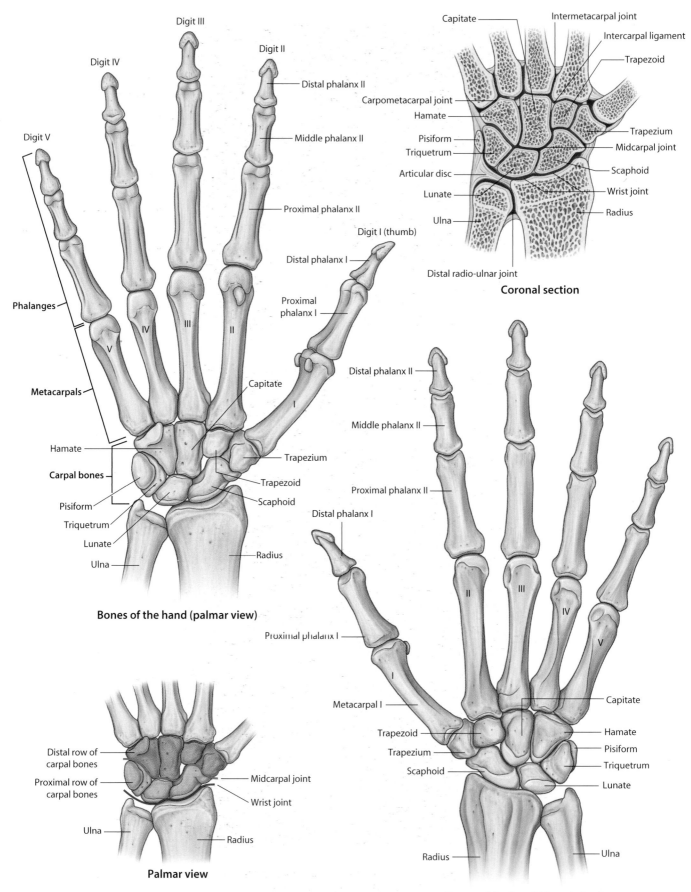

Digit III

Digit IV

Digit II

Distal phalanx II

Middle phalanx II

Digit V

Proximal phalanx II

Digit I (thumb)

Phalanges

Distal phalanx I

Proximal phalanx I

IV

III

II

V

Capitate

Metacarpals

I

Trapezium

Hamate

Trapezoid

Carpal bones

Scaphoid

Pisiform

Triquetrum

Lunate

Ulna

Radius

**Bones of the hand (palmar view)**

Capitate

Intermetacarpal joint

Intercarpal ligament

Trapezoid

Carpometacarpal joint

Hamate

Trapezium

Pisiform

Midcarpal joint

Triquetrum

Scaphoid

Articular disc

Wrist joint

Lunate

Radius

Ulna

Distal radio-ulnar joint

**Coronal section**

Distal phalanx II

Middle phalanx II

Proximal phalanx II

Distal phalanx I

II

III

IV

V

Proximal phalanx I

I

Capitate

Metacarpal I

Hamate

Trapezoid

Pisiform

Trapezium

Triquetrum

Scaphoid

Lunate

Radius

Ulna

**Bones of the hand (dorsal view)**

Distal row of
carpal bones

Proximal row of
carpal bones

Midcarpal joint

Wrist joint

Ulna

Radius

**Palmar view**

392

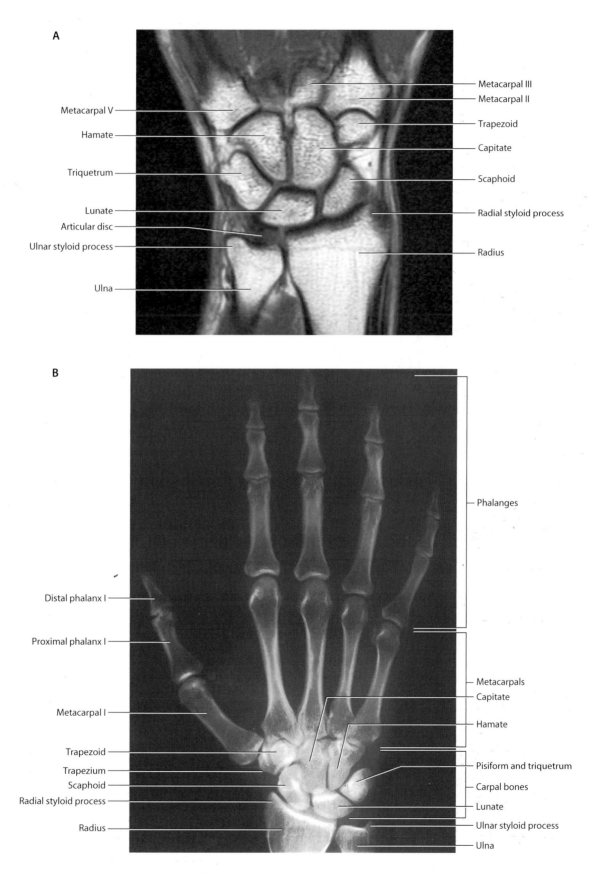

**A**

Metacarpal V

Hamate

Triquetrum

Lunate

Articular disc

Ulnar styloid process

Ulna

Metacarpal III

Metacarpal II

Trapezoid

Capitate

Scaphoid

Radial styloid process

Radius

**B**

Distal phalanx I

Proximal phalanx I

Metacarpal I

Trapezoid

Trapezium

Scaphoid

Radial styloid process

Radius

Phalanges

Metacarpals

Capitate

Hamate

Pisiform and triquetrum

Carpal bones

Lunate

Ulnar styloid process

Ulna

**Imaging of the wrist joint, the carpal bones, and the hand.**
A. T1-weighted MR image in coronal plane
B. Radiograph, AP view

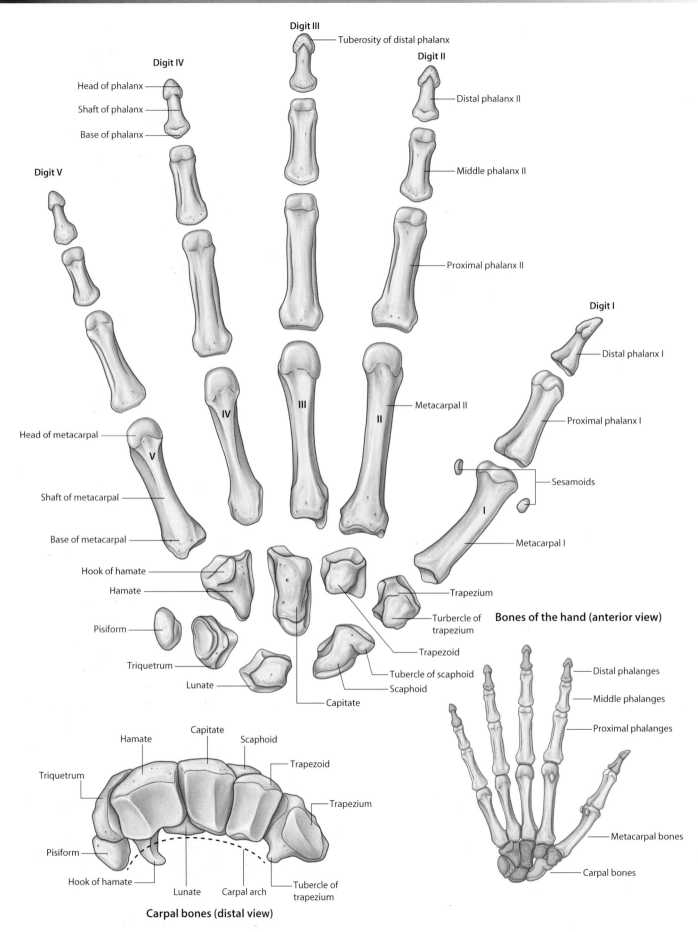

**Digit III**
Tuberosity of distal phalanx

**Digit IV**
Head of phalanx
Shaft of phalanx
Base of phalanx

**Digit II**
Distal phalanx II

Middle phalanx II

**Digit V**

Proximal phalanx II

**Digit I**

Distal phalanx I

Proximal phalanx I

Metacarpal II

Sesamoids

Head of metacarpal

Metacarpal I

Shaft of metacarpal

Base of metacarpal

**Bones of the hand (anterior view)**

Hook of hamate
Hamate

Trapezium

Turbercle of trapezium

Pisiform

Trapezoid

Triquetrum

Tubercle of scaphoid

Lunate

Scaphoid

Capitate

Distal phalanges

Middle phalanges

Proximal phalanges

Hamate

Capitate

Scaphoid

Triquetrum

Trapezoid

Trapezium

Metacarpal bones

Pisiform

Carpal bones

Hook of hamate

Lunate

Carpal arch

Tubercle of trapezium

**Carpal bones (distal view)**

394

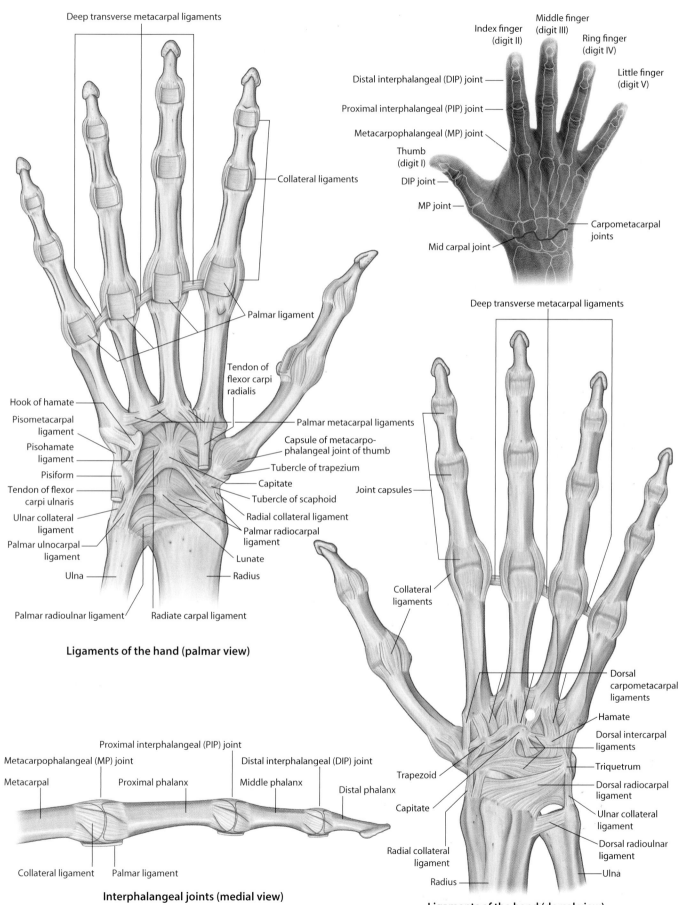

Deep transverse metacarpal ligaments

Collateral ligaments

Palmar ligament

Hook of hamate
Pisometacarpal ligament
Pisohamate ligament
Pisiform
Tendon of flexor carpi ulnaris
Ulnar collateral ligament
Palmar ulnocarpal ligament
Ulna
Palmar radioulnar ligament

Tendon of flexor carpi radialis

Palmar metacarpal ligaments
Capsule of metacarpo-phalangeal joint of thumb
Tubercle of trapezium
Capitate
Tubercle of scaphoid
Radial collateral ligament
Palmar radiocarpal ligament
Lunate
Radius
Radiate carpal ligament

**Ligaments of the hand (palmar view)**

Index finger (digit II)
Middle finger (digit III)
Ring finger (digit IV)
Little finger (digit V)

Distal interphalangeal (DIP) joint
Proximal interphalangeal (PIP) joint
Metacarpophalangeal (MP) joint
Thumb (digit I)
DIP joint
MP joint
Mid carpal joint
Carpometacarpal joints

Deep transverse metacarpal ligaments

Joint capsules

Collateral ligaments

Trapezoid
Capitate
Radial collateral ligament
Radius

Dorsal carpometacarpal ligaments
Hamate
Dorsal intercarpal ligaments
Triquetrum
Dorsal radiocarpal ligament
Ulnar collateral ligament
Dorsal radioulnar ligament
Ulna

**Ligaments of the hand (dorsal view)**

Metacarpophalangeal (MP) joint
Proximal interphalangeal (PIP) joint
Distal interphalangeal (DIP) joint
Metacarpal
Proximal phalanx
Middle phalanx
Distal phalanx

Collateral ligament
Palmar ligament

**Interphalangeal joints (medial view)**

**395**

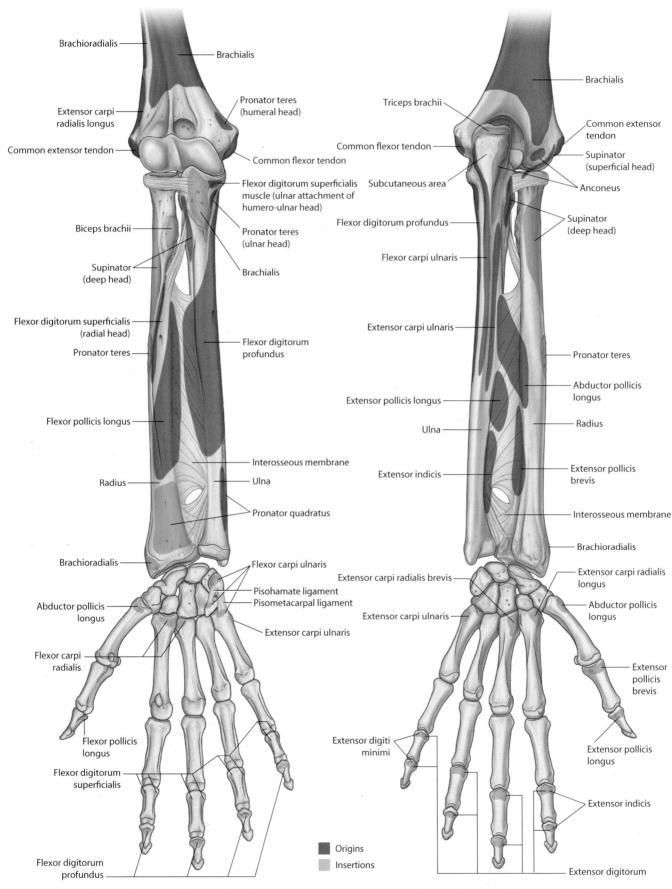

Brachioradialis

Brachialis

Extensor carpi radialis longus

Pronator teres (humeral head)

Common extensor tendon

Common flexor tendon

Flexor digitorum superficialis muscle (ulnar attachment of humero-ulnar head)

Biceps brachii

Pronator teres (ulnar head)

Supinator (deep head)

Brachialis

Flexor digitorum superficialis (radial head)

Pronator teres

Flexor digitorum profundus

Flexor pollicis longus

Interosseous membrane

Radius

Ulna

Pronator quadratus

Brachioradialis

Flexor carpi ulnaris

Pisohamate ligament
Pisometacarpal ligament

Abductor pollicis longus

Extensor carpi ulnaris

Flexor carpi radialis

Flexor pollicis longus

Flexor digitorum superficialis

Flexor digitorum profundus

**Muscle attachments of forearm (anterior view)**

Brachialis

Triceps brachii

Common extensor tendon

Common flexor tendon

Supinator (superficial head)

Subcutaneous area

Anconeus

Flexor digitorum profundus

Supinator (deep head)

Flexor carpi ulnaris

Extensor carpi ulnaris

Pronator teres

Abductor pollicis longus

Extensor pollicis longus

Radius

Ulna

Extensor indicis

Extensor pollicis brevis

Interosseous membrane

Brachioradialis

Extensor carpi radialis brevis

Extensor carpi radialis longus

Abductor pollicis longus

Extensor carpi ulnaris

Extensor pollicis brevis

Extensor digiti minimi

Extensor pollicis longus

Extensor indicis

Extensor digitorum

■ Origins
■ Insertions

**Muscle attachments of forearm (posterior view)**

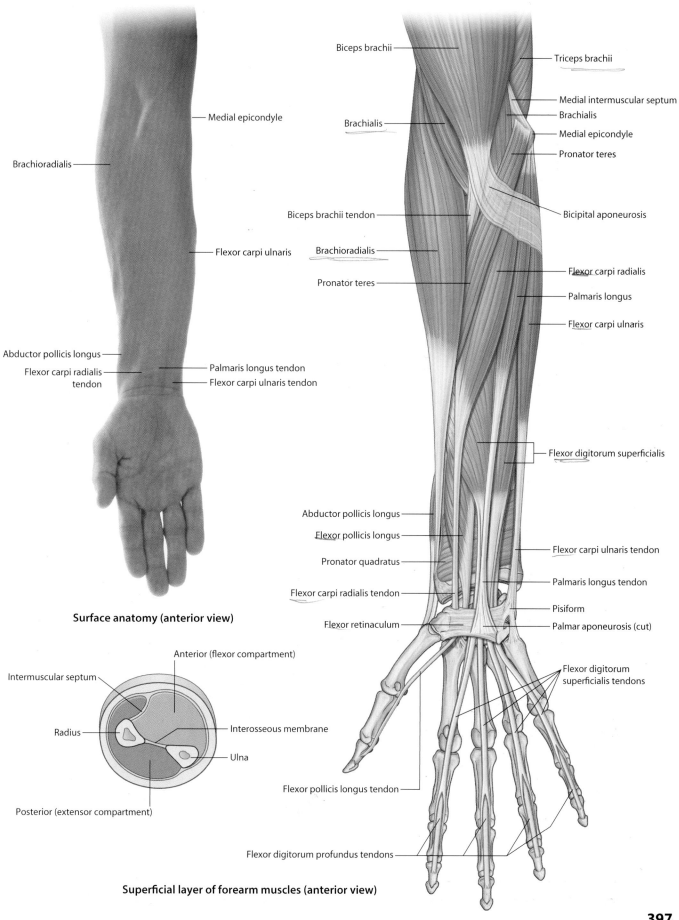

**Surface anatomy (anterior view)**

Brachioradialis

Medial epicondyle

Flexor carpi ulnaris

Abductor pollicis longus

Flexor carpi radialis tendon

Palmaris longus tendon

Flexor carpi ulnaris tendon

Biceps brachii

Triceps brachii

Medial intermuscular septum

Brachialis

Medial epicondyle

Pronator teres

Brachialis

Biceps brachii tendon

Bicipital aponeurosis

Brachioradialis

Flexor carpi radialis

Pronator teres

Palmaris longus

Flexor carpi ulnaris

Flexor digitorum superficialis

Abductor pollicis longus

Flexor pollicis longus

Flexor carpi ulnaris tendon

Pronator quadratus

Palmaris longus tendon

Flexor carpi radialis tendon

Pisiform

Flexor retinaculum

Palmar aponeurosis (cut)

Flexor digitorum superficialis tendons

Flexor pollicis longus tendon

Flexor digitorum profundus tendons

Intermuscular septum

Anterior (flexor compartment)

Radius

Interosseous membrane

Ulna

Posterior (extensor compartment)

**Superficial layer of forearm muscles (anterior view)**

**397**

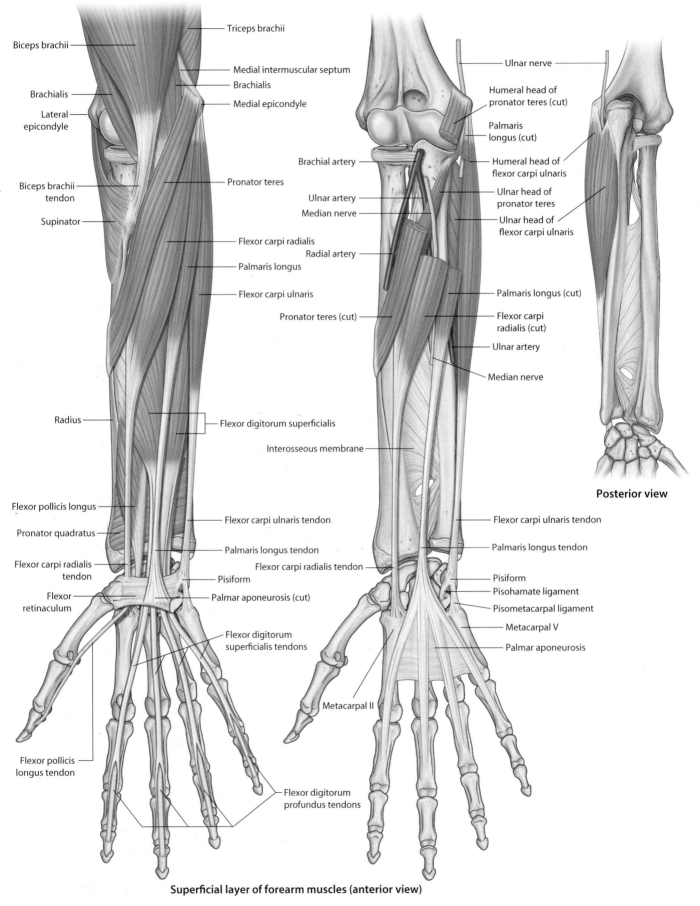

Biceps brachii

Triceps brachii

Medial intermuscular septum

Brachialis

Brachialis

Medial epicondyle

Lateral epicondyle

Ulnar nerve

Humeral head of pronator teres (cut)

Palmaris longus (cut)

Brachial artery

Humeral head of flexor carpi ulnaris

Biceps brachii tendon

Pronator teres

Ulnar artery

Ulnar head of pronator teres

Supinator

Median nerve

Ulnar head of flexor carpi ulnaris

Flexor carpi radialis

Palmaris longus

Radial artery

Palmaris longus (cut)

Flexor carpi ulnaris

Pronator teres (cut)

Flexor carpi radialis (cut)

Ulnar artery

Median nerve

Radius

Flexor digitorum superficialis

Interosseous membrane

Flexor pollicis longus

Pronator quadratus

Flexor carpi ulnaris tendon

Flexor carpi ulnaris tendon

Palmaris longus tendon

Palmaris longus tendon

Flexor carpi radialis tendon

Flexor carpi radialis tendon

Pisiform

Pisiform

Pisohamate ligament

Pisometacarpal ligament

Flexor retinaculum

Palmar aponeurosis (cut)

Metacarpal V

Palmar aponeurosis

Flexor digitorum superficialis tendons

Metacarpal II

Flexor pollicis longus tendon

Flexor digitorum profundus tendons

**Posterior view**

**Superficial layer of forearm muscles (anterior view)**

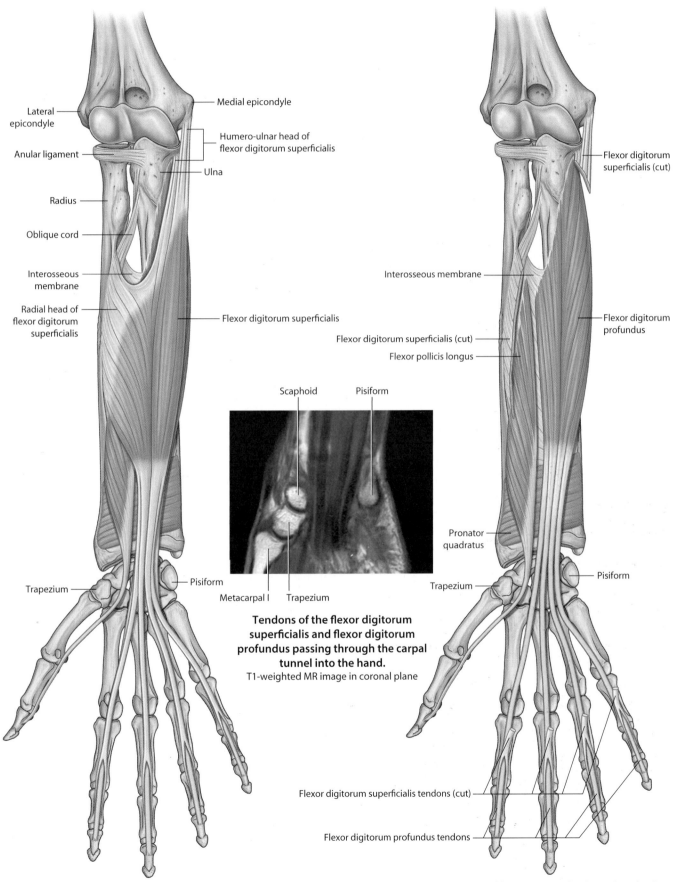

**Intermediate layer of forearm muscles (anterior view)**

Lateral epicondyle

Anular ligament

Radius

Oblique cord

Interosseous membrane

Radial head of flexor digitorum superficialis

Trapezium

Medial epicondyle

Humero-ulnar head of flexor digitorum superficialis

Ulna

Flexor digitorum superficialis

Pisiform

Scaphoid

Pisiform

Metacarpal I

Trapezium

**Tendons of the flexor digitorum superficialis and flexor digitorum profundus passing through the carpal tunnel into the hand.**
T1-weighted MR image in coronal plane

Flexor digitorum superficialis (cut)

Interosseous membrane

Flexor digitorum profundus

Flexor digitorum superficialis (cut)

Flexor pollicis longus

Pronator quadratus

Trapezium

Pisiform

Flexor digitorum superficialis tendons (cut)

Flexor digitorum profundus tendons

**Deep layer of forearm muscles (anterior view)**

Biceps brachii

Posterior cutaneous nerve of forearm (cut) (from radial nerve)

Lateral cutaneous nerve of forearm (cut) (from musculocutaneous nerve)

Biceps brachii tendon

Radial artery

Brachioradialis

Ulnar nerve

Medial cutaneous nerve of forearm (from medial cord of brachial plexus)

Median nerve

Brachial artery

Medial epicondyle

Bicipital aponeurosis

Radial artery

Palmaris longus tendon

Median nerve

Thenar muscles

Palmar branch of median nerve

Palmar aponeurosis

Ulnar artery

Ulnar nerve

Superior ulnar collateral artery

Inferior ulnar collateral artery

Radial collateral artery

**Brachial artery**

Radial recurrent artery

Median nerve

Recurrent interosseous artery

Ulnar nerve

Humeral head of pronator teres (cut)

Posterior interosseous artery

Anterior ulnar recurrent artery

Humeral head of flexor carpi ulnaris

Posterior ulnar recurrent artery

Ulnar head of pronator teres

Ulnar artery

Anterior interosseous nerve

Anterior interosseous artery

**Radial artery**

Interosseous membrane

Flexor digitorum superficialis (cut)

Flexor digitorum profundus

Dorsal branch of ulnar nerve

Flexor carpi ulnaris tendon (cut)

Ulnar nerve

Palmar branch of ulnar nerve

Deep palmar branch of ulnar artery

Deep palmar arch

Superficial palmar arch

Radial nerve

Brachial artery

Lateral epicondyle

Radial recurrent artery

Deep branch radial nerve

Radial artery

Supinator

Superficial branch radial nerve

Common interosseous artery

Posterior interosseous artery

Interosseous membrane

Pronator teres (cut)

Ulnar artery

Perforating branches of anterior interosseous artery

Brachioradialis tendon (cut)

Palmar branch of ulnar nerve

Hypothenar muscles

Median nerve

Flexor carpi radialis tendon (cut)

Flexor retinaculum

Superficial palmar branch of radial artery

Palmar branch of median nerve

Anterior ulnar recurrent artery

Posterior ulnar recurrent artery

Common interosseous artery

Anterior interosseous artery

**Ulnar artery**

Radius

Ulna

Superficial palmar branch of radial artery

Pisiform

Superficial palmar arch

**Arteries and nerves of forearm (anterior view)**

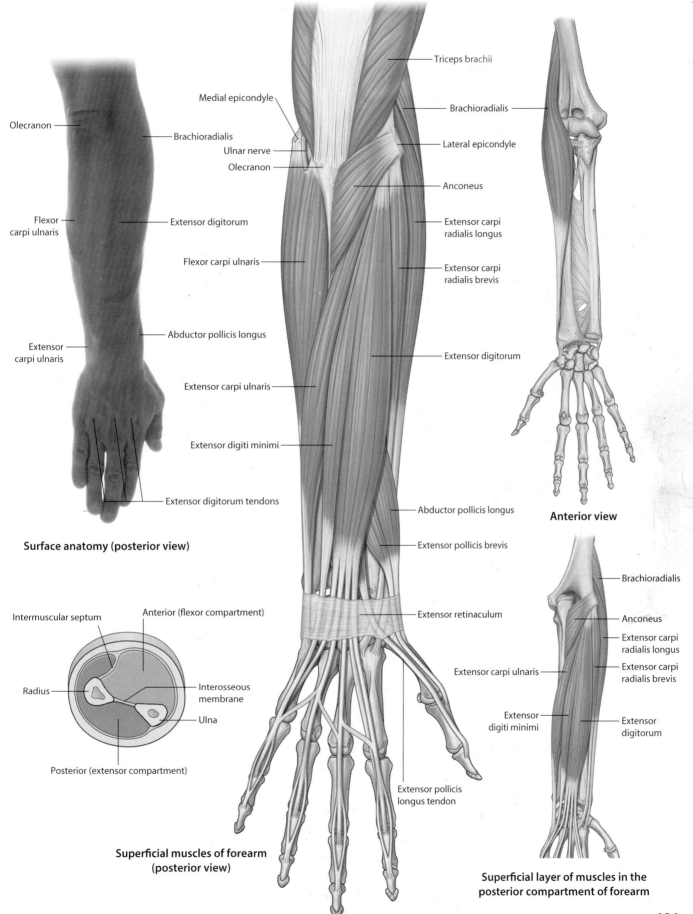

Triceps brachii

Medial epicondyle

Olecranon

Brachioradialis

Ulnar nerve

Olecranon

Brachioradialis

Lateral epicondyle

Anconeus

Extensor carpi radialis longus

Extensor carpi radialis brevis

Extensor digitorum

Flexor carpi ulnaris

Extensor digitorum

Flexor carpi ulnaris

Abductor pollicis longus

Extensor carpi ulnaris

Extensor digiti minimi

Extensor carpi ulnaris

Extensor digitorum tendons

Abductor pollicis longus

Extensor pollicis brevis

**Surface anatomy (posterior view)**

**Anterior view**

Intermuscular septum

Anterior (flexor compartment)

Radius

Interosseous membrane

Ulna

Posterior (extensor compartment)

Extensor retinaculum

Brachioradialis

Anconeus

Extensor carpi radialis longus

Extensor carpi radialis brevis

Extensor carpi ulnaris

Extensor digiti minimi

Extensor digitorum

**Superficial muscles of forearm (posterior view)**

Extensor pollicis longus tendon

**Superficial layer of muscles in the posterior compartment of forearm**

**401**

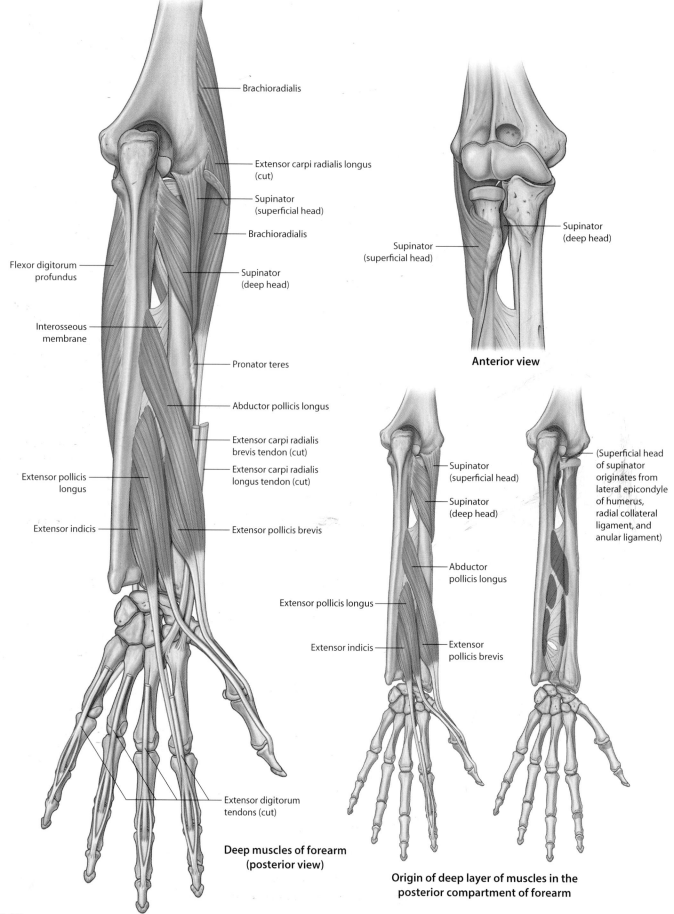

Brachioradialis

Extensor carpi radialis longus (cut)

Supinator (superficial head)

Brachioradialis

Supinator (deep head)

Flexor digitorum profundus

Interosseous membrane

Pronator teres

Abductor pollicis longus

Extensor carpi radialis brevis tendon (cut)

Extensor carpi radialis longus tendon (cut)

Extensor pollicis longus

Extensor indicis

Extensor pollicis brevis

Extensor digitorum tendons (cut)

**Deep muscles of forearm (posterior view)**

Supinator (superficial head)

Supinator (deep head)

Supinator (deep head)

Anterior view

**Anterior view**

Supinator (superficial head)

Supinator (deep head)

(Superficial head of supinator originates from lateral epicondyle of humerus, radial collateral ligament, and anular ligament)

Abductor pollicis longus

Extensor pollicis longus

Extensor indicis

Extensor pollicis brevis

**Origin of deep layer of muscles in the posterior compartment of forearm**

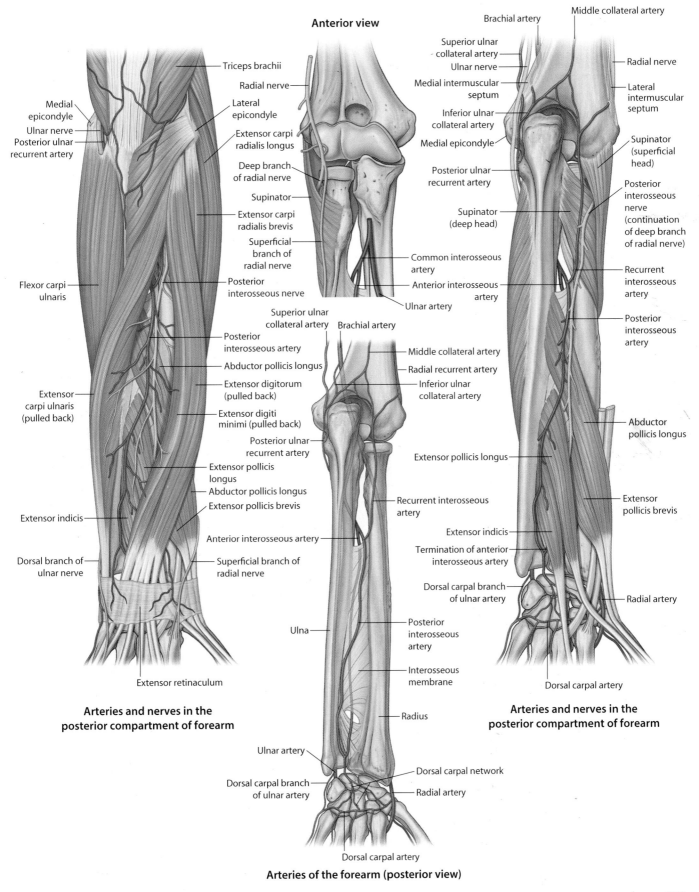

**Anterior view**

Arteries and nerves in the posterior compartment of forearm

Arteries and nerves in the posterior compartment of forearm

Arteries of the forearm (posterior view)

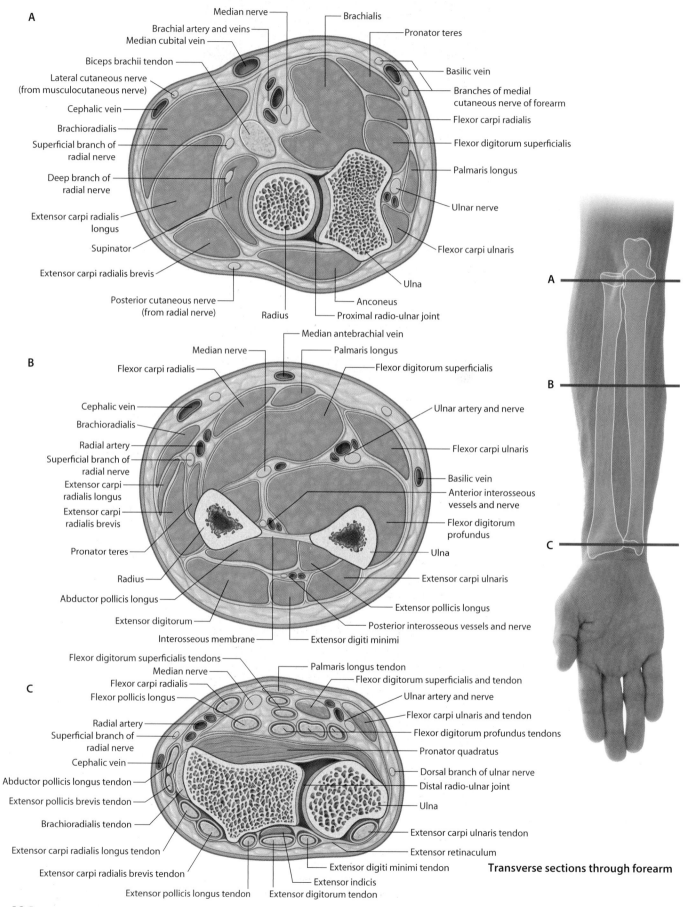

**A**

Median nerve

Brachialis

Brachial artery and veins

Pronator teres

Median cubital vein

Biceps brachii tendon

Basilic vein

Lateral cutaneous nerve
(from musculocutaneous nerve)

Branches of medial
cutaneous nerve of forearm

Cephalic vein

Flexor carpi radialis

Brachioradialis

Flexor digitorum superficialis

Superficial branch of
radial nerve

Palmaris longus

Deep branch of
radial nerve

Ulnar nerve

Extensor carpi radialis
longus

Supinator

Flexor carpi ulnaris

Extensor carpi radialis brevis

Ulna

Posterior cutaneous nerve
(from radial nerve)

Anconeus

Radius

Proximal radio-ulnar joint

**B**

Median antebrachial vein

Median nerve

Palmaris longus

Flexor carpi radialis

Flexor digitorum superficialis

Cephalic vein

Ulnar artery and nerve

Brachioradialis

Flexor carpi ulnaris

Radial artery

Superficial branch of
radial nerve

Basilic vein

Extensor carpi
radialis longus

Anterior interosseous
vessels and nerve

Extensor carpi
radialis brevis

Flexor digitorum
profundus

Pronator teres

Ulna

Radius

Extensor carpi ulnaris

Abductor pollicis longus

Extensor pollicis longus

Extensor digitorum

Posterior interosseous vessels and nerve

Interosseous membrane

Extensor digiti minimi

**C**

Flexor digitorum superficialis tendons

Median nerve

Palmaris longus tendon

Flexor carpi radialis

Flexor digitorum superficialis and tendon

Flexor pollicis longus

Ulnar artery and nerve

Radial artery

Flexor carpi ulnaris and tendon

Superficial branch of
radial nerve

Flexor digitorum profundus tendons

Cephalic vein

Pronator quadratus

Abductor pollicis longus tendon

Dorsal branch of ulnar nerve

Extensor pollicis brevis tendon

Distal radio-ulnar joint

Brachioradialis tendon

Ulna

Extensor carpi radialis longus tendon

Extensor carpi ulnaris tendon

Extensor carpi radialis brevis tendon

Extensor retinaculum

Extensor digiti minimi tendon

Extensor pollicis longus tendon

Extensor indicis

Extensor digitorum tendon

**Transverse sections through forearm**

A

B

C

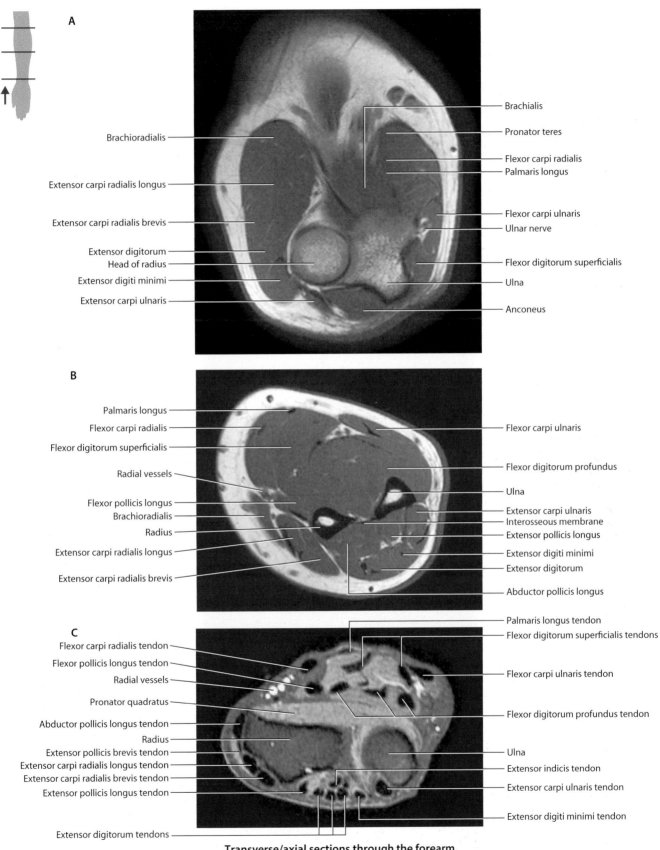

**A**

Brachioradialis

Extensor carpi radialis longus

Extensor carpi radialis brevis

Extensor digitorum

Head of radius

Extensor digiti minimi

Extensor carpi ulnaris

Brachialis

Pronator teres

Flexor carpi radialis
Palmaris longus

Flexor carpi ulnaris

Ulnar nerve

Flexor digitorum superficialis

Ulna

Anconeus

**B**

Palmaris longus

Flexor carpi radialis

Flexor digitorum superficialis

Radial vessels

Flexor pollicis longus

Brachioradialis

Radius

Extensor carpi radialis longus

Extensor carpi radialis brevis

Flexor carpi ulnaris

Flexor digitorum profundus

Ulna

Extensor carpi ulnaris

Interosseous membrane

Extensor pollicis longus

Extensor digiti minimi

Extensor digitorum

Abductor pollicis longus

**C**

Flexor carpi radialis tendon

Flexor pollicis longus tendon

Radial vessels

Pronator quadratus

Abductor pollicis longus tendon

Radius

Extensor pollicis brevis tendon

Extensor carpi radialis longus tendon

Extensor carpi radialis brevis tendon

Extensor pollicis longus tendon

Extensor digitorum tendons

Palmaris longus tendon

Flexor digitorum superficialis tendons

Flexor carpi ulnaris tendon

Flexor digitorum profundus tendon

Ulna

Extensor indicis tendon

Extensor carpi ulnaris tendon

Extensor digiti minimi tendon

**Transverse/axial sections through the forearm.**
**A. Proximal/upper forearm.**
**B. Middle forearm.**
**C. Distal/lower forearm.**
T1-weighted MR image in axial plane

**405**

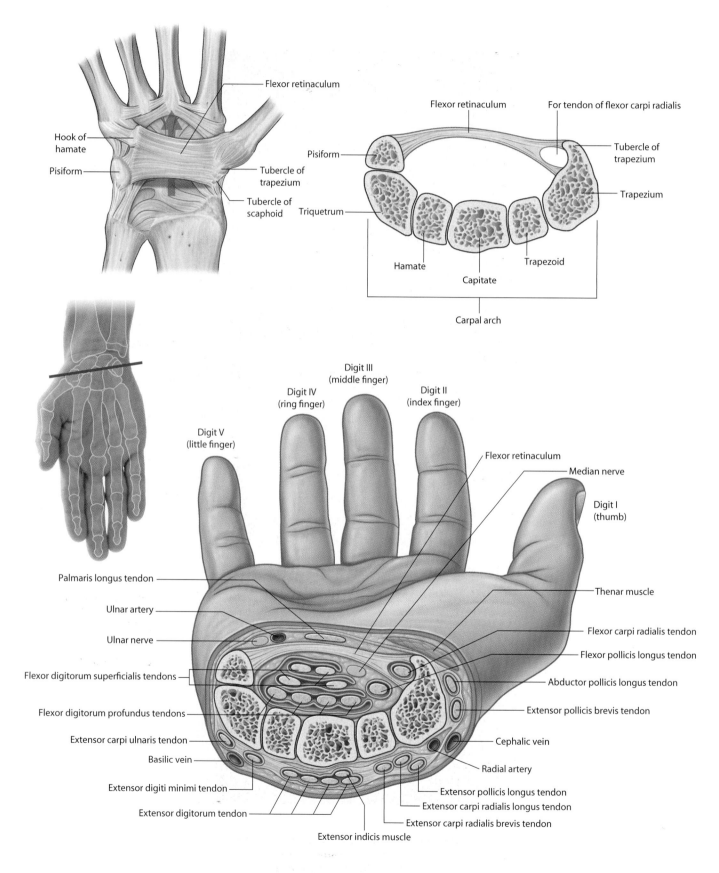

Flexor retinaculum

Hook of hamate

Pisiform

Tubercle of trapezium

Tubercle of scaphoid

Flexor retinaculum

Pisiform

For tendon of flexor carpi radialis

Tubercle of trapezium

Trapezium

Triquetrum

Hamate

Capitate

Trapezoid

Carpal arch

Digit III (middle finger)

Digit IV (ring finger)

Digit II (index finger)

Digit V (little finger)

Flexor retinaculum

Median nerve

Digit I (thumb)

Palmaris longus tendon

Ulnar artery

Ulnar nerve

Flexor digitorum superficialis tendons

Flexor digitorum profundus tendons

Extensor carpi ulnaris tendon

Basilic vein

Extensor digiti minimi tendon

Extensor digitorum tendon

Extensor indicis muscle

Thenar muscle

Flexor carpi radialis tendon

Flexor pollicis longus tendon

Abductor pollicis longus tendon

Extensor pollicis brevis tendon

Cephalic vein

Radial artery

Extensor pollicis longus tendon

Extensor carpi radialis longus tendon

Extensor carpi radialis brevis tendon

**Carpal tunnel, structures and relations**

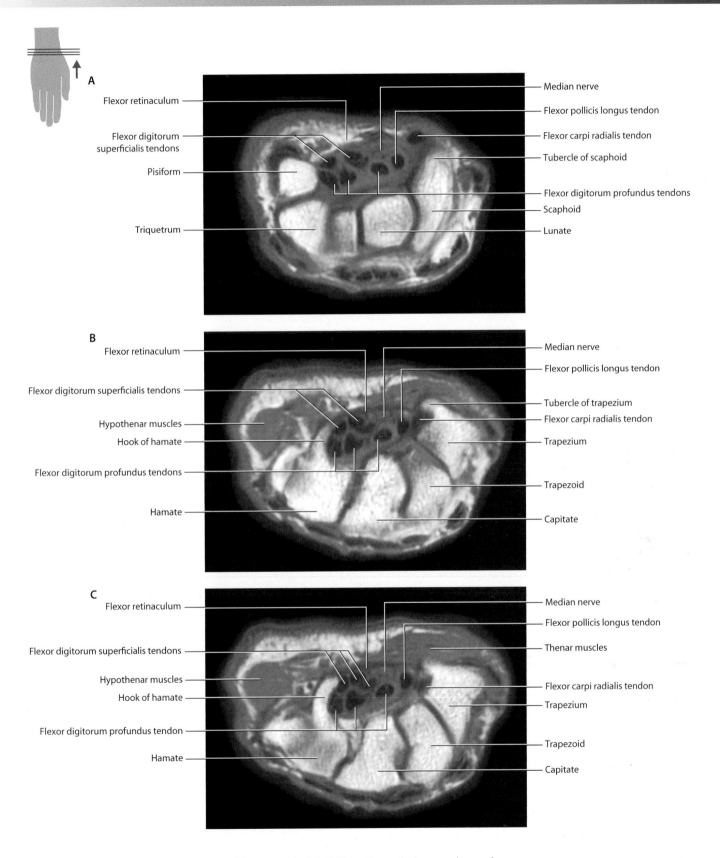

**A**

Flexor retinaculum

Flexor digitorum
superficialis tendons

Pisiform

Triquetrum

Median nerve

Flexor pollicis longus tendon

Flexor carpi radialis tendon

Tubercle of scaphoid

Flexor digitorum profundus tendons

Scaphoid

Lunate

**B**

Flexor retinaculum

Flexor digitorum superficialis tendons

Hypothenar muscles

Hook of hamate

Flexor digitorum profundus tendons

Hamate

Median nerve

Flexor pollicis longus tendon

Tubercle of trapezium

Flexor carpi radialis tendon

Trapezium

Trapezoid

Capitate

**C**

Flexor retinaculum

Flexor digitorum superficialis tendons

Hypothenar muscles

Hook of hamate

Flexor digitorum profundus tendon

Hamate

Median nerve

Flexor pollicis longus tendon

Thenar muscles

Flexor carpi radialis tendon

Trapezium

Trapezoid

Capitate

**Transverse/axial sections through the carpal tunnel.**
**A. Proximal end of carpal tunnel.**
**B. Middle portion of carpal tunnel.**
**C. Distal portion of carpal tunnel.**
T1-weighted MR images in axial plane

**407**

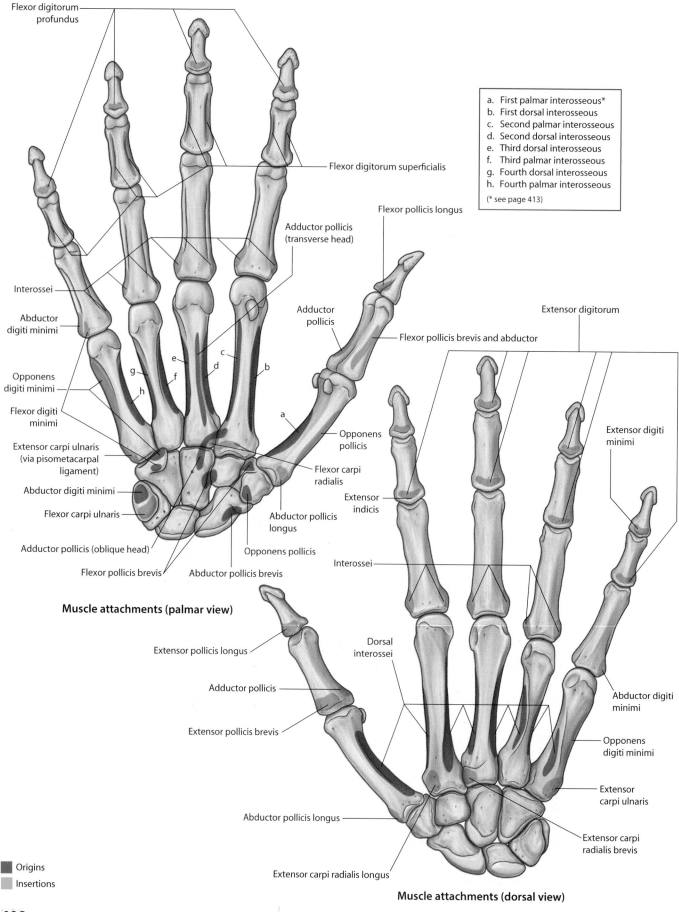

Flexor digitorum profundus

Flexor digitorum superficialis

a. First palmar interosseous*
b. First dorsal interosseous
c. Second palmar interosseous
d. Second dorsal interosseous
e. Third dorsal interosseous
f. Third palmar interosseous
g. Fourth dorsal interosseous
h. Fourth palmar interosseous
(* see page 413)

Adductor pollicis (transverse head)

Flexor pollicis longus

Adductor pollicis

Extensor digitorum

Flexor pollicis brevis and abductor

Interossei

Abductor digiti minimi

Extensor digiti minimi

Opponens digiti minimi

Flexor digiti minimi

Opponens pollicis

Extensor carpi ulnaris (via pisometacarpal ligament)

Flexor carpi radialis

Extensor indicis

Abductor digiti minimi

Flexor carpi ulnaris

Abductor pollicis longus

Adductor pollicis (oblique head)

Opponens pollicis

Interossei

Flexor pollicis brevis

Abductor pollicis brevis

**Muscle attachments (palmar view)**

Extensor pollicis longus

Dorsal interossei

Adductor pollicis

Abductor digiti minimi

Extensor pollicis brevis

Opponens digiti minimi

Abductor pollicis longus

Extensor carpi ulnaris

Extensor carpi radialis brevis

Extensor carpi radialis longus

**Muscle attachments (dorsal view)**

Origins
Insertions

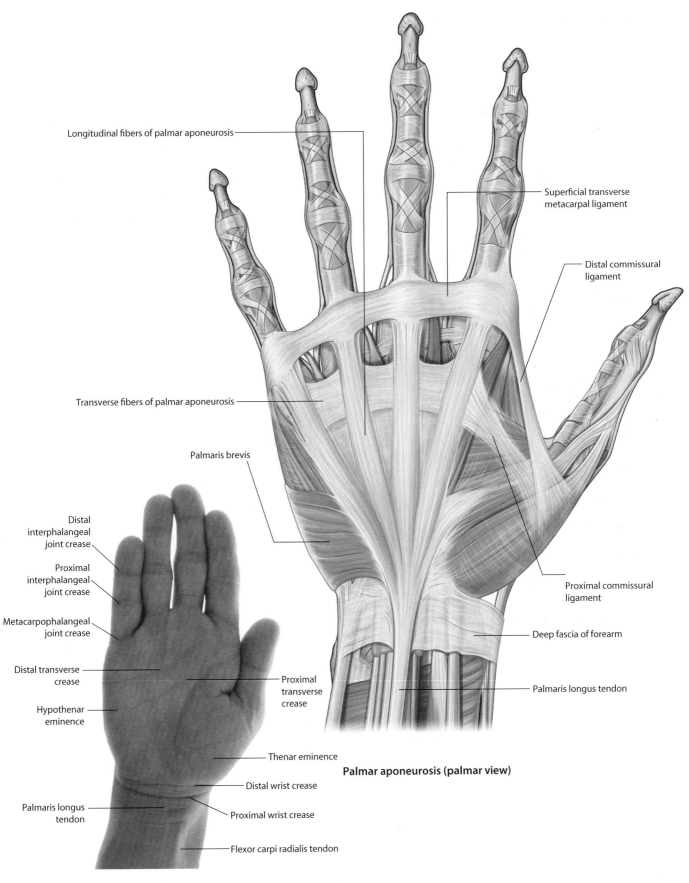

Longitudinal fibers of palmar aponeurosis

Superficial transverse metacarpal ligament

Distal commissural ligament

Transverse fibers of palmar aponeurosis

Palmaris brevis

Distal interphalangeal joint crease

Proximal interphalangeal joint crease

Metacarpophalangeal joint crease

Distal transverse crease

Hypothenar eminence

Proximal transverse crease

Proximal commissural ligament

Deep fascia of forearm

Palmaris longus tendon

Thenar eminence

Palmaris longus tendon

Distal wrist crease

Proximal wrist crease

Flexor carpi radialis tendon

**Palmar aponeurosis (palmar view)**

**Surface anatomy (palmar view)**

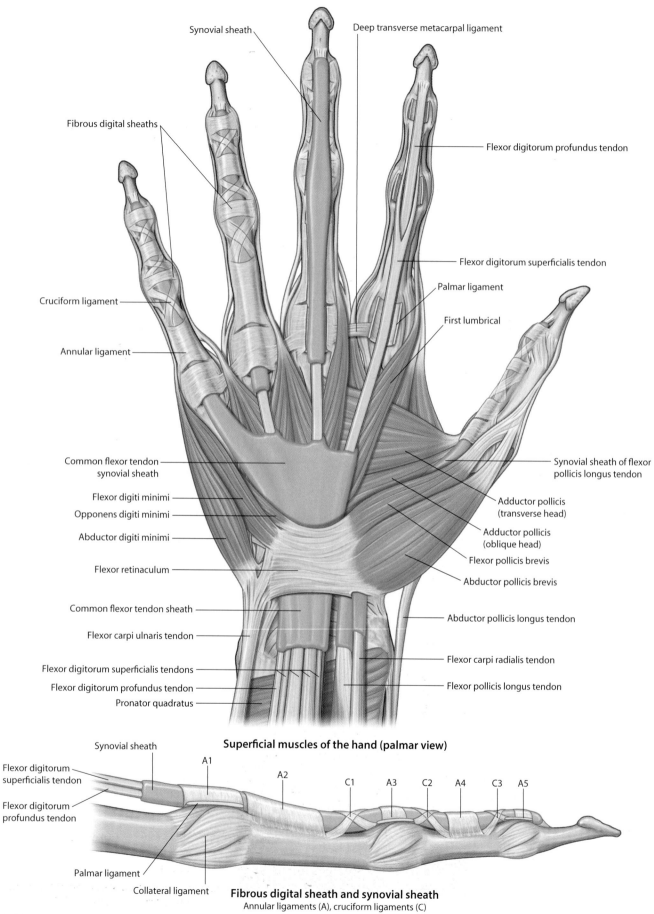

Synovial sheath

Deep transverse metacarpal ligament

Fibrous digital sheaths

Flexor digitorum profundus tendon

Cruciform ligament

Flexor digitorum superficialis tendon

Palmar ligament

First lumbrical

Annular ligament

Common flexor tendon synovial sheath

Synovial sheath of flexor pollicis longus tendon

Flexor digiti minimi

Adductor pollicis (transverse head)

Opponens digiti minimi

Adductor pollicis (oblique head)

Abductor digiti minimi

Flexor pollicis brevis

Flexor retinaculum

Abductor pollicis brevis

Common flexor tendon sheath

Abductor pollicis longus tendon

Flexor carpi ulnaris tendon

Flexor carpi radialis tendon

Flexor digitorum superficialis tendons

Flexor digitorum profundus tendon

Flexor pollicis longus tendon

Pronator quadratus

**Superficial muscles of the hand (palmar view)**

Synovial sheath

A1

Flexor digitorum superficialis tendon

A2

C1 A3 C2 A4 C3 A5

Flexor digitorum profundus tendon

Palmar ligament

Collateral ligament

**Fibrous digital sheath and synovial sheath**
Annular ligaments (A), cruciform ligaments (C)

**410**

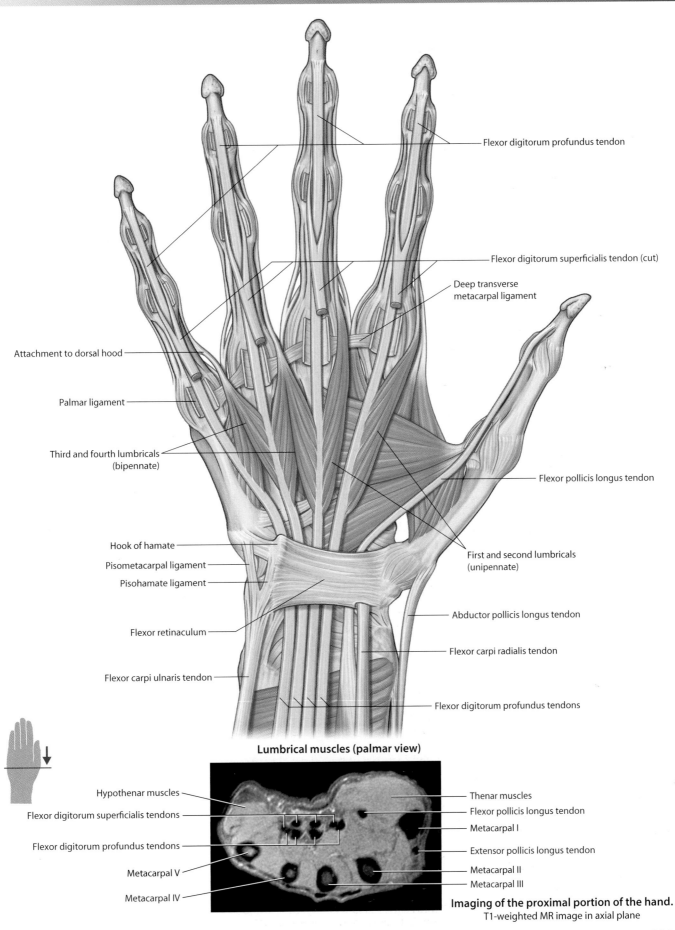

Flexor digitorum profundus tendon

Flexor digitorum superficialis tendon (cut)

Deep transverse metacarpal ligament

Attachment to dorsal hood

Palmar ligament

Third and fourth lumbricals (bipennate)

Flexor pollicis longus tendon

Hook of hamate

Pisometacarpal ligament

Pisohamate ligament

First and second lumbricals (unipennate)

Abductor pollicis longus tendon

Flexor retinaculum

Flexor carpi radialis tendon

Flexor carpi ulnaris tendon

Flexor digitorum profundus tendons

**Lumbrical muscles (palmar view)**

Hypothenar muscles

Thenar muscles

Flexor digitorum superficialis tendons

Flexor pollicis longus tendon

Metacarpal I

Flexor digitorum profundus tendons

Extensor pollicis longus tendon

Metacarpal V

Metacarpal II

Metacarpal IV

Metacarpal III

**Imaging of the proximal portion of the hand.**
T1-weighted MR image in axial plane

**411**

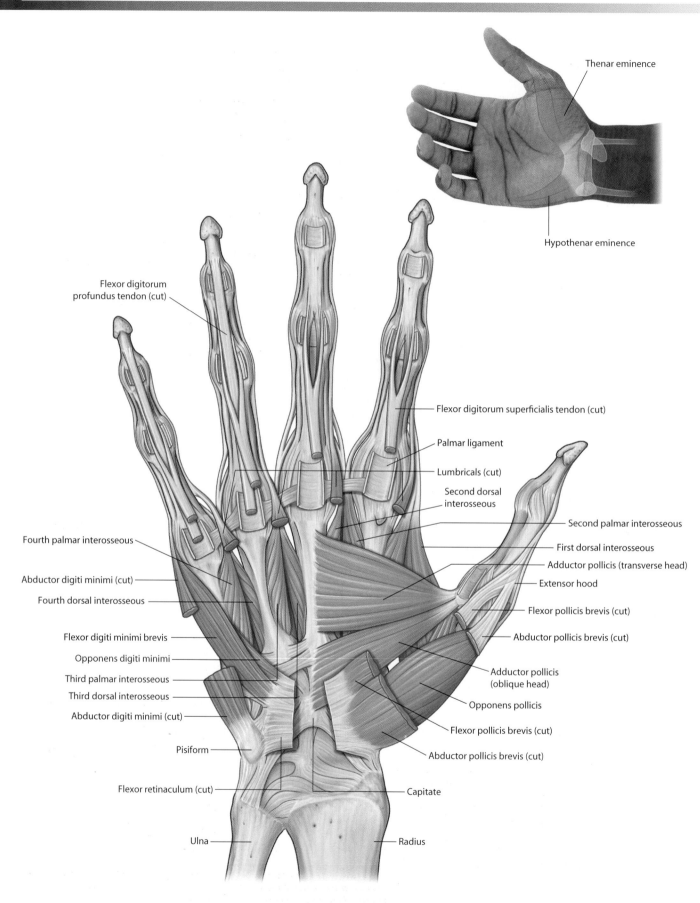

Thenar eminence

Hypothenar eminence

Flexor digitorum profundus tendon (cut)

Flexor digitorum superficialis tendon (cut)

Palmar ligament

Lumbricals (cut)

Second dorsal interosseous

Second palmar interosseous

First dorsal interosseous

Adductor pollicis (transverse head)

Extensor hood

Fourth palmar interosseous

Abductor digiti minimi (cut)

Fourth dorsal interosseous

Flexor pollicis brevis (cut)

Abductor pollicis brevis (cut)

Flexor digiti minimi brevis

Opponens digiti minimi

Third palmar interosseous

Third dorsal interosseous

Abductor digiti minimi (cut)

Adductor pollicis (oblique head)

Opponens pollicis

Flexor pollicis brevis (cut)

Pisiform

Abductor pollicis brevis (cut)

Flexor retinaculum (cut)

Capitate

Ulna

Radius

**Deep muscles of the hand (palmar view)**

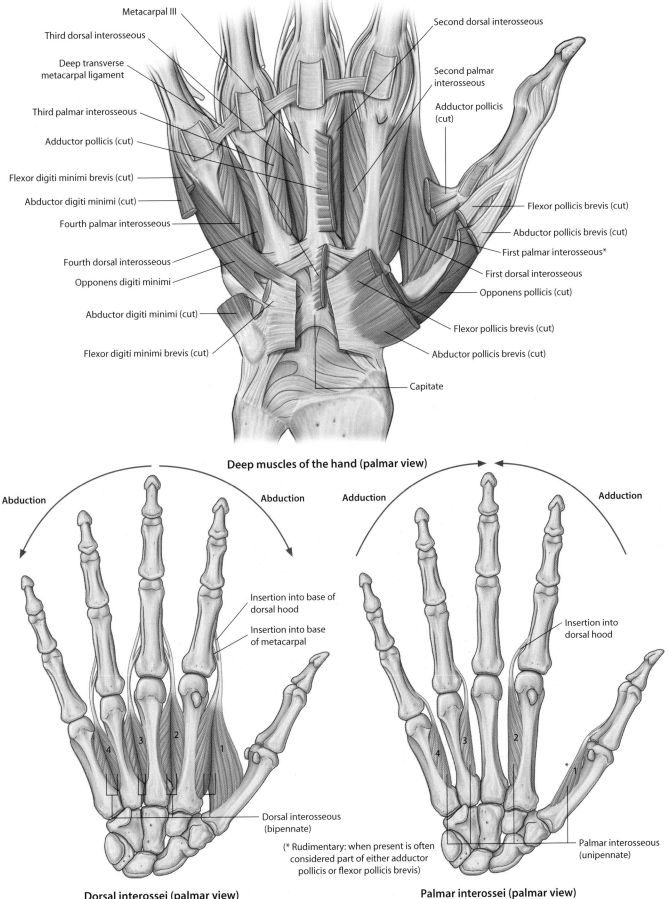

Metacarpal III

Third dorsal interosseous

Deep transverse metacarpal ligament

Third palmar interosseous

Adductor pollicis (cut)

Flexor digiti minimi brevis (cut)

Abductor digiti minimi (cut)

Fourth palmar interosseous

Fourth dorsal interosseous

Opponens digiti minimi

Abductor digiti minimi (cut)

Flexor digiti minimi brevis (cut)

Second dorsal interosseous

Second palmar interosseous

Adductor pollicis (cut)

Flexor pollicis brevis (cut)

Abductor pollicis brevis (cut)

First palmar interosseous*

First dorsal interosseous

Opponens pollicis (cut)

Flexor pollicis brevis (cut)

Abductor pollicis brevis (cut)

Capitate

**Deep muscles of the hand (palmar view)**

Abduction

Abduction

Adduction

Adduction

Insertion into base of dorsal hood

Insertion into base of metacarpal

Insertion into dorsal hood

Dorsal interosseous (bipennate)

Palmar interosseous (unipennate)

(* Rudimentary: when present is often considered part of either adductor pollicis or flexor pollicis brevis)

**Dorsal interossei (palmar view)**

**Palmar interossei (palmar view)**

**413**

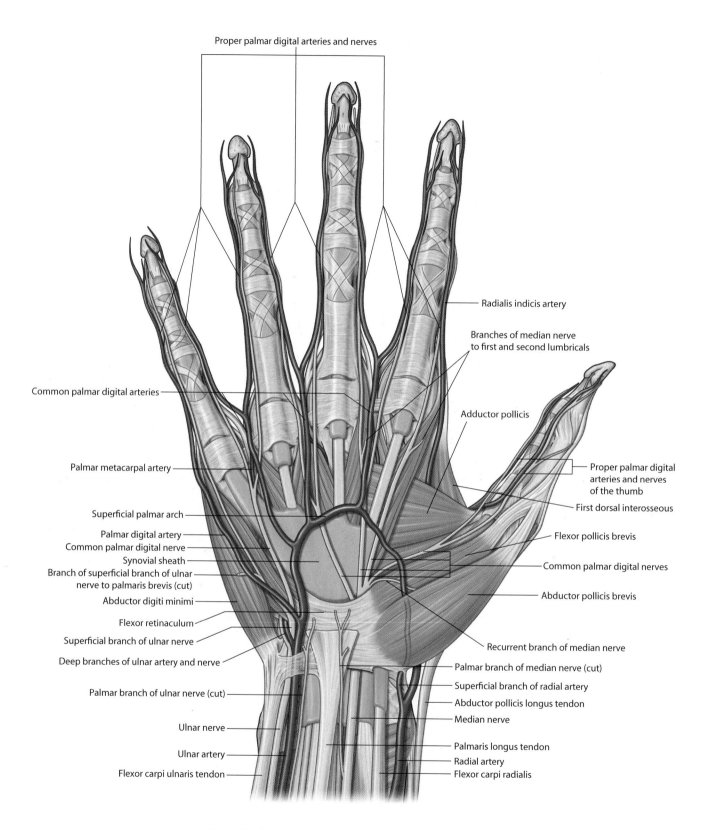

Proper palmar digital arteries and nerves

Radialis indicis artery

Branches of median nerve
to first and second lumbricals

Common palmar digital arteries

Adductor pollicis

Palmar metacarpal artery

Proper palmar digital
arteries and nerves
of the thumb

First dorsal interosseous

Superficial palmar arch

Flexor pollicis brevis

Palmar digital artery
Common palmar digital nerve
Synovial sheath

Common palmar digital nerves

Branch of superficial branch of ulnar
nerve to palmaris brevis (cut)

Abductor pollicis brevis

Abductor digiti minimi

Flexor retinaculum

Superficial branch of ulnar nerve

Recurrent branch of median nerve

Deep branches of ulnar artery and nerve

Palmar branch of median nerve (cut)

Superficial branch of radial artery

Palmar branch of ulnar nerve (cut)

Abductor pollicis longus tendon

Median nerve

Ulnar nerve

Palmaris longus tendon

Ulnar artery

Radial artery

Flexor carpi ulnaris tendon

Flexor carpi radialis

**Superficial arteries and nerves of the hand (palmar view)**

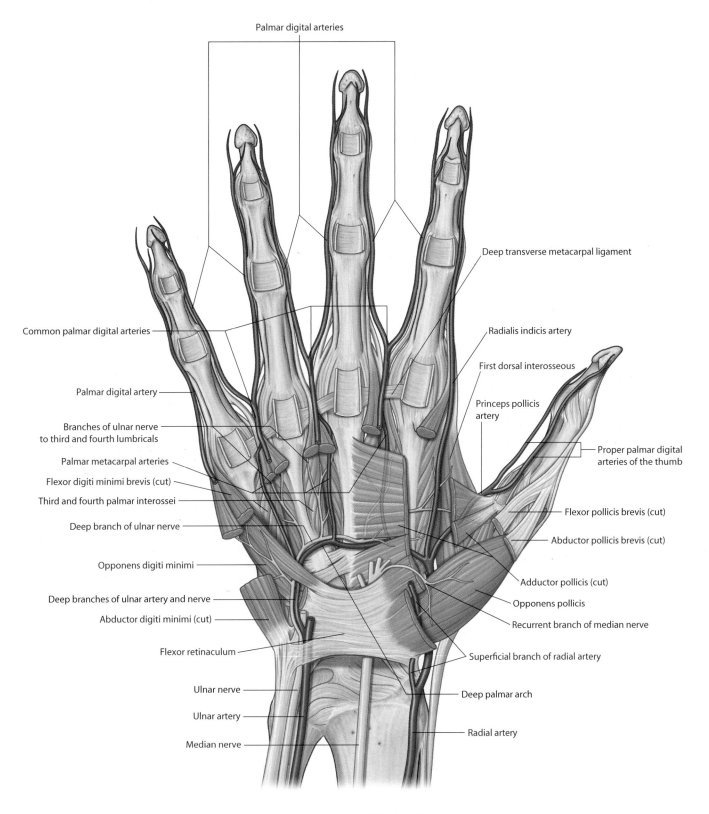

Palmar digital arteries

Deep transverse metacarpal ligament

Common palmar digital arteries

Radialis indicis artery

First dorsal interosseous

Palmar digital artery

Princeps pollicis artery

Branches of ulnar nerve to third and fourth lumbricals

Proper palmar digital arteries of the thumb

Palmar metacarpal arteries

Flexor digiti minimi brevis (cut)

Third and fourth palmar interossei

Flexor pollicis brevis (cut)

Deep branch of ulnar nerve

Abductor pollicis brevis (cut)

Opponens digiti minimi

Adductor pollicis (cut)

Deep branches of ulnar artery and nerve

Opponens pollicis

Abductor digiti minimi (cut)

Recurrent branch of median nerve

Flexor retinaculum

Superficial branch of radial artery

Ulnar nerve

Deep palmar arch

Ulnar artery

Radial artery

Median nerve

**Deep arteries and nerves of the hand (palmar view)**

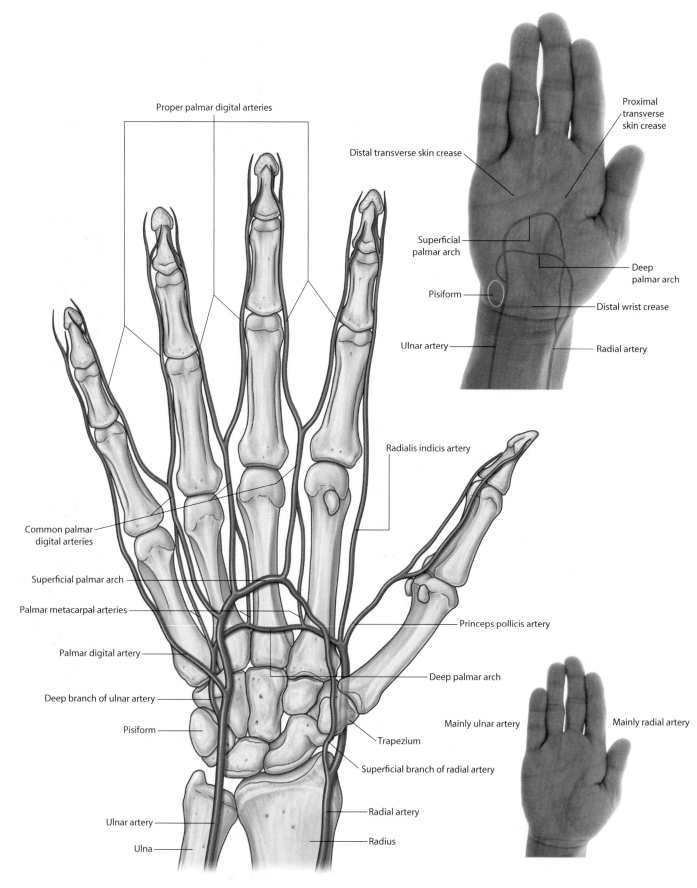

Proper palmar digital arteries

Distal transverse skin crease

Proximal transverse skin crease

Superficial palmar arch

Deep palmar arch

Pisiform

Distal wrist crease

Ulnar artery

Radial artery

Radialis indicis artery

Common palmar digital arteries

Superficial palmar arch

Palmar metacarpal arteries

Princeps pollicis artery

Palmar digital artery

Deep palmar arch

Deep branch of ulnar artery

Mainly ulnar artery

Mainly radial artery

Pisiform

Trapezium

Superficial branch of radial artery

Ulnar artery

Radial artery

Ulna

Radius

**Arteries of the hand (palmar view)**

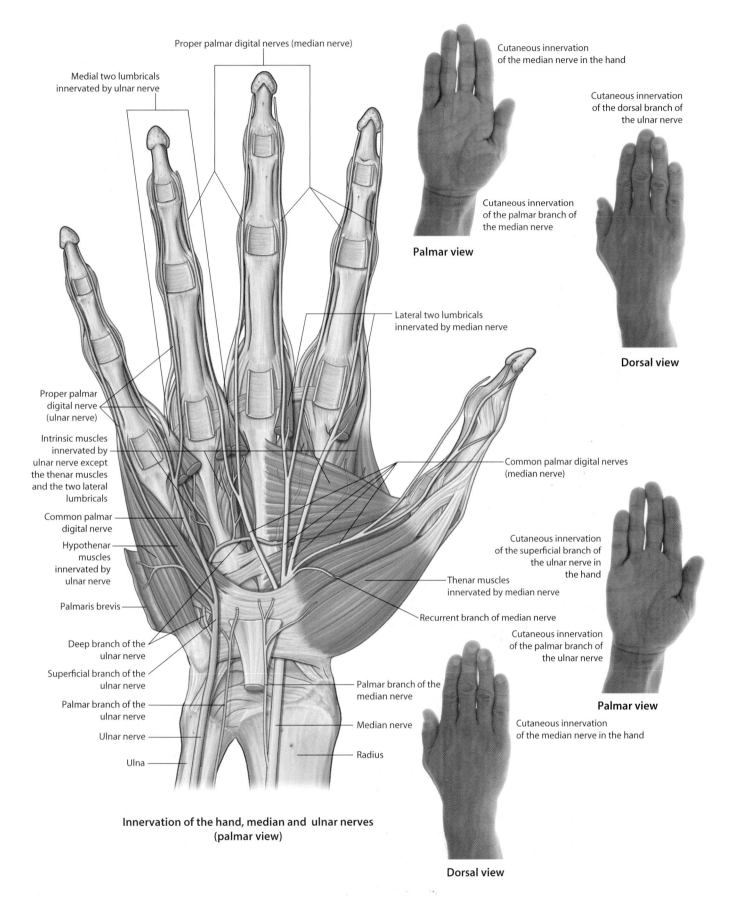

Proper palmar digital nerves (median nerve)

Medial two lumbricals
innervated by ulnar nerve

Cutaneous innervation
of the median nerve in the hand

Cutaneous innervation
of the dorsal branch of
the ulnar nerve

Cutaneous innervation
of the palmar branch of
the median nerve

**Palmar view**

**Dorsal view**

Lateral two lumbricals
innervated by median nerve

Proper palmar
digital nerve
(ulnar nerve)

Intrinsic muscles
innervated by
ulnar nerve except
the thenar muscles
and the two lateral
lumbricals

Common palmar
digital nerve

Hypothenar
muscles
innervated by
ulnar nerve

Palmaris brevis

Deep branch of the
ulnar nerve

Superficial branch of the
ulnar nerve

Palmar branch of the
ulnar nerve

Ulnar nerve

Ulna

Common palmar digital nerves
(median nerve)

Cutaneous innervation
of the superficial branch of
the ulnar nerve in
the hand

Thenar muscles
innervated by median nerve

Recurrent branch of median nerve

Cutaneous innervation
of the palmar branch of
the ulnar nerve

**Palmar view**

Palmar branch of the
median nerve

Median nerve

Radius

Cutaneous innervation
of the median nerve in the hand

**Innervation of the hand, median and ulnar nerves
(palmar view)**

**Dorsal view**

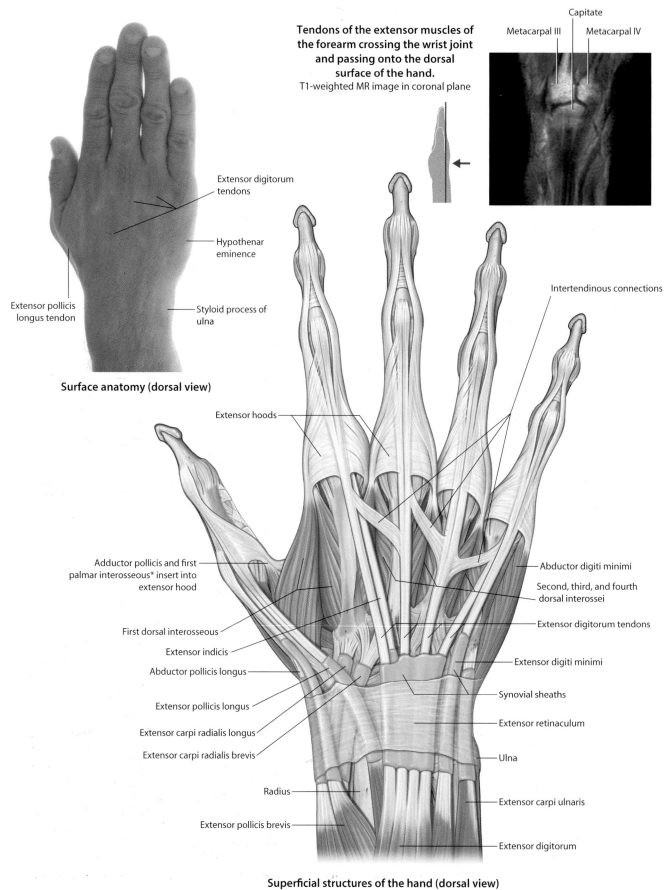

**Tendons of the extensor muscles of the forearm crossing the wrist joint and passing onto the dorsal surface of the hand.**
T1-weighted MR image in coronal plane

Capitate

Metacarpal III    Metacarpal IV

Extensor digitorum tendons

Hypothenar eminence

Styloid process of ulna

Extensor pollicis longus tendon

**Surface anatomy (dorsal view)**

Intertendinous connections

Extensor hoods

Adductor pollicis and first palmar interosseous* insert into extensor hood

First dorsal interosseous

Extensor indicis

Abductor pollicis longus

Extensor pollicis longus

Extensor carpi radialis longus

Extensor carpi radialis brevis

Radius

Extensor pollicis brevis

Abductor digiti minimi

Second, third, and fourth dorsal interossei

Extensor digitorum tendons

Extensor digiti minimi

Synovial sheaths

Extensor retinaculum

Ulna

Extensor carpi ulnaris

Extensor digitorum

**Superficial structures of the hand (dorsal view)**
(* see page 413)

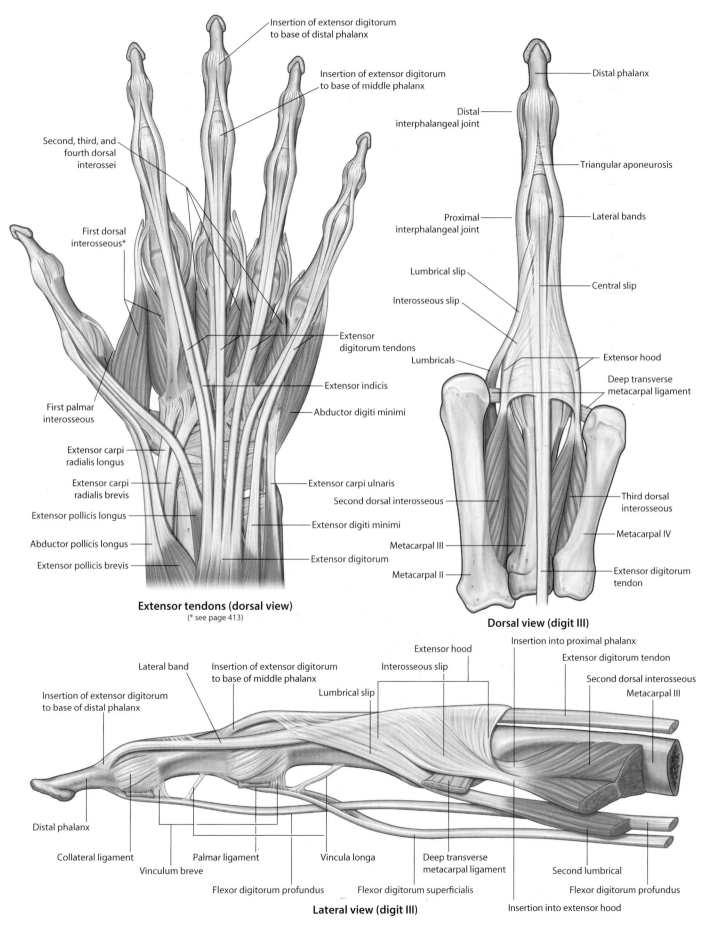

Insertion of extensor digitorum to base of distal phalanx

Insertion of extensor digitorum to base of middle phalanx

Second, third, and fourth dorsal interossei

First dorsal interosseous*

First palmar interosseous

First palmar interosseous

Extensor carpi radialis longus

Extensor carpi radialis brevis

Extensor pollicis longus

Abductor pollicis longus

Extensor pollicis brevis

Extensor digitorum tendons

Extensor indicis

Abductor digiti minimi

Extensor carpi ulnaris

Extensor digiti minimi

Extensor digitorum

**Extensor tendons (dorsal view)**
(* see page 413)

Distal phalanx

Distal interphalangeal joint

Triangular aponeurosis

Proximal interphalangeal joint

Lateral bands

Lumbrical slip

Interosseous slip

Central slip

Lumbricals

Extensor hood

Deep transverse metacarpal ligament

Second dorsal interosseous

Metacarpal III

Metacarpal II

Third dorsal interosseous

Metacarpal IV

Extensor digitorum tendon

**Dorsal view (digit III)**

Lateral band

Insertion of extensor digitorum to base of middle phalanx

Lumbrical slip

Insertion of extensor digitorum to base of distal phalanx

Extensor hood

Interosseous slip

Insertion into proximal phalanx

Extensor digitorum tendon

Second dorsal interosseous

Metacarpal III

Distal phalanx

Collateral ligament

Vinculum breve

Palmar ligament

Flexor digitorum profundus

Vincula longa

Flexor digitorum superficialis

Deep transverse metacarpal ligament

Second lumbrical

Insertion into extensor hood

Flexor digitorum profundus

**Lateral view (digit III)**

**419**

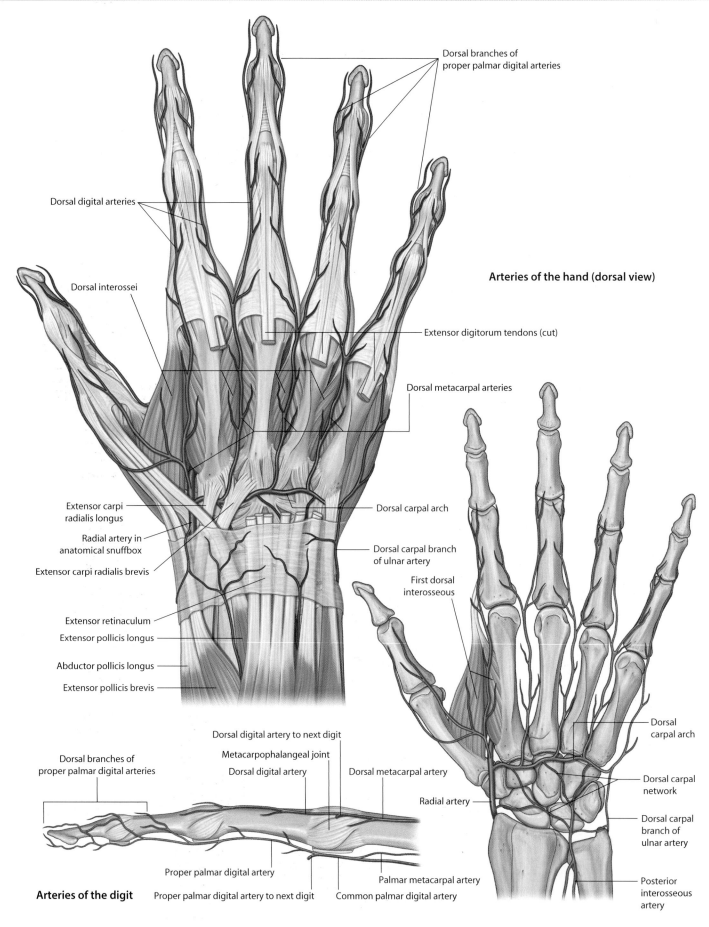

Dorsal branches of proper palmar digital arteries

Dorsal digital arteries

Dorsal interossei

**Arteries of the hand (dorsal view)**

Extensor digitorum tendons (cut)

Dorsal metacarpal arteries

Extensor carpi radialis longus

Radial artery in anatomical snuffbox

Extensor carpi radialis brevis

Dorsal carpal arch

Dorsal carpal branch of ulnar artery

First dorsal interosseous

Extensor retinaculum

Extensor pollicis longus

Abductor pollicis longus

Extensor pollicis brevis

Dorsal carpal arch

Dorsal carpal network

Dorsal carpal branch of ulnar artery

Radial artery

Posterior interosseous artery

Dorsal branches of proper palmar digital arteries

Dorsal digital artery to next digit

Metacarpophalangeal joint

Dorsal digital artery

Dorsal metacarpal artery

Proper palmar digital artery

Palmar metacarpal artery

**Arteries of the digit**

Proper palmar digital artery to next digit

Common palmar digital artery

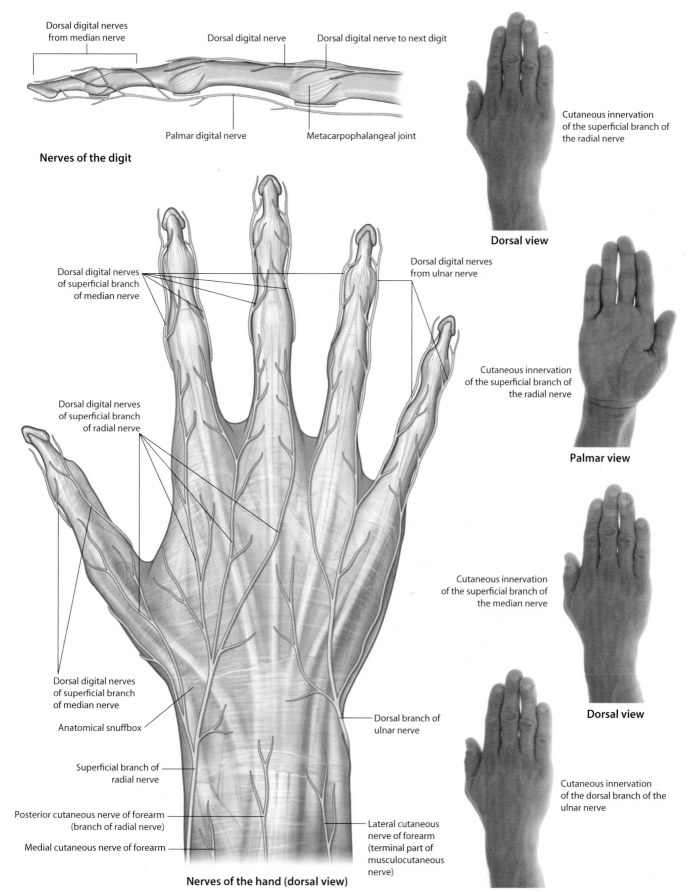

Dorsal digital nerves from median nerve

Dorsal digital nerve

Dorsal digital nerve to next digit

Palmar digital nerve

Metacarpophalangeal joint

**Nerves of the digit**

Cutaneous innervation of the superficial branch of the radial nerve

**Dorsal view**

Dorsal digital nerves of superficial branch of median nerve

Dorsal digital nerves from ulnar nerve

Dorsal digital nerves of superficial branch of radial nerve

Cutaneous innervation of the superficial branch of the radial nerve

**Palmar view**

Dorsal digital nerves of superficial branch of median nerve

Anatomical snuffbox

Dorsal branch of ulnar nerve

Cutaneous innervation of the superficial branch of the median nerve

**Dorsal view**

Superficial branch of radial nerve

Posterior cutaneous nerve of forearm (branch of radial nerve)

Medial cutaneous nerve of forearm

Lateral cutaneous nerve of forearm (terminal part of musculocutaneous nerve)

Cutaneous innervation of the dorsal branch of the ulnar nerve

**Nerves of the hand (dorsal view)**

**Dorsal view**

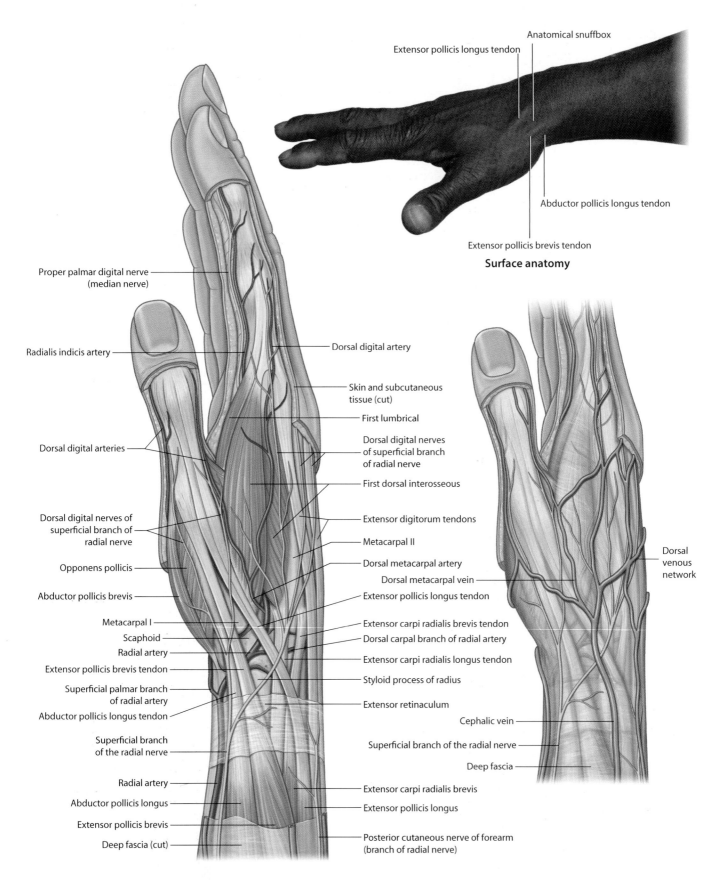

Anatomical snuffbox

Extensor pollicis longus tendon

Abductor pollicis longus tendon

Extensor pollicis brevis tendon

**Surface anatomy**

Proper palmar digital nerve
(median nerve)

Radialis indicis artery

Dorsal digital arteries

Dorsal digital nerves of
superficial branch of
radial nerve

Opponens pollicis

Abductor pollicis brevis

Metacarpal I

Scaphoid

Radial artery

Extensor pollicis brevis tendon

Superficial palmar branch
of radial artery

Abductor pollicis longus tendon

Superficial branch
of the radial nerve

Radial artery

Abductor pollicis longus

Extensor pollicis brevis

Deep fascia (cut)

Dorsal digital artery

Skin and subcutaneous
tissue (cut)

First lumbrical

Dorsal digital nerves
of superficial branch
of radial nerve

First dorsal interosseous

Extensor digitorum tendons

Metacarpal II

Dorsal metacarpal artery

Dorsal metacarpal vein

Extensor pollicis longus tendon

Extensor carpi radialis brevis tendon

Dorsal carpal branch of radial artery

Extensor carpi radialis longus tendon

Styloid process of radius

Extensor retinaculum

Extensor carpi radialis brevis

Extensor pollicis longus

Posterior cutaneous nerve of forearm
(branch of radial nerve)

Dorsal
venous
network

Cephalic vein

Superficial branch of the radial nerve

Deep fascia

**Anatomical snuffbox (lateral view)**

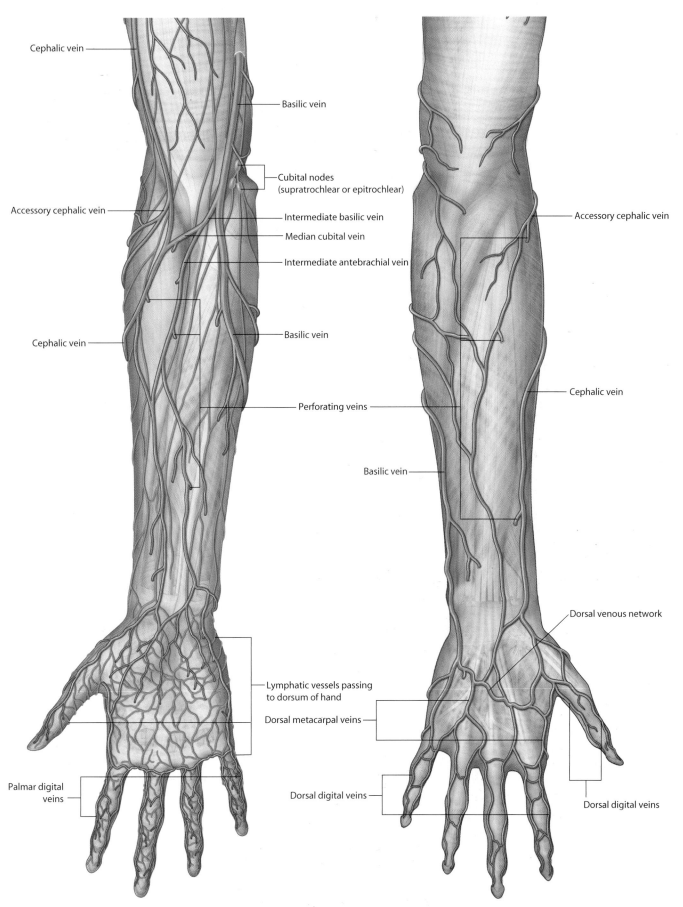

Cephalic vein

Basilic vein

Cubital nodes
(supratrochlear or epitrochlear)

Accessory cephalic vein

Intermediate basilic vein

Median cubital vein

Intermediate antebrachial vein

Cephalic vein

Basilic vein

Accessory cephalic vein

Cephalic vein

Perforating veins

Basilic vein

Dorsal venous network

Lymphatic vessels passing
to dorsum of hand

Dorsal metacarpal veins

Palmar digital
veins

Dorsal digital veins

Dorsal digital veins

**Superficial veins and lymphatics of the forearm (palmar view)**

**Superficial veins  of the forearm (dorsal view)**

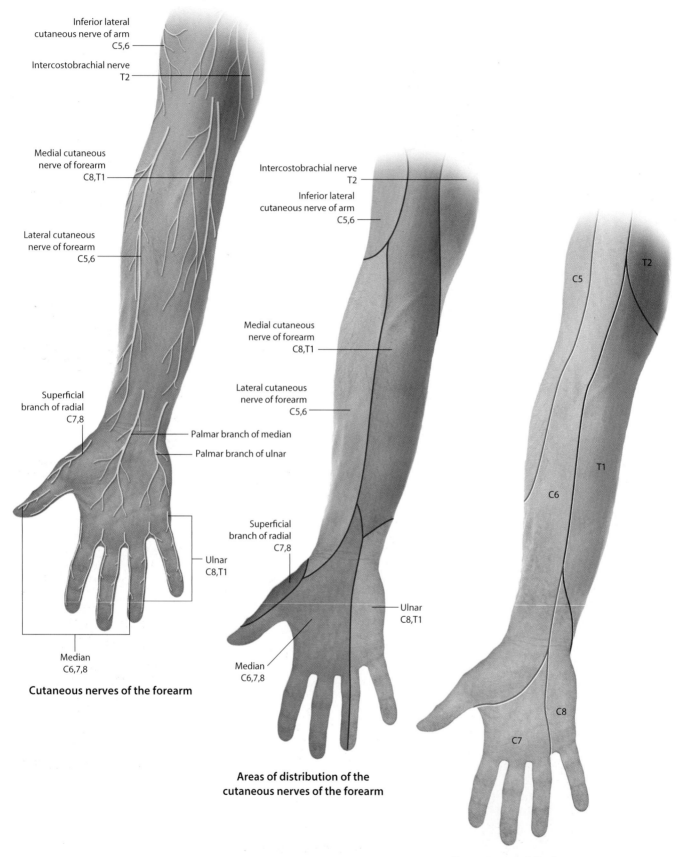

Inferior lateral
cutaneous nerve of arm
C5,6

Intercostobrachial nerve
T2

Medial cutaneous
nerve of forearm
C8,T1

Lateral cutaneous
nerve of forearm
C5,6

Superficial
branch of radial
C7,8

Palmar branch of median

Palmar branch of ulnar

Ulnar
C8,T1

Median
C6,7,8

**Cutaneous nerves of the forearm**

Intercostobrachial nerve
T2

Inferior lateral
cutaneous nerve of arm
C5,6

Medial cutaneous
nerve of forearm
C8,T1

Lateral cutaneous
nerve of forearm
C5,6

Superficial
branch of radial
C7,8

Ulnar
C8,T1

Median
C6,7,8

**Areas of distribution of the
cutaneous nerves of the forearm**

T2

C5

T1

C6

C8

C7

**Dermatomes of the forearm**

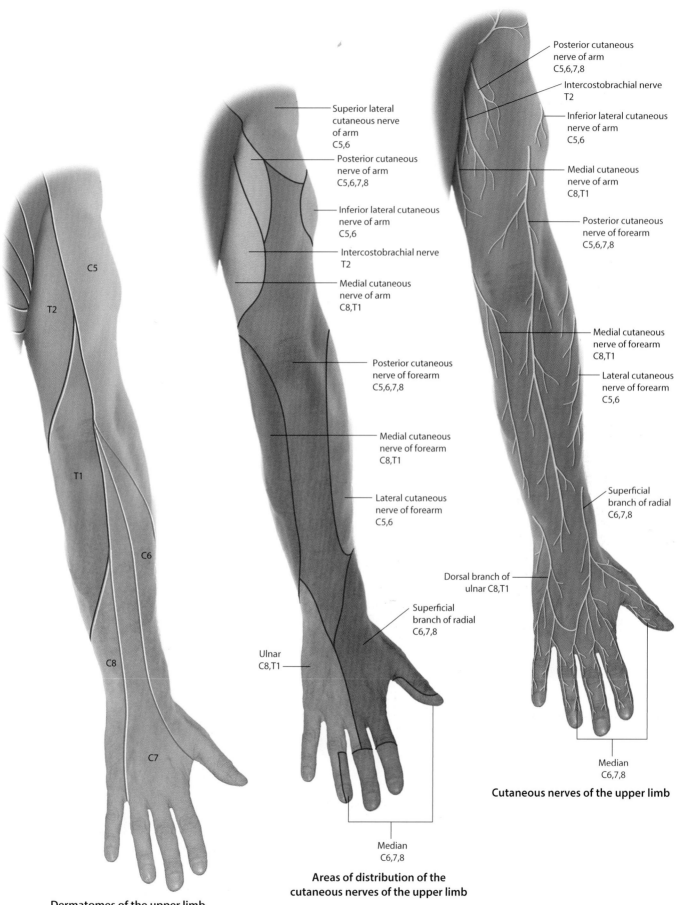

Posterior cutaneous
nerve of arm
C5,6,7,8

Intercostobrachial nerve
T2

Inferior lateral cutaneous
nerve of arm
C5,6

Medial cutaneous
nerve of arm
C8,T1

Posterior cutaneous
nerve of forearm
C5,6,7,8

Medial cutaneous
nerve of forearm
C8,T1

Lateral cutaneous
nerve of forearm
C5,6

Superficial
branch of radial
C6,7,8

Dorsal branch of
ulnar C8,T1

Median
C6,7,8

**Cutaneous nerves of the upper limb**

Superior lateral
cutaneous nerve
of arm
C5,6

Posterior cutaneous
nerve of arm
C5,6,7,8

Inferior lateral cutaneous
nerve of arm
C5,6

Intercostobrachial nerve
T2

Medial cutaneous
nerve of arm
C8,T1

Posterior cutaneous
nerve of forearm
C5,6,7,8

Medial cutaneous
nerve of forearm
C8,T1

Lateral cutaneous
nerve of forearm
C5,6

Superficial
branch of radial
C6,7,8

Ulnar
C8,T1

Median
C6,7,8

**Areas of distribution of the
cutaneous nerves of the upper limb**

C5

T2

T1

C6

C8

C7

**Dermatomes of the upper limb**

# 8 HEAD AND NECK

## CONTENTS

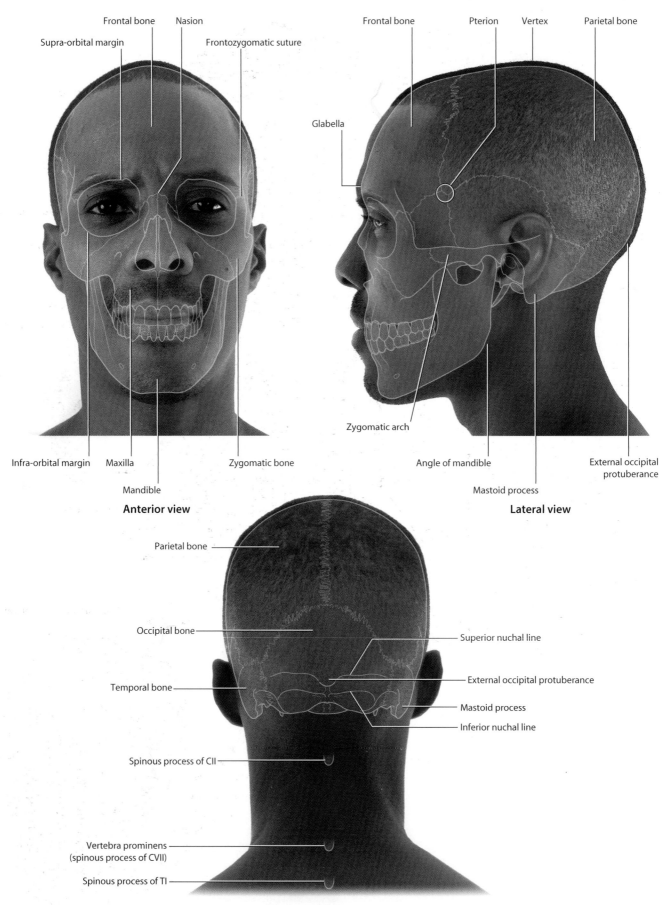

**Anterior view**

Supra-orbital margin
Frontal bone
Nasion
Frontozygomatic suture

Infra-orbital margin
Maxilla
Mandible
Zygomatic bone

**Lateral view**

Frontal bone
Pterion
Vertex
Parietal bone
Glabella

Zygomatic arch
Angle of mandible
Mastoid process
External occipital protuberance

**Posterior view**

Parietal bone
Occipital bone
Temporal bone
Spinous process of CII
Vertebra prominens (spinous process of CVII)
Spinous process of TI

Superior nuchal line
External occipital protuberance
Mastoid process
Inferior nuchal line

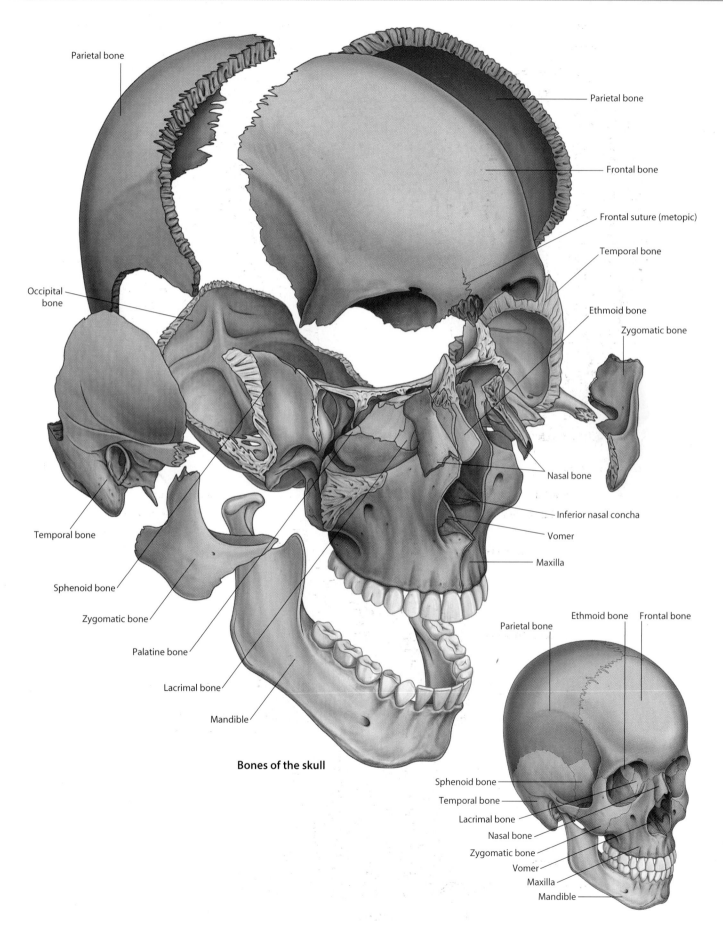

Parietal bone

Parietal bone

Frontal bone

Frontal suture (metopic)

Temporal bone

Occipital bone

Ethmoid bone

Zygomatic bone

Nasal bone

Inferior nasal concha

Vomer

Temporal bone

Maxilla

Sphenoid bone

Zygomatic bone

Palatine bone

Lacrimal bone

Mandible

**Bones of the skull**

Parietal bone

Ethmoid bone    Frontal bone

Sphenoid bone

Temporal bone

Lacrimal bone

Nasal bone

Zygomatic bone

Vomer

Maxilla

Mandible

**429**

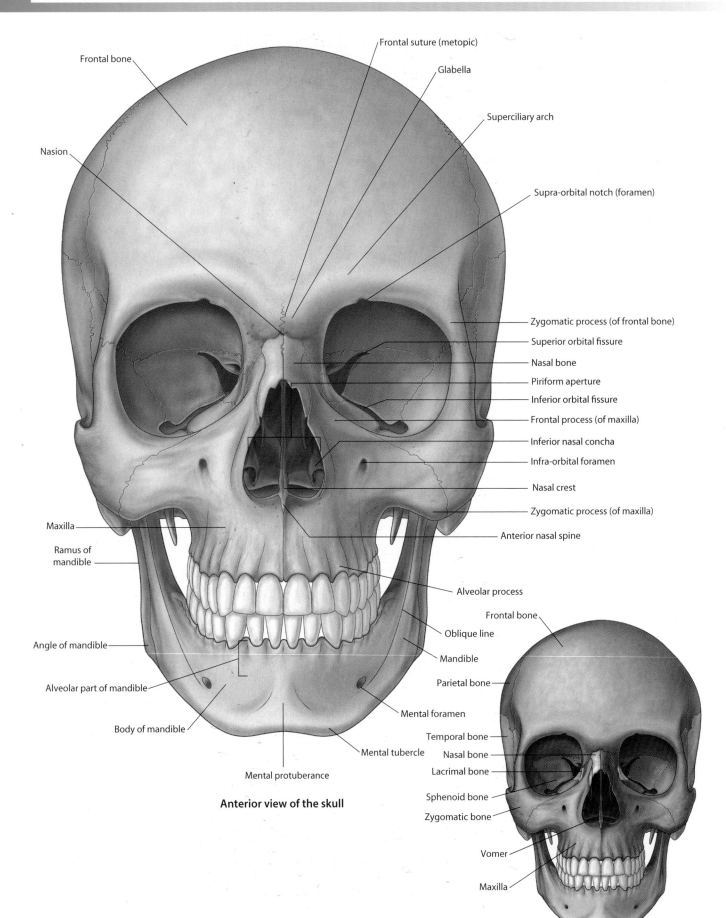

Frontal suture (metopic)

Glabella

Superciliary arch

Supra-orbital notch (foramen)

Frontal bone

Nasion

Zygomatic process (of frontal bone)

Superior orbital fissure

Nasal bone

Piriform aperture

Inferior orbital fissure

Frontal process (of maxilla)

Inferior nasal concha

Infra-orbital foramen

Nasal crest

Zygomatic process (of maxilla)

Anterior nasal spine

Maxilla

Ramus of mandible

Alveolar process

Oblique line

Mandible

Angle of mandible

Parietal bone

Alveolar part of mandible

Mental foramen

Body of mandible

Mental tubercle

Mental protuberance

**Anterior view of the skull**

Frontal bone

Temporal bone

Nasal bone

Lacrimal bone

Sphenoid bone

Zygomatic bone

Vomer

Maxilla

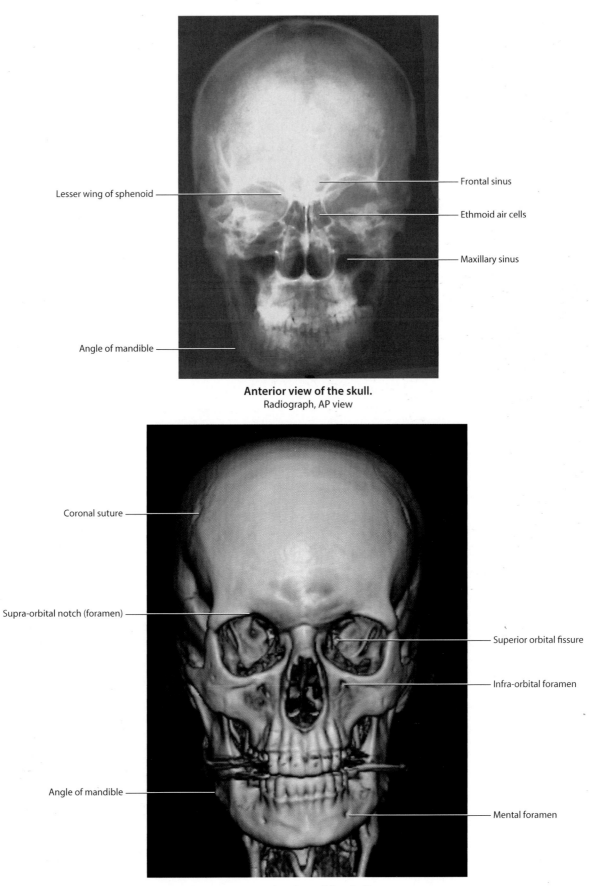

Lesser wing of sphenoid

Frontal sinus

Ethmoid air cells

Maxillary sinus

Angle of mandible

**Anterior view of the skull.**
Radiograph, AP view

Coronal suture

Supra-orbital notch (foramen)

Superior orbital fissure

Infra-orbital foramen

Angle of mandible

Mental foramen

**Anterior view of the skull.**
Volume-rendered anterior view using multidetector computed tomography

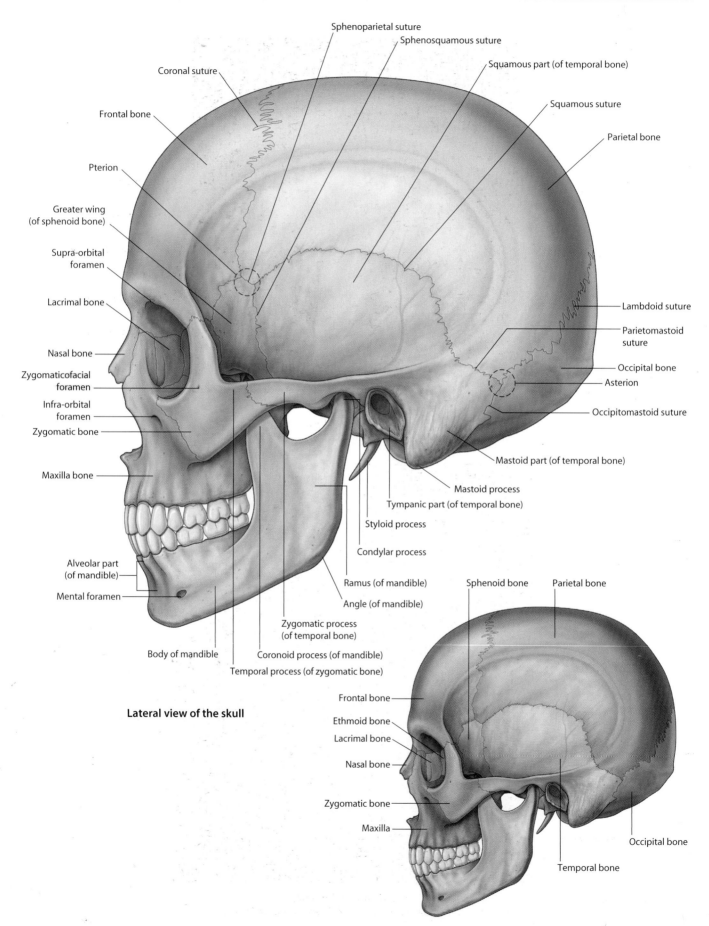

Sphenoparietal suture

Sphenosquamous suture

Squamous part (of temporal bone)

Coronal suture

Squamous suture

Frontal bone

Parietal bone

Pterion

Greater wing
(of sphenoid bone)

Supra-orbital
foramen

Lambdoid suture

Lacrimal bone

Parietomastoid
suture

Nasal bone

Occipital bone

Zygomaticofacial
foramen

Asterion

Infra-orbital
foramen

Occipitomastoid suture

Zygomatic bone

Maxilla bone

Mastoid part (of temporal bone)

Mastoid process

Tympanic part (of temporal bone)

Styloid process

Condylar process

Alveolar part
(of mandible)

Ramus (of mandible)

Mental foramen

Angle (of mandible)

Zygomatic process
(of temporal bone)

Body of mandible

Coronoid process (of mandible)

Temporal process (of zygomatic bone)

**Lateral view of the skull**

Sphenoid bone

Parietal bone

Frontal bone

Ethmoid bone

Lacrimal bone

Nasal bone

Zygomatic bone

Occipital bone

Maxilla

Temporal bone

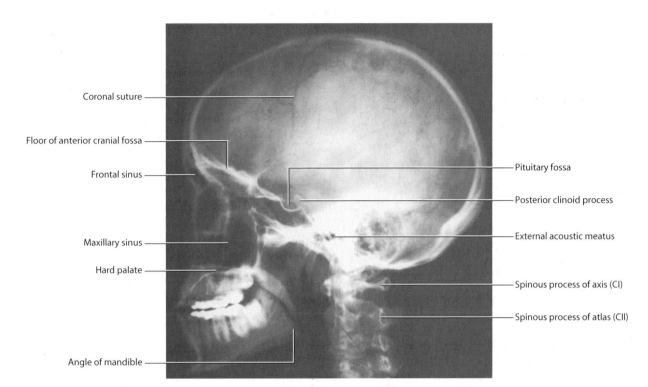

Coronal suture

Floor of anterior cranial fossa

Frontal sinus

Maxillary sinus

Hard palate

Angle of mandible

Pituitary fossa

Posterior clinoid process

External acoustic meatus

Spinous process of axis (CI)

Spinous process of atlas (CII)

**Lateral view of the skull.**
Radiograph, lateral view

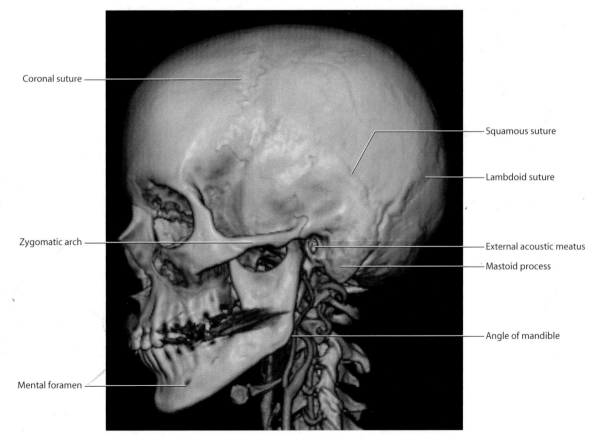

Coronal suture

Zygomatic arch

Mental foramen

Squamous suture

Lambdoid suture

External acoustic meatus

Mastoid process

Angle of mandible

**Lateral view of the skull.**
Volume-rendered lateral view using multidetector computed tomography

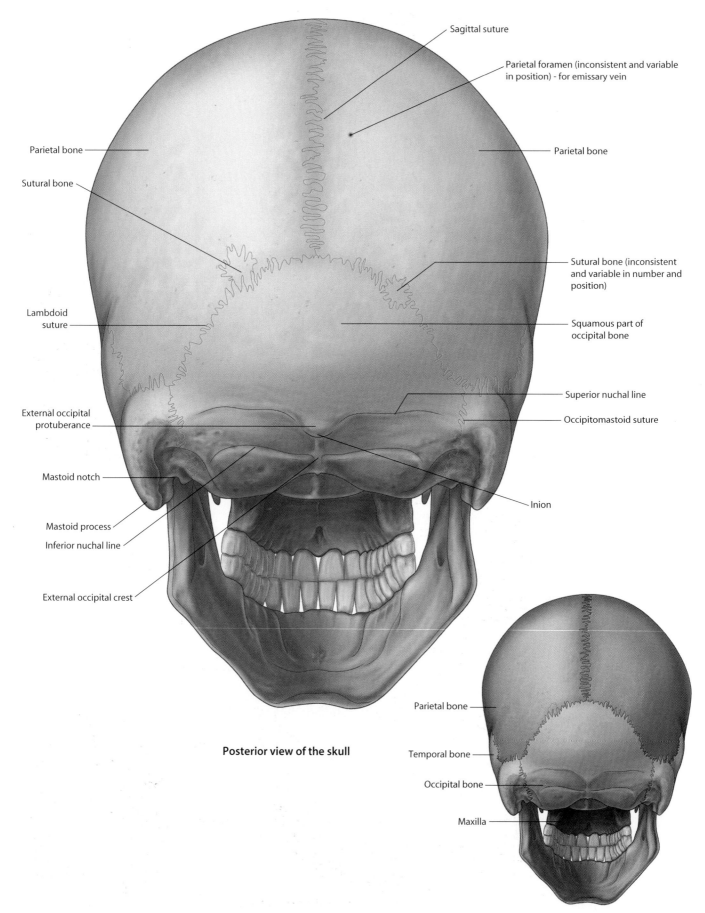

Sagittal suture

Parietal foramen (inconsistent and variable in position) - for emissary vein

Parietal bone

Parietal bone

Sutural bone

Sutural bone (inconsistent and variable in number and position)

Lambdoid suture

Squamous part of occipital bone

External occipital protuberance

Superior nuchal line

Occipitomastoid suture

Mastoid notch

Mastoid process

Inferior nuchal line

Inion

External occipital crest

**Posterior view of the skull**

Parietal bone

Temporal bone

Occipital bone

Maxilla

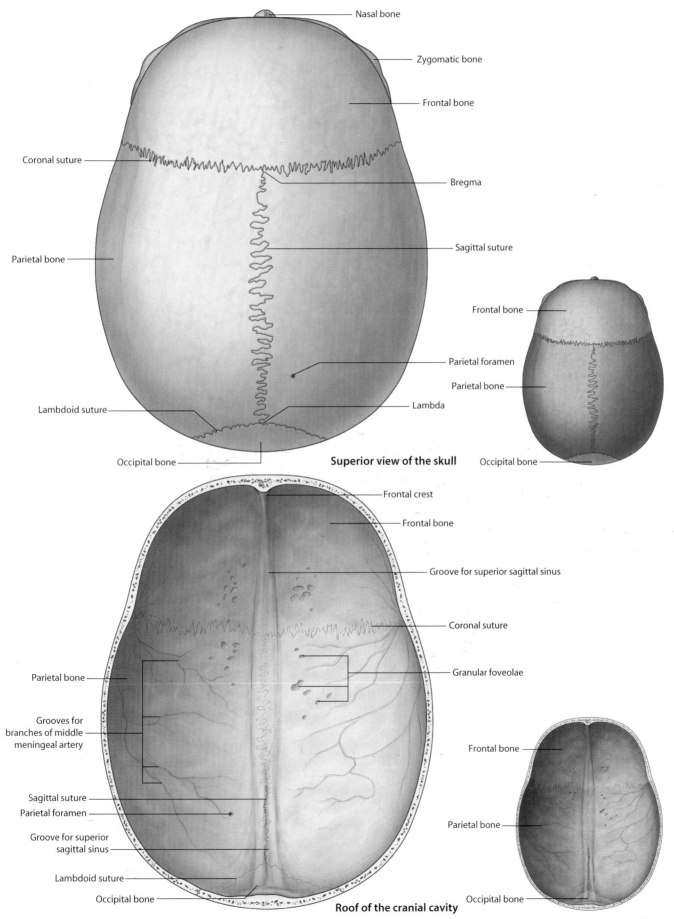

Nasal bone

Zygomatic bone

Frontal bone

Coronal suture

Bregma

Sagittal suture

Parietal bone

Frontal bone

Parietal foramen

Parietal bone

Lambdoid suture

Lambda

Occipital bone

**Superior view of the skull**

Occipital bone

Frontal crest

Frontal bone

Groove for superior sagittal sinus

Coronal suture

Parietal bone

Granular foveolae

Grooves for branches of middle meningeal artery

Frontal bone

Sagittal suture

Parietal foramen

Parietal bone

Groove for superior sagittal sinus

Lambdoid suture

Occipital bone

Occipital bone

**Roof of the cranial cavity**

**435**

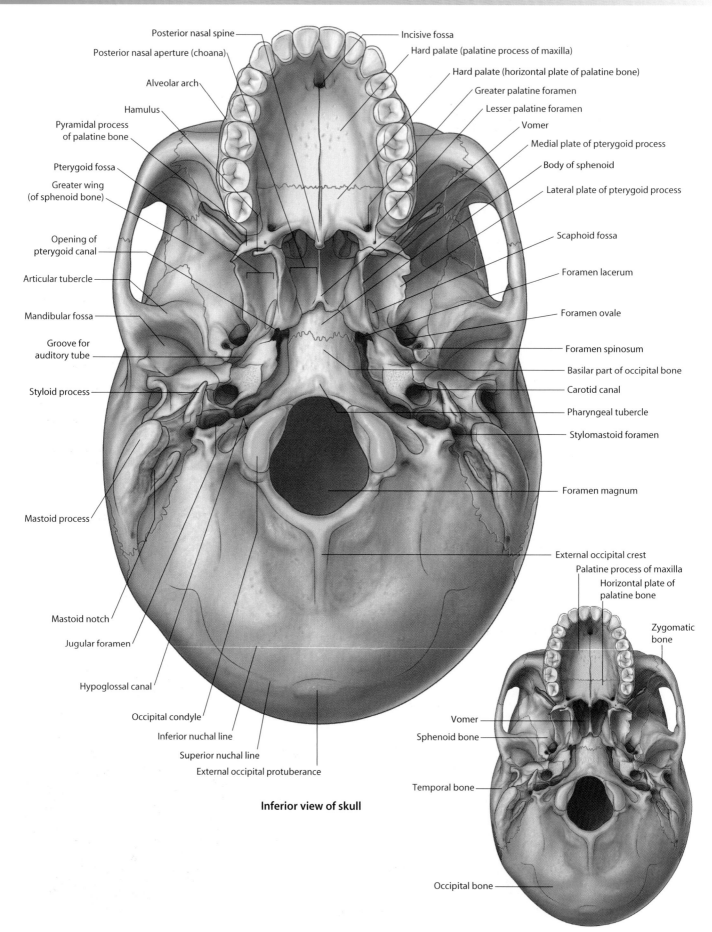

Posterior nasal spine

Posterior nasal aperture (choana)

Alveolar arch

Hamulus

Pyramidal process of palatine bone

Pterygoid fossa

Greater wing (of sphenoid bone)

Opening of pterygoid canal

Articular tubercle

Mandibular fossa

Groove for auditory tube

Styloid process

Mastoid process

Mastoid notch

Jugular foramen

Hypoglossal canal

Occipital condyle

Inferior nuchal line

Superior nuchal line

External occipital protuberance

Incisive fossa

Hard palate (palatine process of maxilla)

Hard palate (horizontal plate of palatine bone)

Greater palatine foramen

Lesser palatine foramen

Vomer

Medial plate of pterygoid process

Body of sphenoid

Lateral plate of pterygoid process

Scaphoid fossa

Foramen lacerum

Foramen ovale

Foramen spinosum

Basilar part of occipital bone

Carotid canal

Pharyngeal tubercle

Stylomastoid foramen

Foramen magnum

External occipital crest

Palatine process of maxilla

Horizontal plate of palatine bone

Zygomatic bone

Vomer

Sphenoid bone

Temporal bone

Occipital bone

**Inferior view of skull**

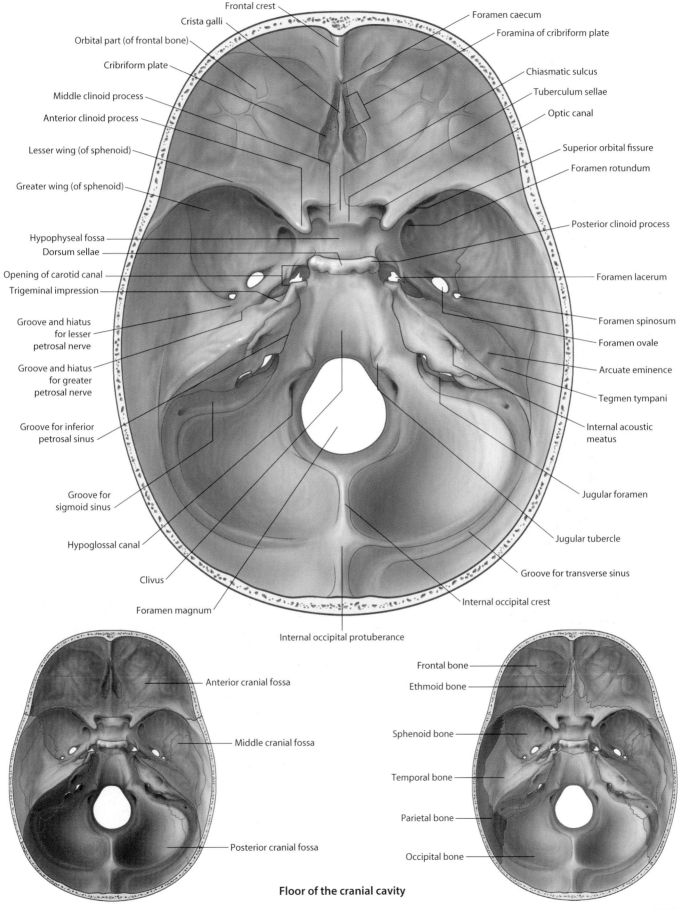

Frontal crest

Crista galli

Orbital part (of frontal bone)

Cribriform plate

Middle clinoid process

Anterior clinoid process

Lesser wing (of sphenoid)

Greater wing (of sphenoid)

Hypophyseal fossa

Dorsum sellae

Opening of carotid canal

Trigeminal impression

Groove and hiatus for lesser petrosal nerve

Groove and hiatus for greater petrosal nerve

Groove for inferior petrosal sinus

Groove for sigmoid sinus

Hypoglossal canal

Clivus

Foramen magnum

Foramen caecum

Foramina of cribriform plate

Chiasmatic sulcus

Tuberculum sellae

Optic canal

Superior orbital fissure

Foramen rotundum

Posterior clinoid process

Foramen lacerum

Foramen spinosum

Foramen ovale

Arcuate eminence

Tegmen tympani

Internal acoustic meatus

Jugular foramen

Jugular tubercle

Groove for transverse sinus

Internal occipital crest

Internal occipital protuberance

Anterior cranial fossa

Middle cranial fossa

Posterior cranial fossa

Frontal bone

Ethmoid bone

Sphenoid bone

Temporal bone

Parietal bone

Occipital bone

**Floor of the cranial cavity**

**437**

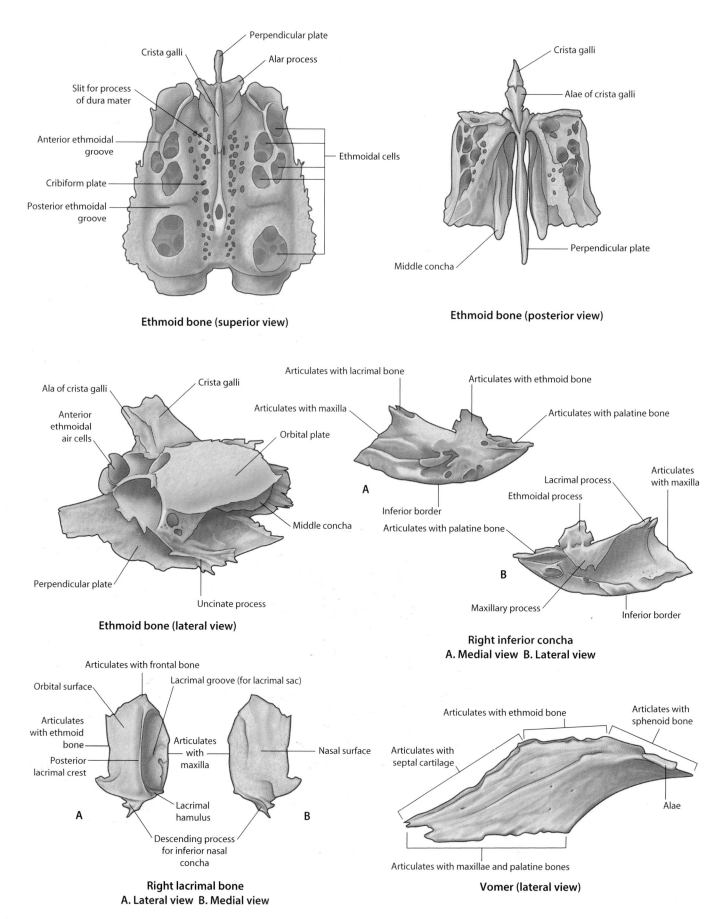

Perpendicular plate

Crista galli

Alar process

Slit for process of dura mater

Anterior ethmoidal groove

Ethmoidal cells

Cribiform plate

Posterior ethmoidal groove

**Ethmoid bone (superior view)**

Crista galli

Alae of crista galli

Middle concha

Perpendicular plate

**Ethmoid bone (posterior view)**

Ala of crista galli

Crista galli

Anterior ethmoidal air cells

Orbital plate

Perpendicular plate

Middle concha

Uncinate process

**Ethmoid bone (lateral view)**

Articulates with lacrimal bone

Articulates with ethmoid bone

Articulates with maxilla

Articulates with palatine bone

Orbital plate

A

Inferior border

Lacrimal process

Articulates with maxilla

Ethmoidal process

Articulates with palatine bone

B

Maxillary process

Inferior border

**Right inferior concha
A. Medial view  B. Lateral view**

Articulates with frontal bone

Orbital surface

Lacrimal groove (for lacrimal sac)

Articulates with ethmoid bone

Articulates with maxilla

Posterior lacrimal crest

Nasal surface

A

Lacrimal hamulus

B

Descending process for inferior nasal concha

**Right lacrimal bone
A. Lateral view  B. Medial view**

Articulates with ethmoid bone

Articlates with sphenoid bone

Articulates with septal cartilage

Alae

Articulates with maxillae and palatine bones

**Vomer (lateral view)**

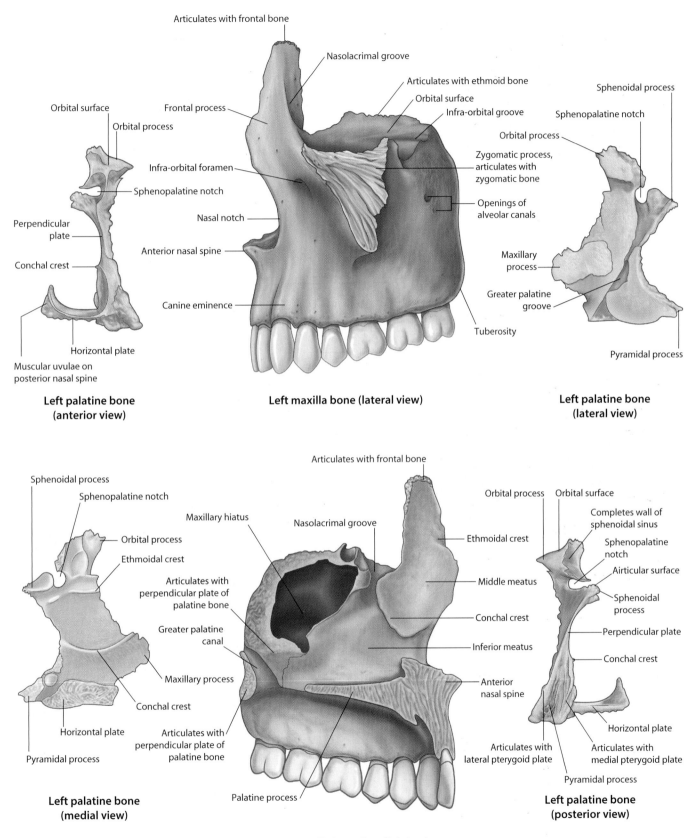

Left palatine bone
(anterior view)

Orbital surface
Orbital process
Perpendicular plate
Conchal crest
Muscular uvulae on posterior nasal spine
Horizontal plate

Left maxilla bone (lateral view)

Articulates with frontal bone
Nasolacrimal groove
Articulates with ethmoid bone
Orbital surface
Infra-orbital groove
Frontal process
Infra-orbital foramen
Sphenopalatine notch
Nasal notch
Anterior nasal spine
Canine eminence
Zygomatic process, articulates with zygomatic bone
Openings of alveolar canals
Tuberosity

Left palatine bone
(lateral view)

Sphenoidal process
Sphenopalatine notch
Orbital process
Maxillary process
Greater palatine groove
Pyramidal process

Left palatine bone
(medial view)

Sphenoidal process
Sphenopalatine notch
Orbital process
Ethmoidal crest
Greater palatine canal
Maxillary process
Conchal crest
Horizontal plate
Pyramidal process
Articulates with perpendicular plate of palatine bone

Left maxilla bone (medial view)

Articulates with frontal bone
Maxillary hiatus
Nasolacrimal groove
Articulates with perpendicular plate of palatine bone
Ethmoidal crest
Middle meatus
Conchal crest
Inferior meatus
Anterior nasal spine
Palatine process

Left palatine bone
(posterior view)

Orbital process
Orbital surface
Completes wall of sphenoidal sinus
Sphenopalatine notch
Airticular surface
Sphenoidal process
Perpendicular plate
Conchal crest
Horizontal plate
Articulates with lateral pterygoid plate
Articulates with medial pterygoid plate
Pyramidal process

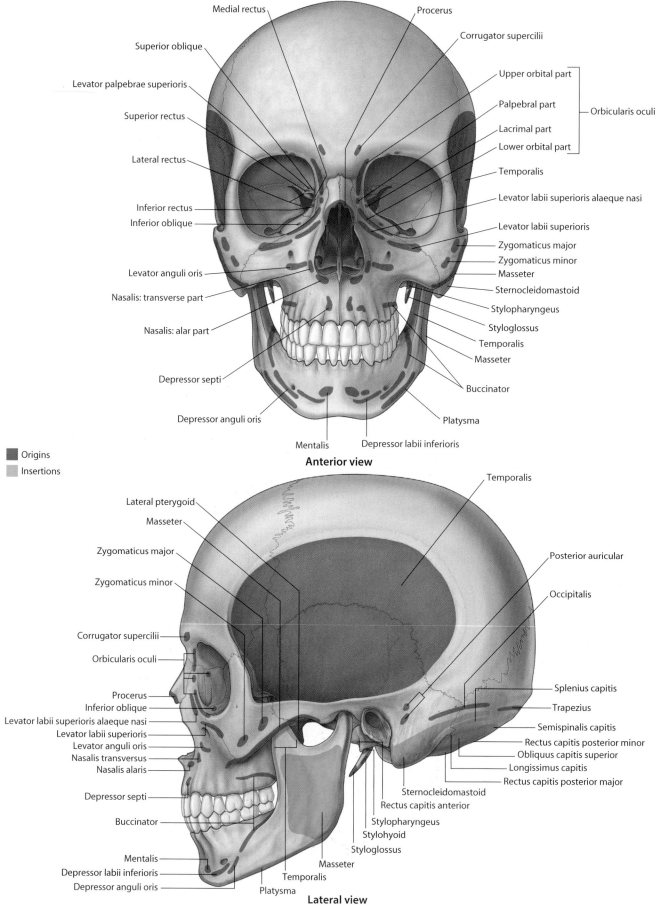

Medial rectus

Procerus

Superior oblique

Corrugator supercilii

Levator palpebrae superioris

Upper orbital part

Superior rectus

Palpebral part

Lacrimal part

Orbicularis oculi

Lateral rectus

Lower orbital part

Temporalis

Levator labii superioris alaeque nasi

Inferior rectus

Levator labii superioris

Inferior oblique

Zygomaticus major

Zygomaticus minor

Masseter

Levator anguli oris

Sternocleidomastoid

Nasalis: transverse part

Stylopharyngeus

Styloglossus

Nasalis: alar part

Temporalis

Masseter

Depressor septi

Buccinator

Depressor anguli oris

Platysma

Mentalis

Depressor labii inferioris

**Anterior view**

■ Origins
□ Insertions

Temporalis

Lateral pterygoid

Masseter

Zygomaticus major

Posterior auricular

Zygomaticus minor

Occipitalis

Corrugator supercilii

Orbicularis oculi

Procerus

Splenius capitis

Inferior oblique

Trapezius

Levator labii superioris alaeque nasi

Semispinalis capitis

Levator labii superioris

Rectus capitis posterior minor

Levator anguli oris

Obliquus capitis superior

Nasalis transversus

Longissimus capitis

Nasalis alaris

Rectus capitis posterior major

Depressor septi

Buccinator

Sternocleidomastoid

Rectus capitis anterior

Mentalis

Stylopharyngeus

Depressor labii inferioris

Stylohyoid

Depressor anguli oris

Styloglossus

Masseter

Temporalis

Platysma

**Lateral view**

440

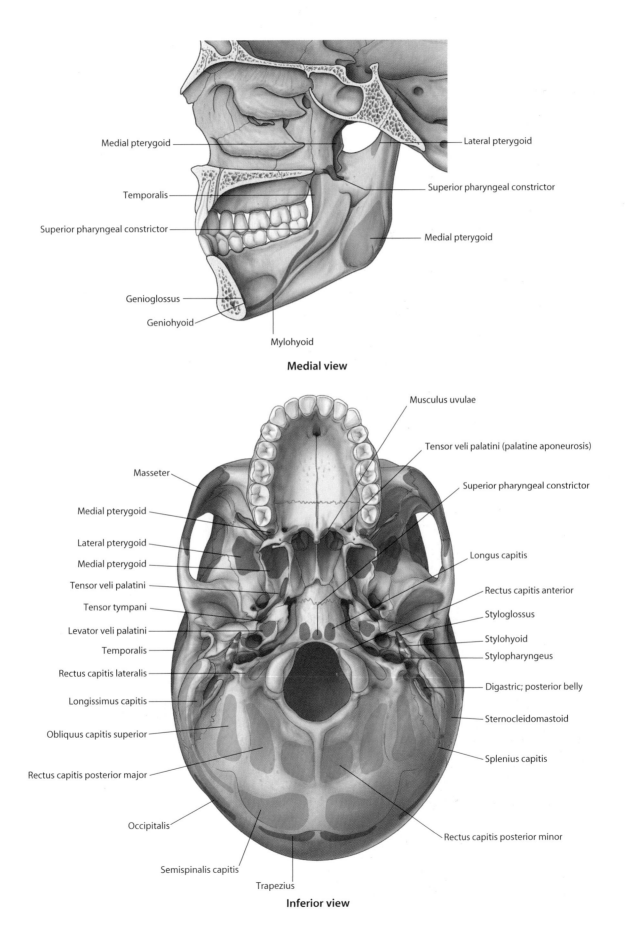

Medial pterygoid

Lateral pterygoid

Temporalis

Superior pharyngeal constrictor

Superior pharyngeal constrictor

Medial pterygoid

Genioglossus

Geniohyoid

Mylohyoid

**Medial view**

Musculus uvulae

Tensor veli palatini (palatine aponeurosis)

Masseter

Superior pharyngeal constrictor

Medial pterygoid

Lateral pterygoid

Longus capitis

Medial pterygoid

Tensor veli palatini

Rectus capitis anterior

Tensor tympani

Styloglossus

Levator veli palatini

Stylohyoid

Temporalis

Stylopharyngeus

Rectus capitis lateralis

Digastric; posterior belly

Longissimus capitis

Sternocleidomastoid

Obliquus capitis superior

Rectus capitis posterior major

Splenius capitis

Rectus capitis posterior minor

Occipitalis

Semispinalis capitis

Trapezius

**Inferior view**

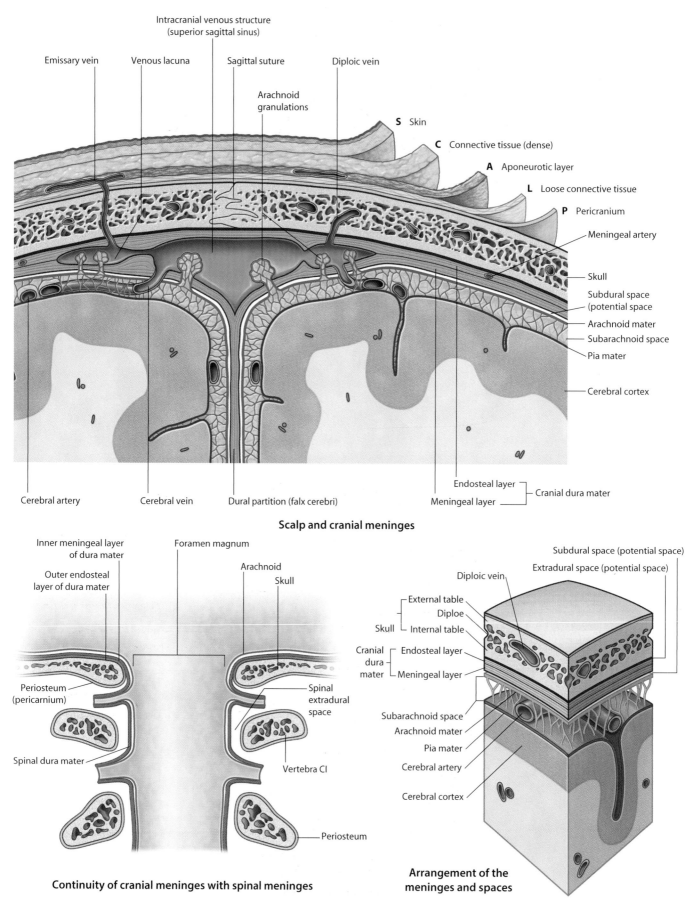

Emissary vein

Venous lacuna

Intracranial venous structure
(superior sagittal sinus)

Sagittal suture

Arachnoid
granulations

Diploic vein

**S** Skin

**C** Connective tissue (dense)

**A** Aponeurotic layer

**L** Loose connective tissue

**P** Pericranium

Meningeal artery

Skull

Subdural space
(potential space

Arachnoid mater

Subarachnoid space

Pia mater

Cerebral cortex

Cerebral artery

Cerebral vein

Dural partition (falx cerebri)

Endosteal layer

Meningeal layer

Cranial dura mater

**Scalp and cranial meninges**

Inner meningeal layer
of dura mater

Outer endosteal
layer of dura mater

Foramen magnum

Arachnoid

Skull

Periosteum
(pericarnium)

Spinal dura mater

Spinal
extradural
space

Vertebra CI

Periosteum

**Continuity of cranial meninges with spinal meninges**

Subdural space (potential space)

Extradural space (potential space)

Diploic vein

External table

Diploe

Skull

Internal table

Cranial
dura
mater

Endosteal layer

Meningeal layer

Subarachnoid space

Arachnoid mater

Pia mater

Cerebral artery

Cerebral cortex

**Arrangement of the
meninges and spaces**

**442**

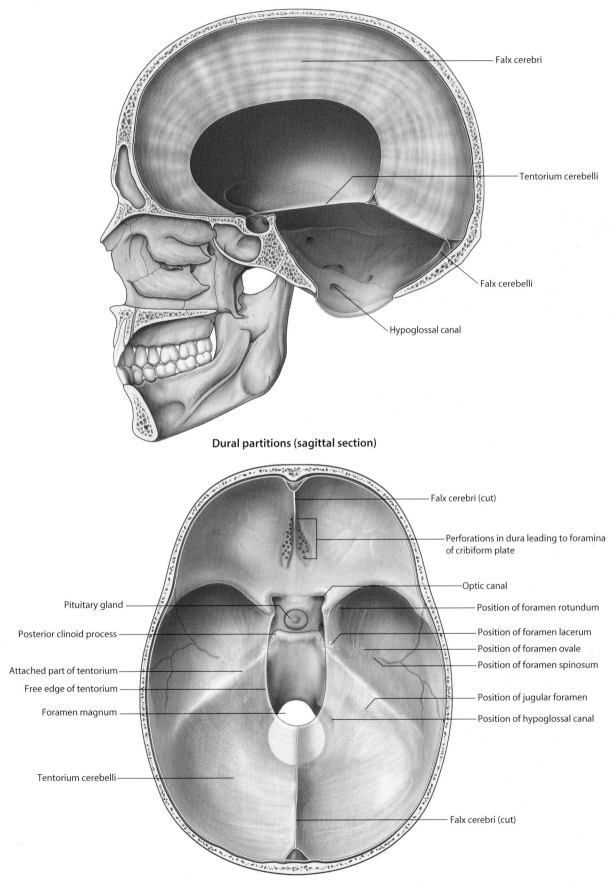

**Dural partitions (sagittal section)**

Falx cerebri

Tentorium cerebelli

Falx cerebelli

Hypoglossal canal

Falx cerebri (cut)

Perforations in dura leading to foramina of cribiform plate

Optic canal

Pituitary gland

Position of foramen rotundum

Posterior clinoid process

Position of foramen lacerum

Position of foramen ovale

Position of foramen spinosum

Attached part of tentorium

Free edge of tentorium

Position of jugular foramen

Foramen magnum

Position of hypoglossal canal

Tentorium cerebelli

Falx cerebri (cut)

**Cranial cavity (superior view)**

**443**

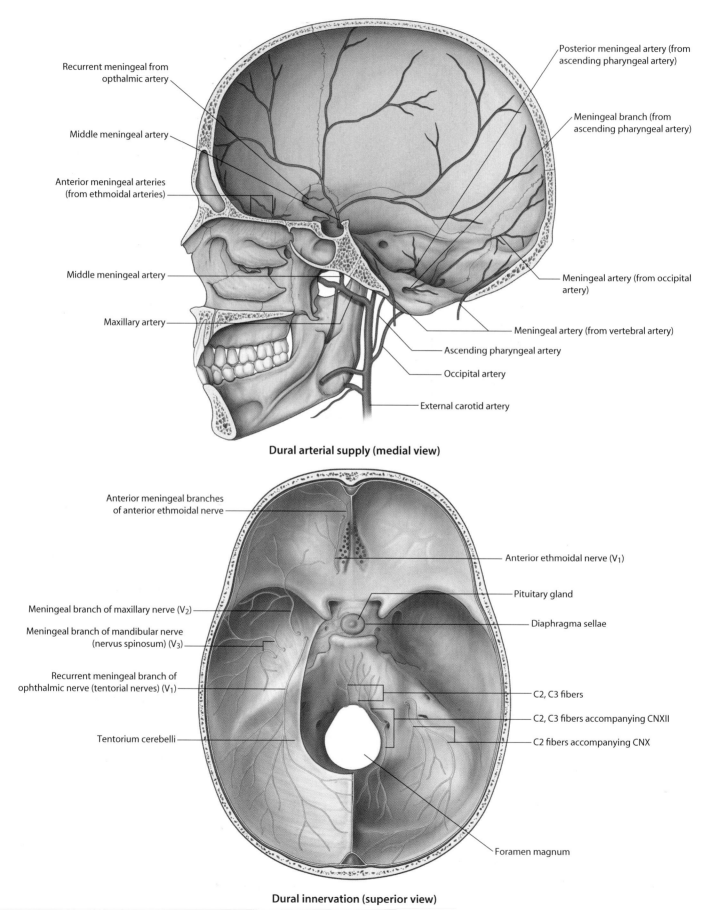

Recurrent meningeal from opthalmic artery

Middle meningeal artery

Anterior meningeal arteries (from ethmoidal arteries)

Middle meningeal artery

Maxillary artery

Posterior meningeal artery (from ascending pharyngeal artery)

Meningeal branch (from ascending pharyngeal artery)

Meningeal artery (from occipital artery)

Meningeal artery (from vertebral artery)

Ascending pharyngeal artery

Occipital artery

External carotid artery

**Dural arterial supply (medial view)**

Anterior meningeal branches of anterior ethmoidal nerve

Meningeal branch of maxillary nerve (V₂)

Meningeal branch of mandibular nerve (nervus spinosum) (V₃)

Recurrent meningeal branch of ophthalmic nerve (tentorial nerves) (V₁)

Tentorium cerebelli

Anterior ethmoidal nerve (V₁)

Pituitary gland

Diaphragma sellae

C2, C3 fibers

C2, C3 fibers accompanying CNXII

C2 fibers accompanying CNX

Foramen magnum

**Dural innervation (superior view)**

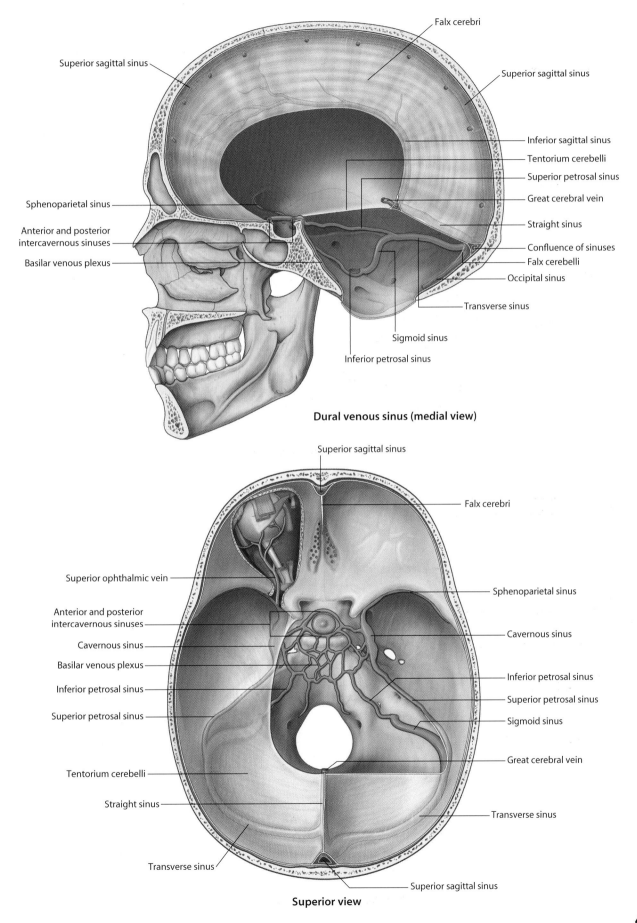

**Dural venous sinus (medial view)**

**Superior view**

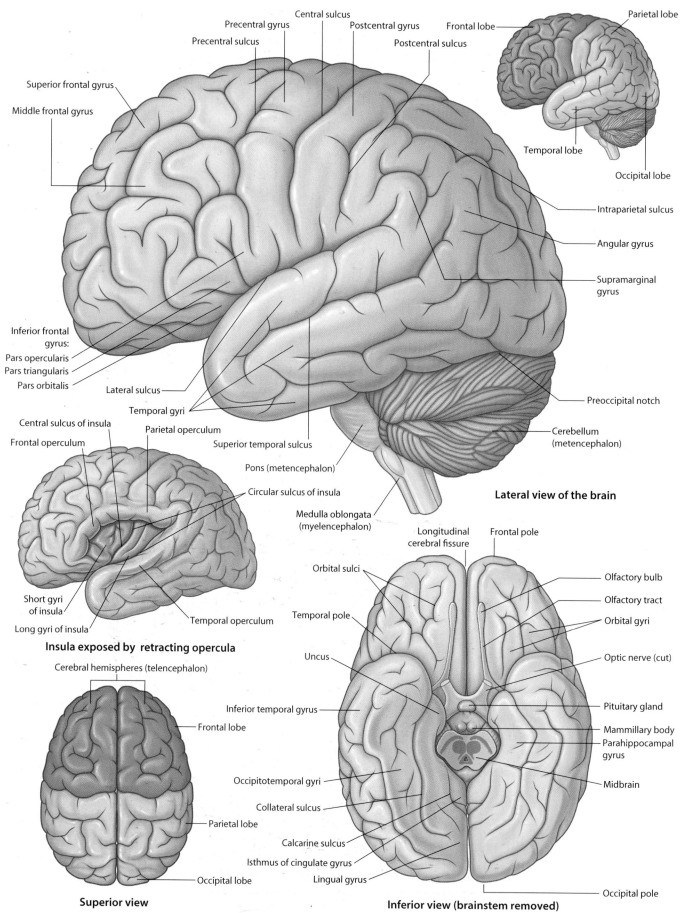

**Lateral view of the brain**

Precentral gyrus
Precentral sulcus
Central sulcus
Postcentral gyrus
Postcentral sulcus
Frontal lobe
Parietal lobe
Superior frontal gyrus
Middle frontal gyrus
Temporal lobe
Occipital lobe
Intraparietal sulcus
Angular gyrus
Supramarginal gyrus
Inferior frontal gyrus:
Pars opercularis
Pars triangularis
Pars orbitalis
Lateral sulcus
Temporal gyri
Superior temporal sulcus
Preoccipital notch
Cerebellum (metencephalon)
Pons (metencephalon)
Medulla oblongata (myelencephalon)

**Insula exposed by retracting opercula**

Central sulcus of insula
Frontal operculum
Parietal operculum
Circular sulcus of insula
Short gyri of insula
Long gyri of insula
Temporal operculum

**Superior view**

Cerebral hemispheres (telencephalon)
Frontal lobe
Parietal lobe
Occipital lobe

**Inferior view (brainstem removed)**

Longitudinal cerebral fissure
Frontal pole
Orbital sulci
Olfactory bulb
Olfactory tract
Orbital gyri
Optic nerve (cut)
Pituitary gland
Mammillary body
Parahippocampal gyrus
Midbrain
Temporal pole
Uncus
Inferior temporal gyrus
Occipitotemporal gyri
Collateral sulcus
Calcarine sulcus
Isthmus of cingulate gyrus
Lingual gyrus
Occipital pole

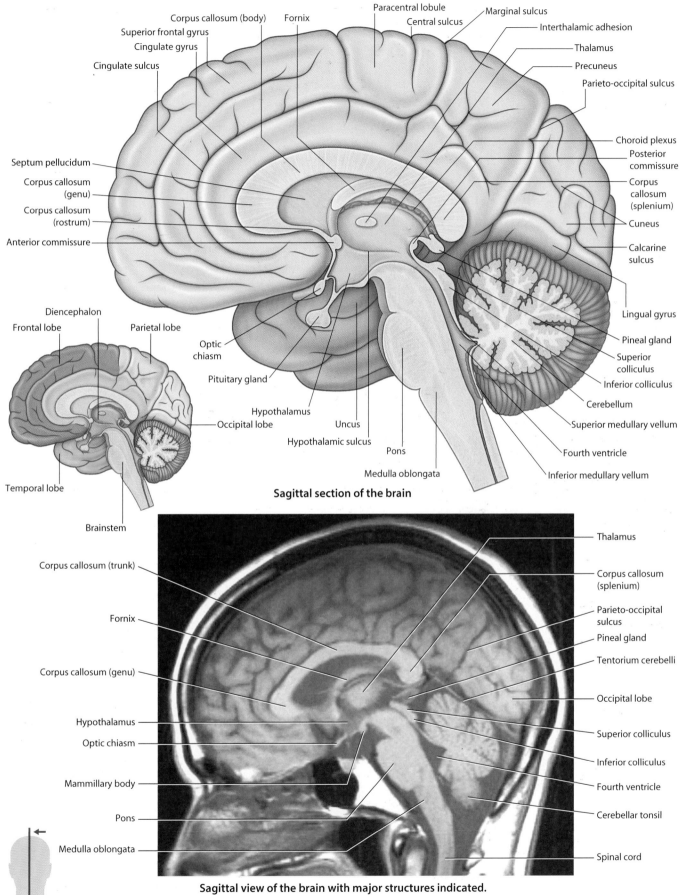

Paracentral lobule
Corpus callosum (body)
Fornix
Central sulcus
Marginal sulcus
Superior frontal gyrus
Interthalamic adhesion
Cingulate gyrus
Thalamus
Cingulate sulcus
Precuneus
Parieto-occipital sulcus
Septum pellucidum
Choroid plexus
Posterior commissure
Corpus callosum (genu)
Corpus callosum (splenium)
Corpus callosum (rostrum)
Cuneus
Anterior commissure
Calcarine sulcus
Diencephalon
Frontal lobe
Parietal lobe
Lingual gyrus
Optic chiasm
Pineal gland
Pituitary gland
Superior colliculus
Inferior colliculus
Hypothalamus
Cerebellum
Occipital lobe
Uncus
Superior medullary vellum
Hypothalamic sulcus
Fourth ventricle
Temporal lobe
Pons
Inferior medullary vellum
Medulla oblongata

**Sagittal section of the brain**

Brainstem

Thalamus
Corpus callosum (trunk)
Corpus callosum (splenium)
Fornix
Parieto-occipital sulcus
Pineal gland
Corpus callosum (genu)
Tentorium cerebelli
Occipital lobe
Hypothalamus
Optic chiasm
Superior colliculus
Inferior colliculus
Mammillary body
Fourth ventricle
Pons
Cerebellar tonsil
Medulla oblongata
Spinal cord

**Sagittal view of the brain with major structures indicated.**
T1-weighted MR image in sagittal plane

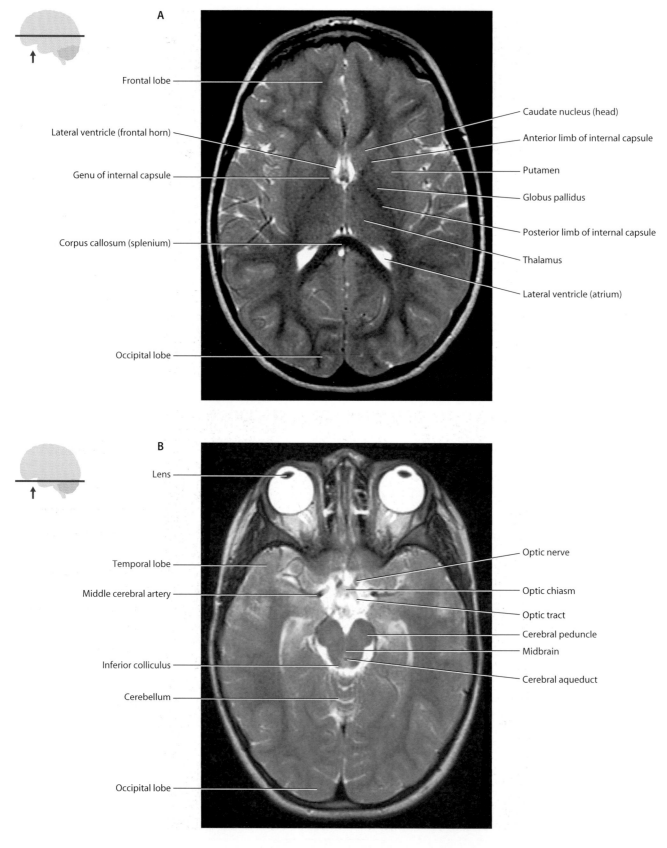

A

Frontal lobe

Lateral ventricle (frontal horn)

Genu of internal capsule

Corpus callosum (splenium)

Occipital lobe

Caudate nucleus (head)

Anterior limb of internal capsule

Putamen

Globus pallidus

Posterior limb of internal capsule

Thalamus

Lateral ventricle (atrium)

B

Lens

Temporal lobe

Middle cerebral artery

Inferior colliculus

Cerebellum

Occipital lobe

Optic nerve

Optic chiasm

Optic tract

Cerebral peduncle

Midbrain

Cerebral aqueduct

Axial or horizontal sections through the brain with major structures indicated.
A. Section showing structures related to the internal capsule.
B. Section showing structures related to the midbrain.
T1-weighted MR image in axial plane

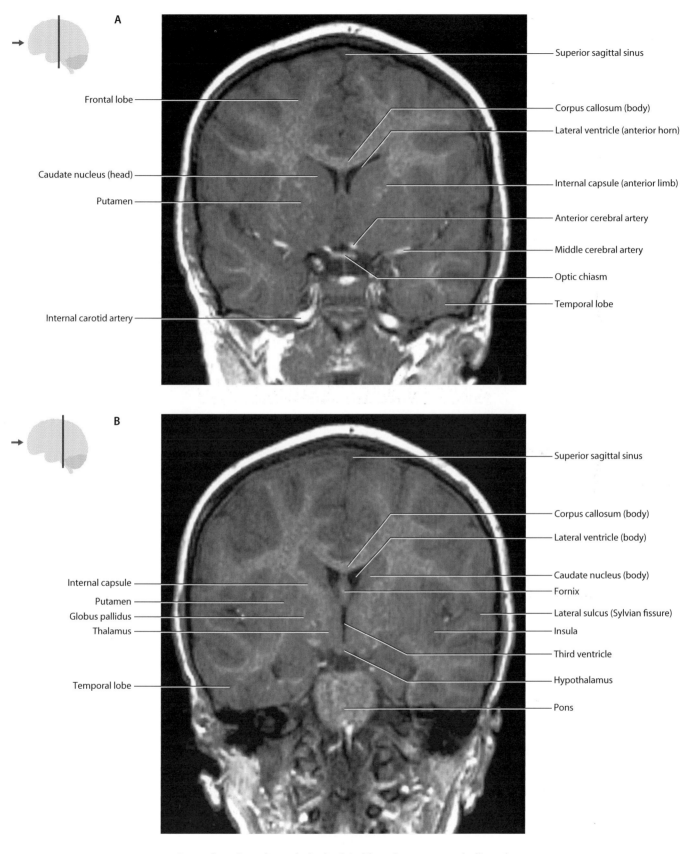

**A**

Frontal lobe

Caudate nucleus (head)

Putamen

Internal carotid artery

Superior sagittal sinus

Corpus callosum (body)

Lateral ventricle (anterior horn)

Internal capsule (anterior limb)

Anterior cerebral artery

Middle cerebral artery

Optic chiasm

Temporal lobe

**B**

Internal capsule

Putamen

Globus pallidus

Thalamus

Temporal lobe

Superior sagittal sinus

Corpus callosum (body)

Lateral ventricle (body)

Caudate nucleus (body)

Fornix

Lateral sulcus (Sylvian fissure)

Insula

Third ventricle

Hypothalamus

Pons

**Coronal sections through the brain with major structures indicated.**
**A. Section showing structures related to the optic chiasm.**
**B. Section showing structures related to the third ventricle.**
T1-weighted MR image in coronal plane

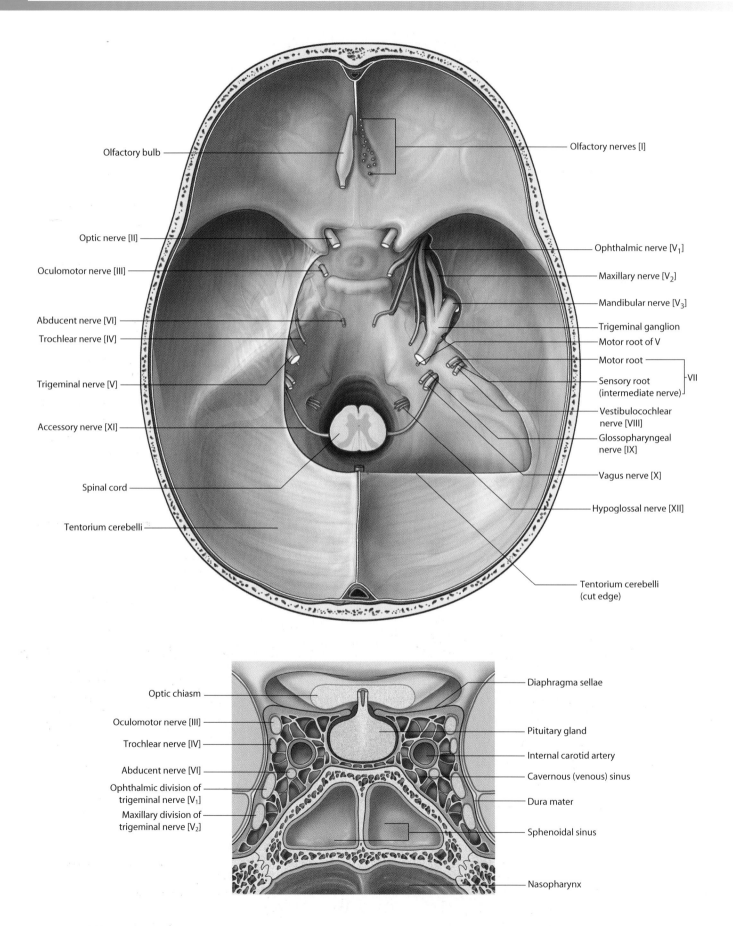

Olfactory bulb

Optic nerve [II]

Oculomotor nerve [III]

Abducent nerve [VI]

Trochlear nerve [IV]

Trigeminal nerve [V]

Accessory nerve [XI]

Spinal cord

Tentorium cerebelli

Olfactory nerves [I]

Ophthalmic nerve [V₁]

Maxillary nerve [V₂]

Mandibular nerve [V₃]

Trigeminal ganglion

Motor root of V

Motor root

Sensory root
(intermediate nerve)

VII

Vestibulocochlear
nerve [VIII]

Glossopharyngeal
nerve [IX]

Vagus nerve [X]

Hypoglossal nerve [XII]

Tentorium cerebelli
(cut edge)

Optic chiasm

Oculomotor nerve [III]

Trochlear nerve [IV]

Abducent nerve [VI]

Ophthalmic division of
trigeminal nerve [V₁]

Maxillary division of
trigeminal nerve [V₂]

Diaphragma sellae

Pituitary gland

Internal carotid artery

Cavernous (venous) sinus

Dura mater

Sphenoidal sinus

Nasopharynx

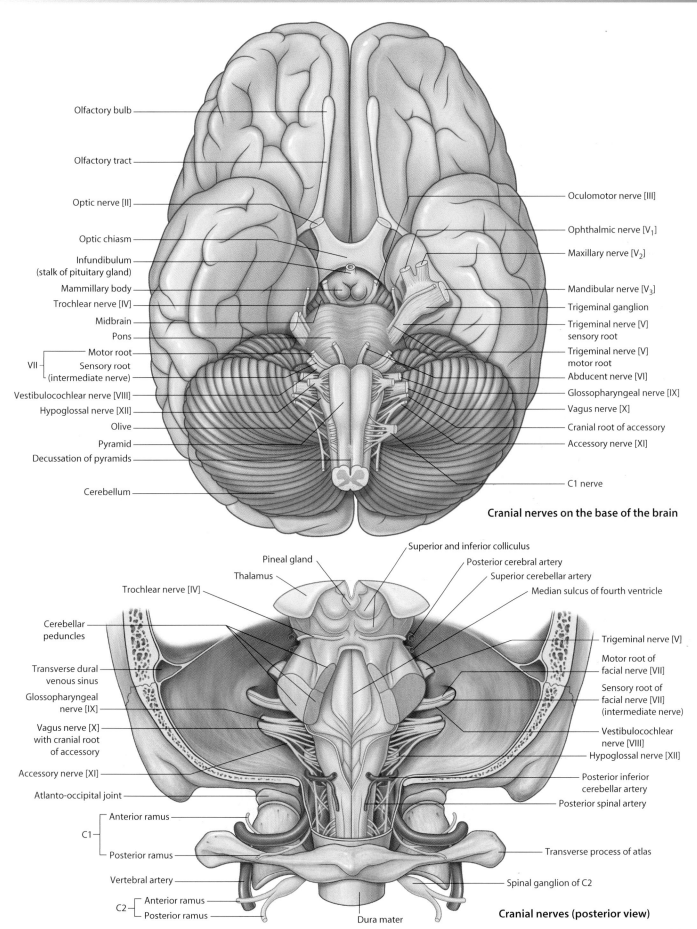

Olfactory bulb

Olfactory tract

Optic nerve [II]

Optic chiasm

Infundibulum
(stalk of pituitary gland)

Mammillary body

Trochlear nerve [IV]

Midbrain

Pons

Motor root

VII

Sensory root
(intermediate nerve)

Vestibulocochlear nerve [VIII]

Hypoglossal nerve [XII]

Olive

Pyramid

Decussation of pyramids

Cerebellum

Oculomotor nerve [III]

Ophthalmic nerve [V₁]

Maxillary nerve [V₂]

Mandibular nerve [V₃]

Trigeminal ganglion

Trigeminal nerve [V]
sensory root

Trigeminal nerve [V]
motor root

Abducent nerve [VI]

Glossopharyngeal nerve [IX]

Vagus nerve [X]

Cranial root of accessory

Accessory nerve [XI]

C1 nerve

**Cranial nerves on the base of the brain**

Superior and inferior colliculus

Pineal gland

Thalamus

Trochlear nerve [IV]

Cerebellar
peduncles

Transverse dural
venous sinus

Glossopharyngeal
nerve [IX]

Vagus nerve [X]
with cranial root
of accessory

Accessory nerve [XI]

Atlanto-occipital joint

Anterior ramus

C1

Posterior ramus

Vertebral artery

C2

Anterior ramus

Posterior ramus

Dura mater

Posterior cerebral artery

Superior cerebellar artery

Median sulcus of fourth ventricle

Trigeminal nerve [V]

Motor root of
facial nerve [VII]

Sensory root of
facial nerve [VII]
(intermediate nerve)

Vestibulocochlear
nerve [VIII]

Hypoglossal nerve [XII]

Posterior inferior
cerebellar artery

Posterior spinal artery

Transverse process of atlas

Spinal ganglion of C2

**Cranial nerves (posterior view)**

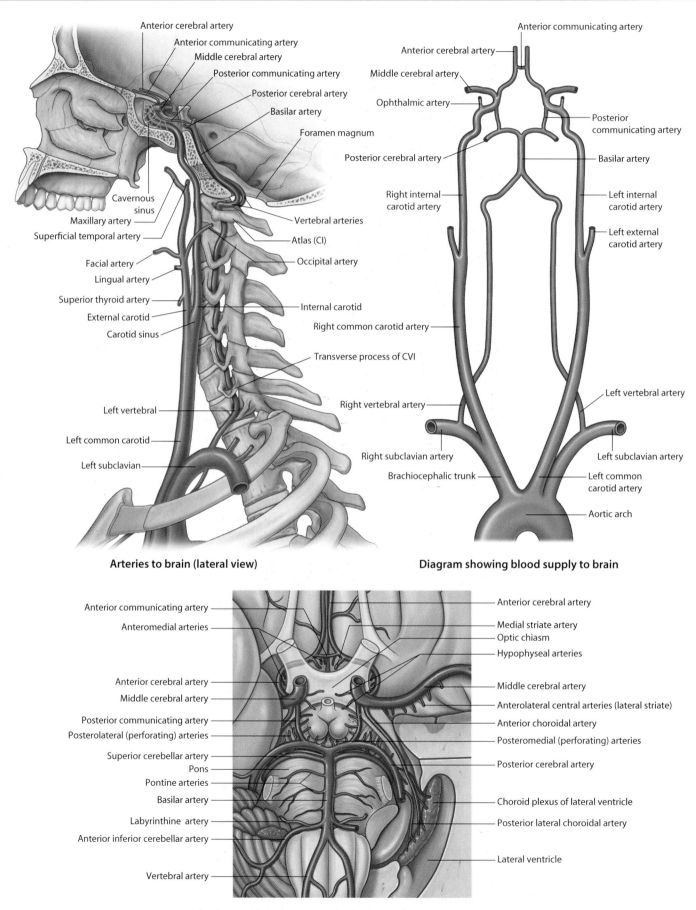

Anterior cerebral artery
Anterior communicating artery
Middle cerebral artery
Posterior communicating artery
Posterior cerebral artery
Basilar artery
Foramen magnum

Cavernous sinus
Maxillary artery
Superficial temporal artery
Facial artery
Lingual artery
Superior thyroid artery
External carotid
Carotid sinus

Vertebral arteries
Atlas (CI)
Occipital artery
Internal carotid
Right common carotid artery
Transverse process of CVI

Left vertebral
Left common carotid
Left subclavian

Right vertebral artery

**Arteries to brain (lateral view)**

Anterior communicating artery
Anterior cerebral artery
Middle cerebral artery
Ophthalmic artery
Posterior cerebral artery
Right internal carotid artery

Anterior cerebral artery

Posterior communicating artery
Basilar artery
Left internal carotid artery
Left external carotid artery
Left vertebral artery

Right subclavian artery
Brachiocephalic trunk

Left subclavian artery
Left common carotid artery
Aortic arch

**Diagram showing blood supply to brain**

Anterior communicating artery
Anteromedial arteries

Anterior cerebral artery
Middle cerebral artery
Posterior communicating artery
Posterolateral (perforating) arteries
Superior cerebellar artery
Pons
Pontine arteries
Basilar artery
Labyrinthine artery
Anterior inferior cerebellar artery

Vertebral artery

Anterior cerebral artery
Medial striate artery
Optic chiasm
Hypophyseal arteries
Middle cerebral artery
Anterolateral central arteries (lateral striate)
Anterior choroidal artery
Posteromedial (perforating) arteries
Posterior cerebral artery
Choroid plexus of lateral ventricle
Posterior lateral choroidal artery
Lateral ventricle

**Cerebral arterial circle (of Willis)**

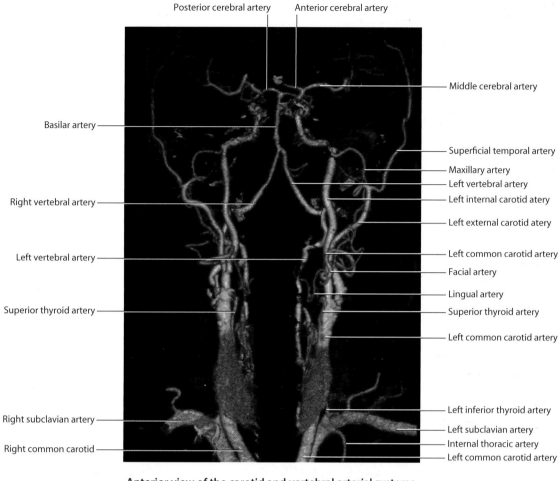

Posterior cerebral artery    Anterior cerebral artery

Middle cerebral artery

Basilar artery

Superficial temporal artery

Maxillary artery

Left vertebral artery

Right vertebral artery

Left internal carotid atery

Left external carotid atery

Left common carotid artery

Left vertebral artery

Facial artery

Lingual artery

Superior thyroid artery

Superior thyroid artery

Left common carotid artery

Left inferior thyroid artery

Right subclavian artery

Left subclavian artery

Internal thoracic artery

Right common carotid

Left common carotid artery

**Anterior view of the carotid and vertebral arterial systems.**
Volume-rendered anterior view using multidetector computed tomography

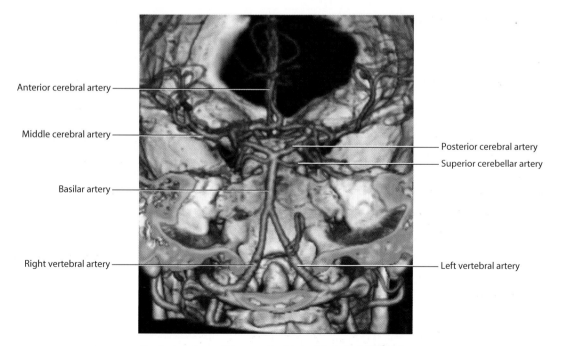

Anterior cerebral artery

Middle cerebral artery

Posterior cerebral artery

Superior cerebellar artery

Basilar artery

Right vertebral artery

Left vertebral artery

**Posterior view of the cerebral arterial circle (of Willis).**
Volume-rendered posterior view using multidetector computed tomography

**453**

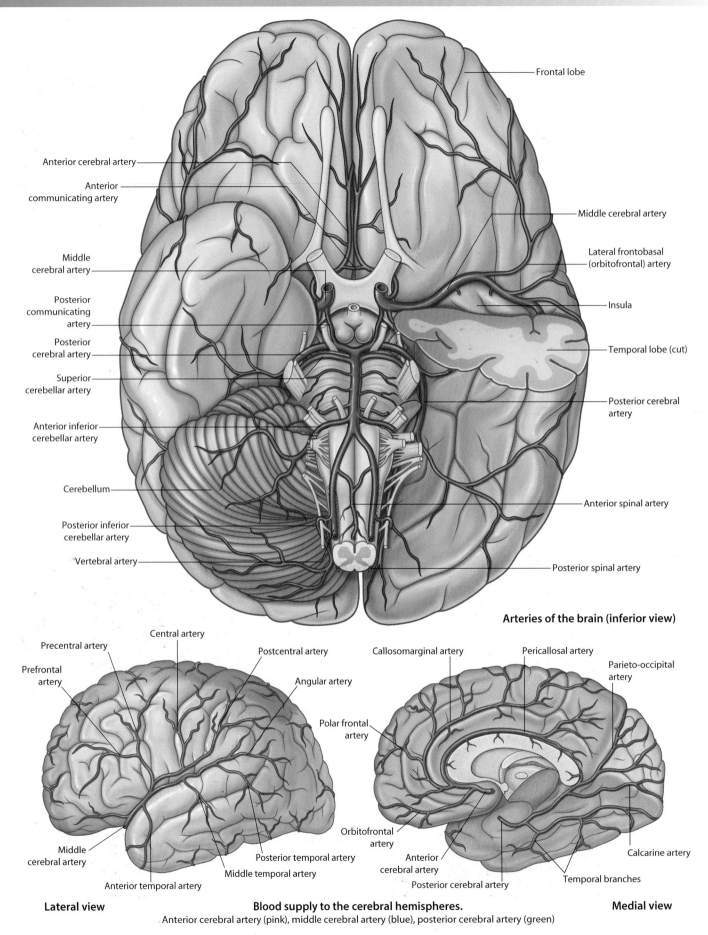

Frontal lobe

Anterior cerebral artery

Anterior communicating artery

Middle cerebral artery

Middle cerebral artery

Lateral frontobasal (orbitofrontal) artery

Posterior communicating artery

Insula

Posterior cerebral artery

Temporal lobe (cut)

Superior cerebellar artery

Posterior cerebral artery

Anterior inferior cerebellar artery

Cerebellum

Anterior spinal artery

Posterior inferior cerebellar artery

Vertebral artery

Posterior spinal artery

**Arteries of the brain (inferior view)**

Central artery

Precentral artery

Postcentral artery

Callosomarginal artery

Pericallosal artery

Parieto-occipital artery

Prefrontal artery

Angular artery

Polar frontal artery

Middle cerebral artery

Posterior temporal artery

Orbitofrontal artery

Calcarine artery

Anterior temporal artery

Middle temporal artery

Anterior cerebral artery

Posterior cerebral artery

Temporal branches

**Lateral view**

**Blood supply to the cerebral hemispheres.**
Anterior cerebral artery (pink), middle cerebral artery (blue), posterior cerebral artery (green)

**Medial view**

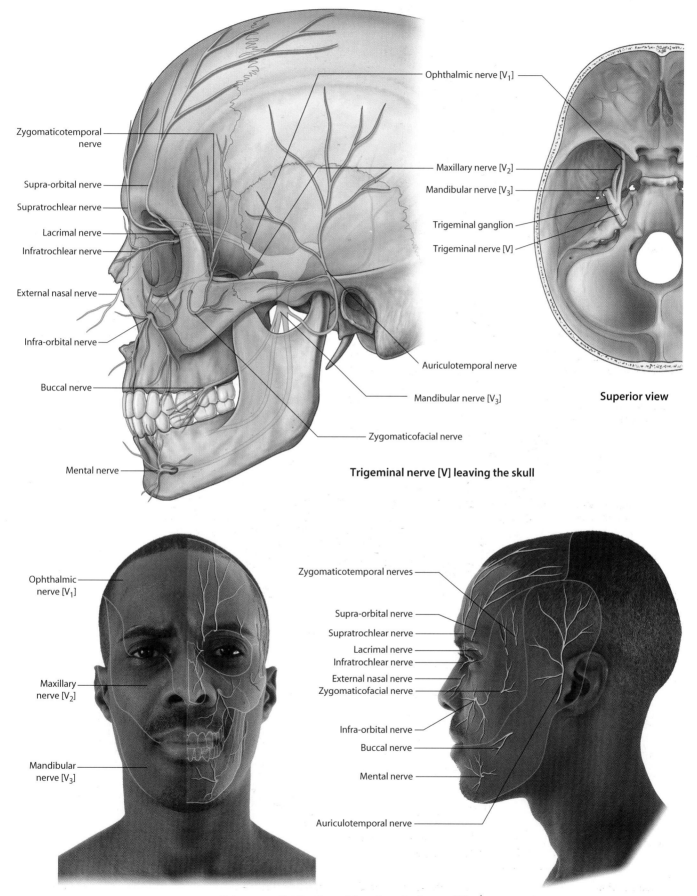

Ophthalmic nerve [V₁]

Zygomaticotemporal nerve

Supra-orbital nerve

Supratrochlear nerve

Lacrimal nerve

Infratrochlear nerve

External nasal nerve

Infra-orbital nerve

Buccal nerve

Mental nerve

Maxillary nerve [V₂]

Mandibular nerve [V₃]

Trigeminal ganglion

Trigeminal nerve [V]

Auriculotemporal nerve

Mandibular nerve [V₃]

Zygomaticofacial nerve

**Superior view**

**Trigeminal nerve [V] leaving the skull**

Ophthalmic nerve [V₁]

Maxillary nerve [V₂]

Mandibular nerve [V₃]

Zygomaticotemporal nerves

Supra-orbital nerve

Supratrochlear nerve

Lacrimal nerve

Infratrochlear nerve

External nasal nerve

Zygomaticofacial nerve

Infra-orbital nerve

Buccal nerve

Mental nerve

Auriculotemporal nerve

**Cutaneous distribution of the trigeminal nerve [V]**

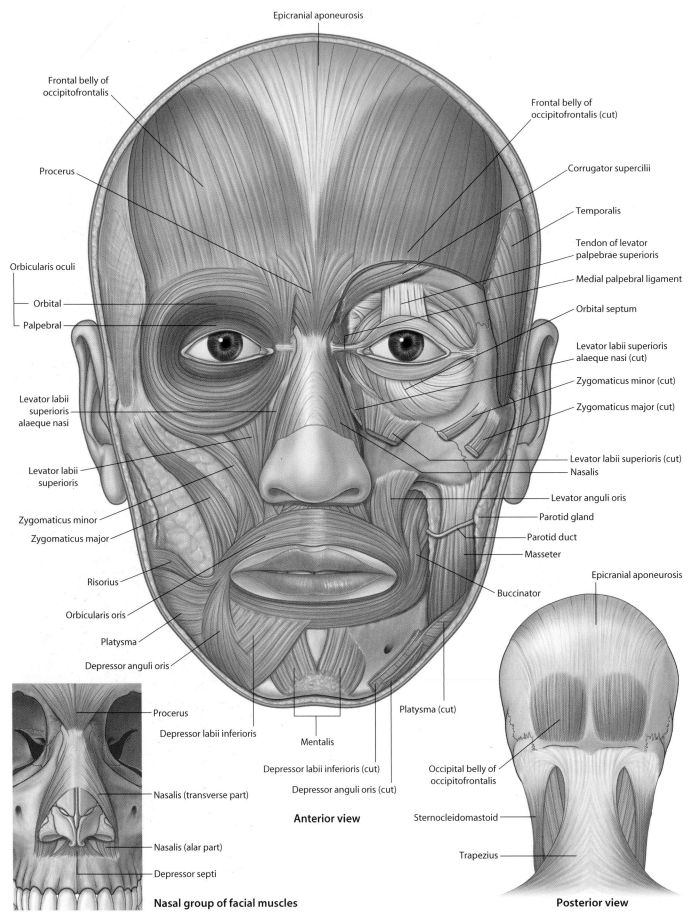

Epicranial aponeurosis

Frontal belly of
occipitofrontalis

Procerus

Orbicularis oculi

Orbital

Palpebral

Levator labii
superioris
alaeque nasi

Levator labii
superioris

Zygomaticus minor

Zygomaticus major

Risorius

Orbicularis oris

Platysma

Depressor anguli oris

Frontal belly of
occipitofrontalis (cut)

Corrugator supercilii

Temporalis

Tendon of levator
palpebrae superioris

Medial palpebral ligament

Orbital septum

Levator labii superioris
alaeque nasi (cut)

Zygomaticus minor (cut)

Zygomaticus major (cut)

Levator labii superioris (cut)

Nasalis

Levator anguli oris

Parotid gland

Parotid duct

Masseter

Buccinator

Platysma (cut)

Procerus

Depressor labii inferioris

Mentalis

Depressor labii inferioris (cut)

Depressor anguli oris (cut)

**Anterior view**

Nasalis (transverse part)

Nasalis (alar part)

Depressor septi

**Nasal group of facial muscles**

Epicranial aponeurosis

Occipital belly of
occipitofrontalis

Sternocleidomastoid

Trapezius

**Posterior view**

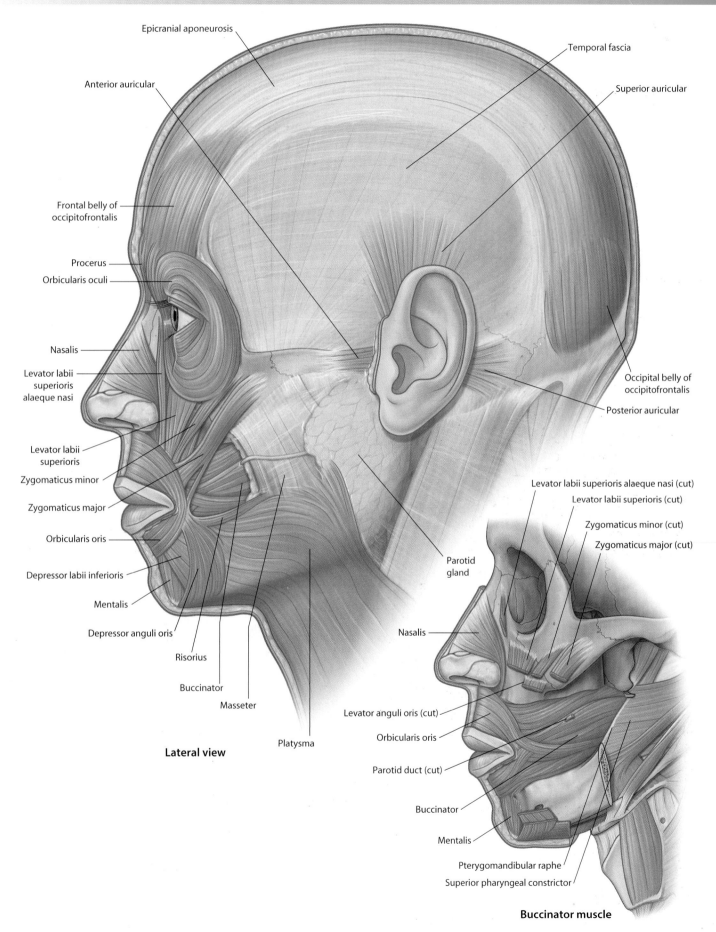

Epicranial aponeurosis

Anterior auricular

Frontal belly of
occipitofrontalis

Procerus

Orbicularis oculi

Nasalis

Levator labii
superioris
alaeque nasi

Levator labii
superioris

Zygomaticus minor

Zygomaticus major

Orbicularis oris

Depressor labii inferioris

Mentalis

Depressor anguli oris

Risorius

Buccinator

Masseter

Platysma

Temporal fascia

Superior auricular

Occipital belly of
occipitofrontalis

Posterior auricular

Parotid
gland

**Lateral view**

Levator labii superioris alaeque nasi (cut)

Levator labii superioris (cut)

Zygomaticus minor (cut)

Zygomaticus major (cut)

Nasalis

Levator anguli oris (cut)

Orbicularis oris

Parotid duct (cut)

Buccinator

Mentalis

Pterygomandibular raphe

Superior pharyngeal constrictor

**Buccinator muscle**

**457**

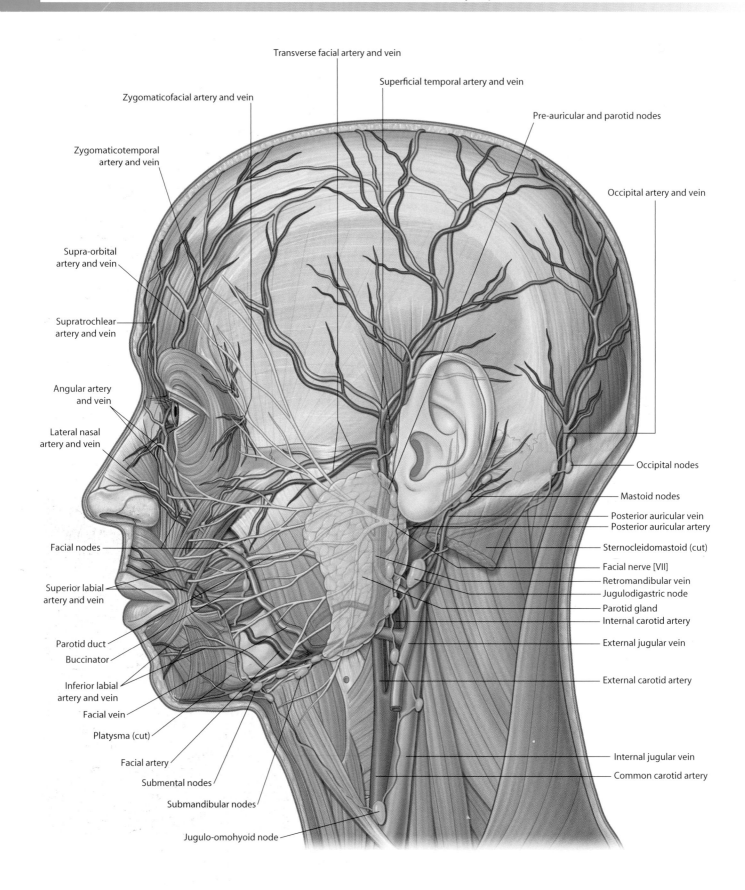

Transverse facial artery and vein

Superficial temporal artery and vein

Pre-auricular and parotid nodes

Zygomaticofacial artery and vein

Zygomaticotemporal artery and vein

Occipital artery and vein

Supra-orbital artery and vein

Supratrochlear artery and vein

Angular artery and vein

Lateral nasal artery and vein

Occipital nodes

Mastoid nodes

Posterior auricular vein
Posterior auricular artery

Facial nodes

Sternocleidomastoid (cut)

Facial nerve [VII]

Superior labial artery and vein

Retromandibular vein
Jugulodigastric node
Parotid gland
Internal carotid artery

Parotid duct

External jugular vein

Buccinator

Inferior labial artery and vein

External carotid artery

Facial vein

Platysma (cut)

Internal jugular vein

Facial artery

Common carotid artery

Submental nodes

Submandibular nodes

Jugulo-omohyoid node

**Vasculature, facial nerve [VII] and lymphatics of the face**

458

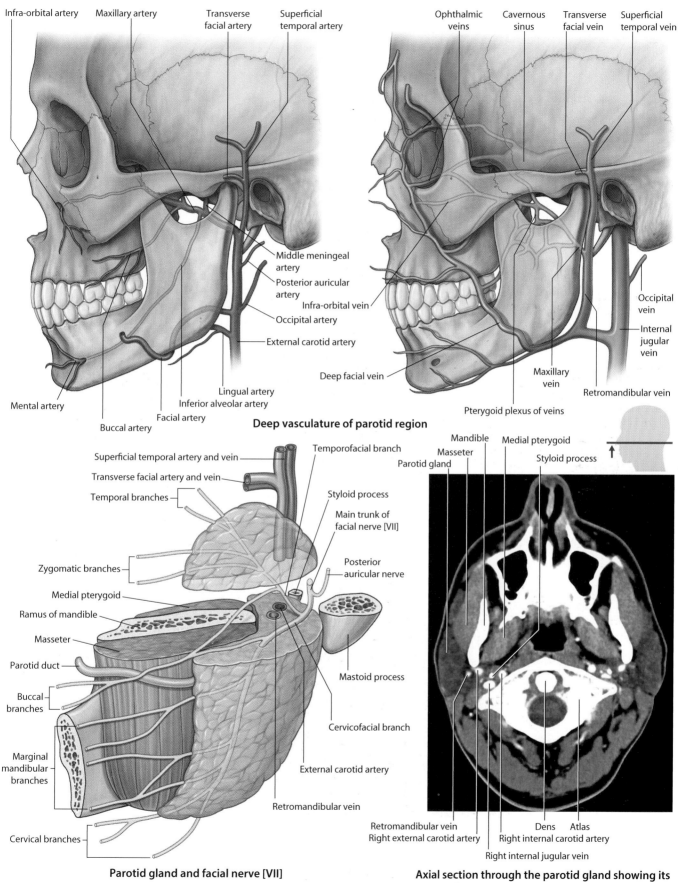

Infra-orbital artery
Maxillary artery
Transverse facial artery
Superficial temporal artery

Middle meningeal artery
Posterior auricular artery
Infra-orbital vein
Occipital artery
External carotid artery

Mental artery
Buccal artery
Facial artery
Inferior alveolar artery
Lingual artery

Ophthalmic veins
Cavernous sinus
Transverse facial vein
Superficial temporal vein

Occipital vein
Internal jugular vein

Deep facial vein
Pterygoid plexus of veins
Maxillary vein
Retromandibular vein

**Deep vasculature of parotid region**

Superficial temporal artery and vein
Transverse facial artery and vein
Temporal branches

Zygomatic branches

Medial pterygoid
Ramus of mandible
Masseter
Parotid duct
Buccal branches

Marginal mandibular branches

Cervical branches

Temporofacial branch
Styloid process
Main trunk of facial nerve [VII]
Posterior auricular nerve

Mastoid process

Cervicofacial branch
External carotid artery
Retromandibular vein

**Parotid gland and facial nerve [VII]**

Parotid gland
Masseter
Mandible
Medial pterygoid
Styloid process

Retromandibular vein
Right external carotid artery
Dens    Atlas
Right internal carotid artery
Right internal jugular vein

**Axial section through the parotid gland showing its relationship to surrounding structures.**
CT image in axial plane

**459**

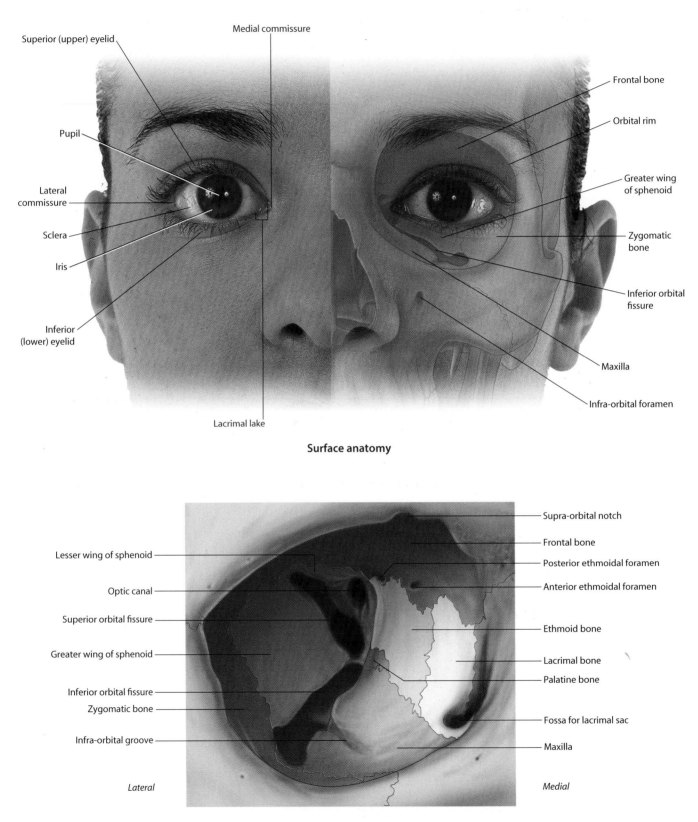

Superior (upper) eyelid

Medial commissure

Frontal bone

Orbital rim

Pupil

Greater wing of sphenoid

Lateral commissure

Zygomatic bone

Sclera

Iris

Inferior orbital fissure

Inferior (lower) eyelid

Maxilla

Infra-orbital foramen

Lacrimal lake

**Surface anatomy**

Lesser wing of sphenoid

Supra-orbital notch

Frontal bone

Optic canal

Posterior ethmoidal foramen

Anterior ethmoidal foramen

Superior orbital fissure

Greater wing of sphenoid

Ethmoid bone

Inferior orbital fissure

Lacrimal bone

Zygomatic bone

Palatine bone

Infra-orbital groove

Fossa for lacrimal sac

Maxilla

*Lateral*

*Medial*

**Bones of the right orbit**

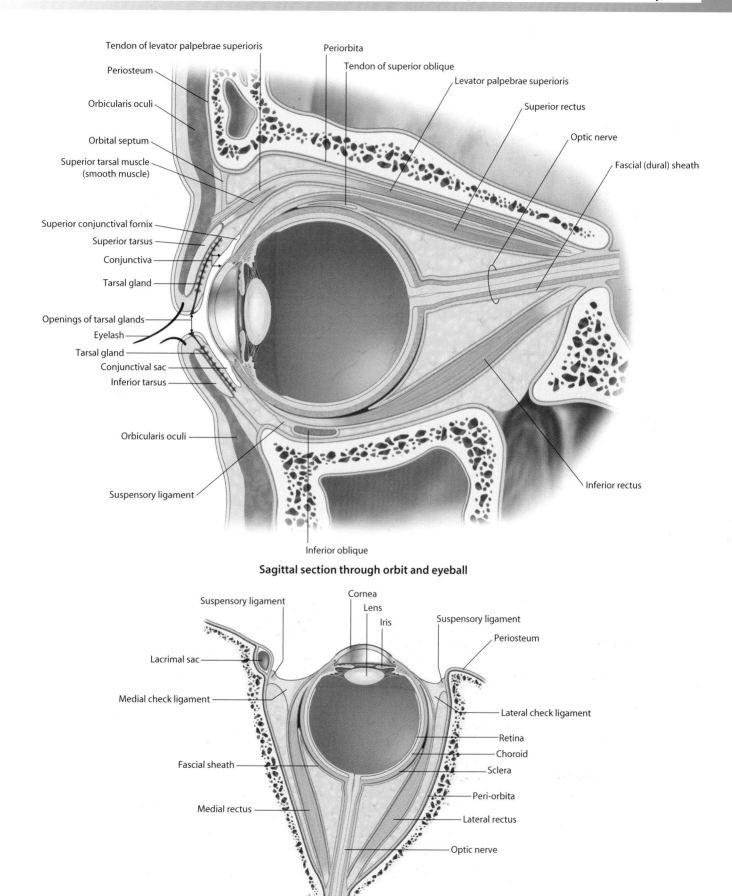

**Sagittal section through orbit and eyeball**

**Horizontal (axial) section through orbit and eyeball**

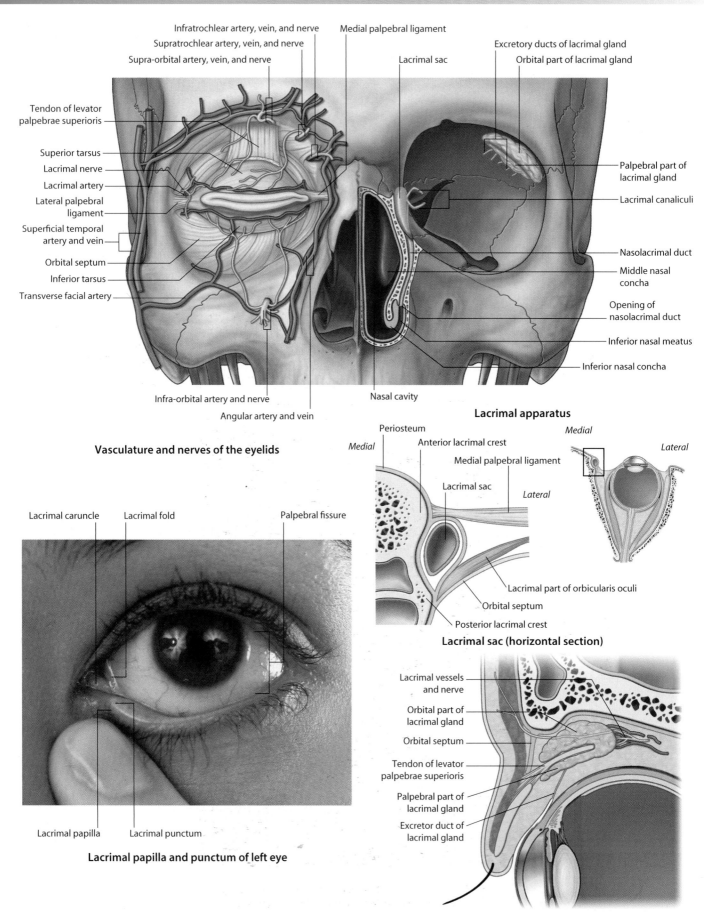

**Vasculature and nerves of the eyelids**

Infratrochlear artery, vein, and nerve
Supratrochlear artery, vein, and nerve
Supra-orbital artery, vein, and nerve
Medial palpebral ligament
Lacrimal sac
Excretory ducts of lacrimal gland
Orbital part of lacrimal gland

Tendon of levator palpebrae superioris
Superior tarsus
Lacrimal nerve
Lacrimal artery
Lateral palpebral ligament
Superficial temporal artery and vein
Orbital septum
Inferior tarsus
Transverse facial artery

Palpebral part of lacrimal gland
Lacrimal canaliculi
Nasolacrimal duct
Middle nasal concha
Opening of nasolacrimal duct
Inferior nasal meatus
Inferior nasal concha

Infra-orbital artery and nerve
Angular artery and vein
Nasal cavity

**Lacrimal papilla and punctum of left eye**

Lacrimal caruncle
Lacrimal fold
Palpebral fissure
Lacrimal papilla
Lacrimal punctum

**Lacrimal apparatus**

**Lacrimal sac (horizontal section)**

Medial
Periosteum
Anterior lacrimal crest
Medial palpebral ligament
Lacrimal sac
Lateral
Lacrimal part of orbicularis oculi
Orbital septum
Posterior lacrimal crest

Medial
Lateral

**Lacrimal gland and levator palpebrae superioris (parasagittal section)**

Lacrimal vessels and nerve
Orbital part of lacrimal gland
Orbital septum
Tendon of levator palpebrae superioris
Palpebral part of lacrimal gland
Excretor duct of lacrimal gland

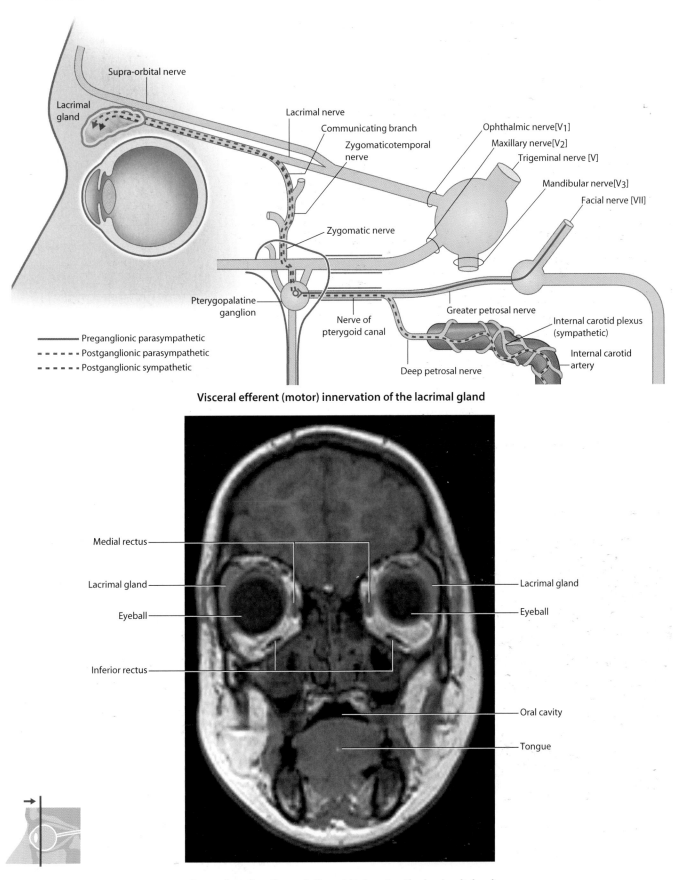

Supra-orbital nerve

Lacrimal gland

Lacrimal nerve

Communicating branch

Zygomaticotemporal nerve

Ophthalmic nerve[V₁]

Maxillary nerve[V₂]

Trigeminal nerve [V]

Mandibular nerve[V₃]

Facial nerve [VII]

Zygomatic nerve

Pterygopalatine ganglion

Nerve of pterygoid canal

Greater petrosal nerve

Internal carotid plexus (sympathetic)

Internal carotid artery

Deep petrosal nerve

———— Preganglionic parasympathetic

- - - - Postganglionic parasympathetic

- - - - Postganglionic sympathetic

**Visceral efferent (motor) innervation of the lacrimal gland**

Medial rectus

Lacrimal gland

Eyeball

Inferior rectus

Lacrimal gland

Eyeball

Oral cavity

Tongue

**Coronal section through the orbit showing the lacrimal gland and its relationship to surrounding structures.**
T1-weighted MR image in coronal plane

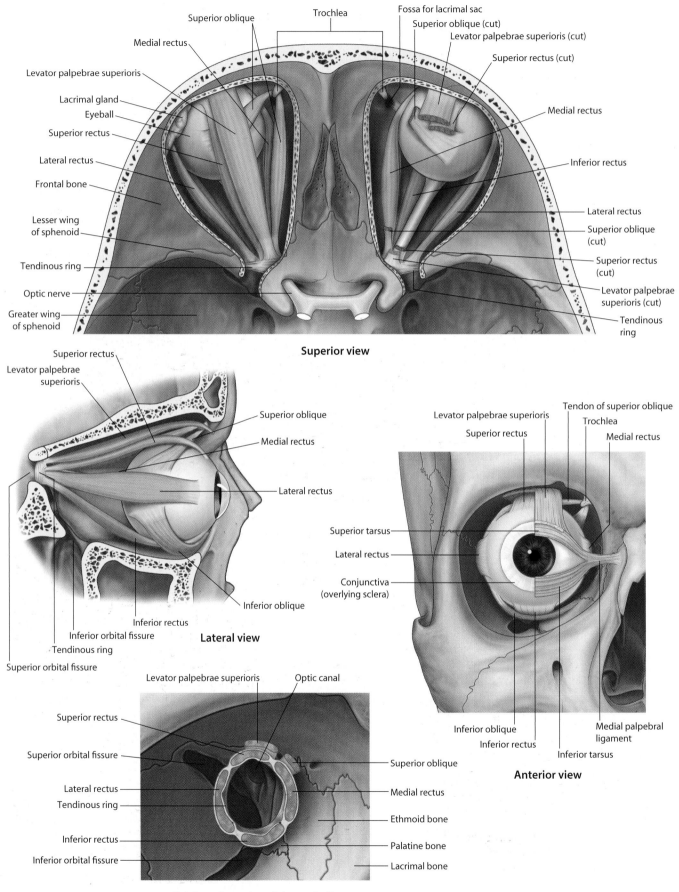

Superior oblique

Trochlea

Fossa for lacrimal sac

Superior oblique (cut)

Levator palpebrae superioris (cut)

Superior rectus (cut)

Medial rectus

Levator palpebrae superioris

Lacrimal gland

Eyeball

Superior rectus

Medial rectus

Lateral rectus

Frontal bone

Inferior rectus

Lesser wing of sphenoid

Lateral rectus

Tendinous ring

Superior oblique (cut)

Optic nerve

Superior rectus (cut)

Greater wing of sphenoid

Levator palpebrae superioris (cut)

Tendinous ring

**Superior view**

Superior rectus

Levator palpebrae superioris

Superior oblique

Medial rectus

Lateral rectus

Inferior oblique

Inferior rectus

Inferior orbital fissure

Tendinous ring

Superior orbital fissure

**Lateral view**

Levator palpebrae superioris

Superior rectus

Tendon of superior oblique

Trochlea

Medial rectus

Superior tarsus

Lateral rectus

Conjunctiva (overlying sclera)

Inferior oblique

Inferior rectus

Medial palpebral ligament

Inferior tarsus

**Anterior view**

Levator palpebrae superioris

Optic canal

Superior rectus

Superior orbital fissure

Superior oblique

Lateral rectus

Medial rectus

Tendinous ring

Ethmoid bone

Inferior rectus

Palatine bone

Inferior orbital fissure

Lacrimal bone

**Origins of muscles of the eyeball**

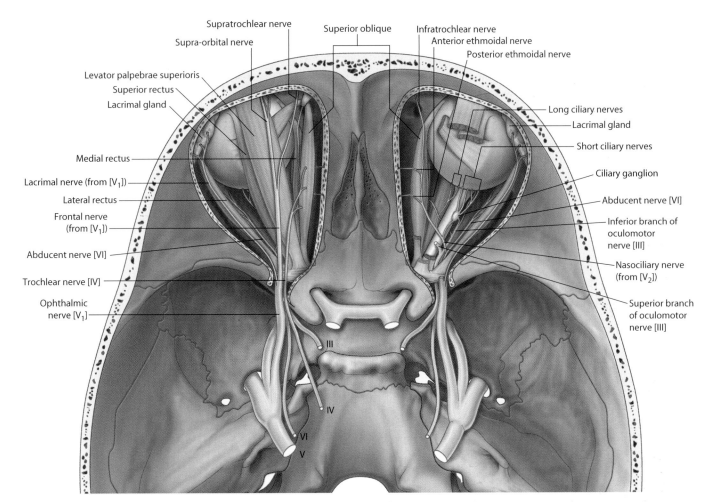

Supratrochlear nerve
Supra-orbital nerve
Levator palpebrae superioris
Superior rectus
Lacrimal gland
Medial rectus
Lacrimal nerve (from [V₁])
Lateral rectus
Frontal nerve (from [V₁])
Abducent nerve [VI]
Trochlear nerve [IV]
Ophthalmic nerve [V₁]

Superior oblique
Infratrochlear nerve
Anterior ethmoidal nerve
Posterior ethmoidal nerve

Long ciliary nerves
Lacrimal gland
Short ciliary nerves
Ciliary ganglion
Abducent nerve [VI]
Inferior branch of oculomotor nerve [III]
Nasociliary nerve (from [V₂])
Superior branch of oculomotor nerve [III]

III
IV
VI
V

**Superior view**

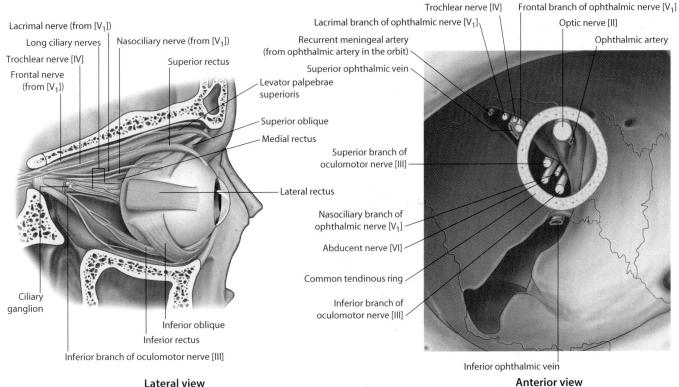

Lacrimal nerve (from [V₁])
Long ciliary nerves
Trochlear nerve [IV]
Frontal nerve (from [V₁])
Nasociliary nerve (from [V₁])
Superior rectus
Levator palpebrae superioris
Superior oblique
Medial rectus
Lateral rectus
Ciliary ganglion
Inferior oblique
Inferior rectus
Inferior branch of oculomotor nerve [III]

**Lateral view**

Trochlear nerve [IV]
Lacrimal branch of ophthalmic nerve [V₁]
Recurrent meningeal artery (from ophthalmic artery in the orbit)
Superior ophthalmic vein
Superior branch of oculomotor nerve [III]
Nasociliary branch of ophthalmic nerve [V₁]
Abducent nerve [VI]
Common tendinous ring
Inferior branch of oculomotor nerve [III]
Frontal branch of ophthalmic nerve [V₁]
Optic nerve [II]
Ophthalmic artery
Inferior ophthalmic vein

**Anterior view**

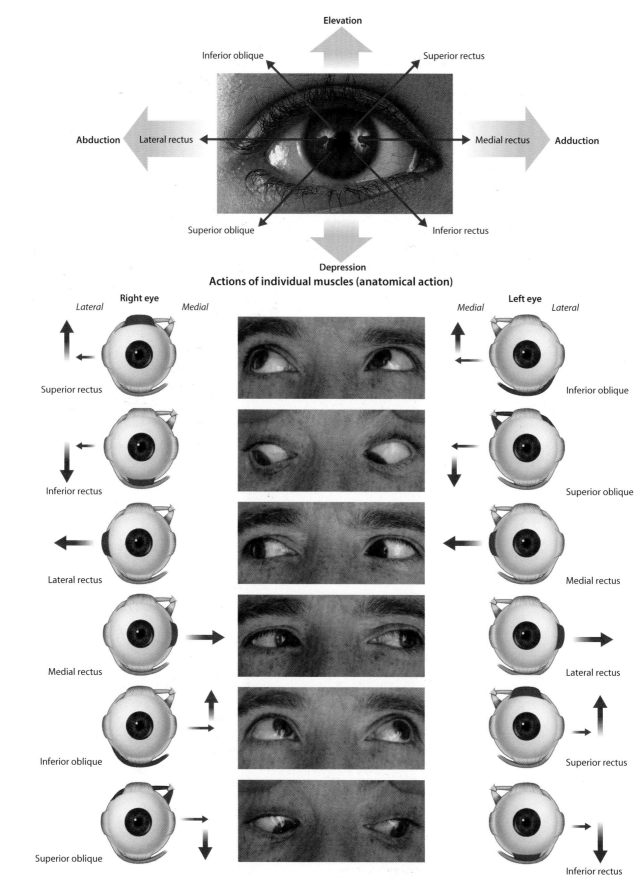

Elevation

Inferior oblique        Superior rectus

Abduction    Lateral rectus        Medial rectus    Adduction

Superior oblique        Inferior rectus

Depression

**Actions of individual muscles (anatomical action)**

Right eye

*Lateral*        *Medial*

Superior rectus

Inferior rectus

Lateral rectus

Medial rectus

Inferior oblique

Superior oblique

Left eye

*Medial*        *Lateral*

Inferior oblique

Superior oblique

Medial rectus

Lateral rectus

Superior rectus

Inferior rectus

**Movement of eyes when testing specific muscle (clinical testing).**

For testing some muscles, a patient is "asked" to first move the eye into a position (small arrow) where the indicated muscle
can best be tested. The large arrow indicates the direction the patient is then "asked" to move the eye to test the muscle

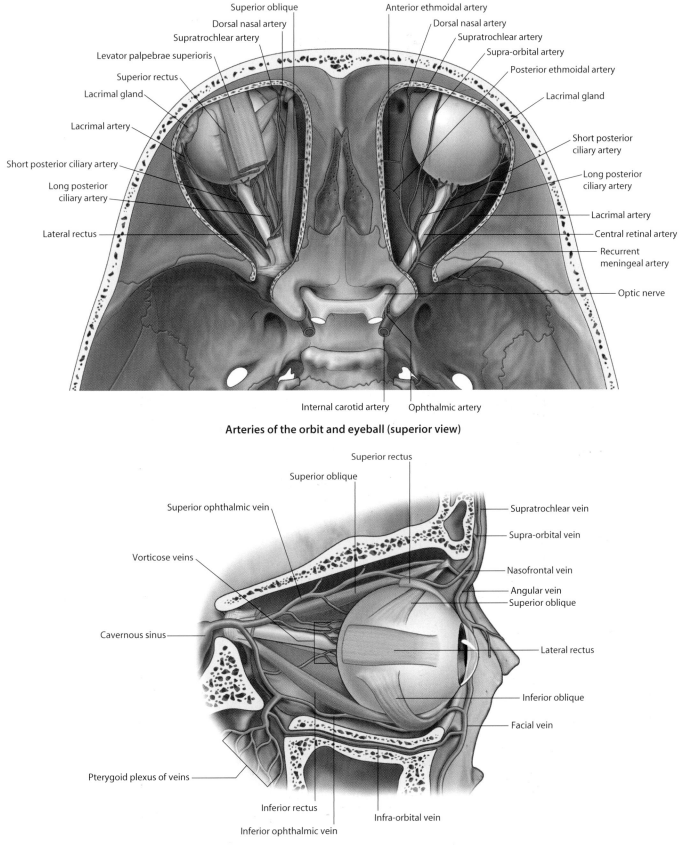

**Arteries of the orbit and eyeball (superior view)**

**Veins of the orbit and eyeball (lateral view)**

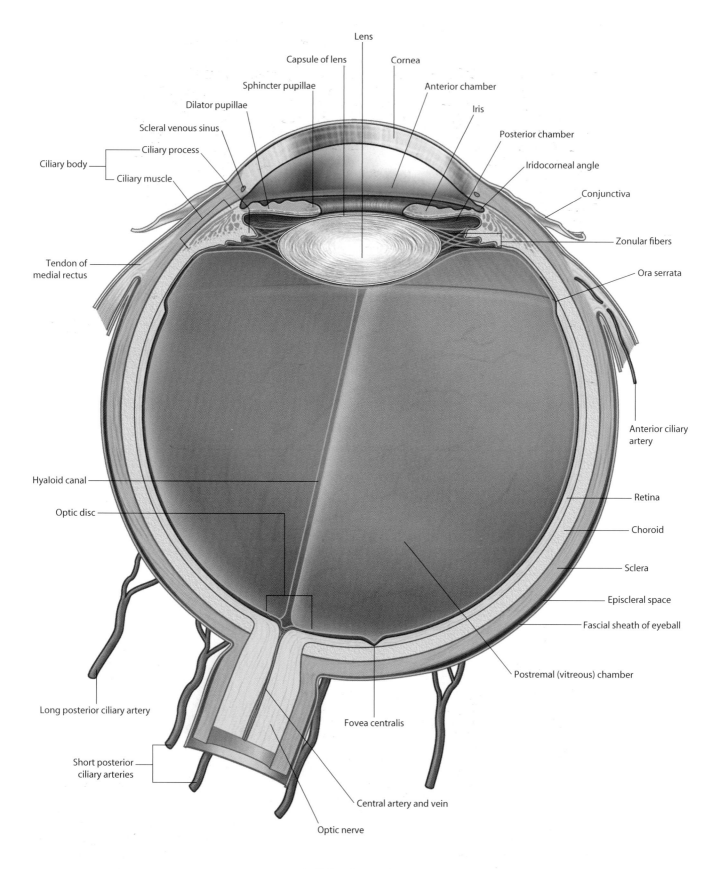

Lens

Capsule of lens

Cornea

Sphincter pupillae

Anterior chamber

Dilator pupillae

Iris

Scleral venous sinus

Posterior chamber

Ciliary process

Ciliary body

Iridocorneal angle

Ciliary muscle

Conjunctiva

Zonular fibers

Tendon of
medial rectus

Ora serrata

Hyaloid canal

Anterior ciliary
artery

Optic disc

Retina

Choroid

Sclera

Episcleral space

Fascial sheath of eyeball

Postremal (vitreous) chamber

Long posterior ciliary artery

Fovea centralis

Short posterior
ciliary arteries

Central artery and vein

Optic nerve

**Eyeball (horizontal section)**

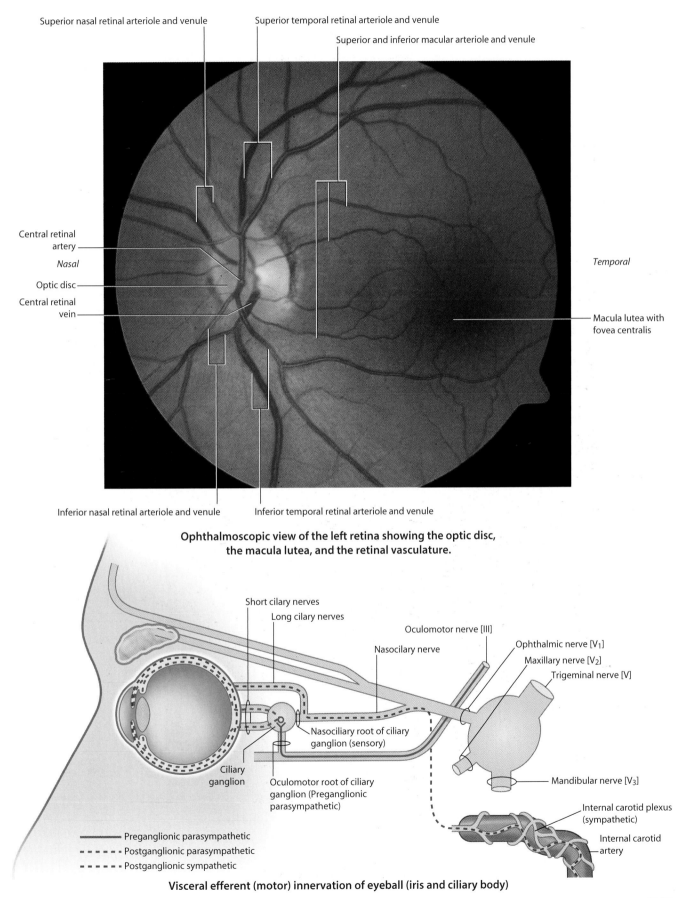

Superior nasal retinal arteriole and venule

Superior temporal retinal arteriole and venule

Superior and inferior macular arteriole and venule

Central retinal artery

*Nasal*

Optic disc

Central retinal vein

*Temporal*

Macula lutea with fovea centralis

Inferior nasal retinal arteriole and venule

Inferior temporal retinal arteriole and venule

**Ophthalmoscopic view of the left retina showing the optic disc, the macula lutea, and the retinal vasculature.**

Short cilary nerves

Long cilary nerves

Nasociliary nerve

Oculomotor nerve [III]

Ophthalmic nerve [V₁]

Maxillary nerve [V₂]

Trigeminal nerve [V]

Nasociliary root of ciliary ganglion (sensory)

Ciliary ganglion

Oculomotor root of ciliary ganglion (Preganglionic parasympathetic)

Mandibular nerve [V₃]

Internal carotid plexus (sympathetic)

Internal carotid artery

——— Preganglionic parasympathetic
- - - - Postganglionic parasympathetic
-- -- -- Postganglionic sympathetic

**Visceral efferent (motor) innervation of eyeball (iris and ciliary body)**

A

B

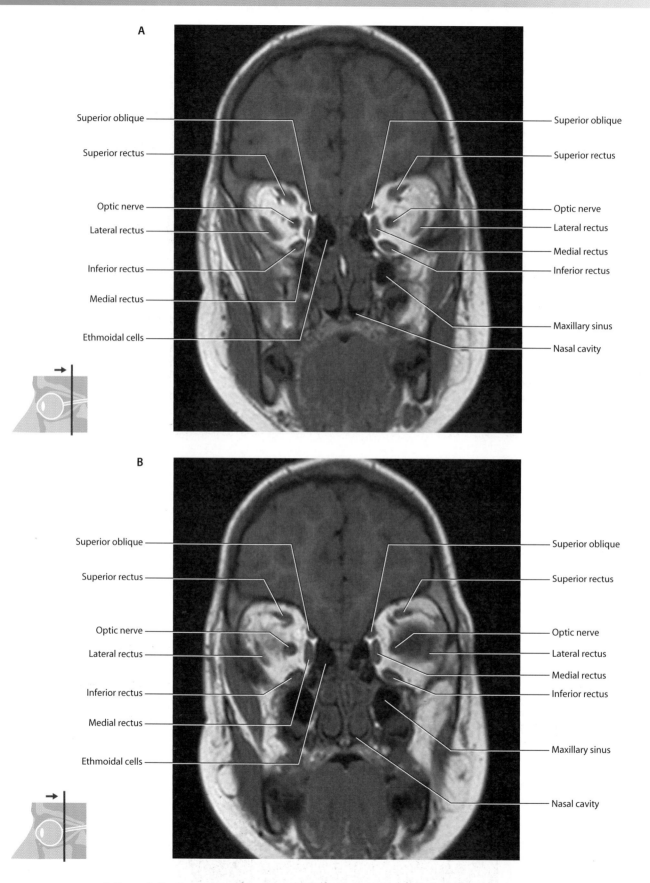

Superior oblique

Superior rectus

Optic nerve

Lateral rectus

Inferior rectus

Medial rectus

Ethmoidal cells

Superior oblique

Superior rectus

Optic nerve

Lateral rectus

Medial rectus

Inferior rectus

Maxillary sinus

Nasal cavity

Superior oblique

Superior rectus

Optic nerve

Lateral rectus

Inferior rectus

Medial rectus

Ethmoidal cells

Superior oblique

Superior rectus

Optic nerve

Lateral rectus

Medial rectus

Inferior rectus

Maxillary sinus

Nasal cavity

**A through D – Coronal sections that pass through the orbit from posterior to anterior showing the extrinsic (extra-ocular) muscles and their relationships with each other and with other structures.**
**T1-weighted MR images in coronal plane**

C

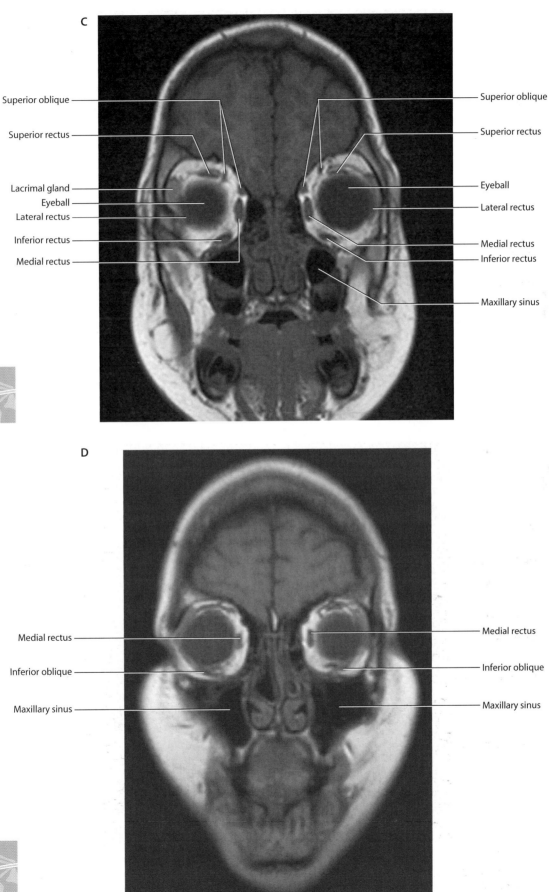

Superior oblique

Superior rectus

Lacrimal gland
Eyeball
Lateral rectus
Inferior rectus
Medial rectus

Superior oblique

Superior rectus

Eyeball

Lateral rectus

Medial rectus
Inferior rectus

Maxillary sinus

D

Medial rectus

Inferior oblique

Maxillary sinus

Medial rectus

Inferior oblique

Maxillary sinus

**471**

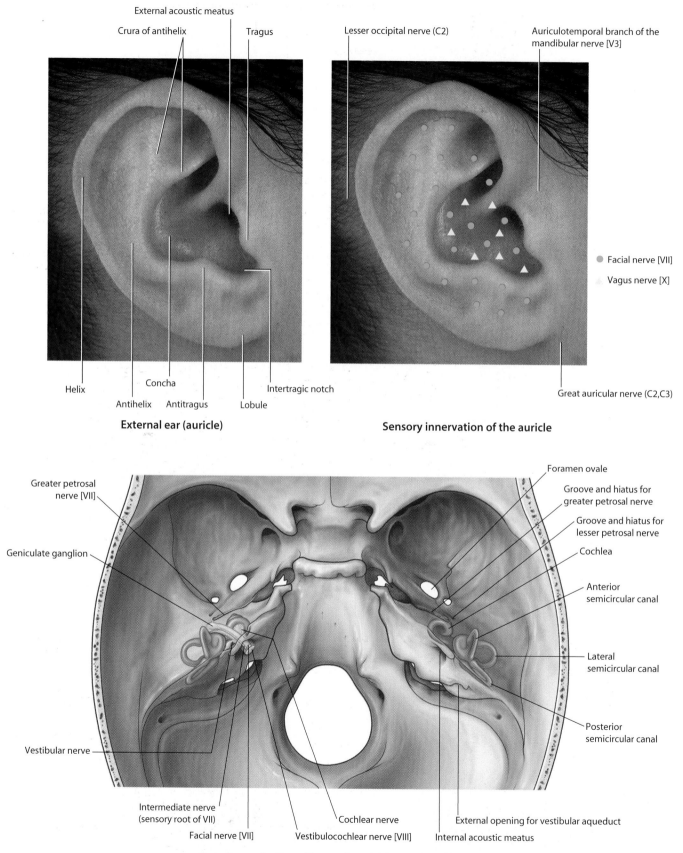

External acoustic meatus

Crura of antihelix

Tragus

Helix

Antihelix  Concha  Antitragus  Lobule

Intertragic notch

**External ear (auricle)**

Lesser occipital nerve (C2)

Auriculotemporal branch of the mandibular nerve [V3]

● Facial nerve [VII]

▲ Vagus nerve [X]

Great auricular nerve (C2,C3)

**Sensory innervation of the auricle**

Greater petrosal nerve [VII]

Geniculate ganglion

Vestibular nerve

Intermediate nerve (sensory root of VII)

Facial nerve [VII]

Vestibulocochlear nerve [VIII]

Cochlear nerve

Foramen ovale

Groove and hiatus for greater petrosal nerve

Groove and hiatus for lesser petrosal nerve

Cochlea

Anterior semicircular canal

Lateral semicircular canal

Posterior semicircular canal

External opening for vestibular aqueduct

Internal acoustic meatus

**Superior projection of internal ear in the temporal bone**

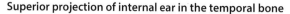

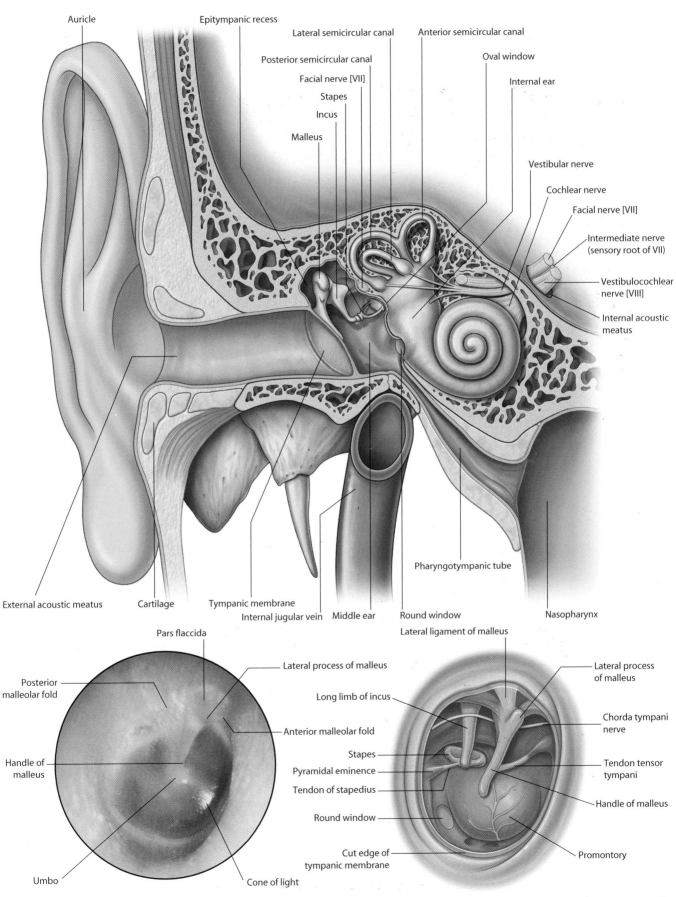

Auricle

Epitympanic recess

Lateral semicircular canal

Anterior semicircular canal

Posterior semicircular canal

Oval window

Facial nerve [VII]

Internal ear

Stapes

Incus

Malleus

Vestibular nerve

Cochlear nerve

Facial nerve [VII]

Intermediate nerve (sensory root of VII)

Vestibulocochlear nerve [VIII]

Internal acoustic meatus

Pharyngotympanic tube

External acoustic meatus

Cartilage

Tympanic membrane

Internal jugular vein

Middle ear

Round window

Nasopharynx

Pars flaccida

Lateral ligament of malleus

Posterior malleolar fold

Lateral process of malleus

Lateral process of malleus

Long limb of incus

Chorda tympani nerve

Handle of malleus

Anterior malleolar fold

Stapes

Tendon tensor tympani

Pyramidal eminence

Tendon of stapedius

Handle of malleus

Round window

Umbo

Cone of light

Cut edge of tympanic membrane

Promontory

**Right tympanic membrane**

**View into right tympanic cavity (tympanic membrane removed)**

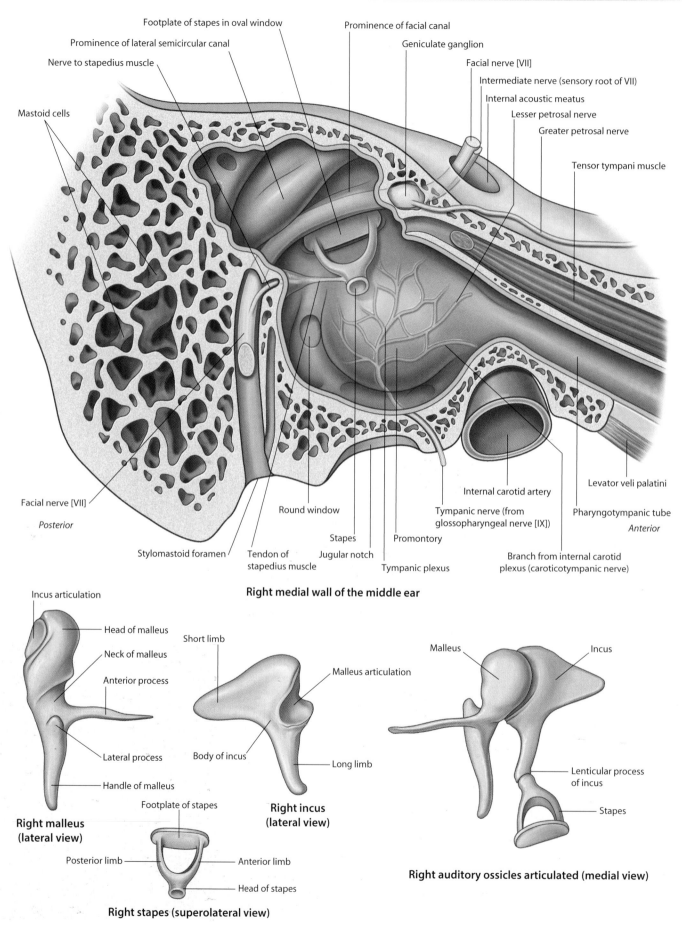

Footplate of stapes in oval window

Prominence of lateral semicircular canal

Nerve to stapedius muscle

Prominence of facial canal

Geniculate ganglion

Facial nerve [VII]

Intermediate nerve (sensory root of VII)

Internal acoustic meatus

Lesser petrosal nerve

Greater petrosal nerve

Tensor tympani muscle

Mastoid cells

Facial nerve [VII]

*Posterior*

Stylomastoid foramen

Tendon of stapedius muscle

Jugular notch

Round window

Stapes

Promontory

Tympanic plexus

Tympanic nerve (from glossopharyngeal nerve [IX])

Internal carotid artery

Branch from internal carotid plexus (caroticotympanic nerve)

Levator veli palatini

Pharyngotympanic tube

*Anterior*

**Right medial wall of the middle ear**

Incus articulation

Head of malleus

Neck of malleus

Anterior process

Lateral process

Handle of malleus

**Right malleus (lateral view)**

Footplate of stapes

Posterior limb

Anterior limb

Head of stapes

**Right stapes (superolateral view)**

Short limb

Malleus articulation

Body of incus

Long limb

**Right incus (lateral view)**

Malleus

Incus

Lenticular process of incus

Stapes

**Right auditory ossicles articulated (medial view)**

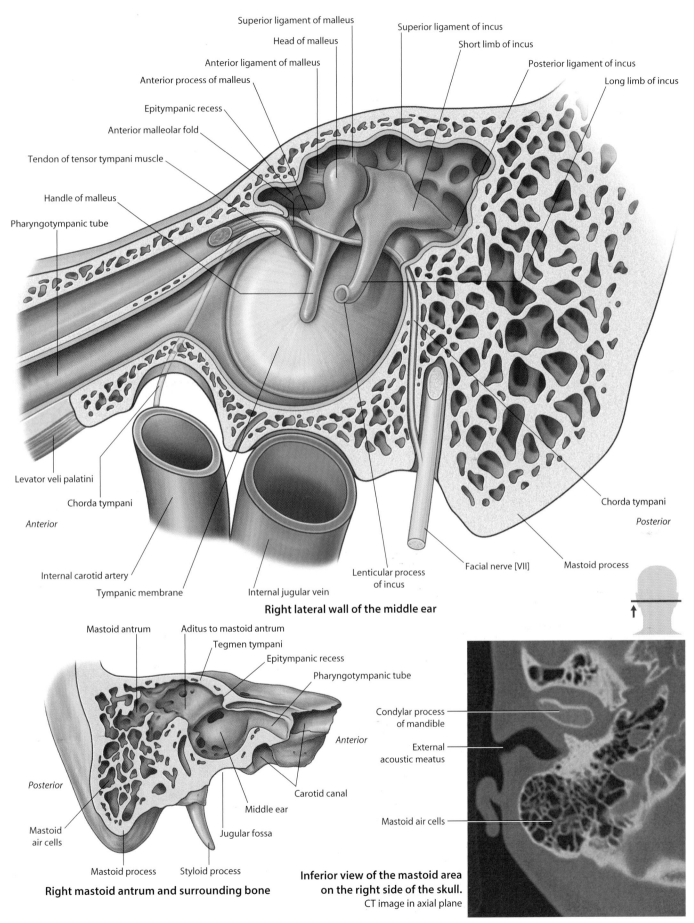

Superior ligament of malleus
Head of malleus
Anterior ligament of malleus
Anterior process of malleus
Epitympanic recess
Anterior malleolar fold
Tendon of tensor tympani muscle
Handle of malleus
Pharyngotympanic tube
Superior ligament of incus
Short limb of incus
Posterior ligament of incus
Long limb of incus
Levator veli palatini
Chorda tympani
*Anterior*
Chorda tympani
*Posterior*
Internal carotid artery
Tympanic membrane
Internal jugular vein
Lenticular process of incus
Facial nerve [VII]
Mastoid process

**Right lateral wall of the middle ear**

Mastoid antrum
Aditus to mastoid antrum
Tegmen tympani
Epitympanic recess
Pharyngotympanic tube
*Anterior*
Carotid canal
Middle ear
Jugular fossa
Styloid process
*Posterior*
Mastoid air cells
Mastoid process

**Right mastoid antrum and surrounding bone**

Condylar process of mandible
External acoustic meatus
Mastoid air cells

**Inferior view of the mastoid area
on the right side of the skull.**
CT image in axial plane

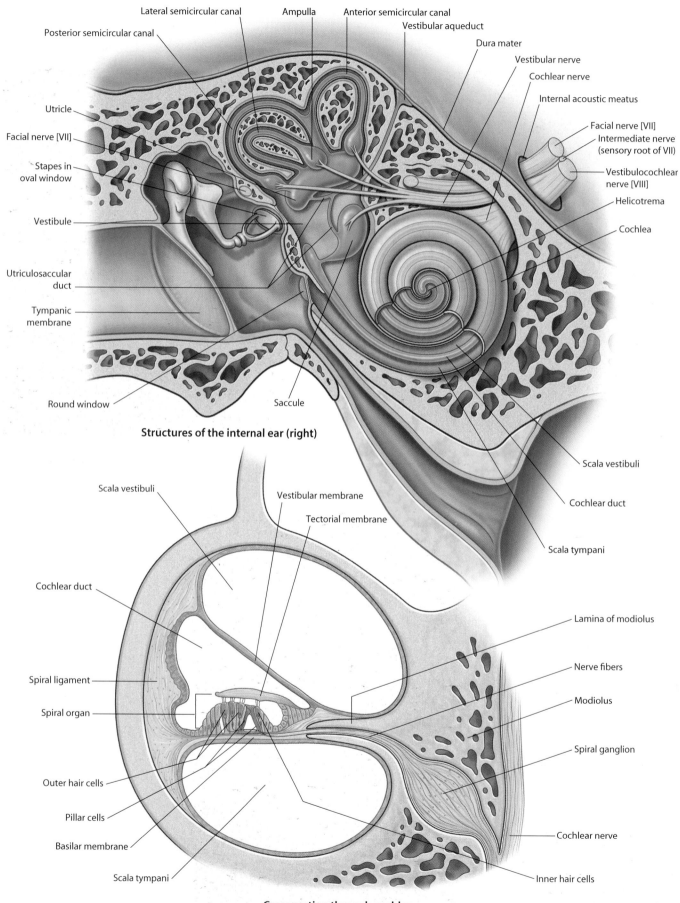

Posterior semicircular canal

Lateral semicircular canal

Ampulla

Anterior semicircular canal

Vestibular aqueduct

Dura mater

Vestibular nerve

Cochlear nerve

Internal acoustic meatus

Facial nerve [VII]

Intermediate nerve (sensory root of VII)

Vestibulocochlear nerve [VIII]

Helicotrema

Cochlea

Utricle

Facial nerve [VII]

Stapes in oval window

Vestibule

Utriculosaccular duct

Tympanic membrane

Round window

Saccule

Scala vestibuli

Cochlear duct

Scala tympani

**Structures of the internal ear (right)**

Scala vestibuli

Vestibular membrane

Tectorial membrane

Cochlear duct

Lamina of modiolus

Nerve fibers

Spiral ligament

Modiolus

Spiral organ

Spiral ganglion

Outer hair cells

Pillar cells

Basilar membrane

Cochlear nerve

Scala tympani

Inner hair cells

**Cross section through cochlea**

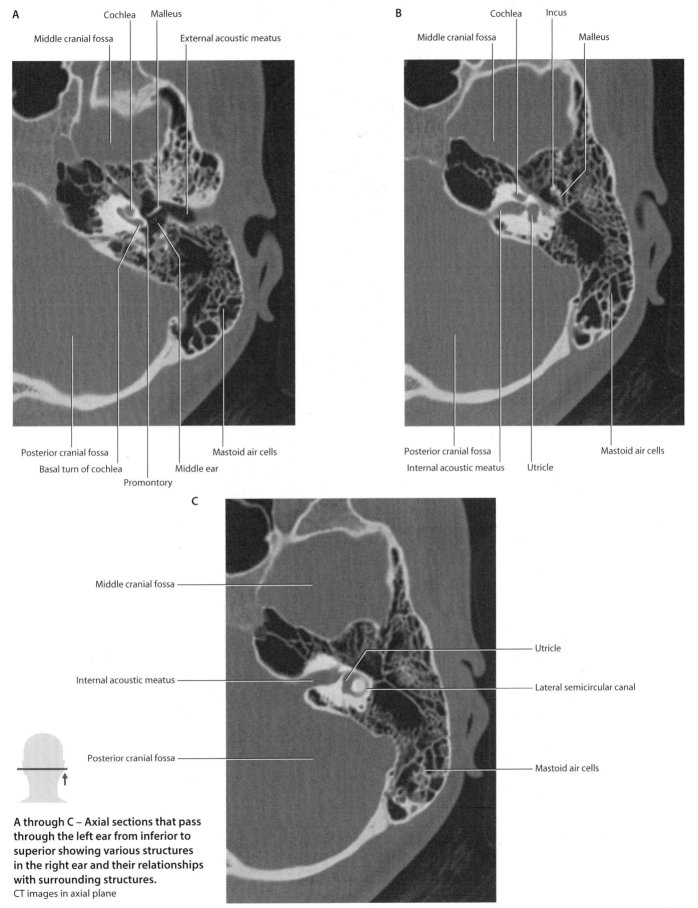

**A**

Middle cranial fossa — Cochlea — Malleus — External acoustic meatus

Posterior cranial fossa — Basal turn of cochlea — Promontory — Middle ear — Mastoid air cells

**B**

Middle cranial fossa — Cochlea — Incus — Malleus

Posterior cranial fossa — Internal acoustic meatus — Utricle — Mastoid air cells

**C**

Middle cranial fossa

Internal acoustic meatus

Posterior cranial fossa

Utricle

Lateral semicircular canal

Mastoid air cells

**A through C – Axial sections that pass through the left ear from inferior to superior showing various structures in the right ear and their relationships with surrounding structures.**
CT images in axial plane

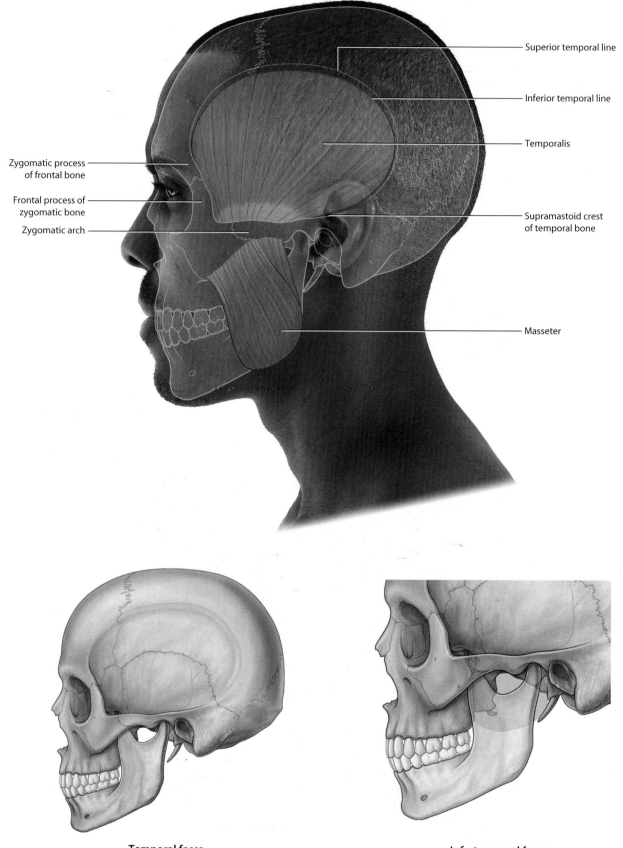

Superior temporal line

Inferior temporal line

Temporalis

Supramastoid crest
of temporal bone

Masseter

Zygomatic process
of frontal bone

Frontal process of
zygomatic bone

Zygomatic arch

**Temporal fossa**

**Infratemporal fossa**

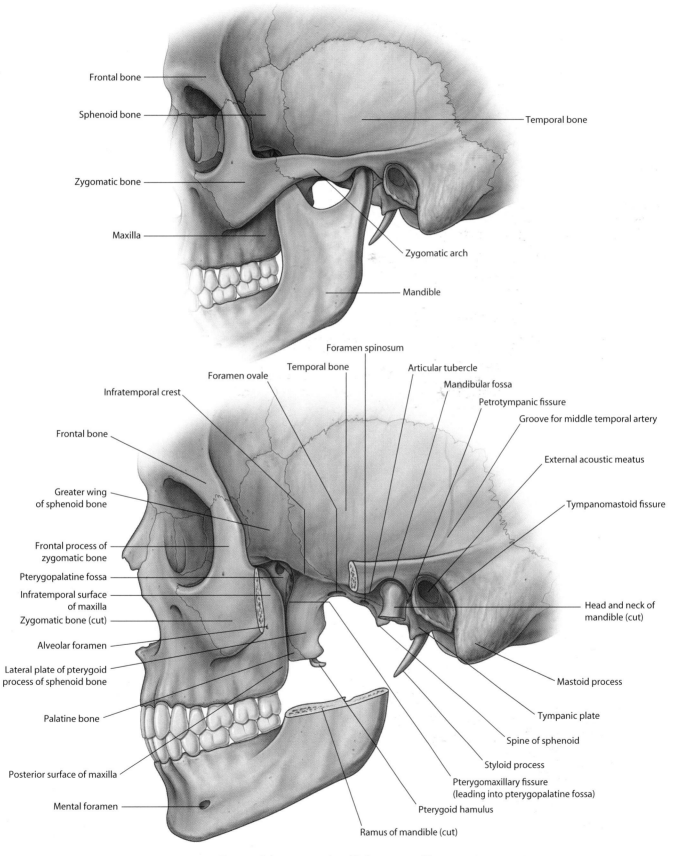

Frontal bone

Sphenoid bone

Temporal bone

Zygomatic bone

Maxilla

Zygomatic arch

Mandible

Foramen spinosum

Temporal bone

Articular tubercle

Mandibular fossa

Foramen ovale

Petrotympanic fissure

Infratemporal crest

Groove for middle temporal artery

Frontal bone

External acoustic meatus

Greater wing
of sphenoid bone

Tympanomastoid fissure

Frontal process of
zygomatic bone

Pterygopalatine fossa

Infratemporal surface
of maxilla

Zygomatic bone (cut)

Head and neck of
mandible (cut)

Alveolar foramen

Lateral plate of pterygoid
process of sphenoid bone

Mastoid process

Palatine bone

Tympanic plate

Spine of sphenoid

Posterior surface of maxilla

Styloid process

Pterygomaxillary fissure
(leading into pterygopalatine fossa)

Mental foramen

Pterygoid hamulus

Ramus of mandible (cut)

**Bones of the temporal band infratemporal fossae**

**479**

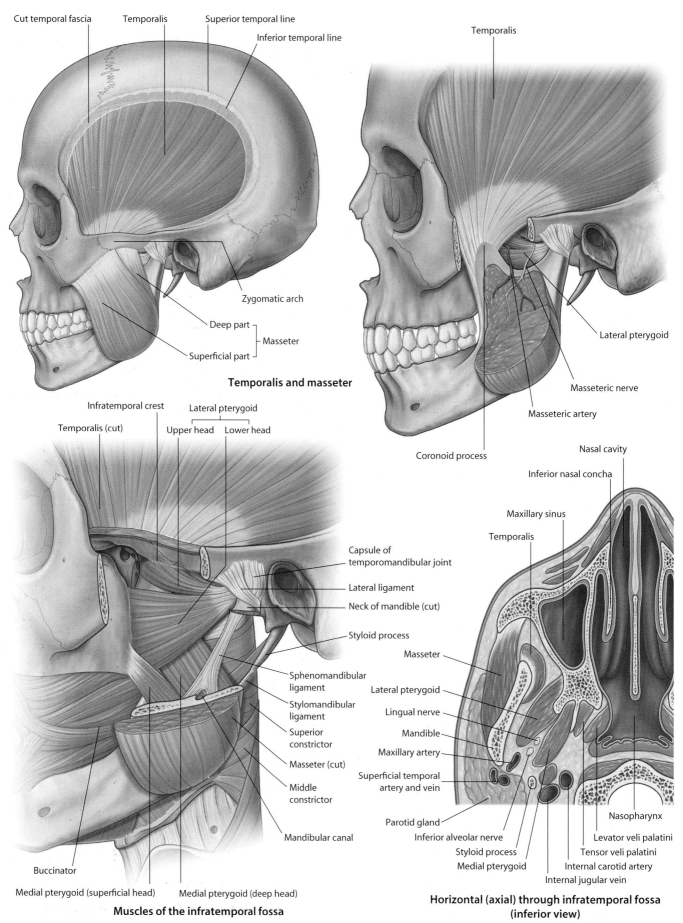

Cut temporal fascia

Temporalis

Superior temporal line

Inferior temporal line

Temporalis

Zygomatic arch

Deep part ⎤
       ⎥ Masseter
Superficial part ⎦

**Temporalis and masseter**

Lateral pterygoid

Masseteric nerve

Masseteric artery

Coronoid process

Infratemporal crest

Temporalis (cut)

Lateral pterygoid

Upper head   Lower head

Capsule of temporomandibular joint

Lateral ligament

Neck of mandible (cut)

Styloid process

Sphenomandibular ligament

Stylomandibular ligament

Superior constrictor

Masseter (cut)

Middle constrictor

Mandibular canal

Buccinator

Medial pterygoid (superficial head)

Medial pterygoid (deep head)

**Muscles of the infratemporal fossa**

Nasal cavity

Inferior nasal concha

Maxillary sinus

Temporalis

Masseter

Lateral pterygoid

Lingual nerve

Mandible

Maxillary artery

Superficial temporal artery and vein

Parotid gland

Inferior alveolar nerve

Styloid process

Medial pterygoid

Internal jugular vein

Nasopharynx

Levator veli palatini

Tensor veli palatini

Internal carotid artery

**Horizontal (axial) through infratemporal fossa (inferior view)**

**480**

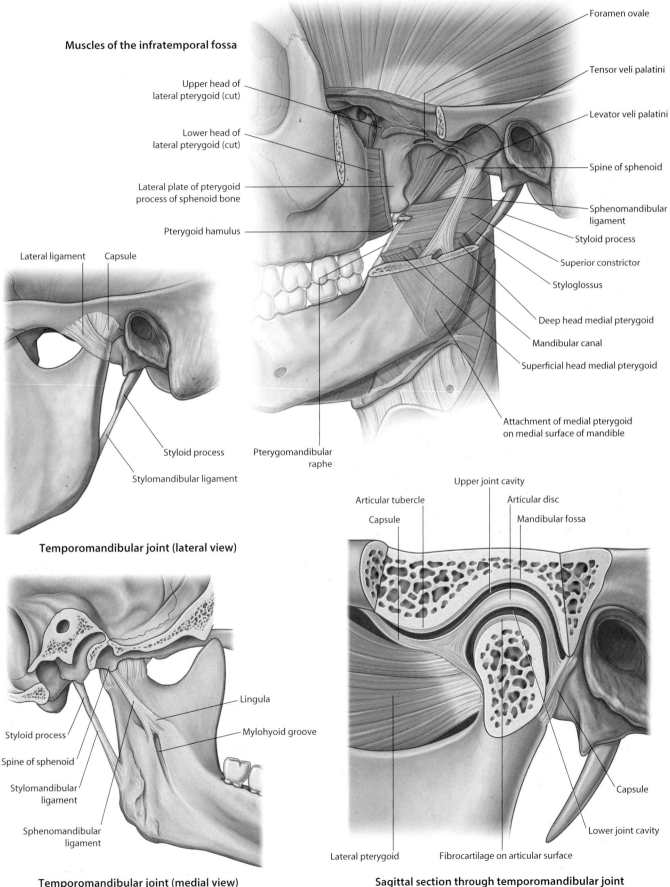

**Muscles of the infratemporal fossa**

Foramen ovale

Tensor veli palatini

Levator veli palatini

Upper head of lateral pterygoid (cut)

Lower head of lateral pterygoid (cut)

Spine of sphenoid

Lateral plate of pterygoid process of sphenoid bone

Sphenomandibular ligament

Styloid process

Pterygoid hamulus

Superior constrictor

Styloglossus

Lateral ligament    Capsule

Deep head medial pterygoid

Mandibular canal

Superficial head medial pterygoid

Styloid process

Stylomandibular ligament

Pterygomandibular raphe

Attachment of medial pterygoid on medial surface of mandible

**Temporomandibular joint (lateral view)**

Upper joint cavity

Articular tubercle

Articular disc

Capsule

Mandibular fossa

Lingula

Mylohyoid groove

Styloid process

Spine of sphenoid

Stylomandibular ligament

Sphenomandibular ligament

Capsule

Lower joint cavity

Lateral pterygoid

Fibrocartilage on articular surface

**Temporomandibular joint (medial view)**

**Sagittal section through temporomandibular joint**

**481**

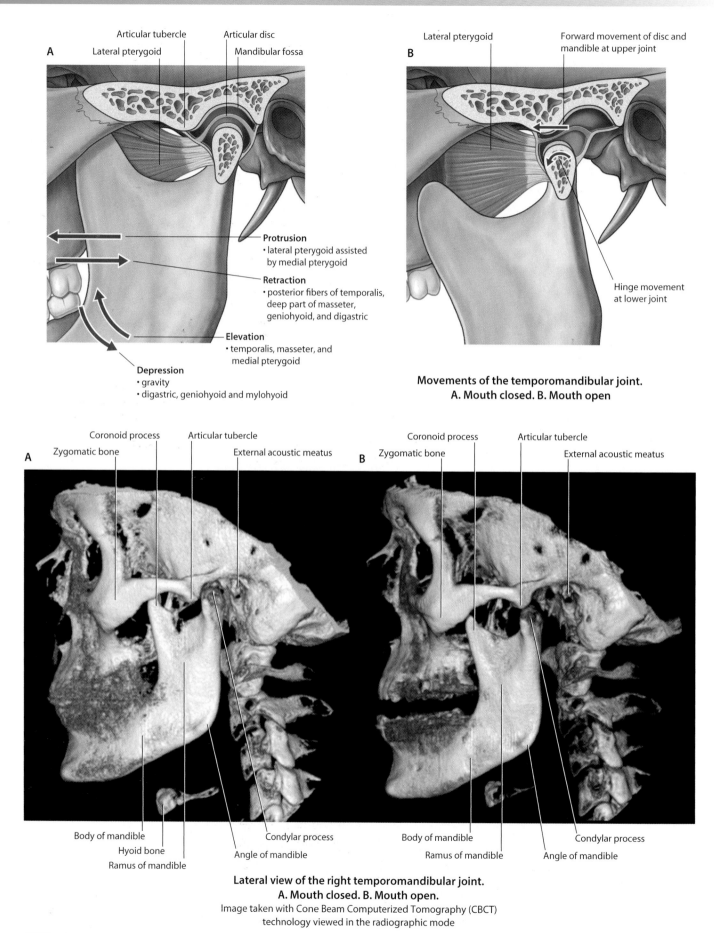

**A**

Articular tubercle
Lateral pterygoid
Articular disc
Mandibular fossa

**Protrusion**
• lateral pterygoid assisted by medial pterygoid

**Retraction**
• posterior fibers of temporalis, deep part of masseter, geniohyoid, and digastric

**Elevation**
• temporalis, masseter, and medial pterygoid

**Depression**
• gravity
• digastric, geniohyoid and mylohyoid

**B**

Lateral pterygoid
Forward movement of disc and mandible at upper joint

Hinge movement at lower joint

**Movements of the temporomandibular joint.**
**A. Mouth closed. B. Mouth open**

**A**

Zygomatic bone
Coronoid process
Articular tubercle
External acoustic meatus

Body of mandible
Hyoid bone
Ramus of mandible
Condylar process
Angle of mandible

**B**

Zygomatic bone
Coronoid process
Articular tubercle
External acoustic meatus

Body of mandible
Ramus of mandible
Condylar process
Angle of mandible

**Lateral view of the right temporomandibular joint.**
**A. Mouth closed. B. Mouth open.**
Image taken with Cone Beam Computerized Tomography (CBCT)
technology viewed in the radiographic mode

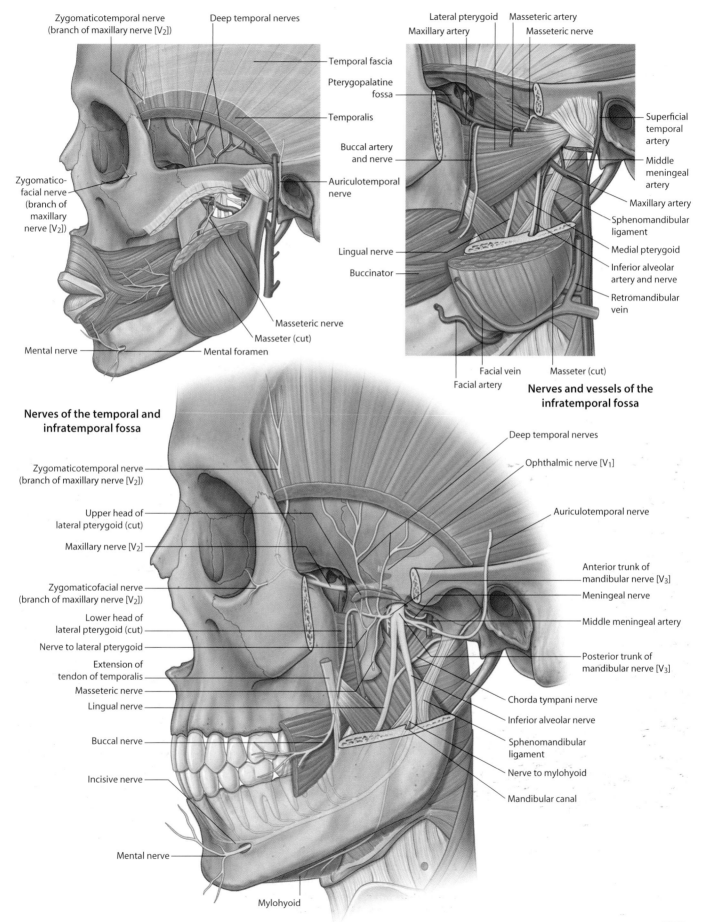

Zygomaticotemporal nerve (branch of maxillary nerve [V₂])

Deep temporal nerves

Temporal fascia

Pterygopalatine fossa

Temporalis

Buccal artery and nerve

Auriculotemporal nerve

Zygomatico-facial nerve (branch of maxillary nerve [V₂])

Lingual nerve

Buccinator

Mental nerve

Mental foramen

Masseteric nerve

Masseter (cut)

Lateral pterygoid   Masseteric artery

Maxillary artery   Masseteric nerve

Superficial temporal artery

Middle meningeal artery

Maxillary artery

Sphenomandibular ligament

Medial pterygoid

Inferior alveolar artery and nerve

Retromandibular vein

Facial vein   Masseter (cut)

Facial artery

**Nerves and vessels of the infratemporal fossa**

**Nerves of the temporal and infratemporal fossa**

Zygomaticotemporal nerve (branch of maxillary nerve [V₂])

Upper head of lateral pterygoid (cut)

Maxillary nerve [V₂]

Zygomaticofacial nerve (branch of maxillary nerve [V₂])

Lower head of lateral pterygoid (cut)

Nerve to lateral pterygoid

Extension of tendon of temporalis

Masseteric nerve

Lingual nerve

Buccal nerve

Incisive nerve

Mental nerve

Mylohyoid

Deep temporal nerves

Ophthalmic nerve [V₁]

Auriculotemporal nerve

Anterior trunk of mandibular nerve [V₃]

Meningeal nerve

Middle meningeal artery

Posterior trunk of mandibular nerve [V₃]

Chorda tympani nerve

Inferior alveolar nerve

Sphenomandibular ligament

Nerve to mylohyoid

Mandibular canal

**483**

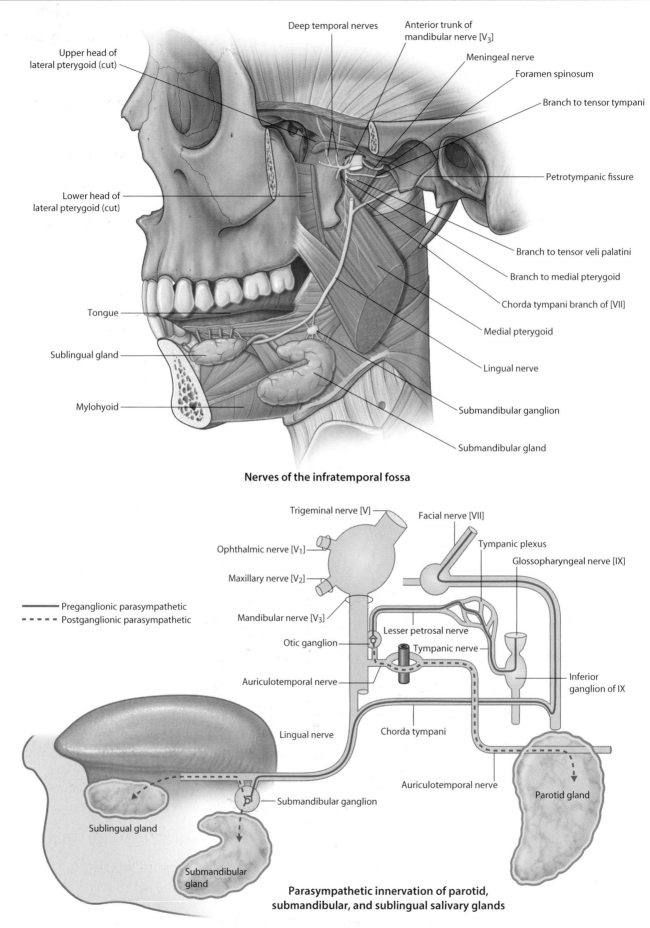

Deep temporal nerves

Anterior trunk of mandibular nerve [V₃]

Meningeal nerve

Foramen spinosum

Branch to tensor tympani

Upper head of lateral pterygoid (cut)

Petrotympanic fissure

Lower head of lateral pterygoid (cut)

Branch to tensor veli palatini

Branch to medial pterygoid

Chorda tympani branch of [VII]

Medial pterygoid

Tongue

Lingual nerve

Sublingual gland

Submandibular ganglion

Mylohyoid

Submandibular gland

**Nerves of the infratemporal fossa**

Trigeminal nerve [V]

Facial nerve [VII]

Tympanic plexus

Ophthalmic nerve [V₁]

Glossopharyngeal nerve [IX]

Maxillary nerve [V₂]

Lesser petrosal nerve

Mandibular nerve [V₃]

Otic ganglion

Tympanic nerve

Auriculotemporal nerve

Inferior ganglion of IX

—— Preganglionic parasympathetic
- - - Postganglionic parasympathetic

Lingual nerve

Chorda tympani

Auriculotemporal nerve

Parotid gland

Submandibular ganglion

Sublingual gland

Submandibular gland

**Parasympathetic innervation of parotid, submandibular, and sublingual salivary glands**

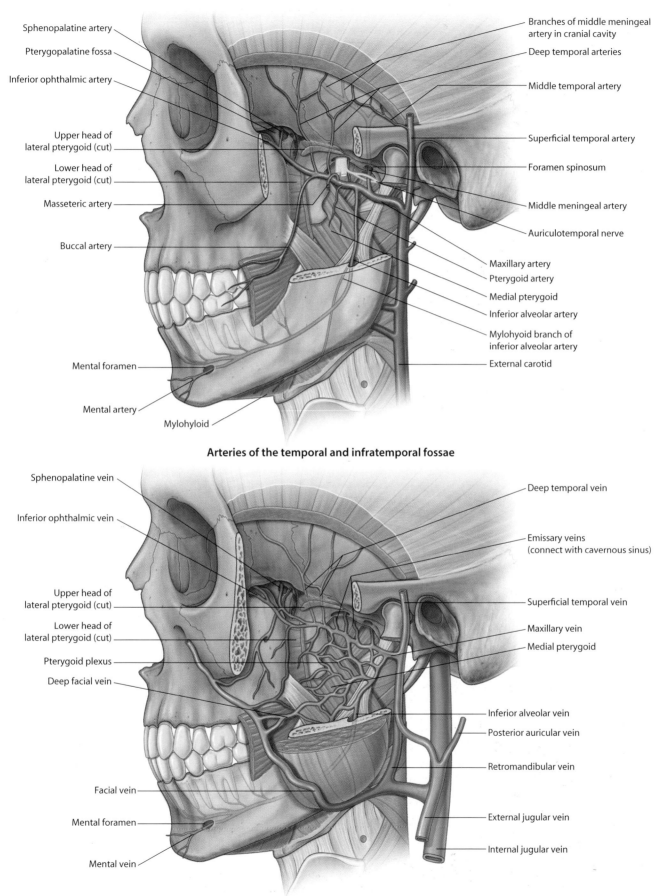

Sphenopalatine artery
Pterygopalatine fossa
Inferior ophthalmic artery
Upper head of lateral pterygoid (cut)
Lower head of lateral pterygoid (cut)
Masseteric artery
Buccal artery
Mental foramen
Mental artery
Mylohyoid

Branches of middle meningeal artery in cranial cavity
Deep temporal arteries
Middle temporal artery
Superficial temporal artery
Foramen spinosum
Middle meningeal artery
Auriculotemporal nerve
Maxillary artery
Pterygoid artery
Medial pterygoid
Inferior alveolar artery
Mylohyoid branch of inferior alveolar artery
External carotid

**Arteries of the temporal and infratemporal fossae**

Sphenopalatine vein
Inferior ophthalmic vein
Upper head of lateral pterygoid (cut)
Lower head of lateral pterygoid (cut)
Pterygoid plexus
Deep facial vein
Facial vein
Mental foramen
Mental vein

Deep temporal vein
Emissary veins (connect with cavernous sinus)
Superficial temporal vein
Maxillary vein
Medial pterygoid
Inferior alveolar vein
Posterior auricular vein
Retromandibular vein
External jugular vein
Internal jugular vein

**Veins of the temporal and infratemporal fossae**

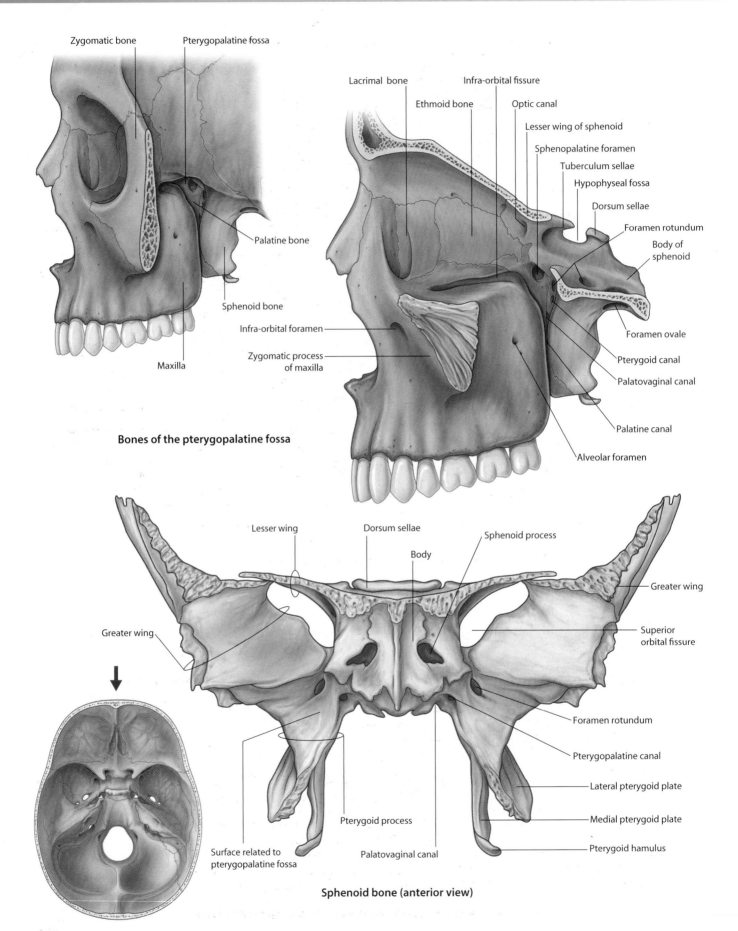

Zygomatic bone

Pterygopalatine fossa

Palatine bone

Sphenoid bone

Maxilla

Infra-orbital foramen

Zygomatic process of maxilla

**Bones of the pterygopalatine fossa**

Lacrimal bone

Ethmoid bone

Infra-orbital fissure

Optic canal

Lesser wing of sphenoid

Sphenopalatine foramen

Tuberculum sellae

Hypophyseal fossa

Dorsum sellae

Foramen rotundum

Body of sphenoid

Foramen ovale

Pterygoid canal

Palatovaginal canal

Palatine canal

Alveolar foramen

Lesser wing

Dorsum sellae

Sphenoid process

Body

Greater wing

Greater wing

Superior orbital fissure

Foramen rotundum

Pterygopalatine canal

Lateral pterygoid plate

Medial pterygoid plate

Pterygoid hamulus

Surface related to pterygopalatine fossa

Pterygoid process

Palatovaginal canal

**Sphenoid bone (anterior view)**

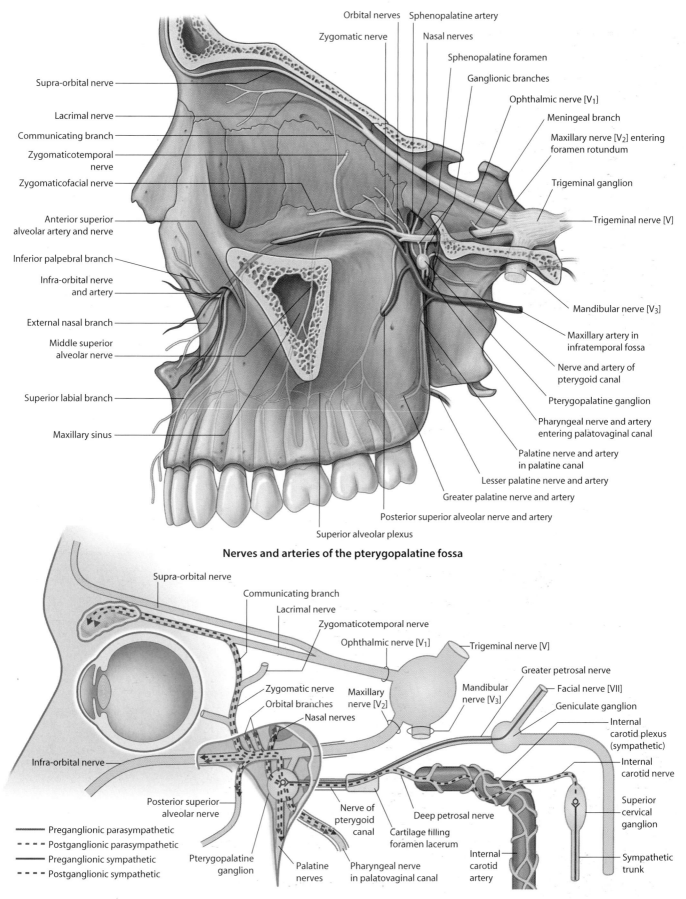

**Nerves and arteries of the pterygopalatine fossa**

**Visceral efferent (motor) pathways through the pterygopalatine fossa**

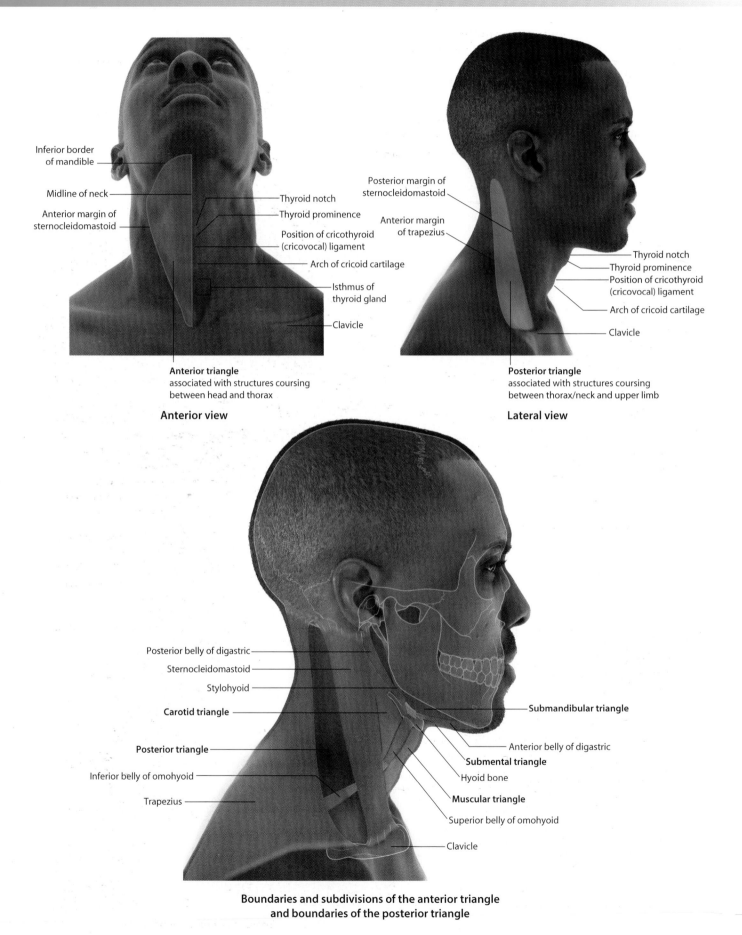

Inferior border of mandible

Midline of neck

Anterior margin of sternocleidomastoid

Thyroid notch

Thyroid prominence

Position of cricothyroid (cricovocal) ligament

Arch of cricoid cartilage

Isthmus of thyroid gland

Clavicle

**Anterior triangle**
associated with structures coursing between head and thorax

**Anterior view**

Posterior margin of sternocleidomastoid

Anterior margin of trapezius

Thyroid notch

Thyroid prominence

Position of cricothyroid (cricovocal) ligament

Arch of cricoid cartilage

Clavicle

**Posterior triangle**
associated with structures coursing between thorax/neck and upper limb

**Lateral view**

Posterior belly of digastric

Sternocleidomastoid

Stylohyoid

**Carotid triangle**

**Posterior triangle**

Inferior belly of omohyoid

Trapezius

**Submandibular triangle**

Anterior belly of digastric

**Submental triangle**

Hyoid bone

**Muscular triangle**

Superior belly of omohyoid

Clavicle

**Boundaries and subdivisions of the anterior triangle
and boundaries of the posterior triangle**

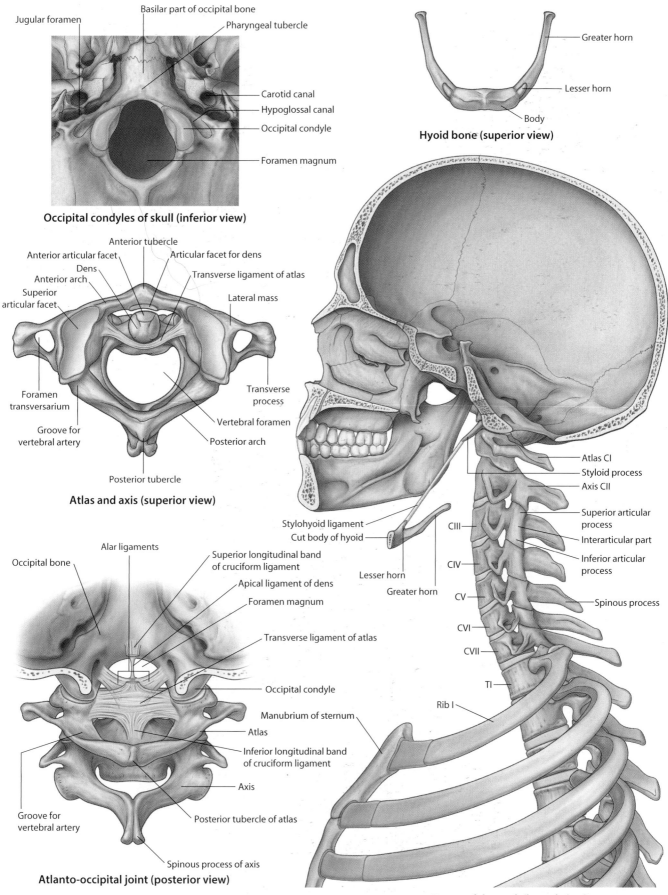

**Occipital condyles of skull (inferior view)**

Jugular foramen

Basilar part of occipital bone

Pharyngeal tubercle

Carotid canal

Hypoglossal canal

Occipital condyle

Foramen magnum

**Hyoid bone (superior view)**

Greater horn

Lesser horn

Body

**Atlas and axis (superior view)**

Anterior tubercle

Anterior articular facet

Articular facet for dens

Dens

Anterior arch

Transverse ligament of atlas

Superior articular facet

Lateral mass

Foramen transversarium

Transverse process

Groove for vertebral artery

Vertebral foramen

Posterior arch

Posterior tubercle

**Atlanto-occipital joint (posterior view)**

Occipital bone

Alar ligaments

Superior longitudinal band of cruciform ligament

Apical ligament of dens

Foramen magnum

Transverse ligament of atlas

Occipital condyle

Atlas

Inferior longitudinal band of cruciform ligament

Axis

Groove for vertebral artery

Posterior tubercle of atlas

Spinous process of axis

**Bones of the neck (lateral view)**

Atlas CI

Styloid process

Axis CII

Superior articular process

Interarticular part

Inferior articular process

Spinous process

Stylohyoid ligament

Cut body of hyoid

Lesser horn

Greater horn

CIII

CIV

CV

CVI

CVII

TI

Rib I

Manubrium of sternum

489

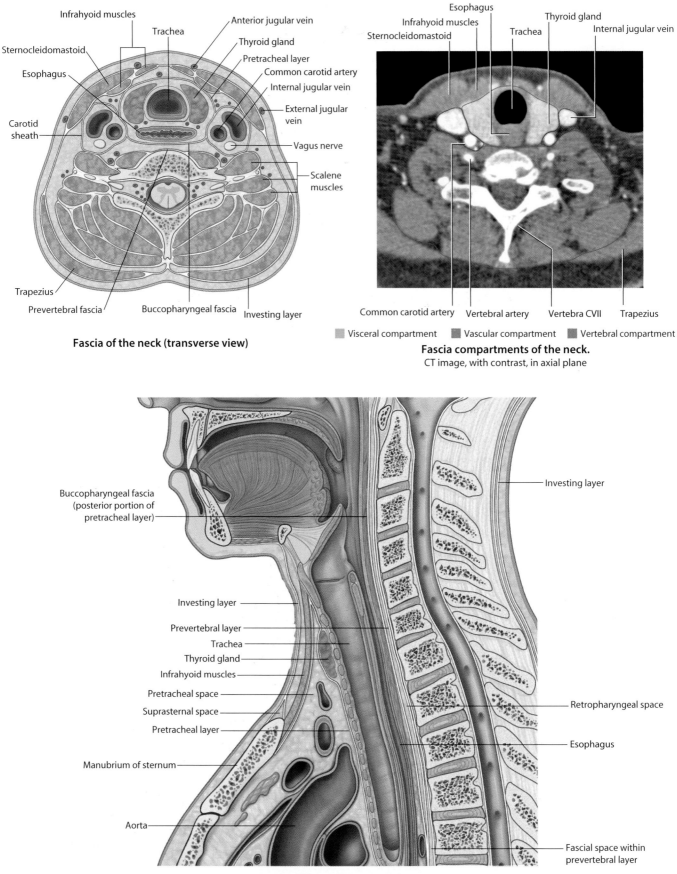

Infrahyoid muscles
Trachea
Sternocleidomastoid
Anterior jugular vein
Thyroid gland
Pretracheal layer
Esophagus
Common carotid artery
Internal jugular vein
External jugular vein
Carotid sheath
Vagus nerve
Scalene muscles
Trapezius
Prevertebral fascia
Buccopharyngeal fascia
Investing layer

**Fascia of the neck (transverse view)**

Esophagus
Infrahyoid muscles
Sternocleidomastoid
Trachea
Thyroid gland
Internal jugular vein

Common carotid artery
Vertebral artery
Vertebra CVII
Trapezius

Visceral compartment    Vascular compartment    Vertebral compartment

**Fascia compartments of the neck.**
CT image, with contrast, in axial plane

Buccopharyngeal fascia
(posterior portion of
pretracheal layer)

Investing layer

Investing layer
Prevertebral layer
Trachea
Thyroid gland
Infrahyoid muscles
Pretracheal space
Suprasternal space
Pretracheal layer
Manubrium of sternum

Retropharyngeal space

Esophagus

Aorta

Fascial space within
prevertebral layer

**Fascia of the neck (sagittal view)**

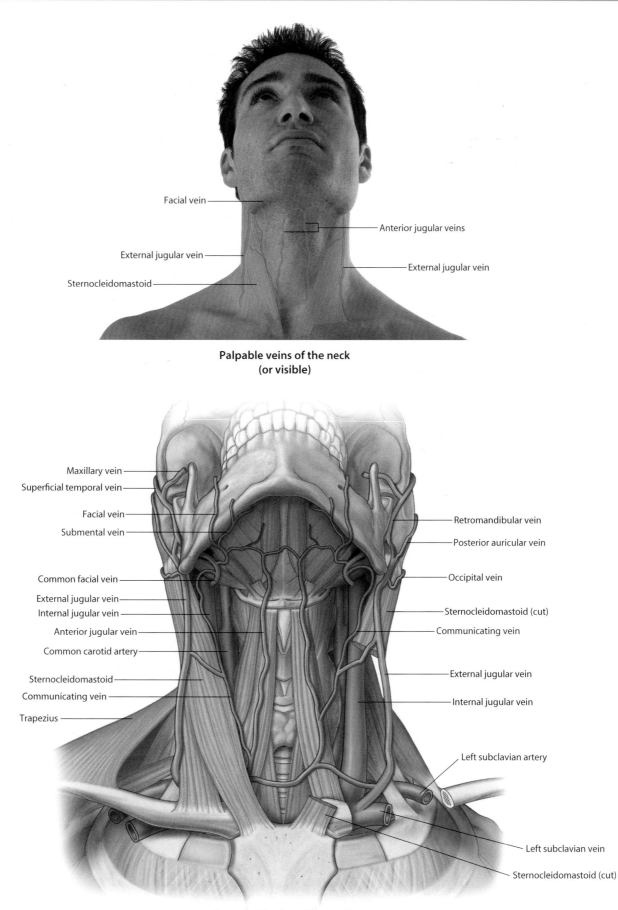

Facial vein

Anterior jugular veins

External jugular vein

External jugular vein

Sternocleidomastoid

**Palpable veins of the neck
(or visible)**

Maxillary vein

Superficial temporal vein

Facial vein

Submental vein

Retromandibular vein

Posterior auricular vein

Occipital vein

Common facial vein

External jugular vein

Internal jugular vein

Anterior jugular vein

Common carotid artery

Sternocleidomastoid (cut)

Communicating vein

External jugular vein

Internal jugular vein

Sternocleidomastoid

Communicating vein

Trapezius

Left subclavian artery

Left subclavian vein

Sternocleidomastoid (cut)

**Superficial veins of the neck**

491

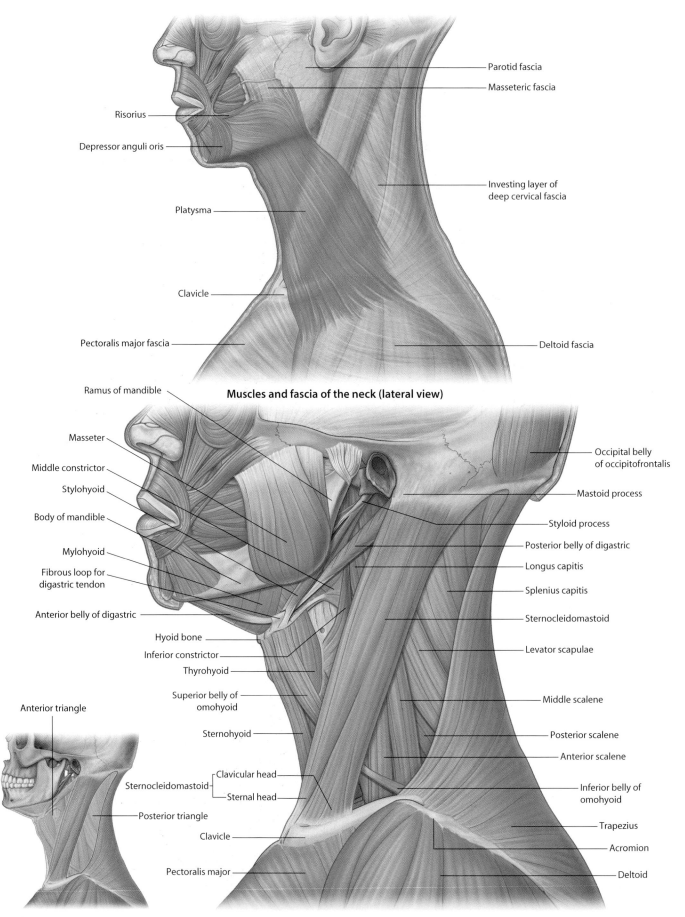

Parotid fascia

Masseteric fascia

Risorius

Depressor anguli oris

Investing layer of
deep cervical fascia

Platysma

Clavicle

Pectoralis major fascia

Deltoid fascia

**Muscles and fascia of the neck (lateral view)**

Ramus of mandible

Masseter

Middle constrictor

Stylohyoid

Body of mandible

Mylohyoid

Fibrous loop for
digastric tendon

Anterior belly of digastric

Hyoid bone

Inferior constrictor

Thyrohyoid

Superior belly of
omohyoid

Sternohyoid

Anterior triangle

Clavicular head

Sternocleidomastoid

Sternal head

Posterior triangle

Clavicle

Pectoralis major

Occipital belly
of occipitofrontalis

Mastoid process

Styloid process

Posterior belly of digastric

Longus capitis

Splenius capitis

Sternocleidomastoid

Levator scapulae

Middle scalene

Posterior scalene

Anterior scalene

Inferior belly of
omohyoid

Trapezius

Acromion

Deltoid

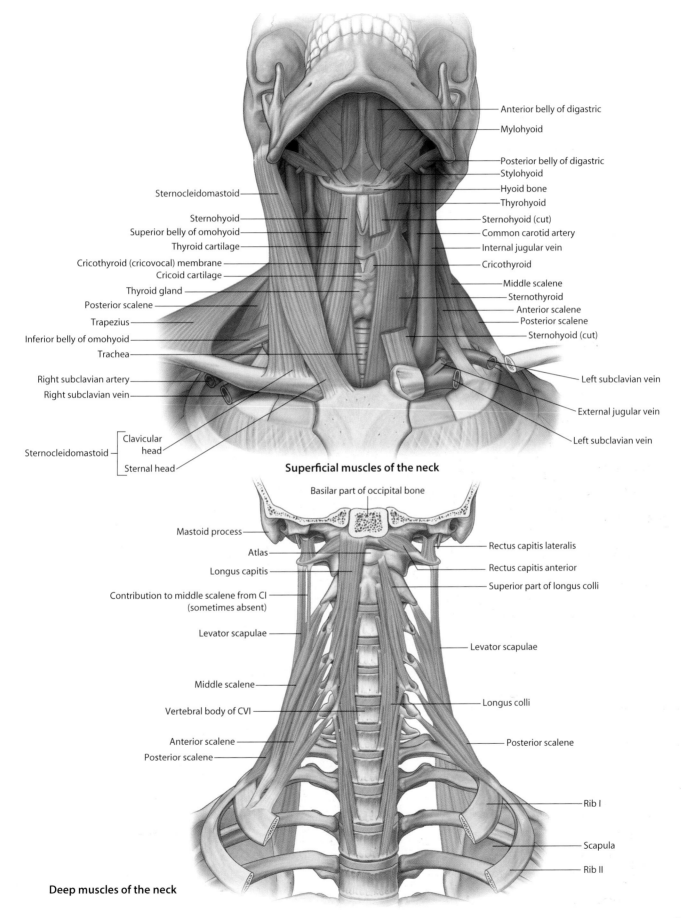

Anterior belly of digastric

Mylohyoid

Posterior belly of digastric

Stylohyoid

Hyoid bone

Thyrohyoid

Sternocleidomastoid

Sternohyoid

Superior belly of omohyoid

Thyroid cartilage

Cricothyroid (cricovocal) membrane

Cricoid cartilage

Thyroid gland

Posterior scalene

Trapezius

Inferior belly of omohyoid

Trachea

Right subclavian artery

Right subclavian vein

Sternohyoid (cut)

Common carotid artery

Internal jugular vein

Cricothyroid

Middle scalene

Sternothyroid

Anterior scalene

Posterior scalene

Sternohyoid (cut)

Left subclavian vein

External jugular vein

Left subclavian vein

Clavicular head

Sternocleidomastoid

Sternal head

**Superficial muscles of the neck**

Basilar part of occipital bone

Mastoid process

Atlas

Longus capitis

Contribution to middle scalene from CI (sometimes absent)

Levator scapulae

Middle scalene

Vertebral body of CVI

Anterior scalene

Posterior scalene

Rectus capitis lateralis

Rectus capitis anterior

Superior part of longus colli

Levator scapulae

Longus colli

Posterior scalene

Rib I

Scapula

Rib II

**Deep muscles of the neck**

**493**

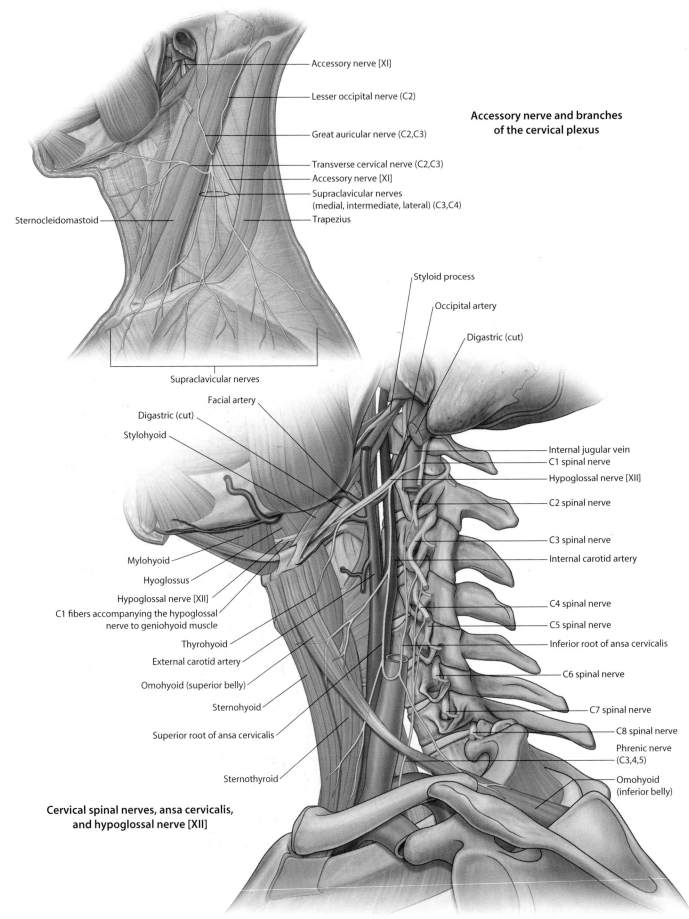

Accessory nerve [XI]

Lesser occipital nerve (C2)

Great auricular nerve (C2,C3)

Transverse cervical nerve (C2,C3)

Accessory nerve [XI]

Supraclavicular nerves
(medial, intermediate, lateral) (C3,C4)

Trapezius

Sternocleidomastoid

**Accessory nerve and branches
of the cervical plexus**

Supraclavicular nerves

Styloid process

Occipital artery

Digastric (cut)

Facial artery

Digastric (cut)

Stylohyoid

Internal jugular vein
C1 spinal nerve

Hypoglossal nerve [XII]

C2 spinal nerve

C3 spinal nerve

Internal carotid artery

Mylohyoid

Hyoglossus

Hypoglossal nerve [XII]

C1 fibers accompanying the hypoglossal
nerve to geniohyoid muscle

Thyrohyoid

External carotid artery

Omohyoid (superior belly)

Sternohyoid

Superior root of ansa cervicalis

Sternothyroid

C4 spinal nerve

C5 spinal nerve

Inferior root of ansa cervicalis

C6 spinal nerve

C7 spinal nerve

C8 spinal nerve

Phrenic nerve
(C3,4,5)

Omohyoid
(inferior belly)

**Cervical spinal nerves, ansa cervicalis,
and hypoglossal nerve [XII]**

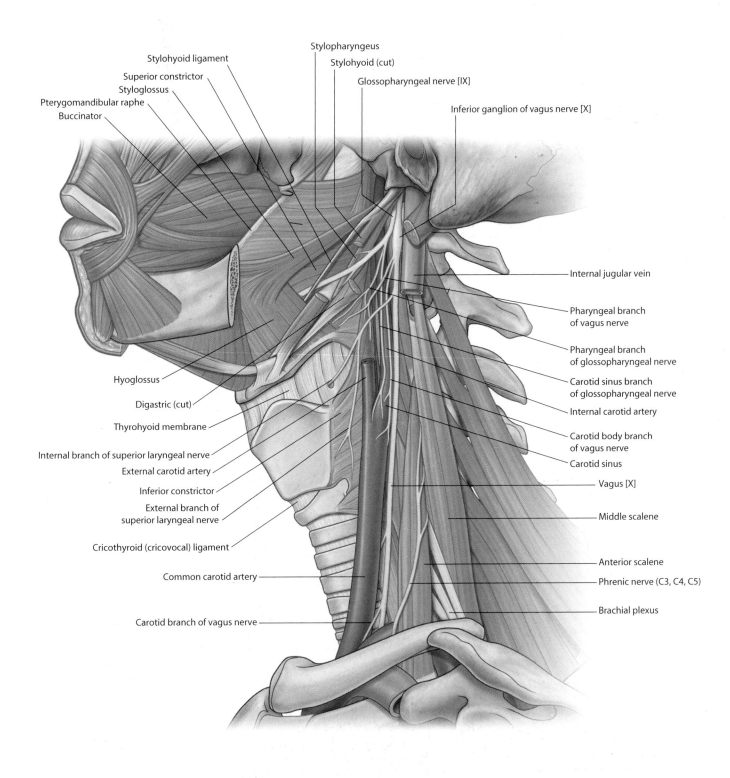

Stylopharyngeus

Stylohyoid (cut)

Glossopharyngeal nerve [IX]

Inferior ganglion of vagus nerve [X]

Stylohyoid ligament

Superior constrictor

Styloglossus

Pterygomandibular raphe

Buccinator

Hyoglossus

Digastric (cut)

Thyrohyoid membrane

Internal branch of superior laryngeal nerve

External carotid artery

Inferior constrictor

External branch of superior laryngeal nerve

Cricothyroid (cricovocal) ligament

Common carotid artery

Carotid branch of vagus nerve

Internal jugular vein

Pharyngeal branch of vagus nerve

Pharyngeal branch of glossopharyngeal nerve

Carotid sinus branch of glossopharyngeal nerve

Internal carotid artery

Carotid body branch of vagus nerve

Carotid sinus

Vagus [X]

Middle scalene

Anterior scalene

Phrenic nerve (C3, C4, C5)

Brachial plexus

**Branches of glossopharyngeal [IX] and vagus nerves [X] in neck**

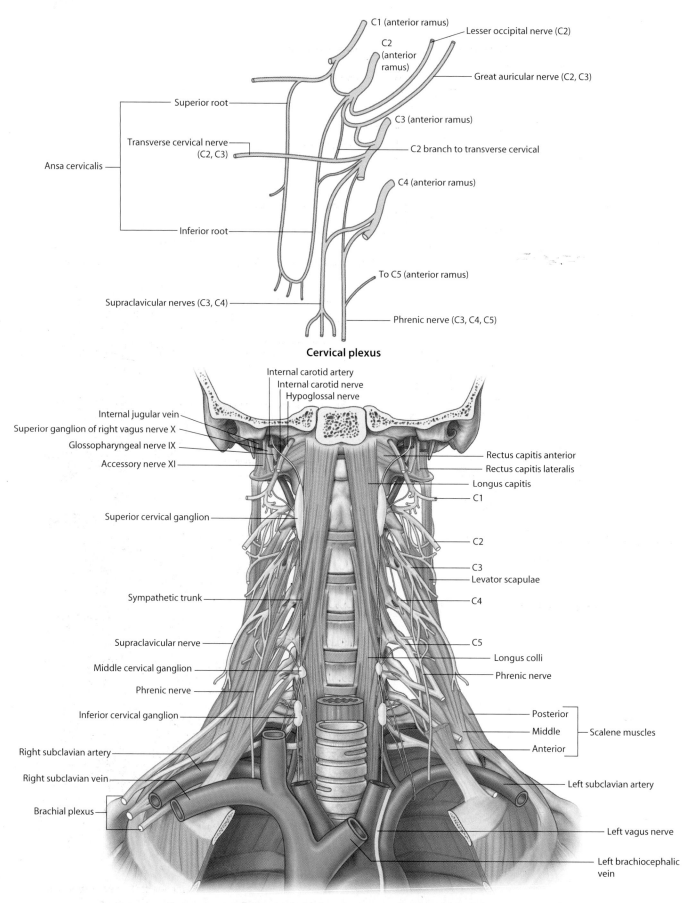

C1 (anterior ramus)

Lesser occipital nerve (C2)

C2 (anterior ramus)

Great auricular nerve (C2, C3)

Superior root

C3 (anterior ramus)

Transverse cervical nerve (C2, C3)

C2 branch to transverse cervical

Ansa cervicalis

C4 (anterior ramus)

Inferior root

To C5 (anterior ramus)

Supraclavicular nerves (C3, C4)

Phrenic nerve (C3, C4, C5)

**Cervical plexus**

Internal carotid artery

Internal carotid nerve

Hypoglossal nerve

Internal jugular vein

Superior ganglion of right vagus nerve X

Glossopharyngeal nerve IX

Accessory nerve XI

Rectus capitis anterior

Rectus capitis lateralis

Longus capitis

C1

Superior cervical ganglion

C2

C3

Levator scapulae

C4

Sympathetic trunk

C5

Supraclavicular nerve

Longus colli

Middle cervical ganglion

Phrenic nerve

Phrenic nerve

Posterior

Inferior cervical ganglion

Middle

Scalene muscles

Anterior

Right subclavian artery

Right subclavian vein

Left subclavian artery

Brachial plexus

Left vagus nerve

Left brachiocephalic vein

**Components of the sympathetic nervous system in the root of the neck**

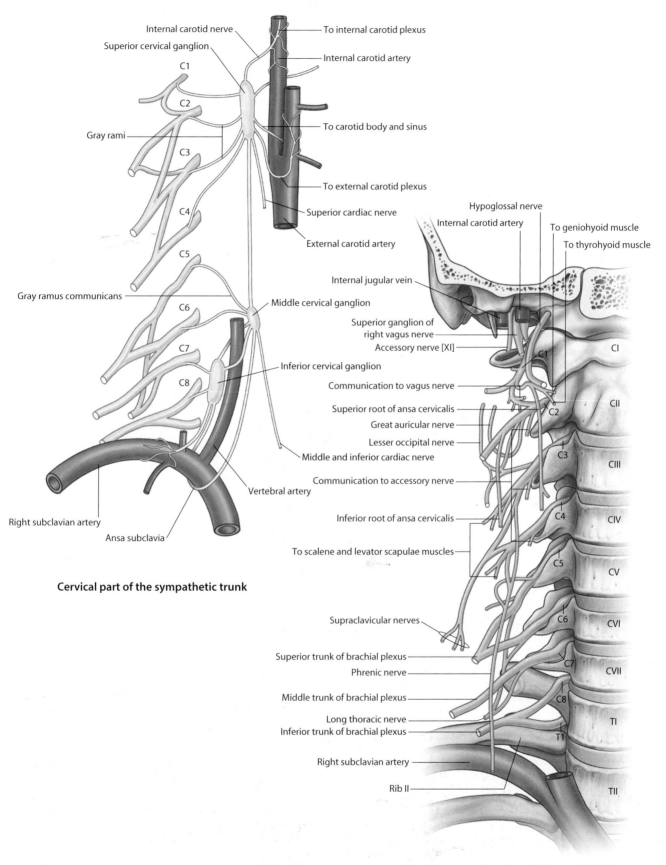

Internal carotid nerve

Superior cervical ganglion

C1

C2

Gray rami

C3

C4

C5

Gray ramus communicans

C6

C7

C8

Right subclavian artery

Ansa subclavia

To internal carotid plexus

Internal carotid artery

To carotid body and sinus

To external carotid plexus

Superior cardiac nerve

External carotid artery

Middle cervical ganglion

Inferior cervical ganglion

Middle and inferior cardiac nerve

Vertebral artery

**Cervical part of the sympathetic trunk**

Hypoglossal nerve

Internal carotid artery

To geniohyoid muscle

To thyrohyoid muscle

Internal jugular vein

Superior ganglion of right vagus nerve

Accessory nerve [XI]

Communication to vagus nerve

Superior root of ansa cervicalis

Great auricular nerve

Lesser occipital nerve

Communication to accessory nerve

Inferior root of ansa cervicalis

To scalene and levator scapulae muscles

Supraclavicular nerves

Superior trunk of brachial plexus

Phrenic nerve

Middle trunk of brachial plexus

Long thoracic nerve

Inferior trunk of brachial plexus

Right subclavian artery

Rib II

CI

CII

CIII

CIV

CV

CVI

CVII

TI

TII

C1

C2

C3

C4

C5

C6

C7

C8

T1

**Branches of the cervical plexus
(rib I removed)**

**497**

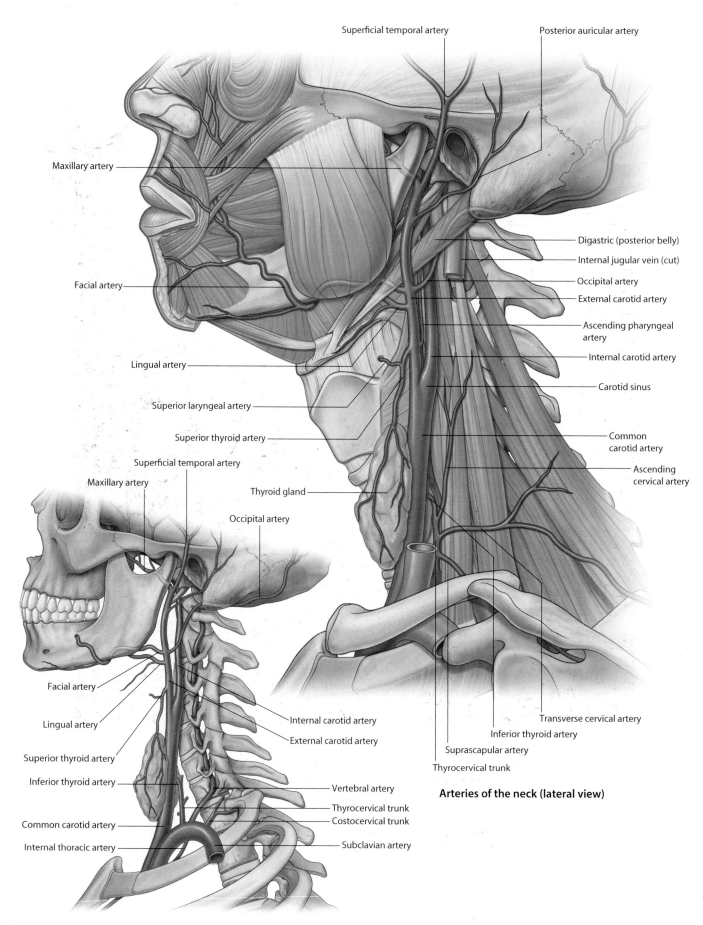

Superficial temporal artery

Posterior auricular artery

Maxillary artery

Facial artery

Lingual artery

Superior laryngeal artery

Superior thyroid artery

Superficial temporal artery

Maxillary artery

Occipital artery

Thyroid gland

Facial artery

Lingual artery

Superior thyroid artery

Inferior thyroid artery

Common carotid artery

Internal thoracic artery

Digastric (posterior belly)

Internal jugular vein (cut)

Occipital artery

External carotid artery

Ascending pharyngeal artery

Internal carotid artery

Carotid sinus

Common carotid artery

Ascending cervical artery

Transverse cervical artery

Inferior thyroid artery

Suprascapular artery

Thyrocervical trunk

Internal carotid artery

External carotid artery

Vertebral artery

Thyrocervical trunk

Costocervical trunk

Subclavian artery

**Arteries of the neck (lateral view)**

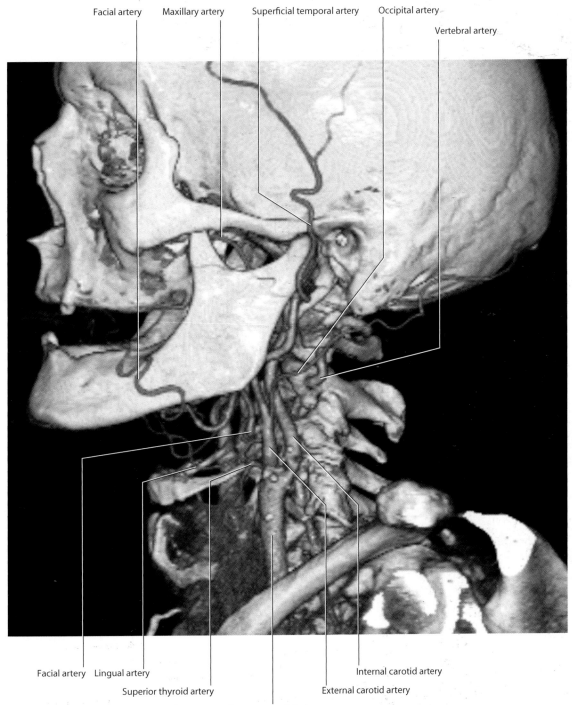

Facial artery  Maxillary artery  Superficial temporal artery  Occipital artery

Vertebral artery

Facial artery  Lingual artery

Superior thyroid artery

Internal carotid artery

External carotid artery

Common carotid artery

**Lateral view of the branches of the external carotid artery.**
Volume-rendered angiographic image with contrast using multidetector CT

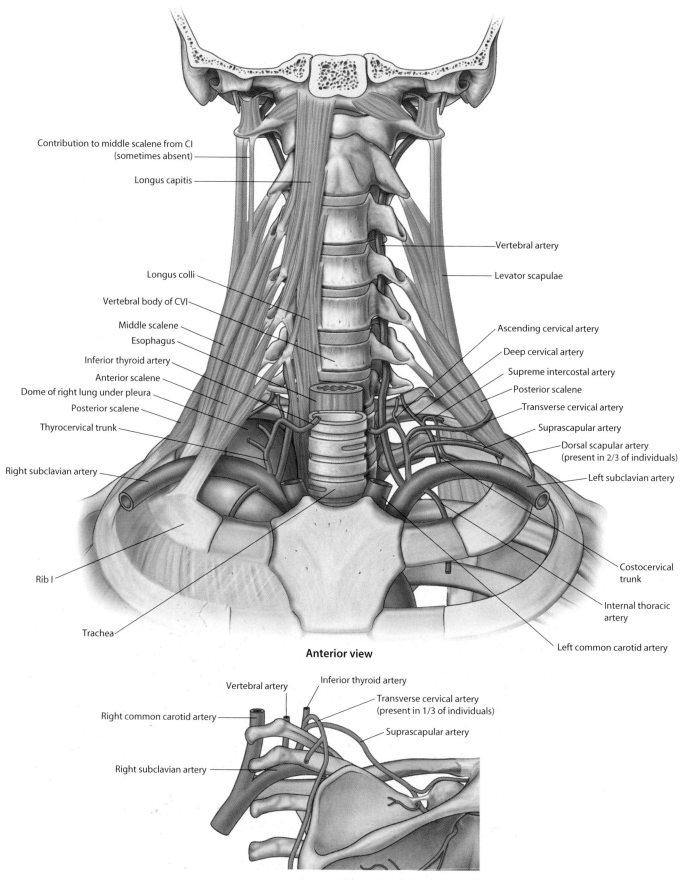

Contribution to middle scalene from CI (sometimes absent)

Longus capitis

Vertebral artery

Levator scapulae

Longus colli

Vertebral body of CVI

Middle scalene

Esophagus

Inferior thyroid artery

Anterior scalene

Dome of right lung under pleura

Posterior scalene

Thyrocervical trunk

Right subclavian artery

Ascending cervical artery

Deep cervical artery

Supreme intercostal artery

Posterior scalene

Transverse cervical artery

Suprascapular artery

Dorsal scapular artery (present in 2/3 of individuals)

Left subclavian artery

Costocervical trunk

Internal thoracic artery

Rib I

Trachea

Left common carotid artery

**Anterior view**

Vertebral artery

Inferior thyroid artery

Right common carotid artery

Transverse cervical artery (present in 1/3 of individuals)

Suprascapular artery

Right subclavian artery

**Posterior view**

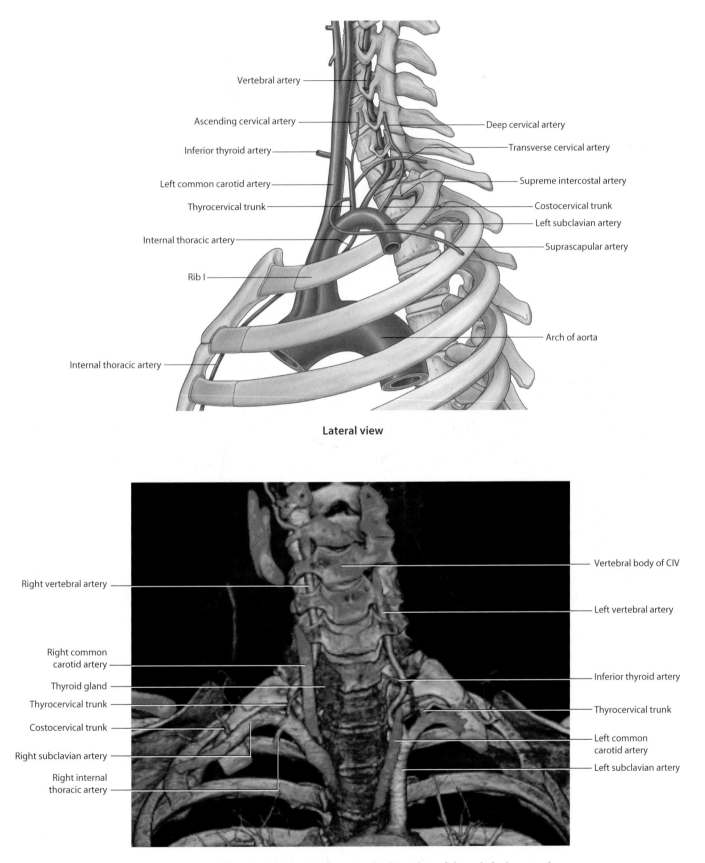

Vertebral artery

Ascending cervical artery

Inferior thyroid artery

Left common carotid artery

Thyrocervical trunk

Internal thoracic artery

Rib I

Internal thoracic artery

Deep cervical artery

Transverse cervical artery

Supreme intercostal artery

Costocervical trunk

Left subclavian artery

Suprascapular artery

Arch of aorta

**Lateral view**

Right vertebral artery

Right common carotid artery

Thyroid gland

Thyrocervical trunk

Costocervical trunk

Right subclavian artery

Right internal thoracic artery

Vertebral body of CIV

Left vertebral artery

Inferior thyroid artery

Thyrocervical trunk

Left common carotid artery

Left subclavian artery

**Anterior view of the root of the neck showing the branches of the subclavian arteries.**
Volume-rendered angiographic image with contrast using multidetector CT

**501**

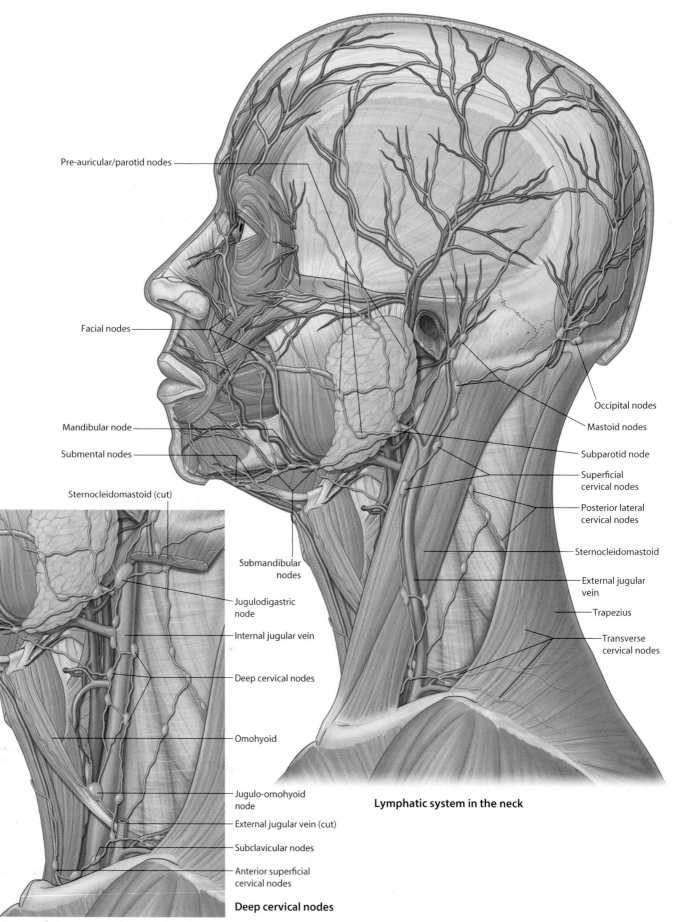

Pre-auricular/parotid nodes

Facial nodes

Mandibular node

Submental nodes

Sternocleidomastoid (cut)

Submandibular nodes

Jugulodigastric node

Internal jugular vein

Deep cervical nodes

Omohyoid

Jugulo-omohyoid node

External jugular vein (cut)

Subclavicular nodes

Anterior superficial cervical nodes

**Deep cervical nodes**

Occipital nodes

Mastoid nodes

Subparotid node

Superficial cervical nodes

Posterior lateral cervical nodes

Sternocleidomastoid

External jugular vein

Trapezius

Transverse cervical nodes

**Lymphatic system in the neck**

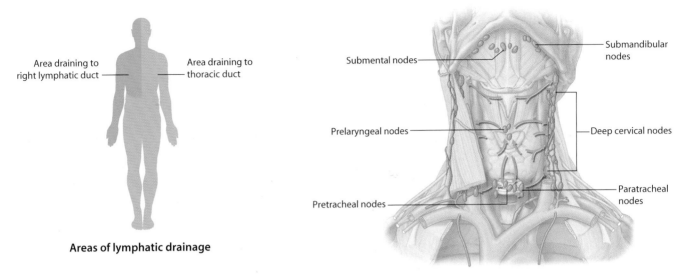

**Areas of lymphatic drainage**

Area draining to right lymphatic duct

Area draining to thoracic duct

Submental nodes

Prelaryngeal nodes

Pretracheal nodes

Submandibular nodes

Deep cervical nodes

Paratracheal nodes

**Lymphatic drainage of the thyroid gland, larynx, and trachea**

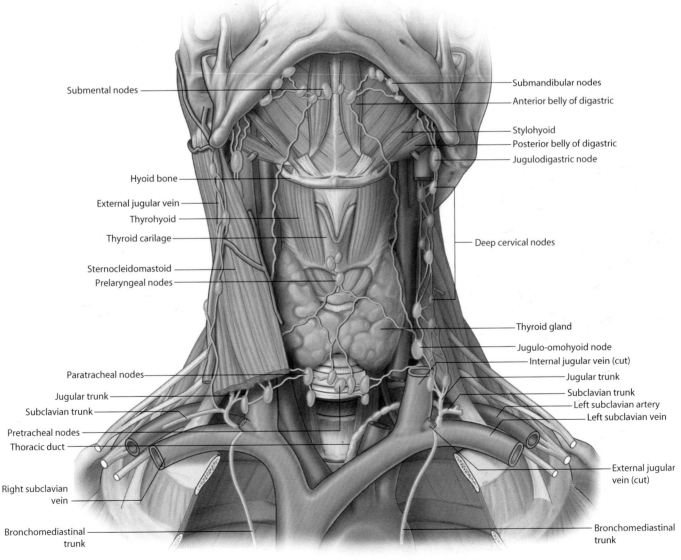

Submental nodes

Hyoid bone

External jugular vein

Thyrohyoid

Thyroid carilage

Sternocleidomastoid

Prelaryngeal nodes

Paratracheal nodes

Jugular trunk

Subclavian trunk

Pretracheal nodes

Thoracic duct

Right subclavian vein

Bronchomediastinal trunk

Submandibular nodes

Anterior belly of digastric

Stylohyoid

Posterior belly of digastric

Jugulodigastric node

Deep cervical nodes

Thyroid gland

Jugulo-omohyoid node

Internal jugular vein (cut)

Jugular trunk

Subclavian trunk

Left subclavian artery

Left subclavian vein

External jugular vein (cut)

Bronchomediastinal trunk

**Lymphatic system in the neck**

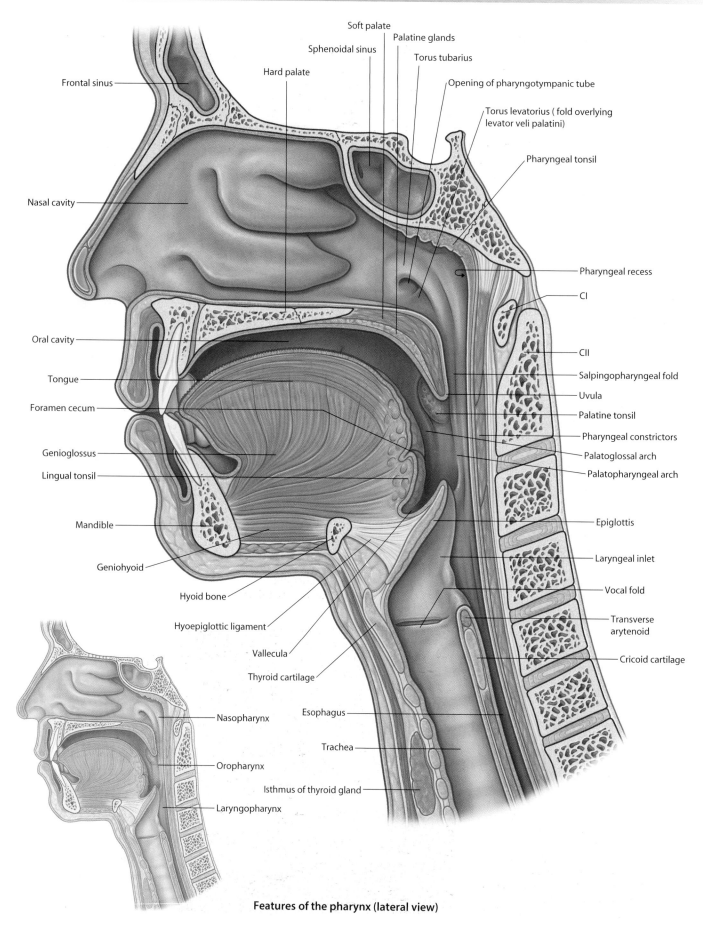

Frontal sinus

Soft palate

Sphenoidal sinus

Palatine glands

Hard palate

Torus tubarius

Opening of pharyngotympanic tube

Torus levatorius ( fold overlying levator veli palatini)

Pharyngeal tonsil

Nasal cavity

Pharyngeal recess

CI

Oral cavity

CII

Tongue

Salpingopharyngeal fold

Foramen cecum

Uvula

Palatine tonsil

Genioglossus

Pharyngeal constrictors

Lingual tonsil

Palatoglossal arch

Palatopharyngeal arch

Mandible

Epiglottis

Geniohyoid

Laryngeal inlet

Hyoid bone

Vocal fold

Hyoepiglottic ligament

Transverse arytenoid

Vallecula

Cricoid cartilage

Thyroid cartilage

Nasopharynx

Esophagus

Oropharynx

Trachea

Isthmus of thyroid gland

Laryngopharynx

**Features of the pharynx (lateral view)**

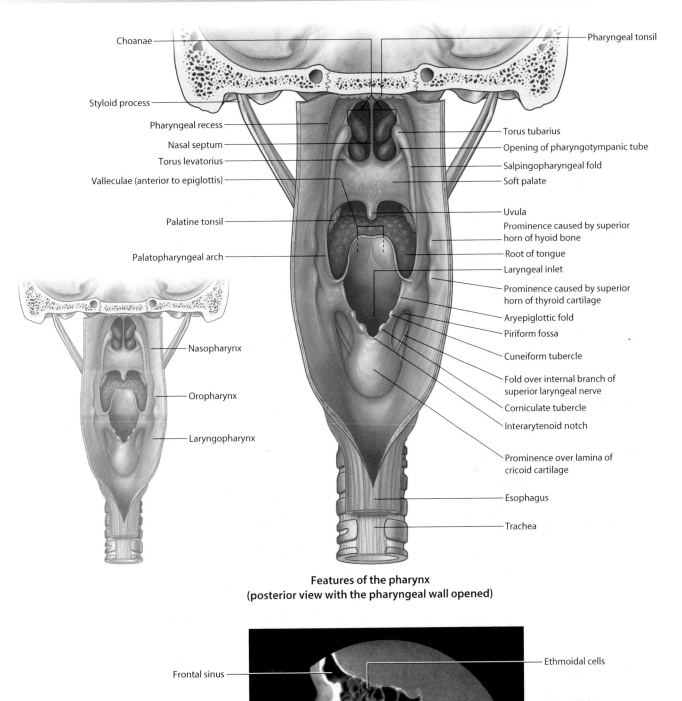

Choanae

Styloid process

Pharyngeal recess

Nasal septum

Torus levatorius

Valleculae (anterior to epiglottis)

Palatine tonsil

Palatopharyngeal arch

Pharyngeal tonsil

Torus tubarius

Opening of pharyngotympanic tube

Salpingopharyngeal fold

Soft palate

Uvula

Prominence caused by superior horn of hyoid bone

Root of tongue

Laryngeal inlet

Prominence caused by superior horn of thyroid cartilage

Aryepiglottic fold

Piriform fossa

Cuneiform tubercle

Fold over internal branch of superior laryngeal nerve

Corniculate tubercle

Interarytenoid notch

Prominence over lamina of cricoid cartilage

Esophagus

Trachea

Nasopharynx

Oropharynx

Laryngopharynx

**Features of the pharynx
(posterior view with the pharyngeal wall opened)**

Frontal sinus

Nasal cavity

Hard palate

Soft palate

Mandible

Ethmoidal cells

Sphenoidal sinus

Nasopharynx

CI

CII

Oropharynx

Epiglottis

Laryngopharynx

**Regions of the pharynx
(mouth closed, teeth together).**
Sagittal image taken with Cone Beam
Computerized Tomography (CBCT)
technology, viewed in the radiographic mode

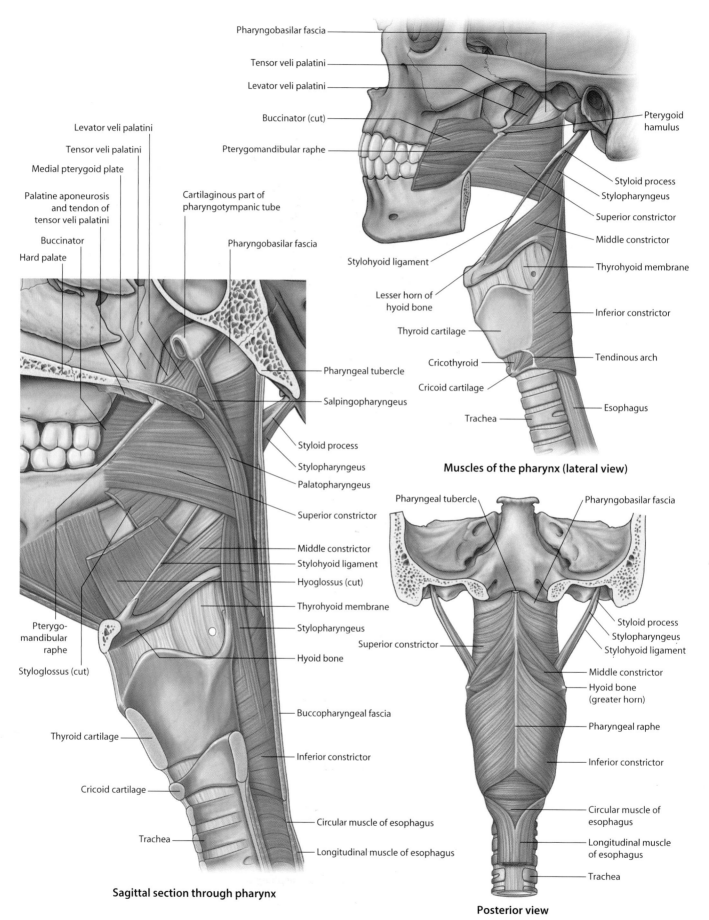

Pharyngobasilar fascia

Tensor veli palatini

Levator veli palatini

Buccinator (cut)

Pterygomandibular raphe

Levator veli palatini

Tensor veli palatini

Medial pterygoid plate

Palatine aponeurosis and tendon of tensor veli palatini

Buccinator

Hard palate

Cartilaginous part of pharyngotympanic tube

Pharyngobasilar fascia

Stylohyoid ligament

Lesser horn of hyoid bone

Thyroid cartilage

Cricothyroid

Cricoid cartilage

Trachea

Pterygoid hamulus

Styloid process

Stylopharyngeus

Superior constrictor

Middle constrictor

Thyrohyoid membrane

Inferior constrictor

Tendinous arch

Esophagus

**Muscles of the pharynx (lateral view)**

Pharyngeal tubercle

Salpingopharyngeus

Styloid process

Stylopharyngeus

Palatopharyngeus

Superior constrictor

Middle constrictor

Stylohyoid ligament

Hyoglossus (cut)

Thyrohyoid membrane

Stylopharyngeus

Hyoid bone

Pterygo-mandibular raphe

Styloglossus (cut)

Thyroid cartilage

Cricoid cartilage

Trachea

Buccopharyngeal fascia

Inferior constrictor

Circular muscle of esophagus

Longitudinal muscle of esophagus

**Sagittal section • through pharynx**

Pharyngeal tubercle

Pharyngobasilar fascia

Superior constrictor

Styloid process

Stylopharyngeus

Stylohyoid ligament

Middle constrictor

Hyoid bone (greater horn)

Pharyngeal raphe

Inferior constrictor

Circular muscle of esophagus

Longitudinal muscle of esophagus

Trachea

**Posterior view**

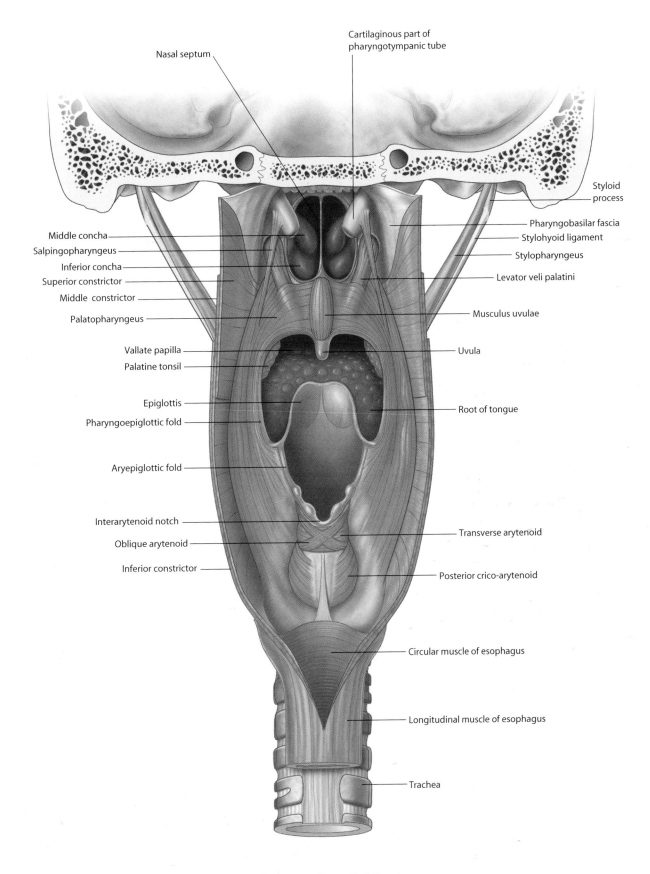

Nasal septum

Cartilaginous part of
pharyngotympanic tube

Styloid
process

Middle concha

Salpingopharyngeus

Inferior concha

Superior constrictor

Middle constrictor

Palatopharyngeus

Pharyngobasilar fascia

Stylohyoid ligament

Stylopharyngeus

Levator veli palatini

Musculus uvulae

Vallate papilla

Palatine tonsil

Uvula

Epiglottis

Pharyngoepiglottic fold

Root of tongue

Aryepiglottic fold

Interarytenoid notch

Oblique arytenoid

Inferior constrictor

Transverse arytenoid

Posterior crico-arytenoid

Circular muscle of esophagus

Longitudinal muscle of esophagus

Trachea

**Muscles of the posterior wall of the pharynx**

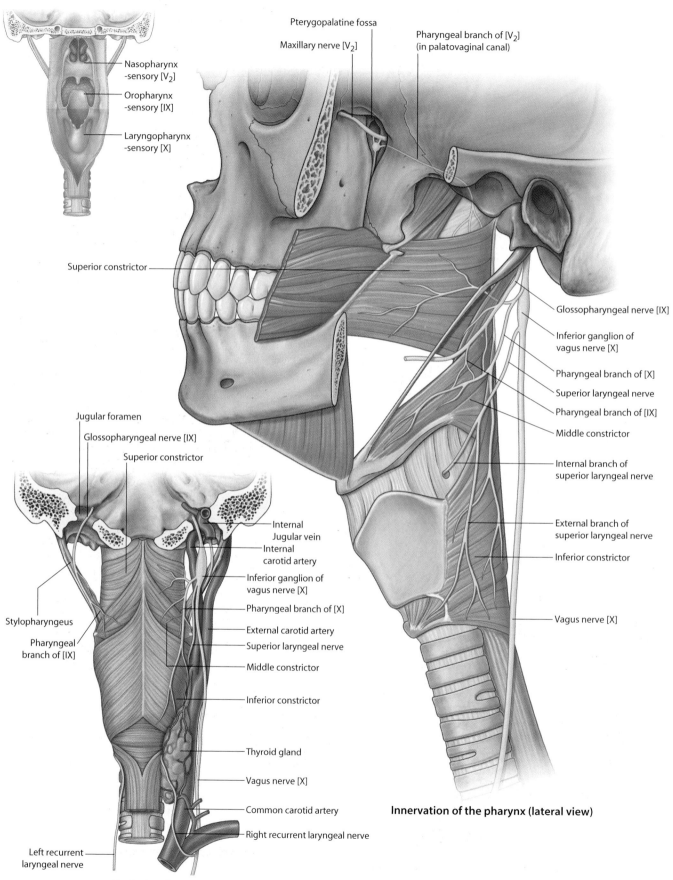

Pterygopalatine fossa

Maxillary nerve [V₂]

Pharyngeal branch of [V₂]
(in palatovaginal canal)

Nasopharynx
-sensory [V₂]

Oropharynx
-sensory [IX]

Laryngopharynx
-sensory [X]

Superior constrictor

Glossopharyngeal nerve [IX]

Inferior ganglion of
vagus nerve [X]

Pharyngeal branch of [X]

Superior laryngeal nerve

Pharyngeal branch of [IX]

Middle constrictor

Internal branch of
superior laryngeal nerve

External branch of
superior laryngeal nerve

Inferior constrictor

Vagus nerve [X]

Jugular foramen

Glossopharyngeal nerve [IX]

Superior constrictor

Internal
Jugular vein

Internal
carotid artery

Inferior ganglion of
vagus nerve [X]

Pharyngeal branch of [X]

External carotid artery

Superior laryngeal nerve

Middle constrictor

Inferior constrictor

Stylopharyngeus

Pharyngeal
branch of [IX]

Thyroid gland

Vagus nerve [X]

Common carotid artery

Right recurrent laryngeal nerve

Left recurrent
laryngeal nerve

**Innervation of the pharynx (lateral view)**

**Posterior view**

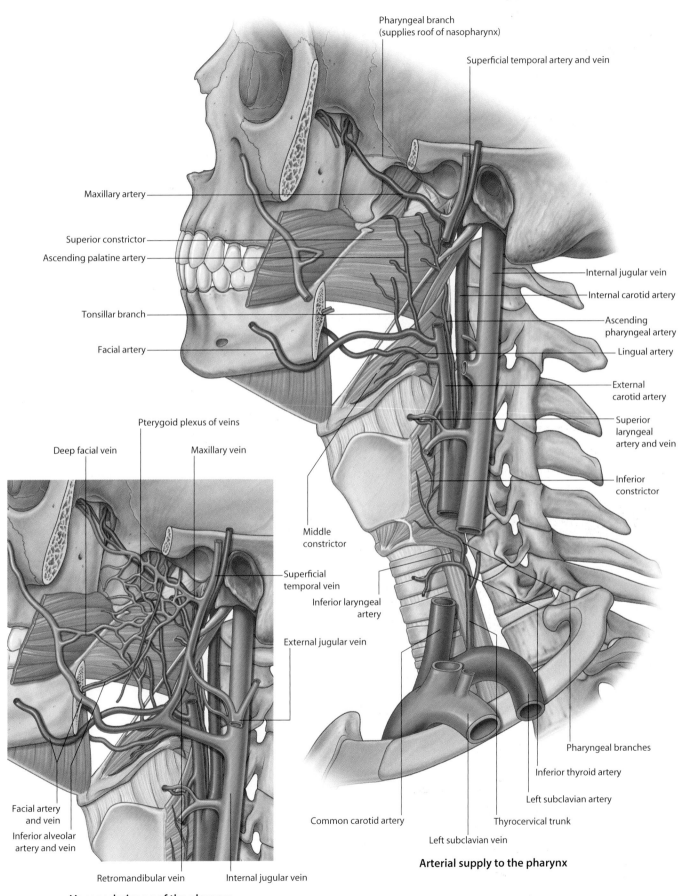

Pharyngeal branch
(supplies roof of nasopharynx)

Superficial temporal artery and vein

Maxillary artery

Superior constrictor

Ascending palatine artery

Tonsillar branch

Facial artery

Internal jugular vein

Internal carotid artery

Ascending
pharyngeal artery

Lingual artery

External
carotid artery

Superior
laryngeal
artery and vein

Inferior
constrictor

Pterygoid plexus of veins

Deep facial vein

Maxillary vein

Middle
constrictor

Superficial
temporal vein

Inferior laryngeal
artery

External jugular vein

Facial artery
and vein

Inferior alveolar
artery and vein

Pharyngeal branches

Inferior thyroid artery

Left subclavian artery

Retromandibular vein

Internal jugular vein

Common carotid artery

Thyrocervical trunk

Left subclavian vein

**Venous drainage of the pharynx**

**Arterial supply to the pharynx**

**509**

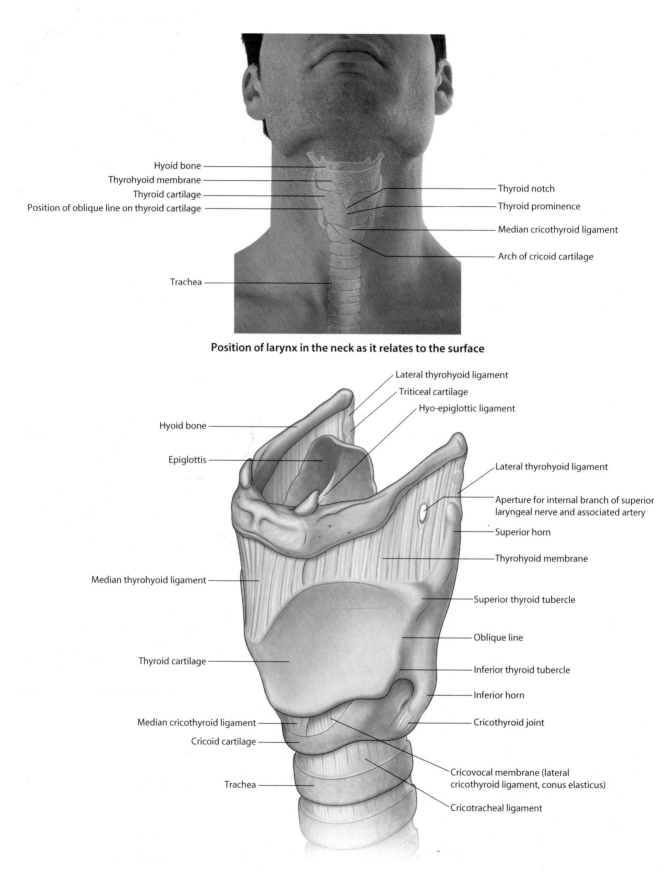

Hyoid bone

Thyrohyoid membrane

Thyroid cartilage

Position of oblique line on thyroid cartilage

Thyroid notch

Thyroid prominence

Median cricothyroid ligament

Arch of cricoid cartilage

Trachea

**Position of larynx in the neck as it relates to the surface**

Lateral thyrohyoid ligament

Triticeal cartilage

Hyo-epiglottic ligament

Hyoid bone

Epiglottis

Lateral thyrohyoid ligament

Aperture for internal branch of superior laryngeal nerve and associated artery

Superior horn

Thyrohyoid membrane

Median thyrohyoid ligament

Superior thyroid tubercle

Oblique line

Inferior thyroid tubercle

Thyroid cartilage

Inferior horn

Cricothyroid joint

Median cricothyroid ligament

Cricoid cartilage

Cricovocal membrane (lateral cricothyroid ligament, conus elasticus)

Trachea

Cricotracheal ligament

**External features of the larynx (anterolateral view)**

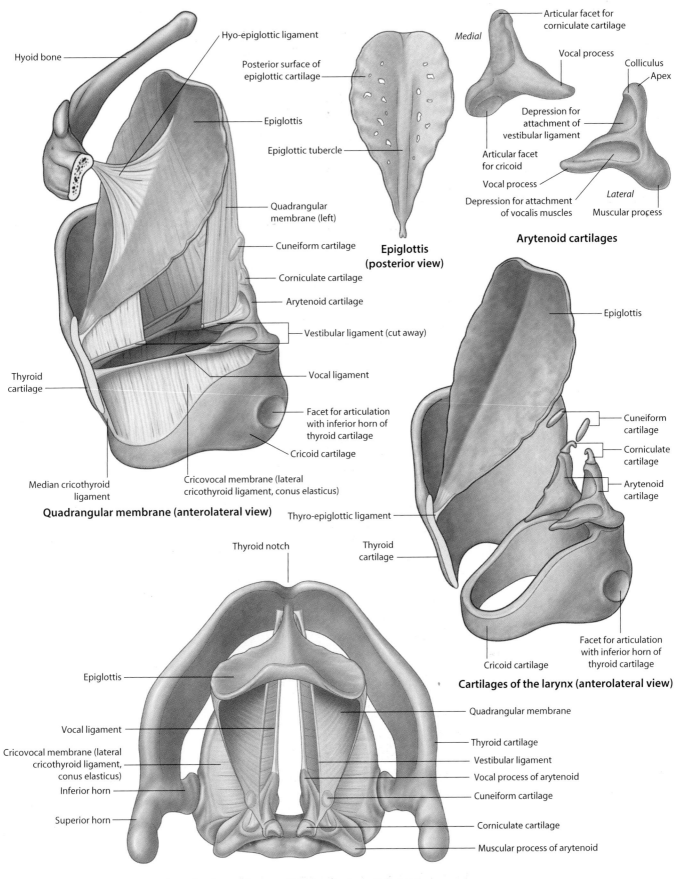

Hyoid bone

Hyo-epiglottic ligament

Posterior surface of
epiglottic cartilage

Epiglottis

Epiglottic tubercle

Quadrangular
membrane (left)

Cuneiform cartilage

Corniculate cartilage

Arytenoid cartilage

Vestibular ligament (cut away)

Vocal ligament

Thyroid
cartilage

Facet for articulation
with inferior horn of
thyroid cartilage

Cricoid cartilage

Median cricothyroid
ligament

Cricovocal membrane (lateral
cricothyroid ligament, conus elasticus)

**Quadrangular membrane (anterolateral view)**

*Medial*

Articular facet for
corniculate cartilage

Vocal process

Colliculus

Apex

Depression for
attachment
of vestibular ligament

Articular facet
for cricoid

Vocal process

Depression for attachment
of vocalis muscles

*Lateral*

Muscular process

**Arytenoid cartilages**

**Epiglottis
(posterior view)**

Epiglottis

Cuneiform
cartilage

Corniculate
cartilage

Arytenoid
cartilage

Thyro-epiglottic ligament

Thyroid
cartilage

Facet for articulation
with inferior horn of
thyroid cartilage

Cricoid cartilage

**Cartilages of the larynx (anterolateral view)**

Thyroid notch

Epiglottis

Vocal ligament

Cricovocal membrane (lateral
cricothyroid ligament,
conus elasticus)

Inferior horn

Superior horn

Quadrangular membrane

Thyroid cartilage

Vestibular ligament

Vocal process of arytenoid

Cuneiform cartilage

Corniculate cartilage

Muscular process of arytenoid

**Fibro-elastic membrane of the larynx (superior view)**

**511**

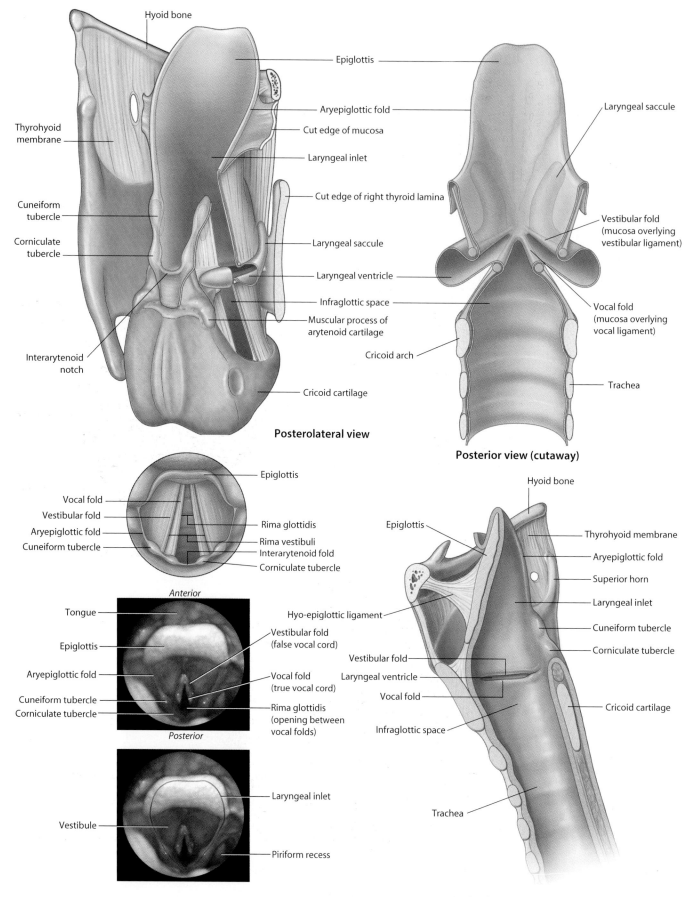

Hyoid bone

Epiglottis

Aryepiglottic fold

Cut edge of mucosa

Laryngeal inlet

Thyrohyoid membrane

Cut edge of right thyroid lamina

Cuneiform tubercle

Laryngeal saccule

Corniculate tubercle

Laryngeal ventricle

Infraglottic space

Muscular process of arytenoid cartilage

Interarytenoid notch

Cricoid cartilage

**Posterolateral view**

Laryngeal saccule

Vestibular fold (mucosa overlying vestibular ligament)

Vocal fold (mucosa overlying vocal ligament)

Cricoid arch

Trachea

**Posterior view (cutaway)**

Epiglottis

Vocal fold

Vestibular fold

Aryepiglottic fold

Cuneiform tubercle

Rima glottidis

Rima vestibuli

Interarytenoid fold

Corniculate tubercle

*Anterior*

Tongue

Vestibular fold (false vocal cord)

Epiglottis

Vocal fold (true vocal cord)

Aryepiglottic fold

Cuneiform tubercle

Rima glottidis (opening between vocal folds)

Corniculate tubercle

*Posterior*

Laryngeal inlet

Vestibule

Piriform recess

**Superior view through the laryngeal inlet**

Hyoid bone

Epiglottis

Thyrohyoid membrane

Aryepiglottic fold

Superior horn

Hyo-epiglottic ligament

Laryngeal inlet

Cuneiform tubercle

Vestibular fold

Corniculate tubercle

Laryngeal ventricle

Vocal fold

Cricoid cartilage

Infraglottic space

Trachea

**Sagittal section through laryngeal cavity**

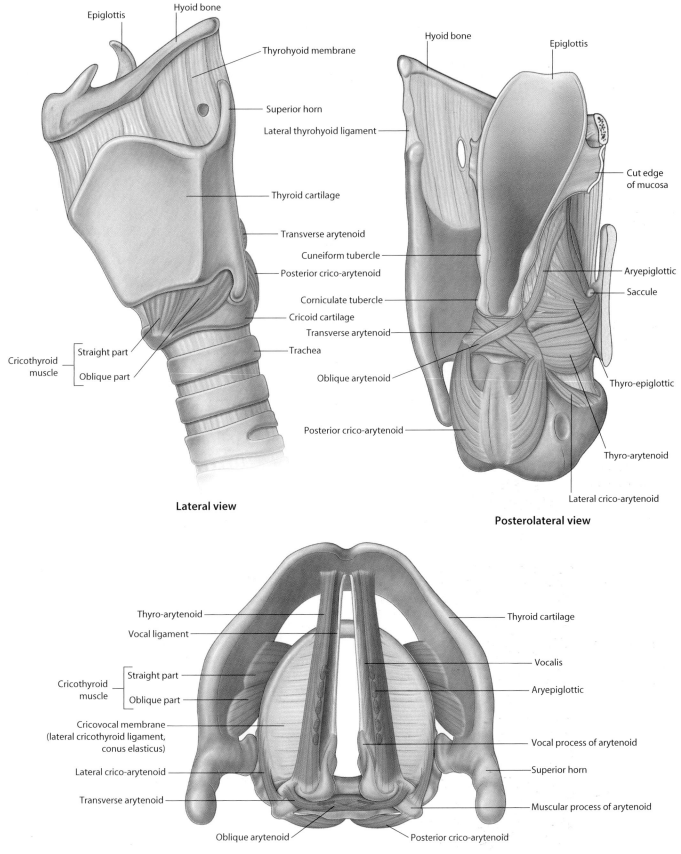

Epiglottis
Hyoid bone
Thyrohyoid membrane
Superior horn
Lateral thyrohyoid ligament
Thyroid cartilage
Transverse arytenoid
Cuneiform tubercle
Posterior crico-arytenoid
Corniculate tubercle
Cricoid cartilage
Transverse arytenoid
Trachea
Oblique arytenoid
Posterior crico-arytenoid
Cricothyroid muscle
Straight part
Oblique part

**Lateral view**

Hyoid bone
Epiglottis
Cut edge of mucosa
Aryepiglottic
Saccule
Thyro-epiglottic
Thyro-arytenoid
Lateral crico-arytenoid

**Posterolateral view**

Thyro-arytenoid
Vocal ligament
Cricothyroid muscle
Straight part
Oblique part
Cricovocal membrane
(lateral cricothyroid ligament,
conus elasticus)
Lateral crico-arytenoid
Transverse arytenoid
Oblique arytenoid
Posterior crico-arytenoid
Thyroid cartilage
Vocalis
Aryepiglottic
Vocal process of arytenoid
Superior horn
Muscular process of arytenoid

**Superior view**

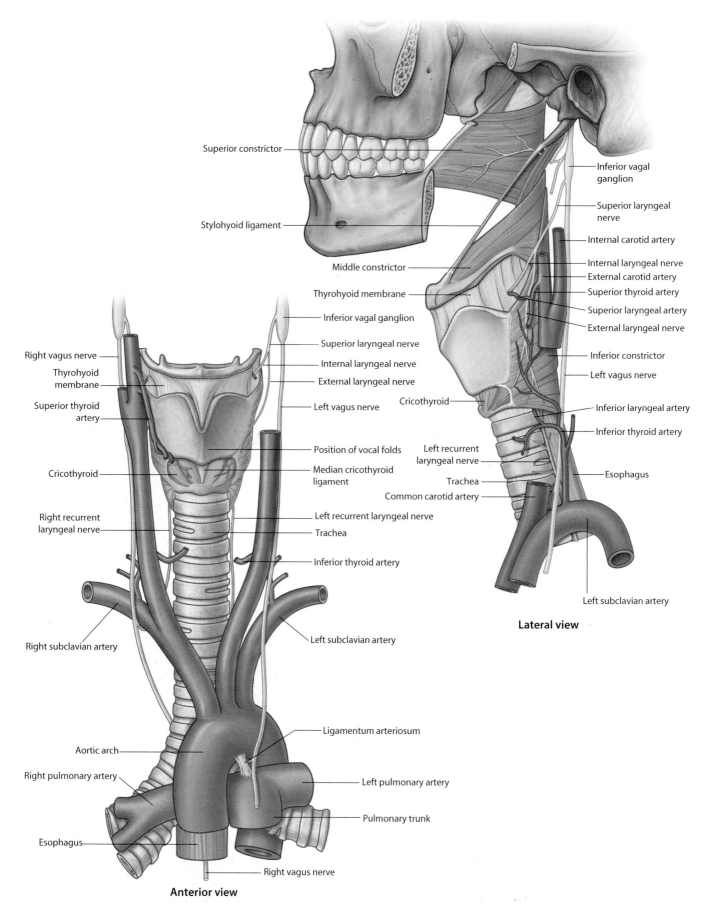

Superior constrictor

Stylohyoid ligament

Middle constrictor

Thyrohyoid membrane

Inferior vagal ganglion

Superior laryngeal nerve

Internal laryngeal nerve

External laryngeal nerve

Left vagus nerve

Position of vocal folds

Median cricothyroid ligament

Left recurrent laryngeal nerve

Trachea

Inferior thyroid artery

Right vagus nerve

Thyrohyoid membrane

Superior thyroid artery

Cricothyroid

Right recurrent laryngeal nerve

Right subclavian artery

Aortic arch

Right pulmonary artery

Esophagus

Right vagus nerve

**Anterior view**

Inferior vagal ganglion

Superior laryngeal nerve

Internal carotid artery

Internal laryngeal nerve

External carotid artery

Superior thyroid artery

Superior laryngeal artery

External laryngeal nerve

Inferior constrictor

Left vagus nerve

Cricothyroid

Inferior laryngeal artery

Inferior thyroid artery

Esophagus

Left recurrent laryngeal nerve

Trachea

Common carotid artery

Left subclavian artery

**Lateral view**

Ligamentum arteriosum

Left pulmonary artery

Pulmonary trunk

Left subclavian artery

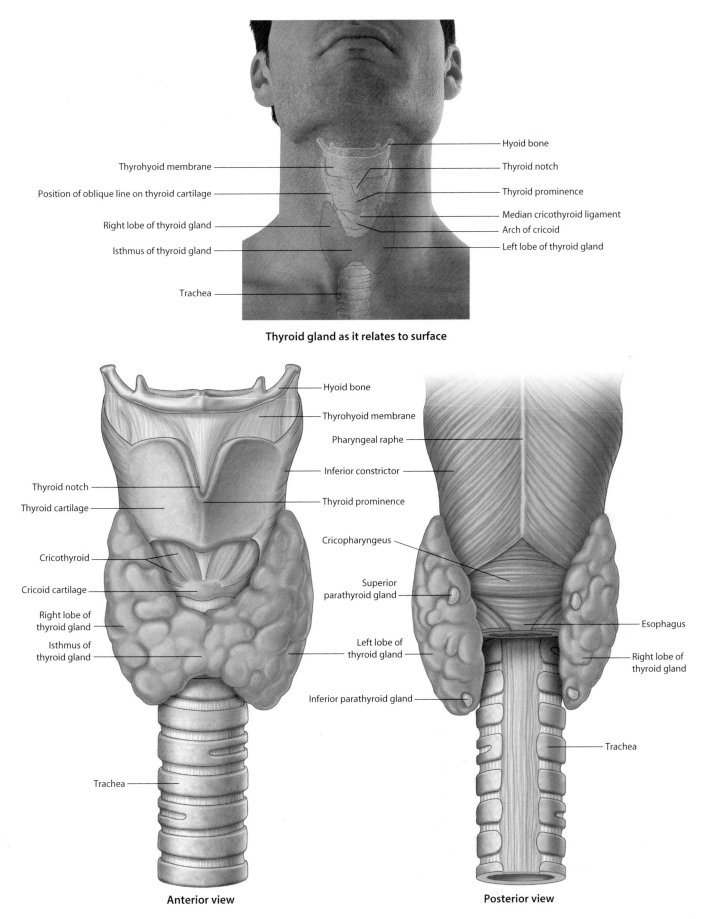

Thyrohyoid membrane

Position of oblique line on thyroid cartilage

Right lobe of thyroid gland

Isthmus of thyroid gland

Trachea

Hyoid bone

Thyroid notch

Thyroid prominence

Median cricothyroid ligament

Arch of cricoid

Left lobe of thyroid gland

**Thyroid gland as it relates to surface**

Hyoid bone

Thyrohyoid membrane

Pharyngeal raphe

Inferior constrictor

Thyroid prominence

Thyroid notch

Thyroid cartilage

Cricothyroid

Cricoid cartilage

Right lobe of thyroid gland

Isthmus of thyroid gland

Trachea

Cricopharyngeus

Superior parathyroid gland

Left lobe of thyroid gland

Inferior parathyroid gland

Esophagus

Right lobe of thyroid gland

Trachea

**Anterior view**

**Posterior view**

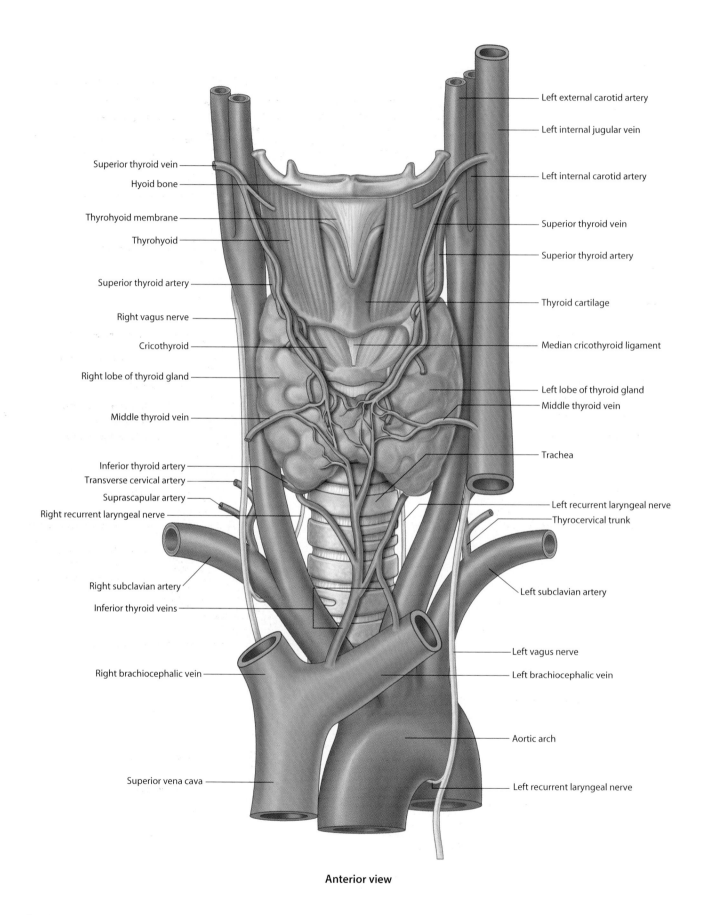

Left external carotid artery

Left internal jugular vein

Left internal carotid artery

Superior thyroid vein

Superior thyroid artery

Thyroid cartilage

Median cricothyroid ligament

Left lobe of thyroid gland

Middle thyroid vein

Trachea

Left recurrent laryngeal nerve

Thyrocervical trunk

Left subclavian artery

Left vagus nerve

Left brachiocephalic vein

Aortic arch

Left recurrent laryngeal nerve

Superior thyroid vein

Hyoid bone

Thyrohyoid membrane

Thyrohyoid

Superior thyroid artery

Right vagus nerve

Cricothyroid

Right lobe of thyroid gland

Middle thyroid vein

Inferior thyroid artery

Transverse cervical artery

Suprascapular artery

Right recurrent laryngeal nerve

Right subclavian artery

Inferior thyroid veins

Right brachiocephalic vein

Superior vena cava

**Anterior view**

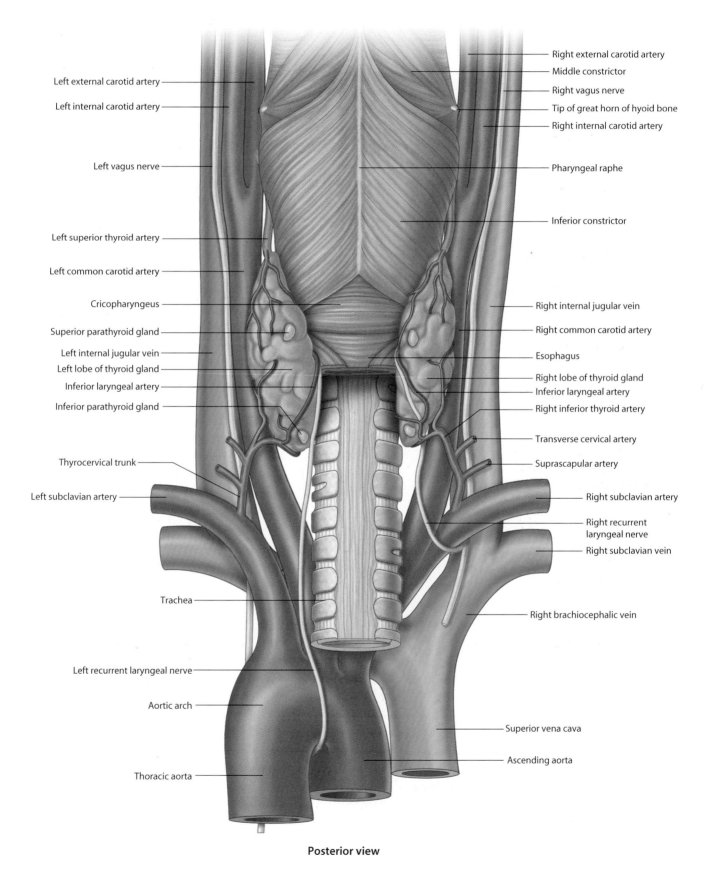

Left external carotid artery

Left internal carotid artery

Left vagus nerve

Left superior thyroid artery

Left common carotid artery

Cricopharyngeus

Superior parathyroid gland

Left internal jugular vein

Left lobe of thyroid gland

Inferior laryngeal artery

Inferior parathyroid gland

Thyrocervical trunk

Left subclavian artery

Trachea

Left recurrent laryngeal nerve

Aortic arch

Thoracic aorta

Right external carotid artery

Middle constrictor

Right vagus nerve

Tip of great horn of hyoid bone

Right internal carotid artery

Pharyngeal raphe

Inferior constrictor

Right internal jugular vein

Right common carotid artery

Esophagus

Right lobe of thyroid gland

Inferior laryngeal artery

Right inferior thyroid artery

Transverse cervical artery

Suprascapular artery

Right subclavian artery

Right recurrent laryngeal nerve

Right subclavian vein

Right brachiocephalic vein

Superior vena cava

Ascending aorta

**Posterior view**

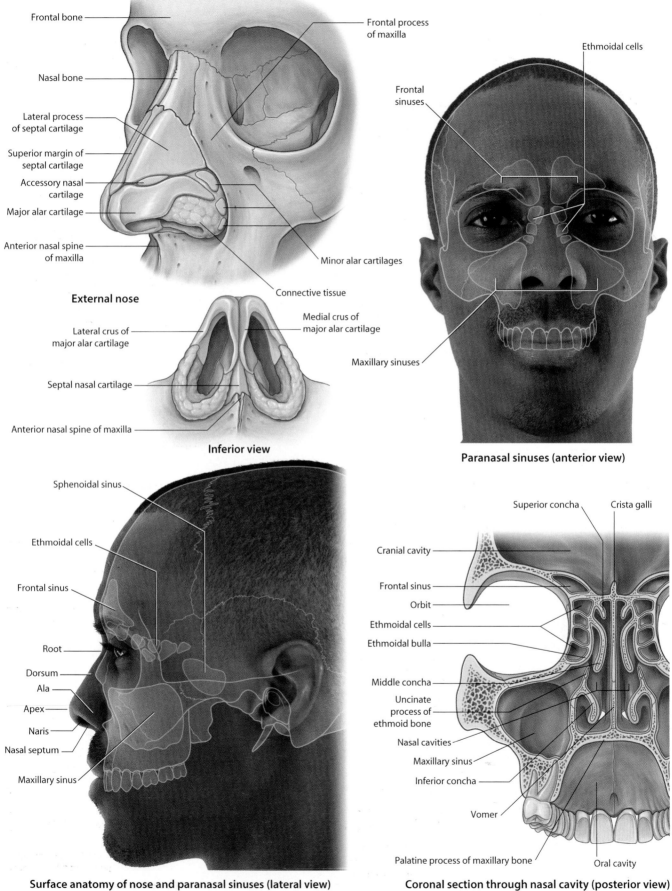

**External nose**

Frontal bone

Nasal bone

Lateral process of septal cartilage

Superior margin of septal cartilage

Accessory nasal cartilage

Major alar cartilage

Anterior nasal spine of maxilla

Frontal process of maxilla

Minor alar cartilages

Connective tissue

**Inferior view**

Lateral crus of major alar cartilage

Medial crus of major alar cartilage

Septal nasal cartilage

Anterior nasal spine of maxilla

**Paranasal sinuses (anterior view)**

Ethmoidal cells

Frontal sinuses

Maxillary sinuses

**Surface anatomy of nose and paranasal sinuses (lateral view)**

Sphenoidal sinus

Ethmoidal cells

Frontal sinus

Root

Dorsum

Ala

Apex

Naris

Nasal septum

Maxillary sinus

**Coronal section through nasal cavity (posterior view)**

Superior concha

Crista galli

Cranial cavity

Frontal sinus

Orbit

Ethmoidal cells

Ethmoidal bulla

Middle concha

Uncinate process of ethmoid bone

Nasal cavities

Maxillary sinus

Inferior concha

Vomer

Palatine process of maxillary bone

Oral cavity

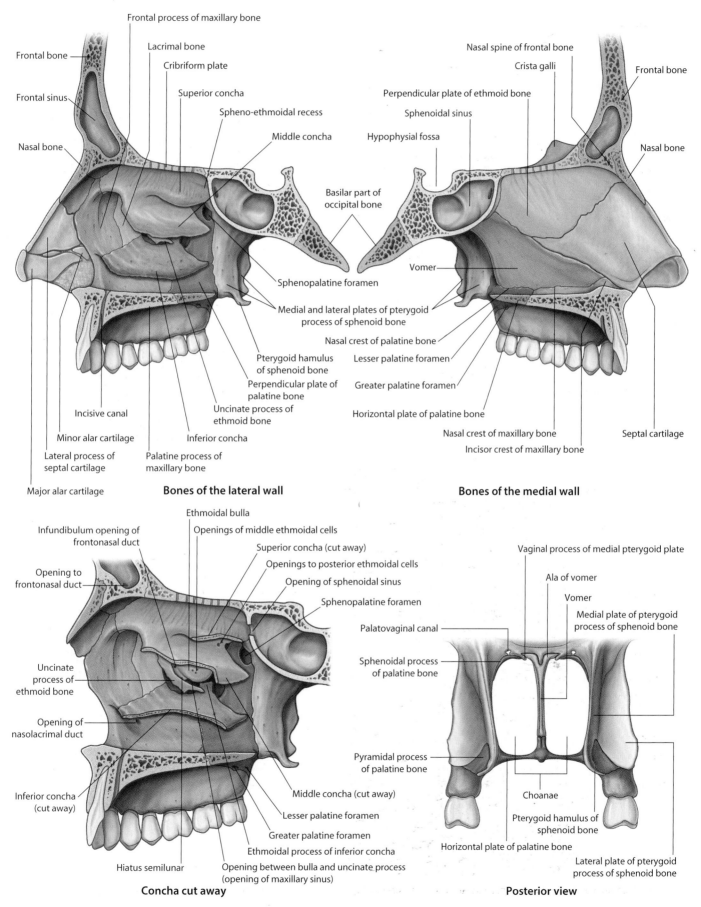

Frontal process of maxillary bone

Lacrimal bone

Cribriform plate

Superior concha

Spheno-ethmoidal recess

Middle concha

Frontal bone

Frontal sinus

Nasal bone

Basilar part of occipital bone

Sphenopalatine foramen

Medial and lateral plates of pterygoid process of sphenoid bone

Pterygoid hamulus of sphenoid bone

Perpendicular plate of palatine bone

Uncinate process of ethmoid bone

Inferior concha

Incisive canal

Minor alar cartilage

Lateral process of septal cartilage

Palatine process of maxillary bone

Major alar cartilage

**Bones of the lateral wall**

Nasal spine of frontal bone

Crista galli

Perpendicular plate of ethmoid bone

Sphenoidal sinus

Hypophysial fossa

Frontal bone

Nasal bone

Vomer

Nasal crest of palatine bone

Lesser palatine foramen

Greater palatine foramen

Horizontal plate of palatine bone

Nasal crest of maxillary bone

Incisor crest of maxillary bone

Septal cartilage

**Bones of the medial wall**

Ethmoidal bulla

Openings of middle ethmoidal cells

Infundibulum opening of frontonasal duct

Superior concha (cut away)

Openings to posterior ethmoidal cells

Opening of sphenoidal sinus

Opening to frontonasal duct

Sphenopalatine foramen

Uncinate process of ethmoid bone

Opening of nasolacrimal duct

Inferior concha (cut away)

Middle concha (cut away)

Lesser palatine foramen

Greater palatine foramen

Ethmoidal process of inferior concha

Hiatus semilunar

Opening between bulla and uncinate process (opening of maxillary sinus)

**Concha cut away**

Vaginal process of medial pterygoid plate

Ala of vomer

Vomer

Medial plate of pterygoid process of sphenoid bone

Palatovaginal canal

Sphenoidal process of palatine bone

Pyramidal process of palatine bone

Choanae

Pterygoid hamulus of sphenoid bone

Horizontal plate of palatine bone

Lateral plate of pterygoid process of sphenoid bone

**Posterior view**

**519**

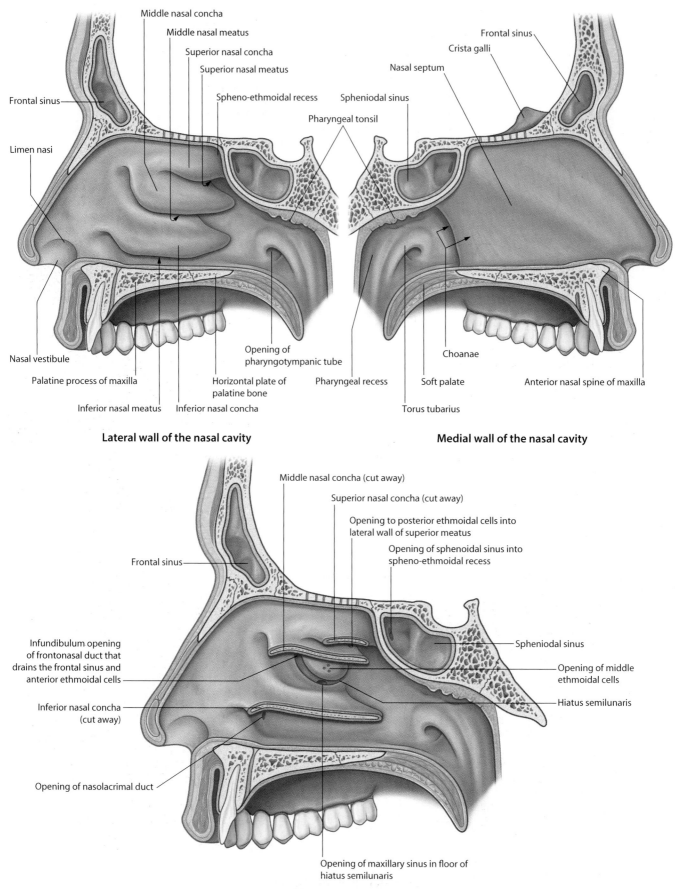

Middle nasal concha

Middle nasal meatus

Superior nasal concha

Superior nasal meatus

Spheno-ethmoidal recess

Nasal septum

Frontal sinus

Crista galli

Frontal sinus

Spheniodal sinus

Pharyngeal tonsil

Limen nasi

Nasal vestibule

Palatine process of maxilla

Opening of
pharyngotympanic tube

Inferior nasal meatus

Horizontal plate of
palatine bone

Inferior nasal concha

Pharyngeal recess

Choanae

Soft palate

Torus tubarius

Anterior nasal spine of maxilla

**Lateral wall of the nasal cavity**

**Medial wall of the nasal cavity**

Middle nasal concha (cut away)

Superior nasal concha (cut away)

Opening to posterior ethmoidal cells into
lateral wall of superior meatus

Opening of sphenoidal sinus into
spheno-ethmoidal recess

Frontal sinus

Infundibulum opening
of frontonasal duct that
drains the frontal sinus and
anterior ethmoidal cells

Spheniodal sinus

Opening of middle
ethmoidal cells

Inferior nasal concha
(cut away)

Hiatus semilunaris

Opening of nasolacrimal duct

Opening of maxillary sinus in floor of
hiatus semilunaris

**Lateral wall of the nasal cavity, concha cut away**

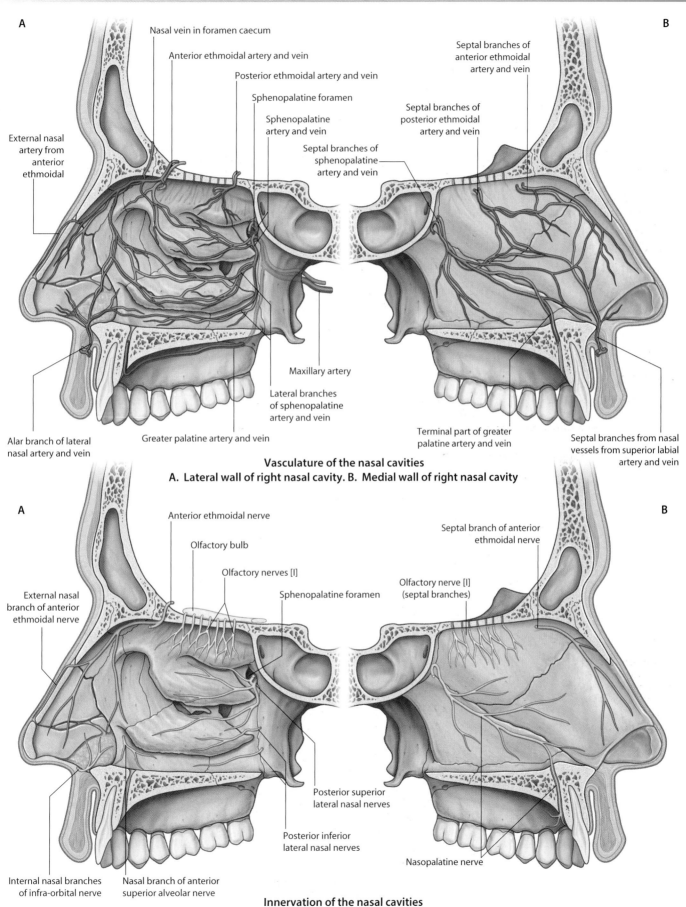

A

Nasal vein in foramen caecum

Anterior ethmoidal artery and vein

Posterior ethmoidal artery and vein

Sphenopalatine foramen

Sphenopalatine artery and vein

Septal branches of sphenopalatine artery and vein

External nasal artery from anterior ethmoidal

Alar branch of lateral nasal artery and vein

Greater palatine artery and vein

Lateral branches of sphenopalatine artery and vein

Maxillary artery

B

Septal branches of anterior ethmoidal artery and vein

Septal branches of posterior ethmoidal artery and vein

Terminal part of greater palatine artery and vein

Septal branches from nasal vessels from superior labial artery and vein

**Vasculature of the nasal cavities**
**A. Lateral wall of right nasal cavity. B. Medial wall of right nasal cavity**

A

Anterior ethmoidal nerve

Olfactory bulb

Olfactory nerves [I]

Sphenopalatine foramen

External nasal branch of anterior ethmoidal nerve

Internal nasal branches of infra-orbital nerve

Nasal branch of anterior superior alveolar nerve

Posterior superior lateral nasal nerves

Posterior inferior lateral nasal nerves

B

Septal branch of anterior ethmoidal nerve

Olfactory nerve [I] (septal branches)

Nasopalatine nerve

**Innervation of the nasal cavities**
**A. Lateral wall of right nasal cavity. B. Medial wall of right nasal cavity**

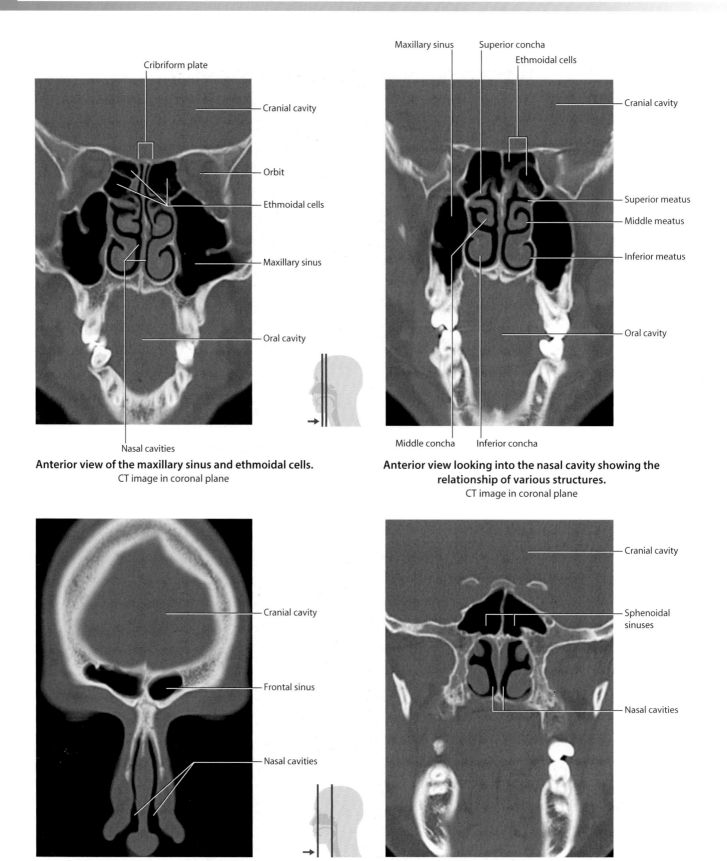

Cribriform plate

Cranial cavity

Orbit

Ethmoidal cells

Maxillary sinus

Oral cavity

Nasal cavities

**Anterior view of the maxillary sinus and ethmoidal cells.**
CT image in coronal plane

Maxillary sinus   Superior concha

Ethmoidal cells

Cranial cavity

Superior meatus

Middle meatus

Inferior meatus

Oral cavity

Middle concha   Inferior concha

**Anterior view looking into the nasal cavity showing the relationship of various structures.**
CT image in coronal plane

Cranial cavity

Frontal sinus

Nasal cavities

**Anterior view of the frontal sinuses.**
CT image in coronal plane

Cranial cavity

Sphenoidal sinuses

Nasal cavities

**Anterior view of the sphenoidal sinuses showing their relationship to the nasal cavity.**
CT image in coronal plane

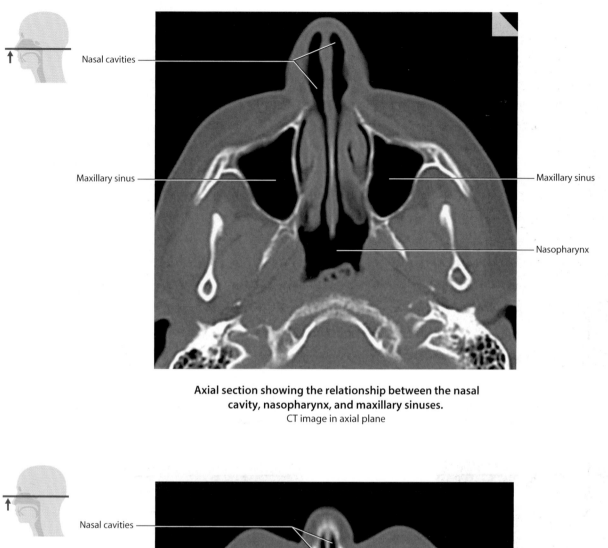

Nasal cavities

Maxillary sinus

Maxillary sinus

Nasopharynx

**Axial section showing the relationship between the nasal cavity, nasopharynx, and maxillary sinuses.**
CT image in axial plane

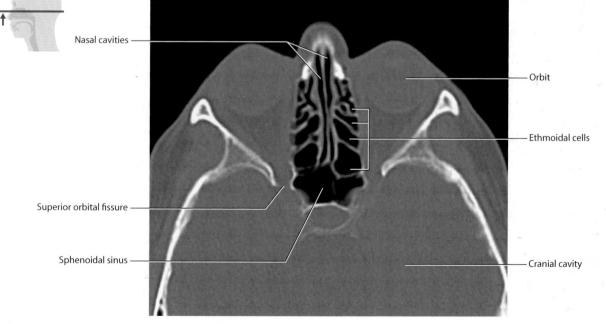

Nasal cavities

Orbit

Ethmoidal cells

Superior orbital fissure

Sphenoidal sinus

Cranial cavity

**Axial section showing the ethmoidal cells and the sphenoidal sinuses and the relationship of these structures to the orbit.**
CT image in axial plane

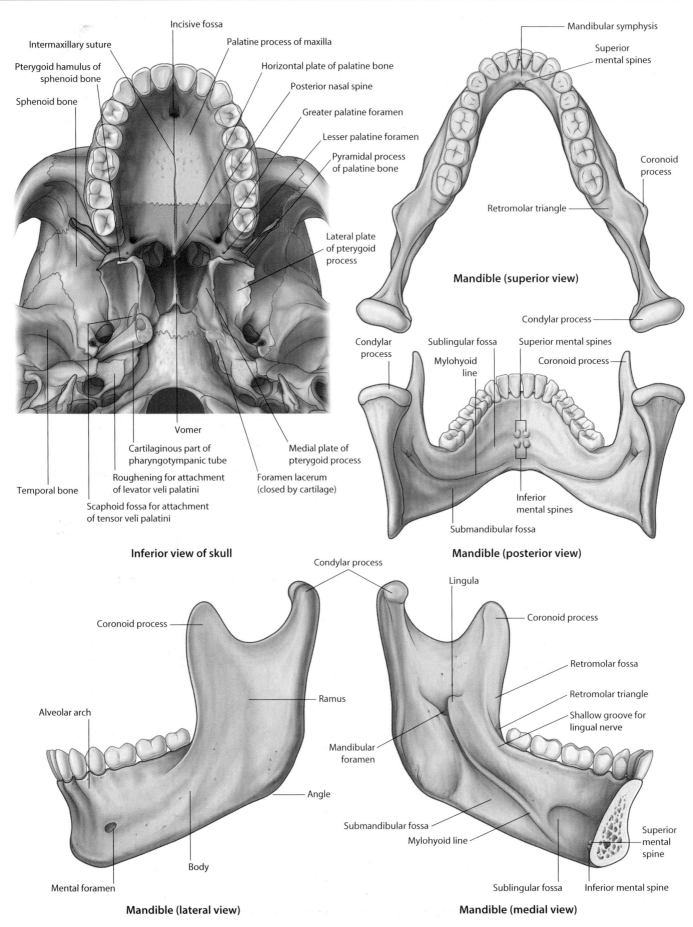

Inferior view of skull

- Incisive fossa
- Intermaxillary suture
- Pterygoid hamulus of sphenoid bone
- Sphenoid bone
- Palatine process of maxilla
- Horizontal plate of palatine bone
- Posterior nasal spine
- Greater palatine foramen
- Lesser palatine foramen
- Pyramidal process of palatine bone
- Lateral plate of pterygoid process
- Vomer
- Cartilaginous part of pharyngotympanic tube
- Roughening for attachment of levator veli palatini
- Scaphoid fossa for attachment of tensor veli palatini
- Temporal bone
- Foramen lacerum (closed by cartilage)
- Medial plate of pterygoid process

**Mandible (superior view)**

- Mandibular symphysis
- Superior mental spines
- Coronoid process
- Retromolar triangle
- Condylar process

**Mandible (posterior view)**

- Condylar process
- Sublingular fossa
- Mylohyoid line
- Superior mental spines
- Coronoid process
- Submandibular fossa
- Inferior mental spines

**Mandible (lateral view)**

- Condylar process
- Coronoid process
- Ramus
- Alveolar arch
- Mandibular foramen
- Angle
- Mental foramen
- Body

**Mandible (medial view)**

- Condylar process
- Lingula
- Coronoid process
- Retromolar fossa
- Retromolar triangle
- Shallow groove for lingual nerve
- Mandibular foramen
- Submandibular fossa
- Mylohyoid line
- Sublingular fossa
- Inferior mental spine
- Superior mental spine

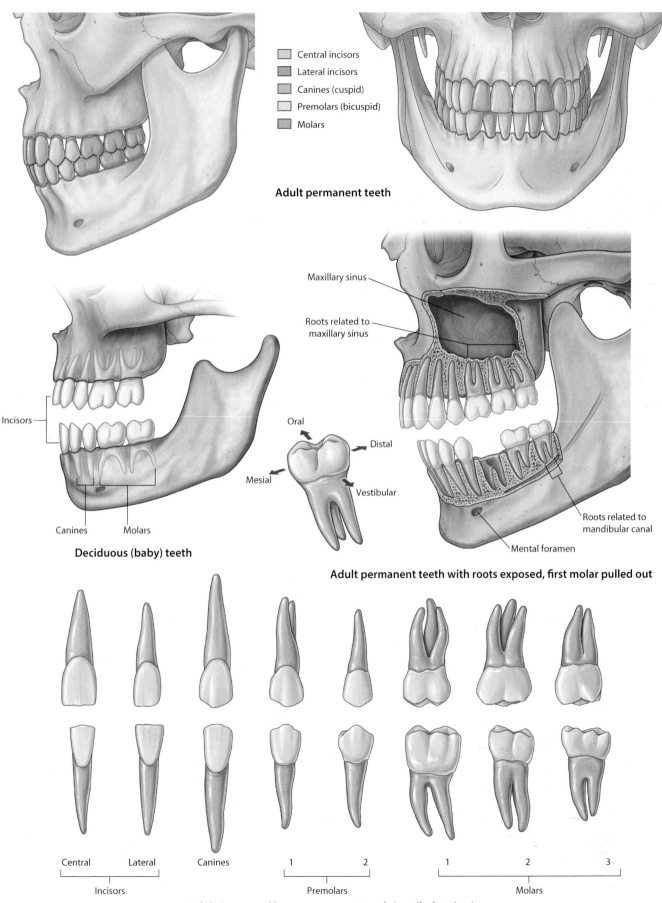

Central incisors
Lateral incisors
Canines (cuspid)
Premolars (bicuspid)
Molars

**Adult permanent teeth**

Maxillary sinus

Roots related to maxillary sinus

Incisors

Oral

Distal

Mesial

Vestibular

Canines

Molars

Roots related to mandibular canal

Mental foramen

**Deciduous (baby) teeth**

**Adult permanent teeth with roots exposed, first molar pulled out**

Central    Lateral    Canines    1    2    1    2    3

Incisors    Premolars    Molars

**Adult upper and lower permanent teeth (vestibular view)**

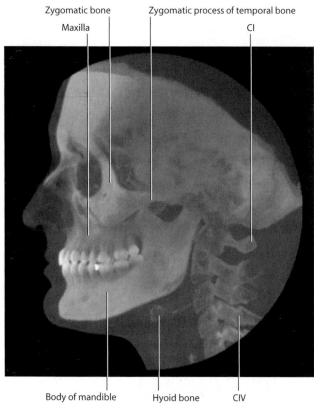

Zygomatic bone
Maxilla
Zygomatic process of temporal bone
CI

Body of mandible          Hyoid bone          CIV

**View of the left side of the face showing the craniofacial
structures including the teeth.**
Image taken with Cone Beam Computerized Tomography (CBCT)
technology, viewed in the Maximum Intensity Projection (MIP) mode,
which combines a radiographic view with a view of surface structures

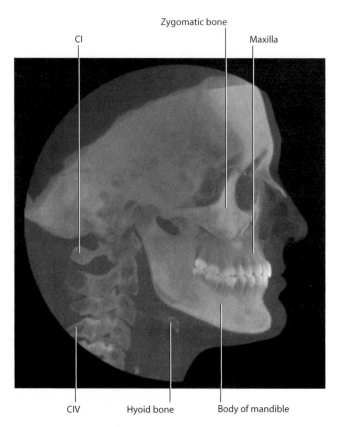

CI
Zygomatic bone
Maxilla

CIV          Hyoid bone          Body of mandible

**View of the right side of the face showing the craniofacial
structures including the teeth.**
Image taken with Cone Beam Computerized Tomography (CBCT)
technology, viewed in the Maximum Intensity Projection (MIP) mode,
which combines a radiographic view with a view of surface structures

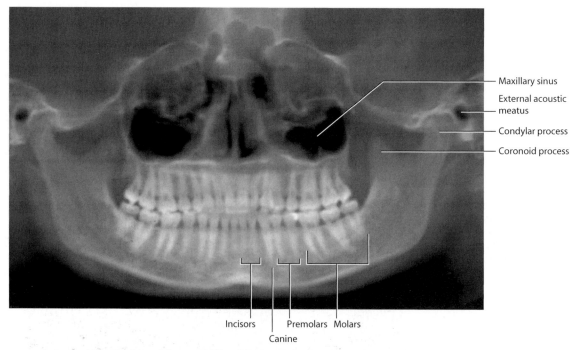

Maxillary sinus

External acoustic
meatus

Condylar process

Coronoid process

Incisors          Premolars   Molars

Canine

**Panoramic view of the teeth (dentition), which also shows the maxillary
sinuses and mandibular condylar processes.**
Image taken with Cone Beam Computerized Tomography (CBCT) technology

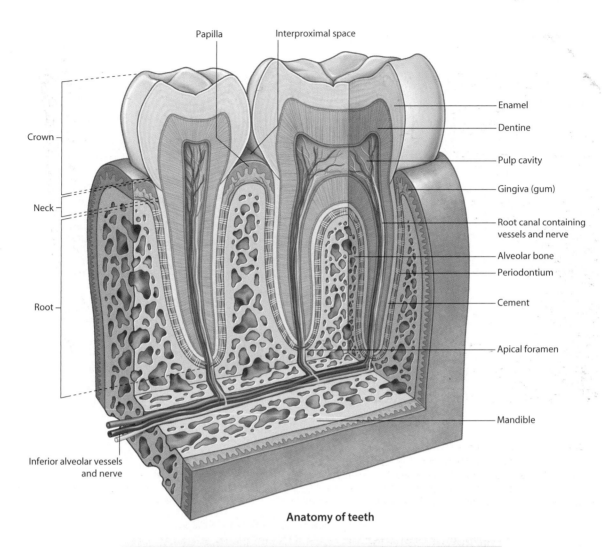

Papilla

Interproximal space

Enamel

Dentine

Pulp cavity

Gingiva (gum)

Root canal containing vessels and nerve

Alveolar bone

Periodontium

Cement

Apical foramen

Crown

Neck

Root

Mandible

Inferior alveolar vessels and nerve

**Anatomy of teeth**

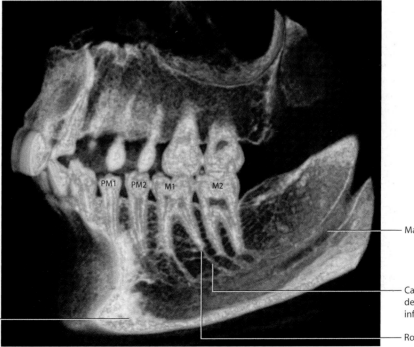

**Inside, lingual  or sagittal view of the right side of the maxillary and mandibular alveolar processes in occlusion (teeth together).**
Image taken with Cone Beam Computerized Tomography (CBCT) technology viewed in the surface mode

PM1  PM2  M1  M2

Mandibular canal

Canals containing the dental branches of the inferior alveolar nerve

Mandible

Root apex

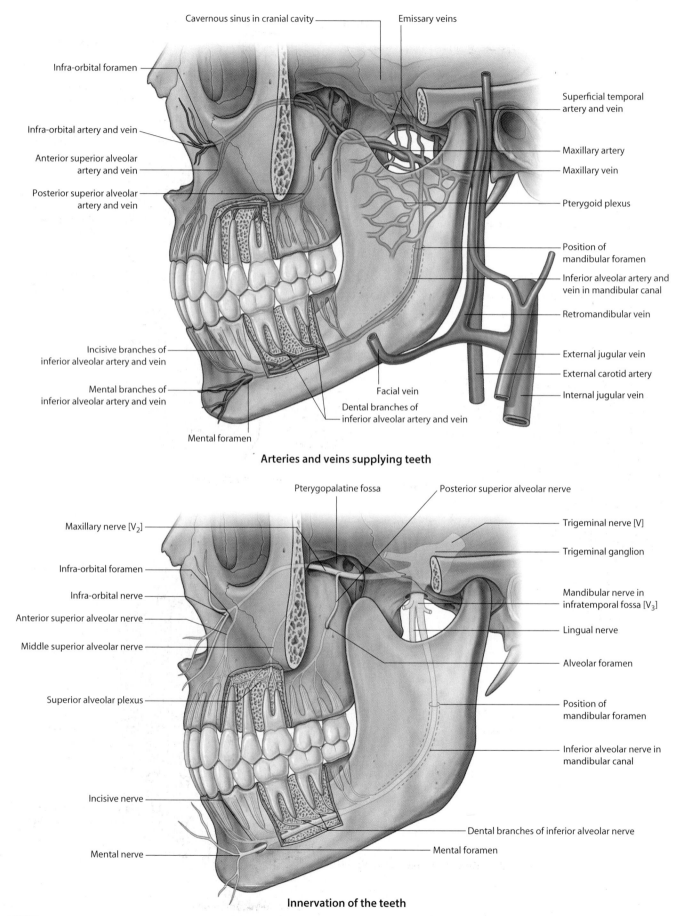

Cavernous sinus in cranial cavity

Emissary veins

Infra-orbital foramen

Infra-orbital artery and vein

Anterior superior alveolar artery and vein

Posterior superior alveolar artery and vein

Superficial temporal artery and vein

Maxillary artery

Maxillary vein

Pterygoid plexus

Position of mandibular foramen

Inferior alveolar artery and vein in mandibular canal

Retromandibular vein

Incisive branches of inferior alveolar artery and vein

Mental branches of inferior alveolar artery and vein

Facial vein

Dental branches of inferior alveolar artery and vein

External jugular vein

External carotid artery

Internal jugular vein

Mental foramen

**Arteries and veins supplying teeth**

Pterygopalatine fossa

Posterior superior alveolar nerve

Maxillary nerve [V₂]

Infra-orbital foramen

Infra-orbital nerve

Anterior superior alveolar nerve

Middle superior alveolar nerve

Superior alveolar plexus

Trigeminal nerve [V]

Trigeminal ganglion

Mandibular nerve in infratemporal fossa [V₃]

Lingual nerve

Alveolar foramen

Position of mandibular foramen

Inferior alveolar nerve in mandibular canal

Incisive nerve

Dental branches of inferior alveolar nerve

Mental nerve

Mental foramen

**Innervation of the teeth**

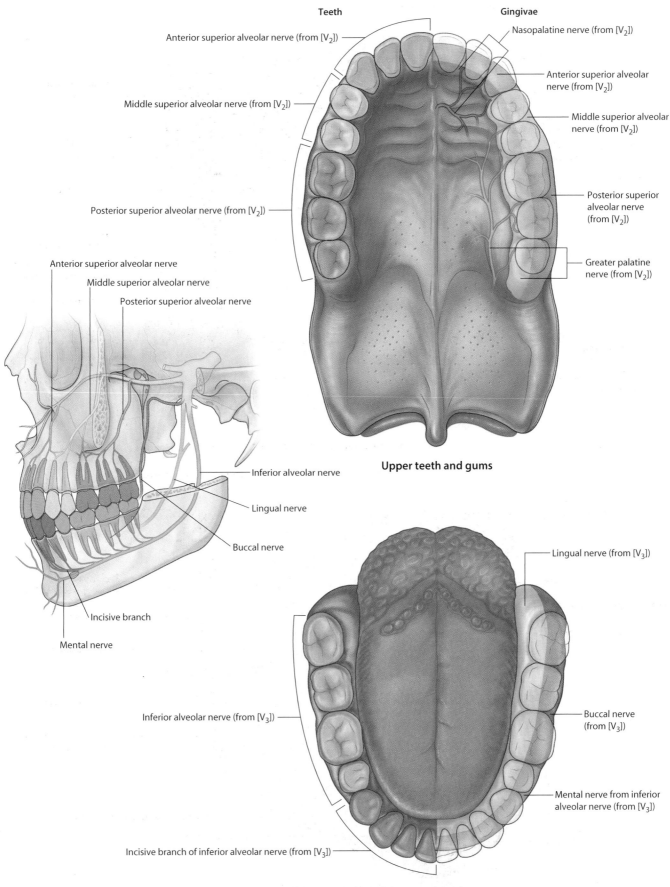

Teeth

Gingivae

Anterior superior alveolar nerve (from [V₂])

Nasopalatine nerve (from [V₂])

Anterior superior alveolar nerve (from [V₂])

Middle superior alveolar nerve (from [V₂])

Middle superior alveolar nerve (from [V₂])

Posterior superior alveolar nerve (from [V₂])

Posterior superior alveolar nerve (from [V₂])

Greater palatine nerve (from [V₂])

Anterior superior alveolar nerve

Middle superior alveolar nerve

Posterior superior alveolar nerve

Inferior alveolar nerve

Lingual nerve

Buccal nerve

Incisive branch

Mental nerve

**Upper teeth and gums**

Lingual nerve (from [V₃])

Inferior alveolar nerve (from [V₃])

Buccal nerve (from [V₃])

Mental nerve from inferior alveolar nerve (from [V₃])

Incisive branch of inferior alveolar nerve (from [V₃])

**Lower teeth and gums**

**529**

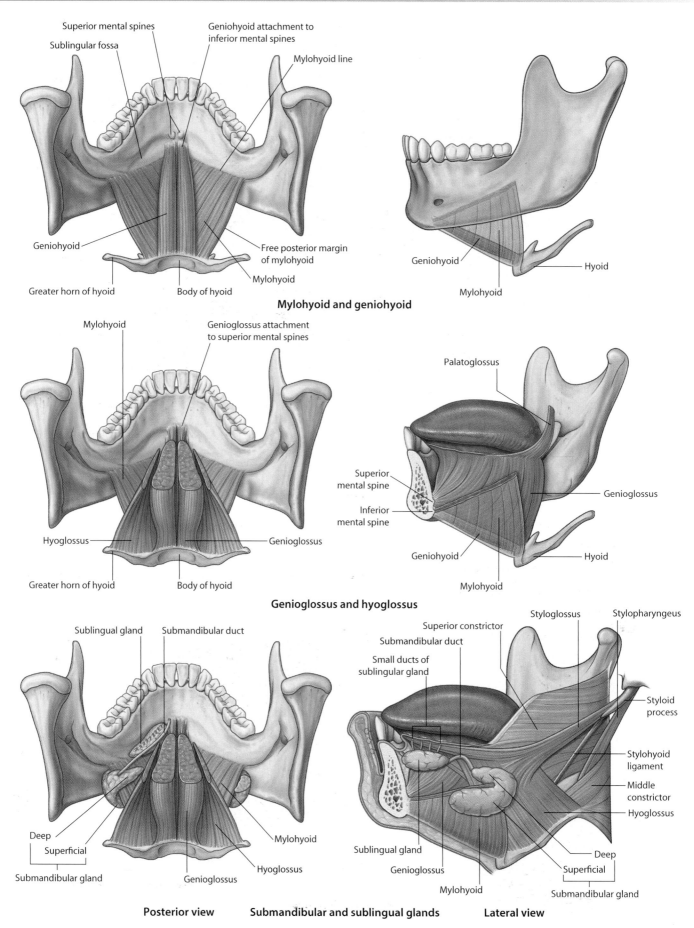

**Mylohyoid and geniohyoid**

Superior mental spines

Geniohyoid attachment to inferior mental spines

Sublingular fossa

Mylohyoid line

Geniohyoid

Free posterior margin of mylohyoid

Mylohyoid

Greater horn of hyoid

Body of hyoid

Geniohyoid

Hyoid

Mylohyoid

**Genioglossus and hyoglossus**

Mylohyoid

Genioglossus attachment to superior mental spines

Hyoglossus

Genioglossus

Greater horn of hyoid

Body of hyoid

Palatoglossus

Superior mental spine

Inferior mental spine

Genioglossus

Geniohyoid

Hyoid

Mylohyoid

**Submandibular and sublingual glands**

Sublingual gland

Submandibular duct

Deep

Superficial

Submandibular gland

Genioglossus

Hyoglossus

Mylohyoid

**Posterior view**

Superior constrictor

Styloglossus

Stylopharyngeus

Submandibular duct

Small ducts of sublingual gland

Styloid process

Stylohyoid ligament

Middle constrictor

Hyoglossus

Sublingual gland

Genioglossus

Mylohyoid

Deep

Superficial

Submandibular gland

**Lateral view**

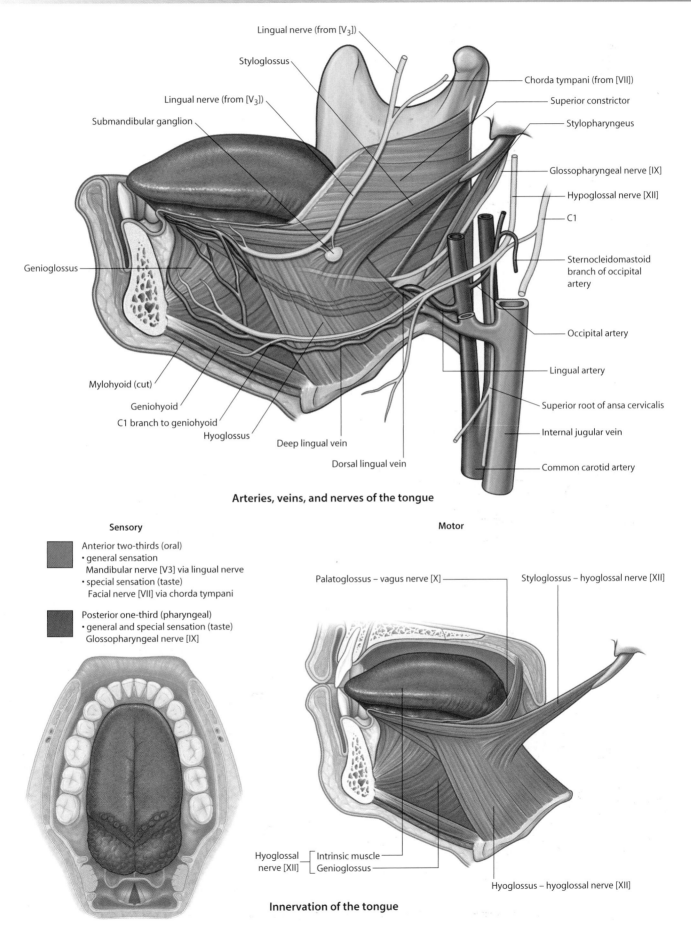

Lingual nerve (from [V₃])

Styloglossus

Lingual nerve (from [V₃])

Submandibular ganglion

Genioglossus

Mylohyoid (cut)

Geniohyoid

C1 branch to geniohyoid

Hyoglossus

Deep lingual vein

Dorsal lingual vein

Chorda tympani (from [VII])

Superior constrictor

Stylopharyngeus

Glossopharyngeal nerve [IX]

Hypoglossal nerve [XII]

C1

Sternocleidomastoid branch of occipital artery

Occipital artery

Lingual artery

Superior root of ansa cervicalis

Internal jugular vein

Common carotid artery

**Arteries, veins, and nerves of the tongue**

Sensory

Anterior two-thirds (oral)
• general sensation
  Mandibular nerve [V3] via lingual nerve
• special sensation (taste)
  Facial nerve [VII] via chorda tympani

Posterior one-third (pharyngeal)
• general and special sensation (taste)
  Glossopharyngeal nerve [IX]

Motor

Palatoglossus – vagus nerve [X]

Styloglossus – hyoglossal nerve [XII]

Hyoglossal nerve [XII]

Intrinsic muscle
Genioglossus

Hyoglossus – hyoglossal nerve [XII]

**Innervation of the tongue**

531

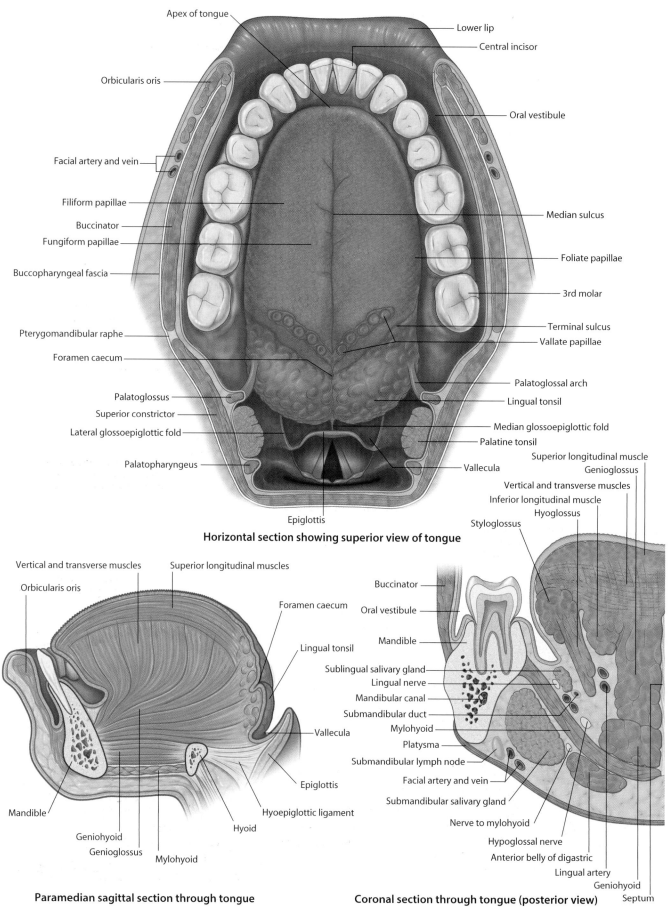

Apex of tongue

Orbicularis oris

Facial artery and vein

Filiform papillae

Buccinator

Fungiform papillae

Buccopharyngeal fascia

Pterygomandibular raphe

Foramen caecum

Palatoglossus

Superior constrictor

Lateral glossoepiglottic fold

Palatopharyngeus

Lower lip

Central incisor

Oral vestibule

Median sulcus

Foliate papillae

3rd molar

Terminal sulcus

Vallate papillae

Palatoglossal arch

Lingual tonsil

Median glossoepiglottic fold

Palatine tonsil

Vallecula

Epiglottis

**Horizontal section showing superior view of tongue**

Vertical and transverse muscles

Orbicularis oris

Superior longitudinal muscles

Foramen caecum

Lingual tonsil

Vallecula

Epiglottis

Hyoepiglottic ligament

Mandible

Geniohyoid

Genioglossus

Mylohyoid

Hyoid

**Paramedian sagittal section through tongue**

Superior longitudinal muscle
Genioglossus
Vertical and transverse muscles
Inferior longitudinal muscle
Hyoglossus
Styloglossus

Buccinator

Oral vestibule

Mandible

Sublingual salivary gland

Lingual nerve

Mandibular canal

Submandibular duct

Mylohyoid

Platysma

Submandibular lymph node

Facial artery and vein

Submandibular salivary gland

Nerve to mylohyoid

Hypoglossal nerve

Anterior belly of digastric

Lingual artery

Geniohyoid

Septum

**Coronal section through tongue (posterior view)**

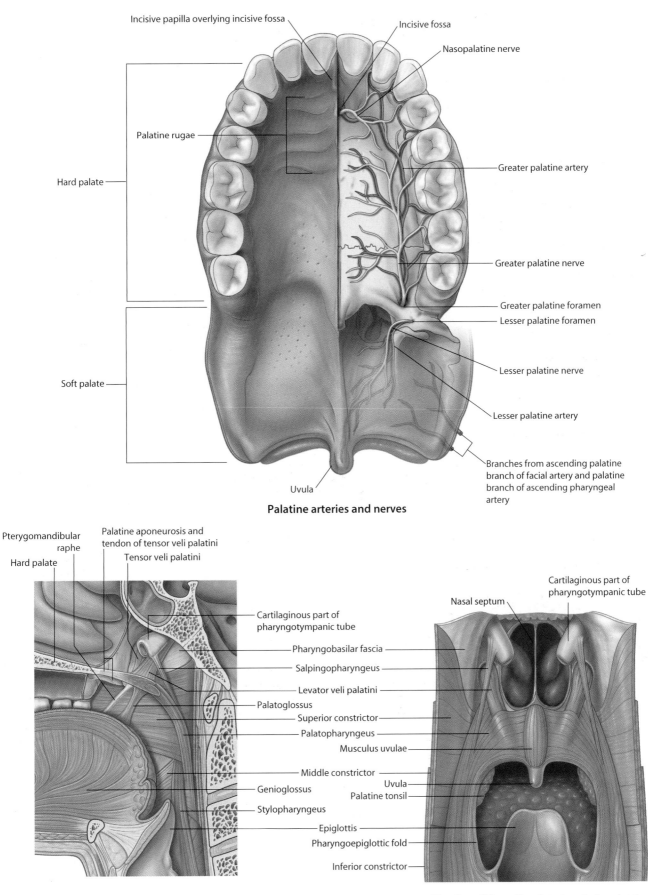

**Palatine arteries and nerves**

Incisive papilla overlying incisive fossa
Incisive fossa
Nasopalatine nerve
Palatine rugae
Greater palatine artery
Hard palate
Greater palatine nerve
Greater palatine foramen
Lesser palatine foramen
Lesser palatine nerve
Soft palate
Lesser palatine artery
Branches from ascending palatine branch of facial artery and palatine branch of ascending pharyngeal artery
Uvula

**Muscles of the soft palate (sagittal section)**

Pterygomandibular raphe
Palatine aponeurosis and tendon of tensor veli palatini
Hard palate
Tensor veli palatini
Cartilaginous part of pharyngotympanic tube
Pharyngobasilar fascia
Salpingopharyngeus
Levator veli palatini
Palatoglossus
Superior constrictor
Palatopharyngeus
Musculus uvulae
Middle constrictor
Genioglossus
Stylopharyngeus
Epiglottis
Pharyngoepiglottic fold
Inferior constrictor

**Muscles of the soft palate (posterior view)**

Nasal septum
Cartilaginous part of pharyngotympanic tube
Uvula
Palatine tonsil

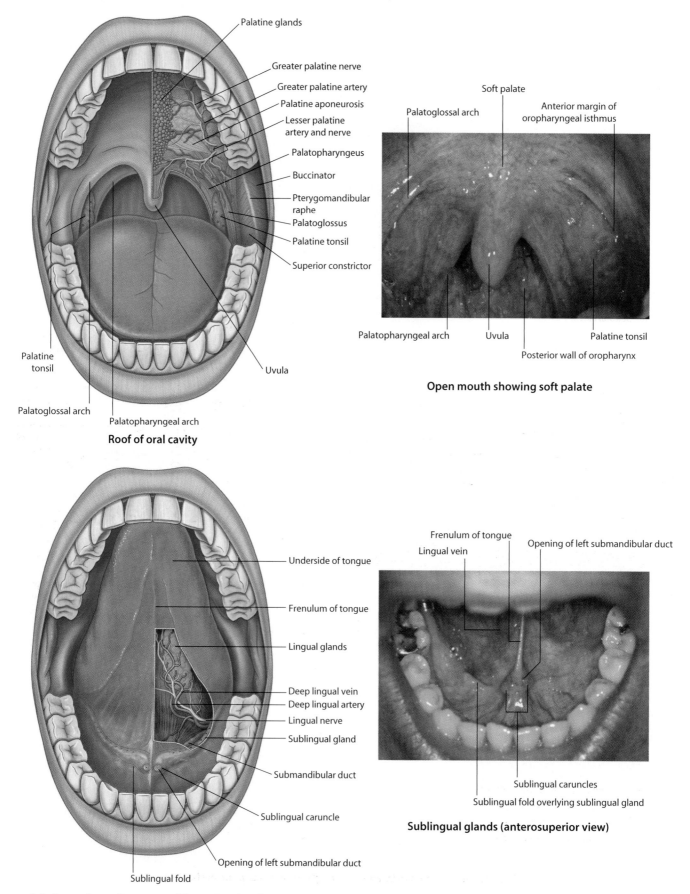

Palatine glands

Greater palatine nerve

Greater palatine artery

Palatine aponeurosis

Lesser palatine artery and nerve

Palatopharyngeus

Buccinator

Pterygomandibular raphe

Palatoglossus

Palatine tonsil

Superior constrictor

Palatine tonsil

Uvula

Palatoglossal arch

Palatopharyngeal arch

**Roof of oral cavity**

Soft palate

Palatoglossal arch

Anterior margin of oropharyngeal isthmus

Palatopharyngeal arch

Uvula

Palatine tonsil

Posterior wall of oropharynx

**Open mouth showing soft palate**

Underside of tongue

Frenulum of tongue

Lingual glands

Deep lingual vein

Deep lingual artery

Lingual nerve

Sublingual gland

Submandibular duct

Sublingual caruncle

Opening of left submandibular duct

Sublingual fold

**Inferior surface of tongue and floor of oral cavity**

Frenulum of tongue

Lingual vein

Opening of left submandibular duct

Sublingual caruncles

Sublingual fold overlying sublingual gland

**Sublingual glands (anterosuperior view)**

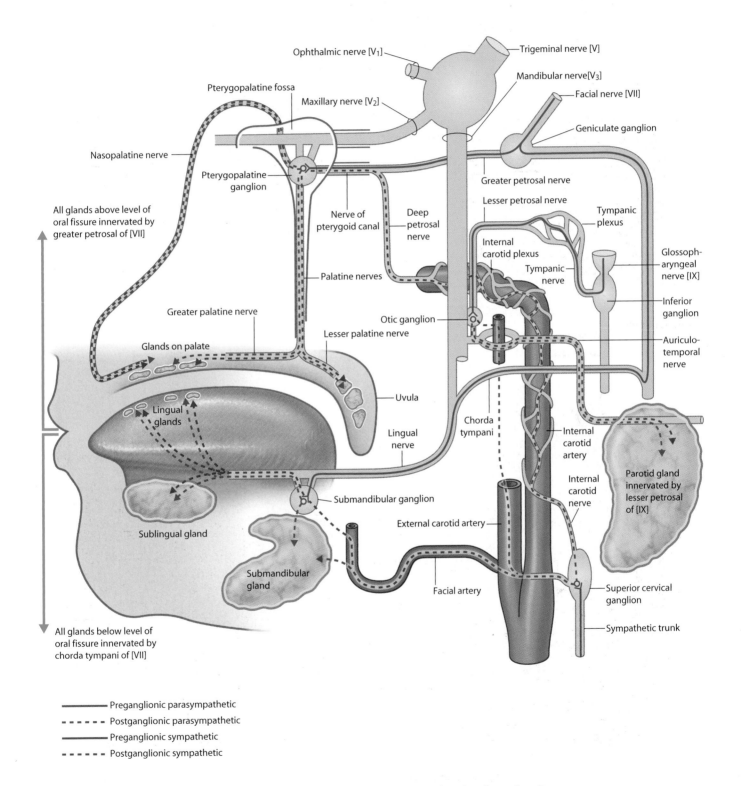

Ophthalmic nerve [V₁]

Trigeminal nerve [V]

Mandibular nerve[V₃]

Facial nerve [VII]

Pterygopalatine fossa

Maxillary nerve [V₂]

Geniculate ganglion

Nasopalatine nerve

Pterygopalatine ganglion

Greater petrosal nerve

Lesser petrosal nerve

Tympanic plexus

All glands above level of oral fissure innervated by greater petrosal of [VII]

Nerve of pterygoid canal

Deep petrosal nerve

Internal carotid plexus

Tympanic nerve

Glossoph- aryngeal nerve [IX]

Palatine nerves

Inferior ganglion

Greater palatine nerve

Otic ganglion

Lesser palatine nerve

Glands on palate

Auriculo- temporal nerve

Lingual glands

Uvula

Lingual nerve

Chorda tympani

Internal carotid artery

Parotid gland innervated by lesser petrosal of [IX]

Submandibular ganglion

Internal carotid nerve

Sublingual gland

External carotid artery

Submandibular gland

Facial artery

Superior cervical ganglion

All glands below level of oral fissure innervated by chorda tympani of [VII]

Sympathetic trunk

——— Preganglionic parasympathetic

- - - - Postganglionic parasympathetic

——— Preganglionic sympathetic

- - - - Postganglionic sympathetic

**Visceral efferent (motor) innervation of glands related to the oral cavity**

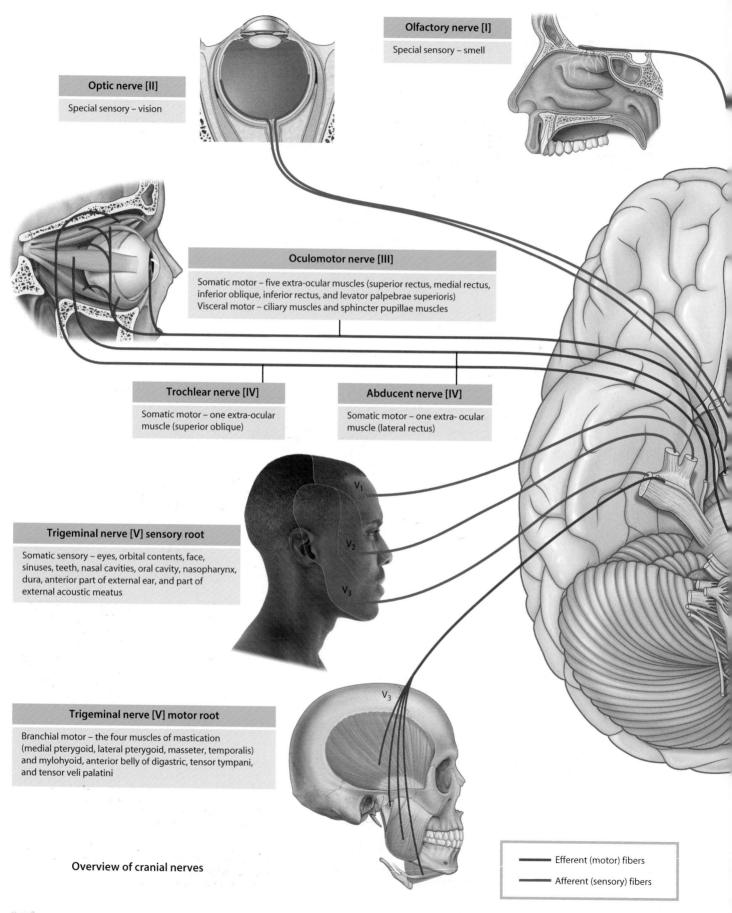

**Olfactory nerve [I]**

Special sensory – smell

**Optic nerve [II]**

Special sensory – vision

**Oculomotor nerve [III]**

Somatic motor – five extra-ocular muscles (superior rectus, medial rectus, inferior oblique, inferior rectus, and levator palpebrae superioris)
Visceral motor – ciliary muscles and sphincter pupillae muscles

**Trochlear nerve [IV]**

Somatic motor – one extra-ocular muscle (superior oblique)

**Abducent nerve [IV]**

Somatic motor – one extra- ocular muscle (lateral rectus)

**Trigeminal nerve [V] sensory root**

Somatic sensory – eyes, orbital contents, face, sinuses, teeth, nasal cavities, oral cavity, nasopharynx, dura, anterior part of external ear, and part of external acoustic meatus

**Trigeminal nerve [V] motor root**

Branchial motor – the four muscles of mastication (medial pterygoid, lateral pterygoid, masseter, temporalis) and mylohyoid, anterior belly of digastric, tensor tympani, and tensor veli palatini

$V_1$

$V_2$

$V_3$

$V_3$

—— Efferent (motor) fibers

—— Afferent (sensory) fibers

**Overview of cranial nerves**

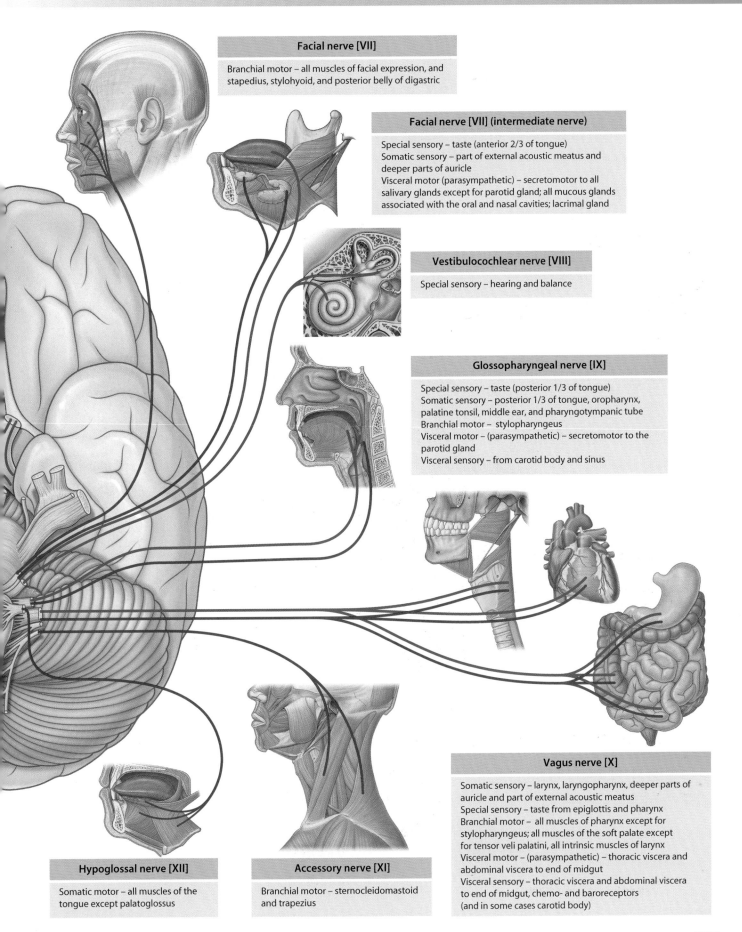

**Facial nerve [VII]**

Branchial motor – all muscles of facial expression, and stapedius, stylohyoid, and posterior belly of digastric

**Facial nerve [VII] (intermediate nerve)**

Special sensory – taste (anterior 2/3 of tongue)
Somatic sensory – part of external acoustic meatus and deeper parts of auricle
Visceral motor (parasympathetic) – secretomotor to all salivary glands except for parotid gland; all mucous glands associated with the oral and nasal cavities; lacrimal gland

**Vestibulocochlear nerve [VIII]**

Special sensory – hearing and balance

**Glossopharyngeal nerve [IX]**

Special sensory – taste (posterior 1/3 of tongue)
Somatic sensory – posterior 1/3 of tongue, oropharynx, palatine tonsil, middle ear, and pharyngotympanic tube
Branchial motor – stylopharyngeus
Visceral motor – (parasympathetic) – secretomotor to the parotid gland
Visceral sensory – from carotid body and sinus

**Hypoglossal nerve [XII]**

Somatic motor – all muscles of the tongue except palatoglossus

**Accessory nerve [XI]**

Branchial motor – sternocleidomastoid and trapezius

**Vagus nerve [X]**

Somatic sensory – larynx, laryngopharynx, deeper parts of auricle and part of external acoustic meatus
Special sensory – taste from epiglottis and pharynx
Branchial motor – all muscles of pharynx except for stylopharyngeus; all muscles of the soft palate except for tensor veli palatini, all intrinsic muscles of larynx
Visceral motor – (parasympathetic) – thoracic viscera and abdominal viscera to end of midgut
Visceral sensory – thoracic viscera and abdominal viscera to end of midgut, chemo- and baroreceptors (and in some cases carotid body)

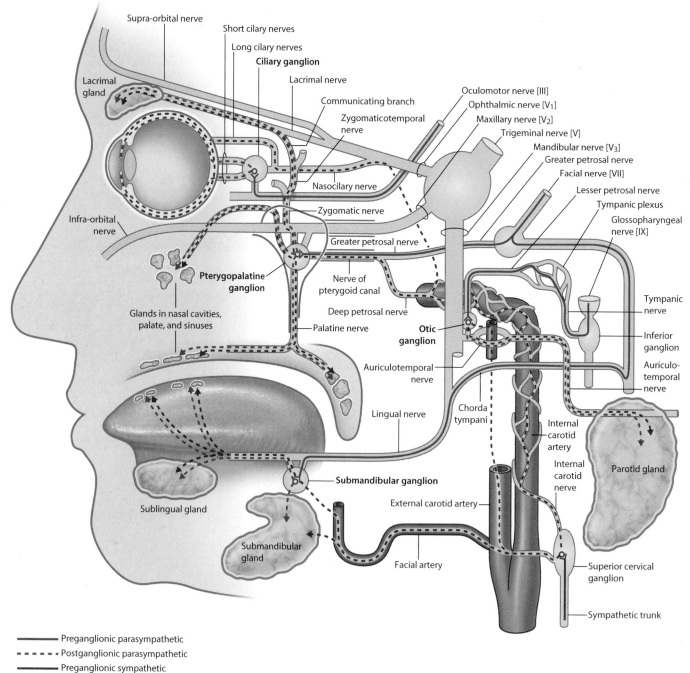

Supra-orbital nerve

Short cilary nerves

Long cilary nerves

**Ciliary ganglion**

Lacrimal nerve

Communicating branch

Zygomaticotemporal nerve

Oculomotor nerve [III]

Ophthalmic nerve [V₁]

Maxillary nerve [V₂]

Trigeminal nerve [V]

Mandibular nerve [V₃]

Greater petrosal nerve

Facial nerve [VII]

Lesser petrosal nerve

Tympanic plexus

Glossopharyngeal nerve [IX]

Lacrimal gland

Nasocilary nerve

Zygomatic nerve

Greater petrosal nerve

Infra-orbital nerve

**Pterygopalatine ganglion**

Nerve of pterygoid canal

Deep petrosal nerve

**Otic ganglion**

Tympanic nerve

Inferior ganglion

Auriculo-temporal nerve

Glands in nasal cavities, palate, and sinuses

Palatine nerve

Auriculotemporal nerve

Lingual nerve

Chorda tympani

Internal carotid artery

Parotid gland

Internal carotid nerve

Sublingual gland

**Submandibular ganglion**

External carotid artery

Submandibular gland

Facial artery

Superior cervical ganglion

Sympathetic trunk

———— Preganglionic parasympathetic

- - - - - Postganglionic parasympathetic

———— Preganglionic sympathetic

- - - - - Postganglionic sympathetic

**Summary of visceral efferent (motor) pathways in the head**

# INDEX

# INDEX